W0079098

# Information Processing in Medical Imaging

# Information Processing in Medical Imaging

Edited by

## C. N. de Graaf

University Hospital Utrecht
Utrecht, The Netherlands

and

## M. A. Viergever

Delft University of Technology
Delft, The Netherlands

Springer Science+Business Media, LLC

Library of Congress Cataloging in Publication Data

International Conference on Information Processing in Medical Imaging (10th: 1987: Utrecht, Netherlands)
    Information processing in medical imaging.

    "Proceedings of the Tenth International Conference on Information Processing in Medical Imaging, held June 22–26, 1987, in Utrecht, The Netherlands"—T.p. verso.
    Includes bibliographies and index.
    1. Diagnostic imaging—Digital techniques—Congresses. 2. Image processing—Congresses. I. Graaf, C. N. de. II. Viergever, M. A. III. Title. [DNM: 1. Diagnosis, Computer Assisted—congresses. 2. Diagnostic Imaging—congresses. 3.Nuclear Medicine—congresses. W3 IN182AF 10th 1987i / WN 200 I598 1987i]
    RC78.7.D53    1987                       616.07′5                          87-36058
    ISBN 978-1-4615-7265-7          ISBN 978-1-4615-7263-3 (eBook)
    DOI 10.1007/978-1-4615-7263-3

Proceedings of the Tenth International Conference on Information Processing in Medical Imaging, held June 22–26, 1987, in Utrecht, The Netherlands

© 1988 Springer Science+Business Media New York
Originally published by Plenum Publishing , New York in 1988
Softcover reprint of the hardcover 1st edition 1988

All rights reserved

No part of this book may be reproduced, stored in a retrieval system, or transmitted in any form or by any means, electronic, mechanical, photocopying, microfilming, recording, or otherwise, without written permission from the Publisher

# PROCEEDINGS OF THE 10th INTERNATIONAL CONFERENCE ON INFORMATION PROCESSING IN MEDICAL IMAGING

Organized by:

C.N. de Graaf          - and -     M.A. Viergever
Institute of Nuclear Medicine      Dept. of Mathematics and Informatics
University Hospital Utrecht         Delft University of Technology
Catharijnesingel 101               PO Box 356
3511 GV Utrecht, The Netherlands   2600 AJ Delft, The Netherlands

Sponsored by:

Un Hospital of Utrecht          Positron Corporation
Mallinckrodt Diagnostica        Bruker Spectrospin
Nucletron                       Elscint
Sopha Médical                   Philips Nederland
Medgenix                        Nodecrest Ltd.
Un of Utrecht Medical Faculty

Scientific Committee:

S.L. Bacharach     M.L. Goris        D.A. Ortendahl
H.H. Barrett       C.N. de Graaf     S.M. Pizer
A.B. Brill         K.H. Höhne        A. Todd-Pokropek
F. Deconinck       J.J. Koenderink   M.A. Viergever
R. Di Paola        C.E. Metz

Local Committee:

M. den Boef            M. Popovits - Visser
C.N. de Graaf          A.E.H. Pronk
A. Hoekstra            P.J.W. Sirba
E.C. Jurg - ten Hove   M.A. Viergever

# Preface

This book summarizes the proceedings of the 10th international conference on Information Processing in Medical Imaging (IPMI-10), held in June, 1987, in Zeist, The Netherlands.

IPMI is a biennial conference, organized alternately in Europe and North America. The subject of the conference is the use of physics, mathematics, computer science, and engineering in the formation, processing and interpretation of medical images. The intent of the conference is to provide a forum where new ideas and results of research in medical imaging can be presented and amply discussed. Accordingly, the programme can comprise only a limited number of papers.

The scientific committee of IPMI-10 selected 41 papers for presentation, although a total of 102 extended abstracts of on the average high quality had been submitted. All selected contributions are included in these proceedings.

During of the preparations of the conference the organizers received the tragic news of the death of François Erbsmann, the initiator of IPMI, and organizer of the first conference in 1969 in Brussels. François always emphasized that the backbone of the IPMI meetings should be promising young and active researchers rather than established scientists in the field. As an appreciation of this idea, and in thankful remembrance of François' stimulating work, the IPMI-board has taken the initiative to present the François Erbsmann prize for the most significant contribution to the conference by a young investigator. At IPMI-10 the prize was awarded to John Gauch, Chapel Hill NC, USA, for his presentation "Multiresolution shape descriptions and their applications in medical imaging".

The success of a meeting primarily depends on the enthusiasm of the participants. It also greatly depends on the financial support as well as on the personal efforts of the programme committee and the local organizing committee. To all who made this conference a success, the organizers wish to express their sincere thanks.

C.N. de Graaf  
M.A. Viergever

Utrecht, September 1987

# Contents

# General Image Processing

# SIGNIFICANCE AND COMPLEXITY IN MEDICAL IMAGES

## -SPACE VARIANT TEXTURE DEPENDENT FILTERING

S. Webb

Joint Section of Physics, Institute of Cancer Research and
Royal Marsden Hospital, Downs Road, Sutton, Surrey
SM2 5PT. U.K.

## BACKGROUND TO THE DIAGNOSTIC PROBLEM

Most medical images, arising from electronic detectors, exist in
digital form as a matrix of pixels. With the exception of optical
reconstruction, all reconstructed images are also matrices of pixels
with specific values. In general such matrices are usually square and
have size the square of 64, 128, 256 or 512. When images are collected
by an analogue detector, for example a film, it is also possible to
produce digital images by scanning densitometry. Other non-medical
images often exist in digital form, for example images from satellites
and spacecraft, from digitised optical cameras etc.

Digital images are particularly suitable for applications of image
processing aimed to improve the clarity of the images and their
diagnostic usefulness. Often these techniques include deconvolution of
the point source response function with constraints to avoid the
amplification of noise. (for example Andrews and Hunt (1977), Webb et
al., (1985), Yanch et al (1987)). Pixellised images are also amenable to
topological analysis and hierarchical image processing techniques (de
Graaf et al. (1984) and also to many other filtering methods including
the application of median window filters (Leach et al. (1984)). In
nuclear medicine, image processing techniques generally aim to optimise
the contrast between the signal from hot or cold regions and the
background distribution.

A general problem arises of quantifying the improvements made by
image processing. This problem often reduces to assessing the
significance of particular pixel values in relation to their neighbours.
In practice this is identically the same problem as posed in the
original unprocessed images. Hence one may generally address the problem
of pixel value significance knowing that whatever techniques and
conclusions arise can be applied equally to processed and unprocessed
images.

The problem of pixel significance is of fundamental importance in
medical imaging. All diagnosis essentially reduces to the question of
deciding whether a pixel value or group of values is significantly
different from its neighbours and whether this is then indicative of
pathology. Generally, in nuclear medicine, it is very difficult to

define what contrast is considered to be significant and the presence of noise (or mottle or speckle), which might be confused with single pixels with small but significant contrast, additionally complicates the problem. In diagnostic radiology, including X-ray CT and NMR images, similar problems arise especially if the abnormality for which a clinician is searching is of small spatial extent.

A number of intuitive practices help the diagnosticians. Firstly they will make use of their previous experience of what is considered to be a normal patient image. Intuitively they are making decisions on the basis of the difference between this normal image in their memory and the image which they are currently searching for abnormalities. It is of course quite impractical to generate such a difference image electronically because of the problems of image registration. In this sense the human mind is doing something which would be extremely difficult if not impossible for a computer to do, namely overlooking the difference in specific size of the region being inspected relative to that being recalled in memory (or inspected in a reference atlas) of a normal. Generally a clinician will need to refer to specific criteria to characterise a significant deviation from normal. Such criteria are necessarily subjective and may be different for different diagnostic tasks.

Also, acting on intuition more than anything else, it has become common practice to smooth images either in real space or Fourier space or, for reconstructed images, during the reconstruction process by application of a suitable filter. Generally this is a considered approach, mindful of the character of noise, but once again the end product is generally selected to be pleasing rather than an image, the significance of whose pixels can be precisely stated.

Against this background it is not surprising that most studies do not address deciding precise methods for determining pixel significance. Techniques are often justified because they lead to known performance for known objects being imaged. For example in nuclear medicine if a technique leads to an increase of contrast without the unacceptable generation of mottle (for a known distribution of activity) then that technique can be said to be valid and can be applied to unknown distributions. A better approach, which also includes the performance of the observer, would be to conduct experiments on image assessment for known distributions and quantify the results, thus leading to a precise statement of what sensitivity and specificity would be achieved in the real diagnostic situation.

It would be unrealistic to expect that the problems of image assessment will suddenly disappear by the introduction of a novel technique. It is however possible to consider images in different ways which can lead to some less empirical methods of image presentation. Some ideas of this kind are developed here. In particular we shall show that considerations of the significance to be attached to individual pixel values has led to the development of two independent techniques for non-linear picture processing which are presented in sections 3 and 4 of this paper.

## A simple example illustrating pixel significance

Consider the scene in figure 1 which is a childlike drawing of a sunflower and a house. Imagine that the image has been digitised into pixels of some size 's'. The sunflower is thin on the scale of s, perhaps only a couple of pixels thick for its stalk whilst the house, which has been drawn greyer, encompasses many pixels. We are used to

4

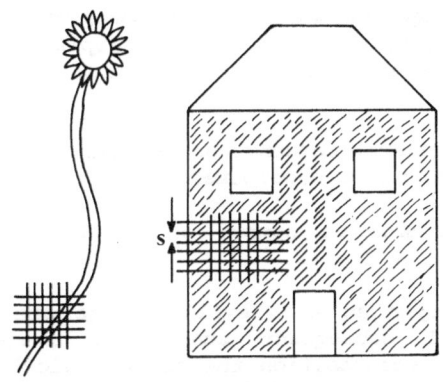

Fig.1 A simple illustrative image showing the relation between pixel size and size of structure.

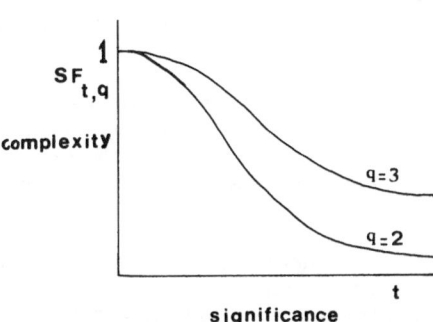

Fig.2 A typical complexity-significance curve.

representing images as matrices of pixels all equal in size and this has been done here. The reason for this practice is that most equipment generates images in this way and most display devices are conveniently fed by images of this type. It is obvious however that the house in figure 1 does not require such small pixels. In the region of the house larger pixels would serve the same purpose. One cannot however sweep through the image replacing small pixels by larger ones because then the image of the sunflower will suffer. In the region of the sunflower small pixels are needed. One might argue that even smaller pixels than size 's' are needed as the digitised stem would have unrealistic steps even at the pixel size shown. We are therefore drawn to the notion that a variable pixel size would be acceptable for such an image. If however the image were noisy, whether large pixels could replace smaller ones would depend on decisions based on the relative sizes of signal and noise contributions to the image. With this in mind we shall formulate some concept of pixel significance based on the simplest (stack) method of image decomposition.


IMAGE DECOMPOSITION

Methodology

Imagine the following series of operations are applied to the digitised image at pixel size 's'. Let the original image have dimension NxN.

1. The image is subdivided into $(N/2)^2$ larger superpixels of size $2^2$ and the mean of each superpixel is found.

2. For each of the superpixels, each of the $2^2$ members are compared with the mean for that superpixel. If the absolute difference between each contributor and the mean is less than some value 't' for ALL contributors, then all contributors are replaced by that mean for the superpixel. (This will be referred to as 'pixel merging' or 'pixel compression'). These two steps will be referred to as a level 2 decomposition of the image.

3. The two processes are now repeated by subdivision into $(N/4)^2$ larger superpixels of size $4^2$ using the same value of 't'. If the absolute departure from the mean of all 16 contributors to a superpixel is

less than t, all values are replaced by the mean. This process will be referred to as a level 3 decomposition. Any group of superpixels which survived merger at the level 2 stage are excluded from the level 3 stage.

4. Steps 1 and 2 are repeated with the general sequence as follows. For the $q^{th}$ level of decomposition there are M superpixels of size a where $a = 2^{q-1}$ and $M = (N/a)^2$.
It can therefore be seen that the maximum number of levels of decomposition for an NxN image is $Q = 1 + \log_2 N$.

Any superpixels which survive merger at the level q stage are excluded from the $(q+1)^{th}$ and all subsequent stages of image decomposition. At the $Q^{th}$ level of decomposition the image could be just a single superpixel. This would however be totally adequate for an entirely uniform field.

After these operations, the resulting image will appear to have a variable pixel size. Returning to our simple demonstration image we would observe that for groups of pixels within the region of the house, pixel merging will have occurred whereas, near the stem of the sunflower, pixels will have survived at the original pixel size 's'.

## Properties of the image formed by decomposition

The resulting image is naturally less familiar to our experience. It contains large and small pixels and many sharp edges between regions where pixel compression has occurred, and regions where pixels have survived compression. In that sense it would almost certainly be rejected as an 'improved' image in terms of its visual appearance.

The resulting image is however giving direct information on the significant structure of the original image. No information has been lost; in fact information has been gained, because, if the original and the decomposed image are displayed side by side, a comparison shows where insignificant detail has been removed. Confidence in the significance of the remaining detail is thus increased.

How much detail survives the image decomposition depends entirely on the parameter 't' in the scheme described above. 't' may be thought of as expressing the level of minimum significance, since if detail of significance less than 't' existed it was removed, and vice-versa.

Returning to our illustrative example, let us imagine that the original process of digitisation introduced some noise into the image. Now if 't' was set very small in relation to such noise even pixels within the region of the house, which was supposed to be of a uniform grey level in the absence of noise, would survive merger and the image decomposition would achieve nothing. Now as 't' were increased, more and more pixels would fail to survive merger. When 't' was above the level of the noise introduced by digitisation then only those pixels which genuinely represent true small scale detail (for example the sunflower stalk) will be retained at the smallest pixel size 's'.

## The Complexity-significance curve

These comments intuitively lead to what we will call a complexity-significance curve. Let $SF_{t,q}$ represent the fraction of pixels surviving merger at the $q^{th}$ level when the threshold of significance is 't' . A graph of this quantity may be plotted for any image as a function of 't'. Each level of decomposition will give a separate curve on the graph for a particular image. The graph for figure 1 might look like figure 2. The graph has the following general properties:

a) For a fixed level of decomposition, (and generally only the first few levels will be of interest) $SF_{t,q}$ decreases as t increases. In absurdum if t is set ridiculously high, all pixels will merge and $SF_{t,q}$ will be zero. Equally when t is set to zero no pixels will merge and $SF_{t,q}$ will be unity. The abcissa may thus be thought of as representing pixel significance.

b) At a fixed significance 't', $SF_{t,q}$ will increase as q increases.

c) The exact shape of the curve is itself a parameter of the image. The quantity $SF_{t,q}$ may be thought of as the image 'complexity'. If an image is very complex the value of $SF_{t,q}$ will be high for some significance 't'. For example a chequerboard of black and white pixels of size 's' would survive merger at all levels and all thresholds below that representing the difference between black and white! $SF_{t,q}$ would be unity everywhere. This is the most complex image. On the other hand an entirely uniform image would lead to zero $SF_{t,q}$ at all levels and all thresholds. This is the least complex image. Complexity might be thought of as the opposite of uniformity in this sense.

d) It is important to stress that complexity is not the same as real detail. Artefacts and indeed image noise are a form of complexity and have indistinguishable contributions from real detail or signal to this diagram. It is only by prior knowledge of the value of the expected noise that one can attempt to perform image decomposition to the point of retaining only 'significant complexity'.

e) The image decomposition scheme is a space variant technique operating differently on areas of the image with different correlation structure. In this sense it is quite unlike a Fourier method of image filtering by which operations on the image are globally performed in the frequency domain; any operation, for example smoothing, performed in F-space affects all of the image equally.

Figure 3 further clarifies the information carried by the complexity- significance diagram provided a true threshold significance ($t_T$)can be identified. With $t = t_T$, the information in the image is presented so as to display no false detail. The observer would see only detail which is significant and displayed at different pixel sizes as appropriate to the differing components of the image. If instead t had been set $<t_T$ the shaded region would show the 'false survivors' at each level of decomposition. (solid squares are for level 2 and open triangles are for level 3). Conversely if t had been set $>t_T$ there would have been a number of 'casualty pixels', namely those which have been merged but which would have survived had the true threshold significance been set, (eg. solid circles are for level 2).

## Clinical examples of image decomposition

The unknown parameter in the image decomposition scheme described above is the value to assign for 't' for a given imaging system or modality. If one knew 't', then pixel merging at several levels with this known value would give an image whose unique property was that only significant detail had survived. There would be absolutely no confusion that a feature was in some way not real. Unfortunately the character of image noise precludes such an identification. For a Gaussian distribution with infinitely extending tails there is always a chance an apparently significant departure from the mean could arise by chance.

However it is intuitive that it ought to be possible to identify a threshold significance 't' allowing pixel merging to reduce a large part of the noise contribution.

Figure 4 shows the complexity-significance diagram for a pelvic NMR scan (N=256) where the original image has been normalised to the range 0-255 and the values of 't' are the percentage of the maximum value occuring. Curves of SF for levels 2- 4 are shown for t in the range 0-16%. One would for example note that less than 50% of the pixels survive merger at level 2 at the 1% threshold significance. Less than 30% survive level 3 merger at 2% threshold significance etc. The true significance is not known but a level 4 decomposition at 4% shows much pixel merging in the bladder and the heads of the femur with retention of detail at the original pixel size in the gut (Figure 5). At this threshold significance only 10% of the pixels have survived at the original pixel size, 8% have survived at the next largest pixel size and 7% have survived at the second largest pixel size. 75% of the pixels are three sizes larger than the original.

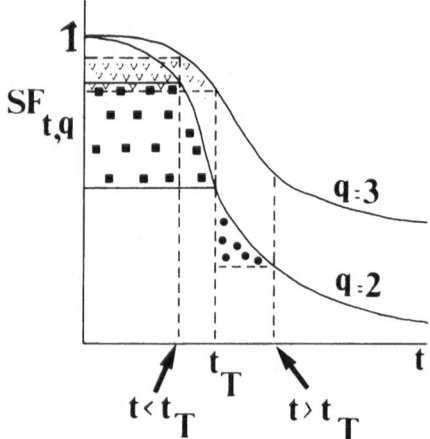

Figure 3 Showing 'casualty pixels' and 'false survivors' in the complexity- significance diagram if the threshold is wrongly set.

Figure 6 shows a complexity-significance diagram for an abnormal liver SPECT image (N=64) also normalised to the range 0-255. Notice that the curves are generally higher than the corresponding curves for the NMR scan for each level and each threshold significance. This implies the complexity of the SPECT scan is greater than that of the NMR scan but beware this complexity may be unreal noise or artefact. Also on figure 6 are the curves for a liver SPECT image after constrained deconvolution of the point spread function by the techniques described by Webb (1986) . The curves for the surviving fraction are higher reflecting the complexity introduced by deconvolution. A successful image processing technique is one which should lead to a raising of the SF curve in this way.

## An analytic example: image decomposition for a noise distribution

An NxN matrix of pixels has been generated which have the nominal value V but are generated such that a pixel value is given by $V+r\chi\sqrt{V}$ where r is a Gaussianly distributed random number. The distribution is a noise pattern with $\sigma = \sqrt{V}$. The complexity significance curves for level 2-4 image merging are shown in figure 7 for N=64 where the scheme has been modified so that the test of pixel deviation is made against V rather than against the mean of the pixels comprising the enlarged superpixels.

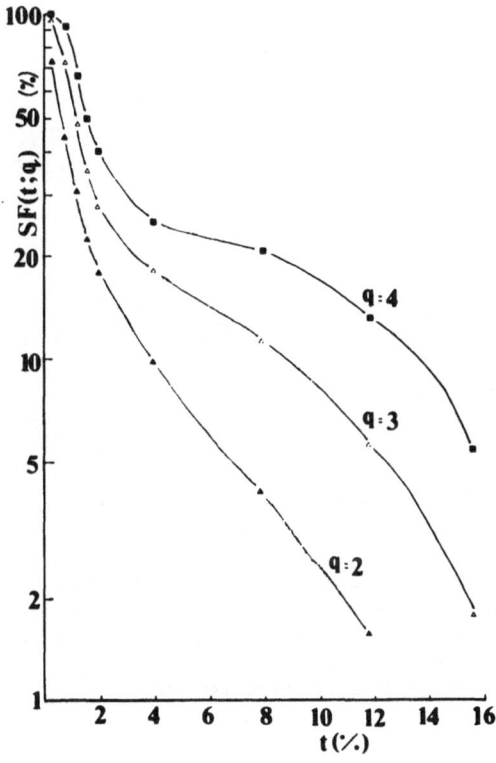

Figure 4  Complexity significance diagram for a pelvic NMR image.

These curves can of course be predicted analytically as follows: The probability of a single pixel lying within $\pm b.\sigma$ is erf $(b/\sigma)$ where erf is the integral error function (see eg Barford page 91). Hence the probability of x pixels lying in this range is $(\text{erf }(b/\sigma))^x$. Hence the probability of these x pixels surviving with a significance threshold of $b.\sigma$ is $1 - (\text{erf }(b/\sigma))^x$. Using the fact that there are $2^{2q-2}$ pixels in each superpixel at the q-th level of decomposition, we have the analytic expression that

$$SF_{b.\sigma, q} = 1 - (erf(b/\sigma))^{2^{2q-2}} \qquad (1)$$

This expression has also been plotted in figure 7 agreeing with the experimental values almost exactly. The small residual disagreement is entirely due to the finite number of pixels in the image.

## Pixel merger based on neighbourhood comparisons

It has proved difficult to identify a value of 't' which is an inherent property of each imaging modality. Probably a global value over an image is not physically significant since, if we think again of a

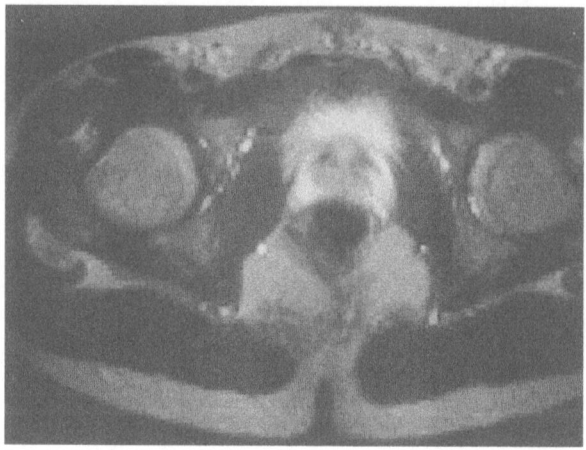

Figure 5 Image decomposition up to level 4 for a pelvic NMR image with t=4% of the pixel maximum. (note enlargement on a monitor is really necessary to appreciate the variable pixel size). The original image before decompositon is figure 12a.

nuclear medicine image, different parts of the image may well contain pixels of very different count densities. The noise error attached to the measurement is related to this count density and thus a global $t_T$ might not be appropriate.

Suppose instead of some absolute value 't' we replace the criterion 't' by b.$\sigma$ where $\sigma$ is now the standard deviation of the pixels which are being considered for merger. The advantage of this is that the criterion for significance becomes itself locally variable. Repeating the methodology, ALL pixels in a group being considered for merger are merged if they are all within b.$\sigma$ of their mean. Instead of $SF_{t,q}$ we now above criterion.

It is immediately obvious that for b=1, merger can never occur. There is always at least one pixel in a group which departs from the mean of the group by more than one standard deviation, by definition. Hence we know immediately that $SF_{1,q} = 1$ for all levels q. More than this, one can predict exactly the value of b for which $SF_{b,q}$ becomes zero. If we consider a group of x pixels in which all but one are zero, this represents the most skew distribution of x pixels. Suppose the single non-zero value is k, then the mean is k/x and the standard

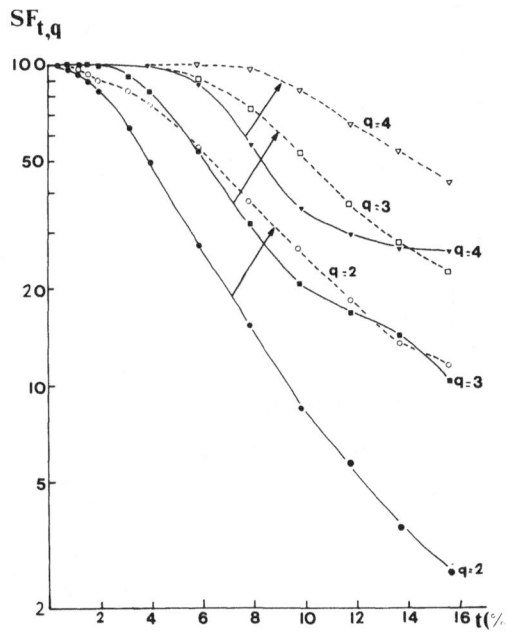

Figure 6 Complexity-significance curve for an abnormal liver SPECT image; solid curves are for reconstructed image; dotted curves for the deconvolved image.

deviation is $k.\sqrt{(x-1)}/x$. The largest departure from the mean is $k(x-1)/x$. The largest departure from the mean is thus $\sqrt{(x-1)}$ times the standard deviation. Hence x pixels can always be merged if b is greater than $\sqrt{(x-1)}$. We can write this formally (using the number of pixels in each sub- pixel at the q-th level) as

$$SF_{b>b_c, q} = 0$$

where

$$b_c = \sqrt{(2^{2q-2}-1)}$$

In particular $SF_{1.7321,2} = 0$. This analytic theory was checked by generating a very large number of groups of 4 pixel values with a random distribution and plotting the survival fraction for a range of b between 1 and 1.7321. The results are shown in figure 8. The limits with b=1 and 1.7321 are indeed reproduced. Additionally in figure 8, $SF_{b,2}$ has been plotted for the NMR image and for the SPECT image discussed earlier. The curves are almost identical to those of random noise. This is making a

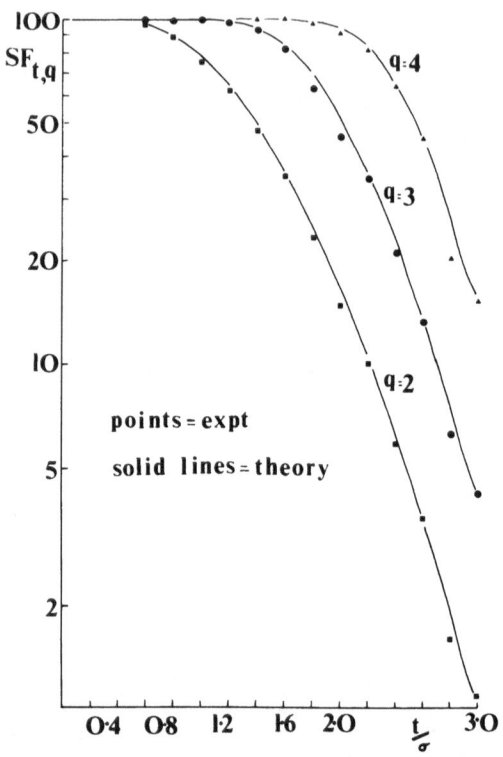

Figure 7 Complexity-significance diagram for an experimental noise distribution (solid points) with the analytic prediction (curves).

very significant statement. It is saying that the information carried within a picture is little different from noise if the pixels are considered only within their 2nd level context, i.e. the context of their immediately nearest neighbour. The following statements say the same thing in different ways:

If one scanned the image with a mask having a 2x2 opening only and obscuring the rest of the image, then it would be exceedingly difficult to identify the image and discriminate it from a pure noise distribution.

12

An image of pixels is more than the sum of its parts. The contextual information or 'glue holding the pixels together' contains most of the information. In sections 3 and 4, image filtering methods are developed which specifically use the local context information in a space-variant manner.

The departure of the curves for the clinical images from those for noise reflect the structure of the image at that level.

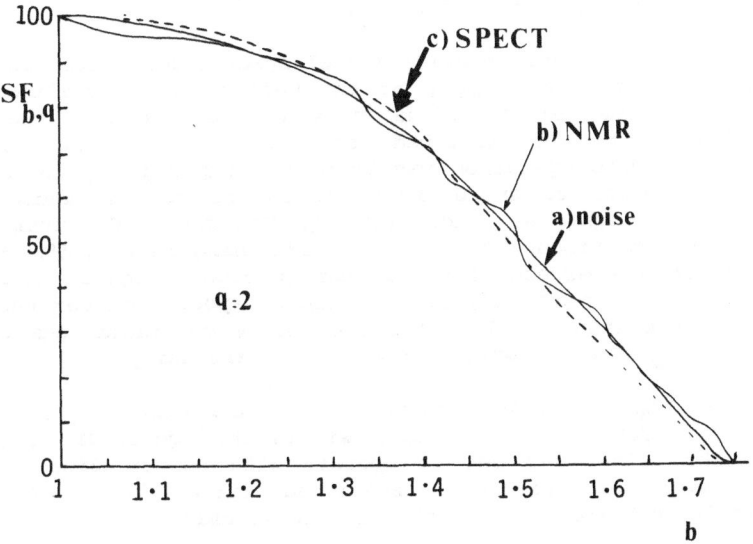

Figure 8 Complexity-significance diagram for pure noise (curve a), an NMR image (curve b) and an abnormal liver SPECT image (curve c) at the 2nd level of decomposition.

## A SIGNIFICANCE DRIVEN IMAGE-PROCESSING FILTER

### Details of the non-linear filter

It is apparent that although the macroscopic collective behaviour $SF_{b,q}$ for an image is not carrying information which is easily interpreted, nevertheless the local value of each departure from the mean expressed in terms of the standard deviation for constituent pixels at the stage of contemplating merger does carry meaningful information on the local complexity. Against this background a new and more flexible methodology emerges in which the point by point complexity may be preserved during an image processing technique which reduces the visual impact of insignificant structure. Moreover the restriction of level-by-level generation of ever larger superpixels is removed. Images processed in this way display not just significant detail but in a conventionally acceptable manner. The methodology is as follows:

1. The mean and standard deviation of a square region of interest surrounding each pixel was computed and the departure of that pixel value from the mean was expressed in units of the standard deviation. This value is called the weight $w_{i,j}$ of the pixel $a_{i,j}$. The weight $w_{i,j}$ is generated for all pixels $(i,j)$ in the image. A map of these weights when displayed shows the regions in the image where local changes in pixel value are of significance, large weights arising for such pixels. Conversely regions of an image which are almost uniform would generate small weights. The smallest weight which can occur is zero (all pixel values in the square ROI are equal). The largest weight which could arise is $\sqrt{(x-1)}$ where x pixels comprise the ROI as shown in section 2.6. We shall refer to this ROI as the feature kernel.

2. The weights were used to drive a real space image filter as follows. Firstly the reciprocal $p_{i,j}$ of the weights was normalised to the range 0-1. The lowest value p = 0 thus implies the highest significance to be ascribed to the corresponding pixel and vice-versa. This operation was however 'tempered' by an additional constraint aimed to avoid oversmoothing of regions where $w_{i,j}$ is small. All weights $w_{i,j}$ less than $C_w$ were set to $C_w$. This step was taken prior to producing $p_{i,j}$ and normalising in 0-1. The result is to increase the effect of the filter at other weights. $C_w$ becomes a free parameter in the filter. One would expect, however that values of $w_{i,j}$ less than 1 will arise from noise considerations alone and that thus $C_w$ should always be set to at least unity.

3. The means $NN_k$ of the k-th nearest neighbours were computed for each pixel $a_{i,j}$ for those neighbours within the square ROI surrounding $a_{i,j}$. The filter was set to operate with contributions from only those neighbours within a specified filter kernel (which was generally much smaller than the feature kernel).

4. Each value $a_{i,j}$ in the image was replaced by the value

$$[1 - p_{i,j}/2] \, a_{i,j} + \sum_{k=1}^{K} \left[ 2 \sum_{k=1}^{K} (1/d_k) \right]^{-1} p_{i,j} \, NN_k / d_k \qquad (2)$$

where $d_k$ is the distance to the k-th nearest neighbour in units of the pixel side size.

This filter has the following properties:

a)  The coefficient multiplying the central term is equal to the sum of the coefficients multiplying the nearest neighbour means, when the maximum filtering occurs (minimum pixel weight $w_{i,j} = C_w$) (ie $p_{i,j}=1$).

b)  When $p_{i,j} = 0$ no filtering occurs since this represents the maximum significance to the pixel $a_{i,j}$ .

c)  The contribution from the nearest neighbour means is inversely proportional to their distance from the central pixel.

d) The filter is a space dependent filter driven by the value of $P_{i,j}$ with the extremes expressed in (a) and (b) above.

A more general filter relaxing properties (a) and (c) is to replace $a_{i,j}$ by

$$[1 - P_{i,j} \sum_{k=1}^{K} c_k] a_{i,j} \quad + \quad \sum_{k=1}^{K} c_k P_{i,j} \, NN_k \tag{3}$$

where $c_k$ is the coefficient to be multiplied into the k-th nearest neighbour mean. The coefficients in the constrained version of the filter (eq(2)) are explicitly $c_1 = 0.1662, c_2 = 0.1175, c_3 = 0.0831, c_4 = 0.0743, c_5 = 0.0570$ for a 5x5 filter kernel and $c_1 = 0.293, c_2 = 0.207$ for a 3x3 filter kernel.

Equation (2) derives from equation (3) by requiring

$$\sum_{k}^{K} c_k = 1/2 \text{ and } c_k \ \alpha \ 1/d_k.$$

With a completely free choice of $c_k$ it is apparent that the filter could be made to behave very badly! Indeed if $c_k$ are chosen such that the sum of $c_k$ over all k=1....K becomes greater than 1, the central term can be completely swamped by the contributions from the nearest neighbours. It was for this reason that the more constrained filter in equation (2) was found more suitable.

In step (1) the generation of the weight is not restricted to a consideration within the superpixels of the type considered in section 2.6 which expanded in size in integral multiples of 2 and tesellated in the field. The feature kernel is centred on each pixel and may have any size. The filtering technique will operate best when the structure one is attempting to highlight has small spatial extent compared with the size of the feature kernel used to elucidate the weight to be attached to a pixel and priming the filtering of that pixel. If the feature-kernel is increased in size the method is improved. Increasing the size of the feature kernel does however carry some penalty in terms of increased computational time and for this reason numerous commercial companies are manufacturing array- processor based image processing equipment for when real-space operations of this kind are to be performed.

Display of the image feature 'driving' the filter

Bearing in mind the free choice which is allowed by the filter, it is clear that a single starting image can give rise to any number of filtered images. The filter coefficients are chosen so that a desired amount of smoothing takes place for those regions where it is deemed

that smoothing shall occur. The methodology ensures differential smoothing such that significant detail receives less smoothing than insignificant structure, but the whole scale of smoothing can be varied by the choice of coefficients $c_k$.

Even with the less arbitrary first scheme in which the coefficients are constrained to give the filter extra properties, the free choice introduced with the weight cutoff $C_w$ still retains this sliding scale of filtration.

Because of this flexibility, it has been found useful to display the map of the reciprocal weights $p_{i,j}$ found in step 2 as an image. This is the space variant feature which has been extracted to 'drive' the filter. When this is displayed adjacent to the original and the filtered image it is possible to glance from one to the other and develop a stronger impression than from just inspecting original or filtered images.

It has also proved useful to inspect the number of weights falling below $C_w$ which represents the number receiving maximum smoothing and also to display the histogram of the weights and the histogram of the reciprocal weights as the cutoff was varied. Somewhat similar techniques have been employed by Bamber and Daft (1986) and Bamber and Cook-Martin (1987) for investigating texture in ultrasonic B-scan images, when more than one feature may be extracted and used vectorially to control image processing.

## Illustrative example for a noise pattern

Consider again for a moment the noise distribution introduced in section 2.5. This was a matrix of 4096 pixels with a nominal value of V and standard deviation of 10% V.

Using a 5x5 feature kernel and setting $C_w = 1$, 2961 weights were found to be below this limit. That is (2961/4096) = 0.72 of the pixels are within 1 standard deviation of the mean of the 5x5 ROI surrounding them. If we made the assumption that the mean of 25 Gaussian numbers is close to the mean of the full set we would expect (from considerations in section 7) that this fraction should have been erf (1)= 0.68. The results are consistent with this, the difference being that each pixel value was tested for departure from the local not the global mean.

## Illustrative example for a signal buried in noise

Figure 9a shows a small (2x2) region of pixels of signal 30% above background with 10% noise added to the entire field. There is no difficulty seeing the central region in this case. When the methodology in section 3.1 was applied to this image using a 13x13 feature kernel with $C_w = 2$ and filtering equation (2), the result, shown in figure 9b, is much less mottled and shows the central region even more clearly. Other pixels which have randomly occurred more than 2 standard deviations from the mean of the background are also made more prominent.

## A perception experiment to evaluate non-linear filtering

A 64x64 matrix of pixels, each of value B = 1000 units was constructed. The values within the pixels were then varied by the addition of Gaussian noise with a standard deviation of N% of 1000 using the Hanning algorithm. Between one and sixteen (selected randomly) 4x4 fields of equal increased intensity S were then buried in the image

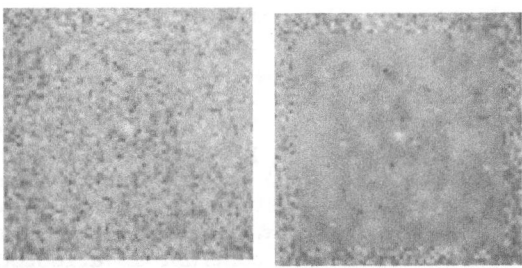

Figure 9 A 2x2 signal buried in a 64x64 noise field. a) before image filtering b) after image filtering.

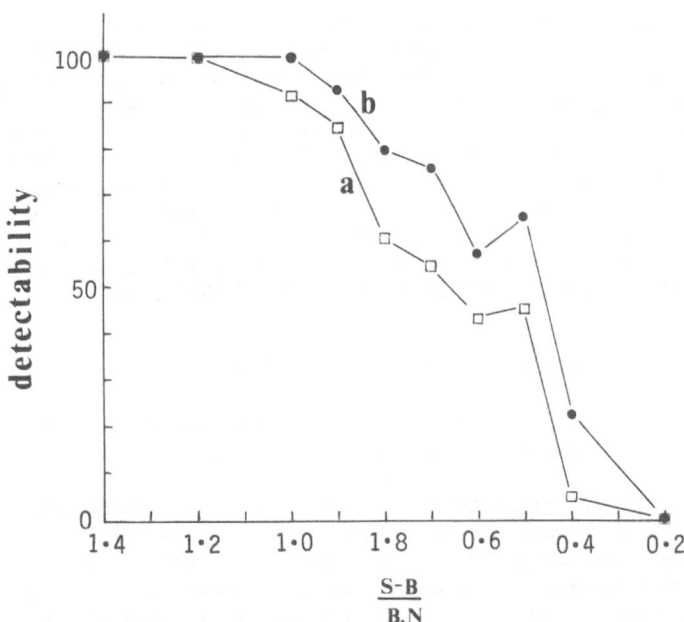

Figure 10 Detectability versus contrast for small signals in noisy background curve a is for unprocessed images; curve b is for processed images.

without the observer knowing their locations (which were stored in a file for later reference). A single observer was then asked to state how many small fields were present and their locations. The detectability of the fields was scored as the ratio of the number of correctly located fields to the total present. Altogether 69 frames of data were observed with 340 fields. (The reason the average number of fields per frame was not half of sixteen was that the computer could choose the same location more than once without penalty). The graph of detectability versus $(S-B)/B.N$ is shown in figure 10. The same 69 frames were then put through the non-linear filtering process and the blind experiment repeated. From the result (curve b) we can conclude that detectability has been improved by non-linear filtering especially where the signal intensity is less than one standard deviation above background. It is appreciated that the measurement of contrast is affected by the transfer function of the monitor used for display but the experiment was performed on the approximately linear part of this curve and contrast measurements should be meaningful.

Illustrative clinical images

Figure 11 shows an abnormal liver SPECT image before and after processing with the non-linear filter using a 13x13 feature kernel. Figure 12 shows a part of a pelvic NMR image before and after filtering in the same way  In order to generate these images the image of the inverse weights has been inspected and the cutoff $C_w$ has been varied until the processed image was satisfactory. The histogram of the inverse weights was also used. Similar image processing has been applied to tomographic data from the Royal Marsden Hospital prototype Multiwire Proportional Counter Positron Camera (MUPPET) and will be reported elsewhere (Webb et al, 1987).

A possible limitation of the technique is that it is essentially designed for enhancing the presence of a structure against a background which is large compared with both the structure and also the size of the feature kernel. That is the gross background must not itself vary greatly within the kernel. Fortunately, at least in nuclear medicine, one is generally interested in attempting to identify tumours as small scale hot or cold regions within more or less uniform uptake. The potential problem of a gross structural boundary lying within the feature kernel leads us to suggest a quite different method of non-linear filtering which is not affected by this problem as it has an inbuilt mechanism to detect gross structural changes.

TEXTURE DEPENDENT NON LINEAR IMAGE FILTERING

This filtering technique uses a quite different methodology to that described in section 3. It is as follows:

Each pixel is compared with the mean of its neighbours up to and including the n th nearest neighbour (n.n) in the plane. n begins at 1 and increases sequentially to embrace ever wider contexts for each pixel. If the absolute value of the difference between the pixel and this mean exceeds a preset value, the pixel 'survives'. If it does not exceed this value then it is replaced by the mean. The image is inspected at each cycle labelled by n; thus after considering comparisons with the mean of just the first n.n.'s, the comparison proceeds for each pixel with the mean of the 1st and 2nd n.n.'s together and so on. If a pixel is replaced at some level 'n' it goes on to be considered for replacement at the next highest level (n+1). If however it survives replacement at some level 'n' it receives no further

18

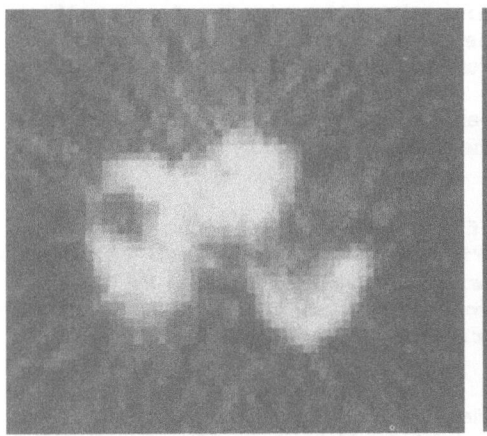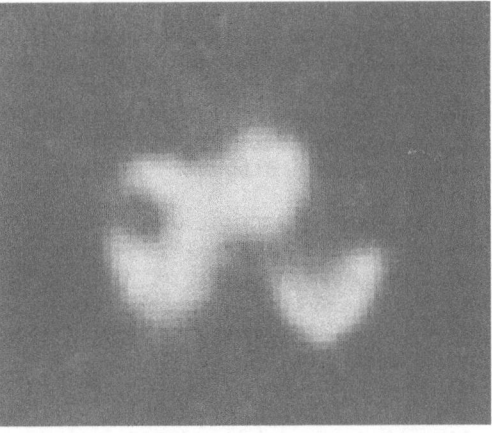

Figure 11 Abnormal liver SPECT image. a) before image filtering; b) after image filtering.

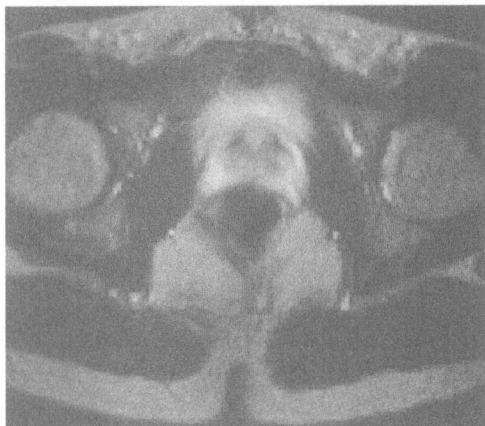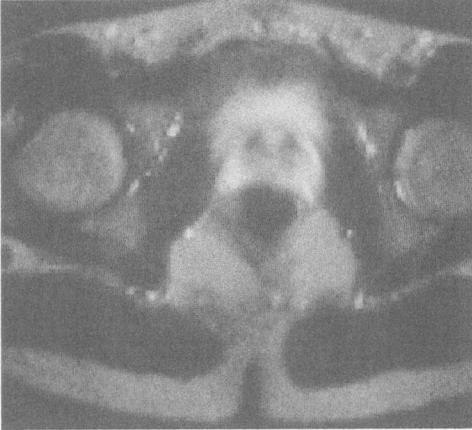

Figure 12 Pelvic NMR image a) before image filtering b) after image filtering.

consideration.

This scheme allows for the possibility that the texture in the image is space-variant because the pixel will survive replacement earlier (ie at lower values of n) where the texture is fine but will be replaced at higher values of n where the structure is coarser. In particular when a boundary is encountered, it is self-evident that the current value for a pixel will thereafter survive and no attempt to cross the boundary and include neighbours, from what is a different region, in the replacing mean will be made. Similar philosophy has been discussed by McGeehan et al (1985) but not in the context of image processing. A biproduct of the method is the confidence which arises from watching the diminishing change in the image as ever higher values of n are considered. As an aside we note that we did consider replacing, by the mean, all pixels used to comprise the mean, in a 'region growing scheme' , but this was not found to be so successful as single pixel replacement as it reintroduced unwanted sharp boundaries.

Software to achieve this texture-dependent filtering has been constructed for SPECT, PET and NMR data, the format of which is different in our centre. In common with the image decomposition methodology discussed earlier, it is clear that the significance of pixels is controlled by the free parameter on the comparison (with the mean) of pixel deviation from the mean. Ideally one would like to have this predicted from the physics of the imaging modality but this is not easy as we have discussed earlier.

Figure 13 illustrates the use of the technique for the same liver SPECT image considered previously (Fig 11a). The comparison criterion was set equal to 15% of the maximum pixel value. Figure 14 shows a thyroid phantom, before and after processing with the same conditions, imaged with the prototype PET scanner. The processing considered up to the 10th n.n's.

This method is readily extendable to include neighbours from adjacent tomographic planes and in principle this is much more logical than considering 'in-plane' image processing alone. For SPECT,PET and NMR data software has been constructed to achieve this. Necessarily this software is much more slow to run. We illustrate the technique in figure 15 which are the results of this 3D texture-dependent non-linear filtering method for the same planes of date shown after 2D filtering in figures 13 and 14. Again up to the 10th n.n's were considered with the criterion for comparison set at 15% of the maximum pixel count.

SUMMARY

All methods of image processing convert one image into another whose diagnostic usefulness is considered greater. In this paper the diagnostic process has been analysed and stated in terms of ascribing a significance to a pixel in relation to its contextual neighbours. Image decomposition into a field whose pixels vary in size has been simply achieved by a stacking algorithm. It has been shown that if the noise

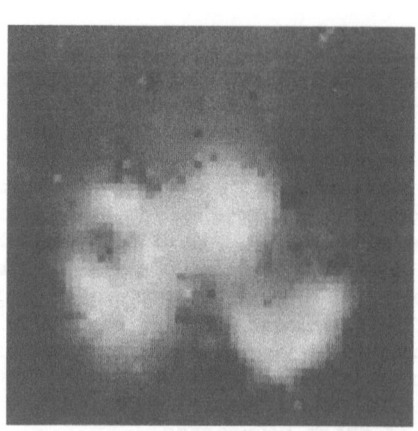

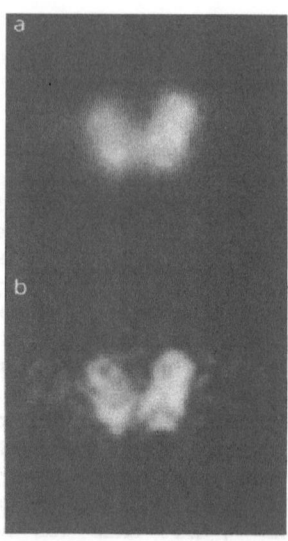

Figure 13 Abnormal liver SPECT image after texture dependent filtering.

Figure 14 Thyroid PET image before (a) and after (b) filtering

level in an image could be specified, such images would display only significant structure. The generation of a complexity-significance diagram gives a quantitative expression for the fraction of data in the original image which should be represented by pixels of differing sizes. When the decomposition is governed by local significance criteria, it has been shown that the significant data is encapsulated in the departure of the complexity-significance diagram from that for pure noise. Additionally this method of considering images clearly demonstrated that most of the useful information in an image is stored in the context of pixels rather than in the values of the pixels as a string.

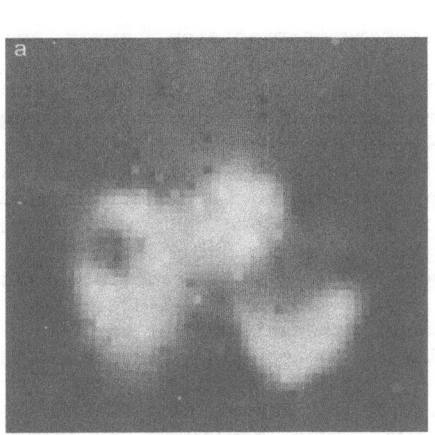 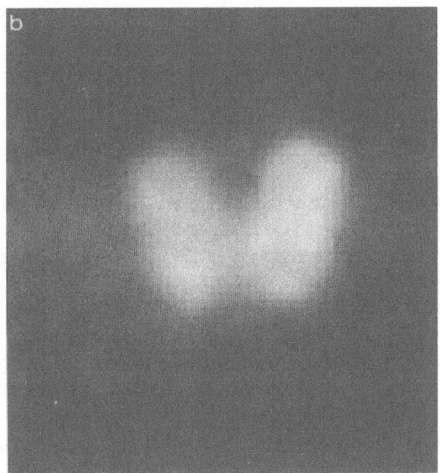

Figure 15 a) Abnormal liver SPECT image and b) thyroid phantom PET image after 3D texture dependent filtering.

The significance of a pixel in relation to its neighbours has been used as a feature to prime a non-linear space-variant filter. The filtered image retains significant detail whilst differentially smoothing noise. The size of the feature kernel may be varied and, provided it does not encompass more than one gross structure, it has been shown that the feature strength increases as this size is increased relative to the size of the small-scale structure it is desired to highlight. The filter may be interactively tuned by observing, as an image, the windowed feature. The method was illustrated with clinical examples from SPECT and NMR and a simple perception experiment.

A second image filter was presented which takes account of the local changes in image texture and which has been implemented in both a 2D and 3D manner. Clinical examples from SPECT and PET were presented.

In this paper we have concentrated on methodology with clinical illustration. It is intended to evaluate the filtering techniques via a more substantial clinical study.

ACKNOWLEDGEMENTS

I should like to acknowledge the clinical data supplied by my colleagues, in particular Drs Bob Ott and Paul Marsden (PET), Dr. Maggie Flower (SPECT) and Dr. Martin Leach (NMR) and for much discussion of image processing with them. I am grateful to Dr Roy Bentley for providing the image processing facilities (VAX 750 and SIGMEX ARGS 7000 display for this work).

REFERENCES

Andrews, H.C., and Hunt, B.R., 1977, Digital image restoration (Prentice-Hall, Englewood Cliffs, NJ).

Bamber, J.C., and Cook-Martin, G.,1987, Texture analysis and speckle reduction in medical echography. SPIE Symposium on pattern recognition and acoustical imaging. Newport Beach C.A. Feb 1987 SPIE publication 768.

Bamber, J.C., and Daft, C., 1986, Adaptive filtering for reduction of speckle in ultrasonic pulse-echo images. Ultrasonics Jan 1986 41-46.

Barford, N.C., 1967, "Experimental measurements:precision, error and truth", pub. Addison-Wesley.

de Graaf, C.N., Toet, A., Koenderink, J.J. and Zuidema, P., 1984, Some applications of hierarchical image processing algorithms. in "Image Processing in Medical Imaging", 343-369 pub Martinus Nijhoff.

Leach, M.O., Flatman, W.D., Webb, S., Flower, M.A. and Ott, R.J., 1984, The application of variable median window filtering to computerised tomography in "Image Processing in Medical Imaging", 130-150 pub Martinus Nijhoff.

McGeechan, C.S., Gemmell, H.G. and Dendy, P.P., 1985, Texture analysis in radionuclide liver imaging. Phys Med Biol 30 669-676.

Webb, S., 1986, Comparison of data processing techniques for the improvement of contrast in SPECT liver tomograms. Phys.Med.Biol.30, 1077-1086.

Webb, S., Long, A.P., Ott, R.J., Leach, M.O. and Flower, M.A., 1985, Constrained deconvolution of SPECT liver tomograms by direct digital image restoration, Medical Physics 12 53-58.

Webb, S., Ott, R.J., Marsden, P.K., Flower, M.A., 1987, Image enhancement in PET scanning with Royal Marsden MWPC camera. Proc. of the International Symposium on the use of Wire Chambers in Medical Imaging. Corsondonk, Belgium June 1987.

Yanch, J.C., Webb, S., Flower, M.A. and Irvine, A.T., 1987, Constrained deconvolution to remove resolution degradation caused by scatter in SPECT.

# TOWARD A NOTION OF FEATURE EXTRACTION FOR PLANE MAPPINGS

Fred L. Bookstein

Center for Human Growth and Development
University of Michigan
Ann Arbor, MI 48109 USA

## INTRODUCTION

My concern is the delineation of features for plane mappings as they express the relation of two biological images. Perhaps one picture represents a statistical norm for an organ, the other the form observed in an individual patient; or perhaps one represents an organ prior to a treatment, the other the same after treatment or after growth. I and my colleagues have argued elsewhere (Bookstein, 1986a, 1986b; Bookstein et al., 1985) that the crux of the quantitative analysis of biological form is the representation of its variation by means of such mappings: this is the mathematical model of shape change as **deformation**. The idea is not new—it is most often associated with the name of the great British natural philosopher D'Arcy Thompson—but it is not familiar in the context of "feature extraction" as currently applied in medical imaging. It is usual instead for features to pertain to images considered one at a time. In this paper I continue the elaboration of quantitative features for a pair of images viewed as corresponding biological scenes.

My earlier work has emphasized the representation of biological form by a finite number of discrete, individually identifiable points, the **landmarks**. These are presumed to be "homologous," to correspond from form to form, according to evolutionary or developmental evidence that is not our concern here. When forms are related by landmarks in this way, the mappings between them may be represented for statistical purposes as a finite-dimensional vector space over the complex numbers (Bookstein, 1987c), and the "features" of those mappings are just the ordinary statistical features of such a finite-dimensional vector space: separations of group means, directions of change, clusters.

But there is more information in a set of biological images than can be encoded in the locations of one single roster of discretely labeled points. Especially when data arise from fully three-dimensional representations, much of the information underlying diagnosis of abnormal forms is derived directly from features of curving form in-between the landmarks. But when, for instance, one attempts to represent curves explicitly as additional dimensions of the "feature" space, as by their identification with a space of functions of arc-length, one rapidly "loses the picture" of the mapping. The feature space is now so far removed from the object geometry of the organism as to sever quantification from understanding (see, for example, the discussion in Sec. 2.3 of Bookstein et al., 1985).

The present essay somewhat speculatively pursues an alternative approach. Working within a function space of arbitrarily high dimension, I provide a semigraphical method for selecting low-dimensional representations of particular deformations in terms of systems of "pseudolandmarks" finite in number but, in general, different from comparison to comparison. There is a whole series of these function spaces, each of a different finite dimension: one involving correspondences of three landmarks only, the next of four, the next of five, and so on. We pass upward along this sequence of steadily larger subspaces, at each step adding one degree of complexity to the "feature space," until we have adequately archived the comparison of images before us, in a sense to be explained presently. At each stage we select the least informative function consistent with the given pairing of the images. This tactic guarantees that in the resulting analysis the somewhat arbitrary assignments of homologues between landmarks, in the areas where there are no data, has the least possible effect upon image interpretation.

## THIN-PLATE SPLINES

To drive this hierarchical inspection of multiple function subspaces one needs a geometric machine for interpolating maps under constraints of diverse style: specification of the values of functions, but also specifications of certain functionals of their derivatives. A suitable technology may be borrowed wholesale from a neighboring field, interpolation theory. One particular method of interpolating scattered data, the **thin-plate spline**, incorporates a quasilinear theory of "local information" which can be applied to our needs. (I am indebted to David Ragozin of the University of Washington for explaining this literature to me and for insisting, correctly, that it exactly suits the application to mappings.) This approach to interpolation was introduced by Duchon—"le principe des plaques minces"—in a series of reports in the middle 1970's, and was later formalized by Jean Meinguet (1979a, 1979b, 1984) in a very general mathematical setting. Franke (1982) and Wahba and Wendelberger (1980) describe some earlier applications. To my knowledge these splines had not been considered for use in the analysis of plane mappings prior to Bookstein (1987a, 1987b). The remainder of this section comprises a terse overview of the crux of the thin-plate method. For details, see the sources cited above.

Let $P_1 = (x_1, y_1)$, $P_2 = (x_2, y_2)$, ..., $P_n = (x_n, y_n)$ be $n$ points in the ordinary Euclidean plane according to any convenient Cartesian coordinate system. We will be concerned with functions $f$ taking specified values at the points $P_i$; should certain pairs or triples of $P$'s be closely adjacent, the effect is that of specifying derivatives of $f$ as well as values. Write $r_{ij} = |P_i - P_j|$ for the distance between points $i$ and $j$.

The function $U(0) = 0$, $U(r) = r^2 \log r$ is, up to a multiplicative constant of $8\pi$, the fundamental solution of the iterated Laplacian $\Delta^2$. That is,

$$\Delta^2 U = \left[\frac{\partial^2}{\partial x^2} + \frac{\partial^2}{\partial y^2}\right]^2 U$$

is a multiple of the delta-function $\delta_{0,0}$ nonzero everywhere except at the origin.

This differential expression underlies the theory of elasticity of a thin metal plate subject to normal displacements: hence the name of the spline functions to be developed with its aid.

Define matrices

$$K = \begin{bmatrix} 0 & U(r_{12}) & \cdots & U(r_{1n}) \\ U(r_{21}) & 0 & \cdots & U(r_{2n}) \\ \cdots & \cdots & \cdots & \cdots \\ U(r_{n1}) & U(r_{n2}) & \cdots & 0 \end{bmatrix}, \ n \times n;$$

$$P = \begin{bmatrix} 1 & x_1 & y_1 \\ 1 & x_2 & y_2 \\ \cdots & \cdots & \cdots \\ 1 & x_n & y_n \end{bmatrix}, \ 3 \times n;$$

and

$$L = \left[\begin{array}{c|c} K & P \\ \hline P^T & 0 \end{array}\right], \ (n+3) \times (n+3),$$

where $^T$ is the matrix transpose operator and $0$ is a $3 \times 3$ matrix of $0$'s.

Let $V = (v_1, \ldots, v_n)$ be any $n$-vector, and write $Y = (V \mid 0\ 0\ 0)^T$, a column vector of length $n+3$. Define the vector $W = (w_1, \ldots, w_n)$ and the coefficients $a_1$, $a_x$, $a_y$ by the equation

$$L^{-1}Y = (W \mid a_1\ a_x\ a_y)^T.$$

Use the elements of $L^{-1}Y$ to define a function $f(x,y)$ everywhere in the plane:

$$f(x,y) = a_1 + a_x x + a_y y + \sum_{i=1}^{n} w_i U(\,|P_i - (x,y)|\,).$$

Then the following three propositions hold:

1. $f(x_i, y_i) = v_i$, all $i$.

2. The function $f$ minimizes the nonnegative quantity

$$I_f = \iint_{\mathbf{R}^2} \left[\; \left[\frac{\partial^2 f}{\partial x^2}\right]^2 + 2\left[\frac{\partial^2 f}{\partial x \partial y}\right]^2 + \left[\frac{\partial^2 f}{\partial y^2}\right]^2 \;\right]$$

over the class of such interpolants. Call this the "integral quadratic variation" or the "integral bending norm."

3. The value of $I_f$ is proportional to

$$WKW^T = V(L_n^{-1} K L_n^{-1}) V^T,$$

where $L_n^{-1}$ is the upper left $n \times n$ subblock of $L^{-1}$. This integral is zero only when all the components of $W$ are zero: in this case, the computed map is $f(x,y) = a_1 + a_x x + a_y y$, a linear or <u>uniform</u> transformation.

In the present application we take $V$ to be the $2 \times n$ matrix

$$V = \begin{bmatrix} x'_1 & y'_1 \\ x'_2 & y'_2 \\ \cdots & \cdots \\ x'_n & y'_n \end{bmatrix}$$

where each $(x'_i, y'_i)$ is a point "homologous to" $(x_i, y_i)$ in another copy of $\mathbf{R}^2$.

The resulting function $f$ is now vector-valued: it maps each point $(x_i, y_i)$ to its homologue $(x'_i, y'_i)$ and is smoothest (according to the measure $I_f$, integral quadratic variation over all $\mathbf{R}^2$, computed separately for real and imaginary parts of $f$ and summed) of all such functions. These vector-valued functions $f(x,y)$ are the **thin-plate spline mappings** of this paper.

To accomodate the relaxation procedure described below, we must slightly extend the usual algebra in a direction somewhat different from that of the statistical splining of Wahba and Wendelberger (1980) or Silverman (1985).

Suppose we allow certain of the homologues $(x_i',y_i')$ to vary along straight lines. That is, we allow the homologue $(x_i',y_i')$ to be any point of the form

$$(x_i',y_i') = ([x_i']_0 + t_i r_i,\ [y_i']_0 + t_i s_i)$$

where $r_i$ and $s_i$ are direction cosines of the line along which $(x_i',y_i')$ is varying, and the value of $t_i$ is to be determined. If $k$ homologues are freed to "slide" along lines in this way, the matrix $V$ actually covers an affine $k$-flat ($k$-dimensional vector subspace shifted away from the origin):

$$V = V(t_{j_1},\ ...,\ t_{j_k}) = \begin{bmatrix} x_1' & y_1' \\ \cdots & \cdots \\ [x_{j_1}']_0 + t_{j_1} r_{j_1} & [y_{j_1}']_0 + t_{j_1} s_{j_1} \\ \cdots & \cdots \\ [x_{j_k}']_0 + t_{j_k} r_{j_k} & [y_{j_k}']_0 + t_{j_k} s_{j_k} \\ \cdots & \cdots \\ x_n' & y_n' \end{bmatrix}.$$

Then as the $t_{j_l}$ vary, the integral $I_f = I_f(t_{j_1},\ ...,\ t_{j_k})$ varies about a nonnegative minimum as a positive-semidefinite quadratic form in $t_{j_1}\ ...\ t_{j_k}$. The minimizing of $I_f(t_{j_1},\ ...,\ t_{j_k})$ is numerically very tractable for $k \le n - 3$.


FEATURE EXTRACTION AS EIGENANALYSIS OF THE INTEGRAL $I_f$

The value of the integral $I_f$ is zero for mappings which yield a zero vector for $W$. These are just the affine transformations or uniform shears that leave parallel lines parallel. From the point of view of biological shape analysis, these mappings have no localizable "features": rather, each is characterized wholly by a single global tensor descriptor the biometrics of which are by now quite well worked-out (Bookstein, 1986b). We will attempt to identify local information in mappings by the deviation of $I_f$ from this minimum of zero. In doing so we exploit the second characterization of the thin-plate spline map $f(x,y)$ as the mapping of lowest $I_f$ among all those satisfying a certain finite set of point-correspondences; as a consequence, our estimate of this net local information is as conservative as it can possibly be.

Consider, for instance, the mapping $f$ shown in Figure 1. It relates four landmark points $(x_i,y_i)$ having the form of a square (left) to four homologues $(x_i',y_i')$ having the different form shown at the right. For this map, the value of $I_f$ (labelled "integral bending norm" in these figures) is exactly zero—the map is uniform. This $f$ maps the starting square into an exact rhombus on the right, and

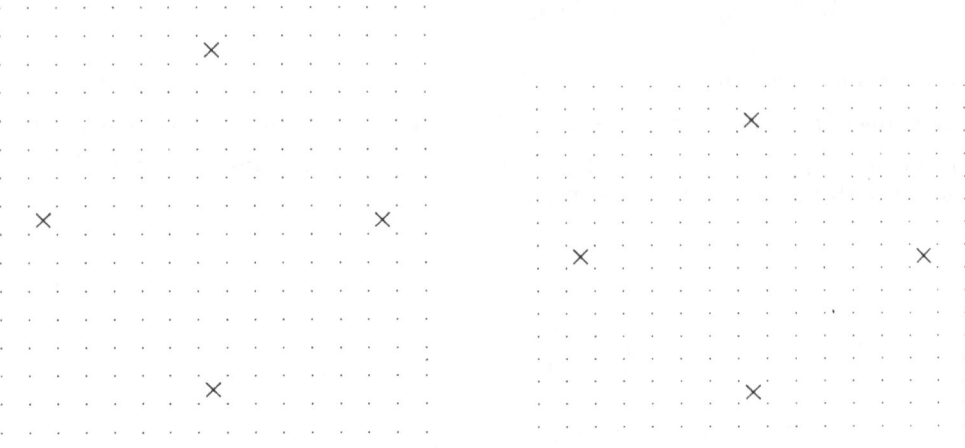

Integral bending norm     0.0000

Figure 1

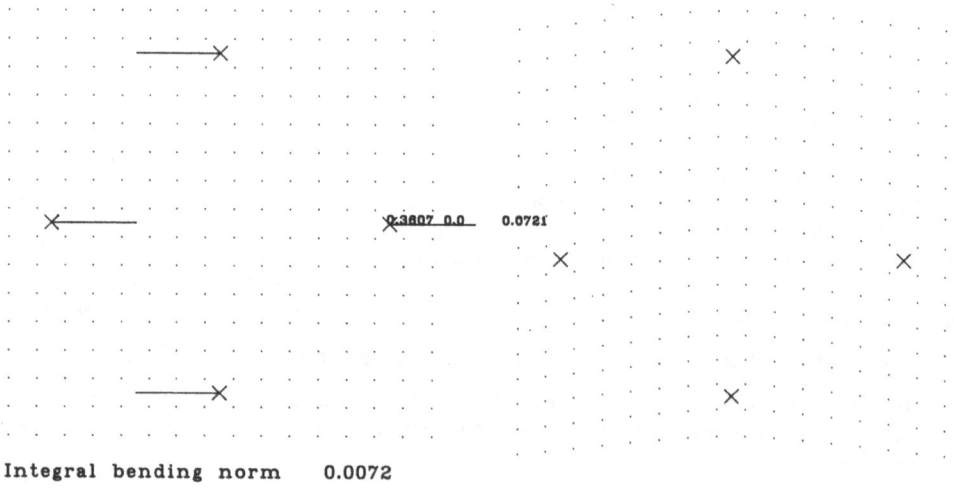

Integral bending norm     0.0072

Figure 2

its action is the same in each of the little squares of the grid.

In Figure 2, we have mapped this same square onto a form which is no longer a parallelogram, so that the grid on the right is no longer uniform. The "features" of this mapping are its projections on the eigenvectors of the matrix $L_n^{-1}KL_n^{-1}$ which operates upon the matrix of coordinates $(x_i', y_i')$ of points in the right-hand image to generate a net measure of nonlinearity, a "deformation norm" that is zero for all uniform transformations, whether isotropic or not. The matrix $L_n^{-1}KL_n^{-1}$ always has three zero eigenvalues, corresponding to the three degrees of freedom $a_1$, $a_x$, $a_y$ of the uniform transformations in each Cartesian coordinate. For $n=4$ landmarks, as here, there remains one degree of freedom per coordinate, one nontrivial eigenvector, the loadings of which may be represented by scalars at each landmark as shown on the left in Figure 2. [In the graphic convention I have chosen, these displacements have only signs, not directions. In later figures there will be up to four of these eigenvectors shown at angles of 0° (or 180°), 30° (or 210°), 60° (or 240°), and 90° (or 270°) to the horizontal. Segments drawn away from landmarks in opposite directions correspond to loadings of opposite sign.] The eigenvector applies separately to the x-and y-components of the transformation, the separate columns of $V$.

The symmetry of the eigenvector in Figure 2 implies that even for transformations of four landmarks—at least, four in the form of a square—shape change cannot be localized: there is only one available feature of nonlinearity, a feature which can be represented as any of the four displacements shown in the figure. (The reader may convince himself, for instance, that the deformation which consists in moving the leftmost landmark upward by some extent is equivalent, up to an affine transformation, to that moving the rightmost landmark upward, and to those moving either the uppermost or the lowermost landmark downward.)

Choosing one right-hand landmark arbitrarily (here, the one at the top), we may ask, direction by direction, how far this landmark must be moved to minimize the deviation from uniformity. If we move this topmost landmark straight down, the minimum of $I_f$ is achieved at the value 0, corresponding to a function $f$ for which $W = 0$, no nonlinearity at all. The $X$ along the straight line in Figure 3 lies exactly at the location previously encountered in Figure 1. But along a direction not passing through that exact zero of $I_f$ (and, in general, there will not be such a direction), the minimum of $I_f$ lies somewhat above zero. For instance, in Figure 4 the top landmark is constrained to move toward the southwest instead, and the minimum of bending (Figure 5) is now some 40% of the initial value, achieved where this tangent line passes closest to the position of no inhomogeneity shown in Figures 1 and 3. This minimum is a composite of contributions to $I_f$ from the x-coordinate and the y-coordinate of deformation separately. That from the x-coordinate decreases for a while under displacement toward the southwest, whereas that of the y-coordinate was at zero to begin with, owing to symmetry of the starting configuration, and increases consistently.

For four-landmark forms not beginning in the form of a square, the term for inhomogeneity does not involve all the landmarks equally. Figure 6, for instance, shows the single eigenvector of nonzero eigenvalue for the quadratic form $I_f$ corresponding to a landmark configuration with three landmarks collinear. The

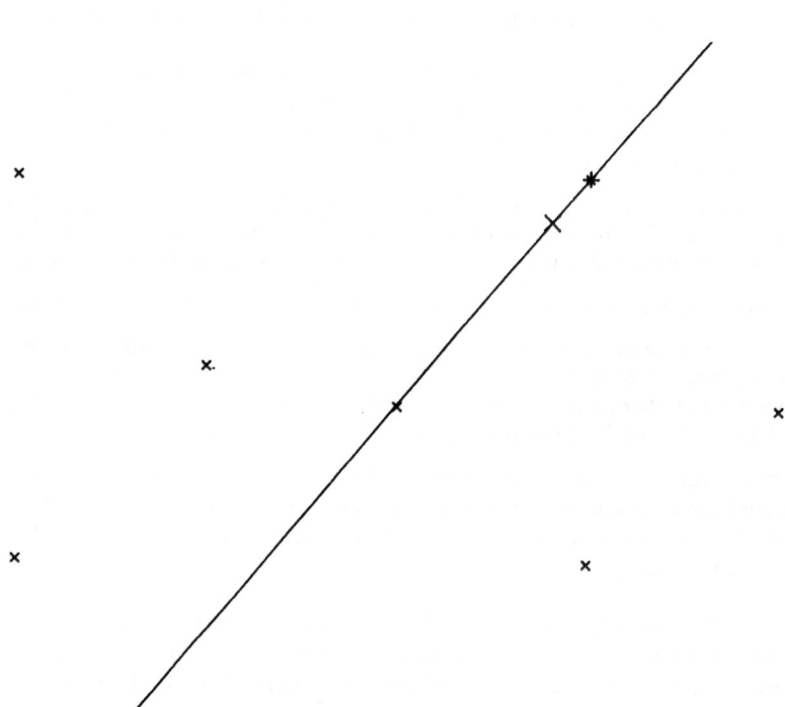

Figure 3

Figure 4

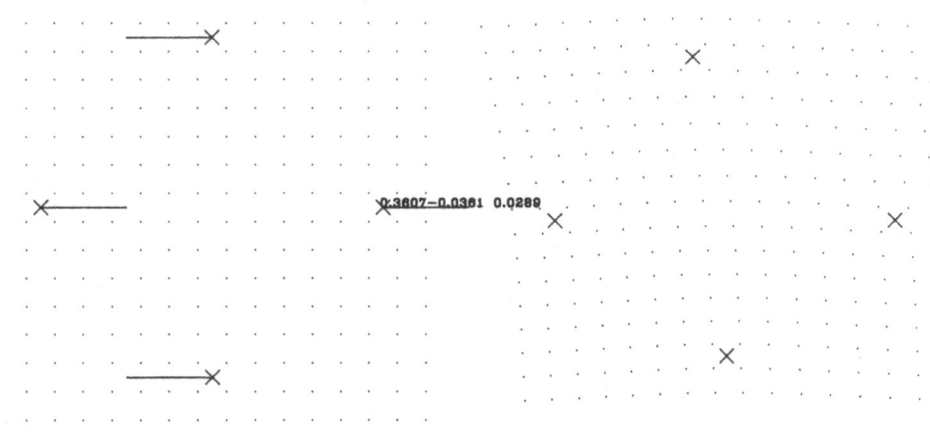

Integral bending norm    0.0030

Figure 5

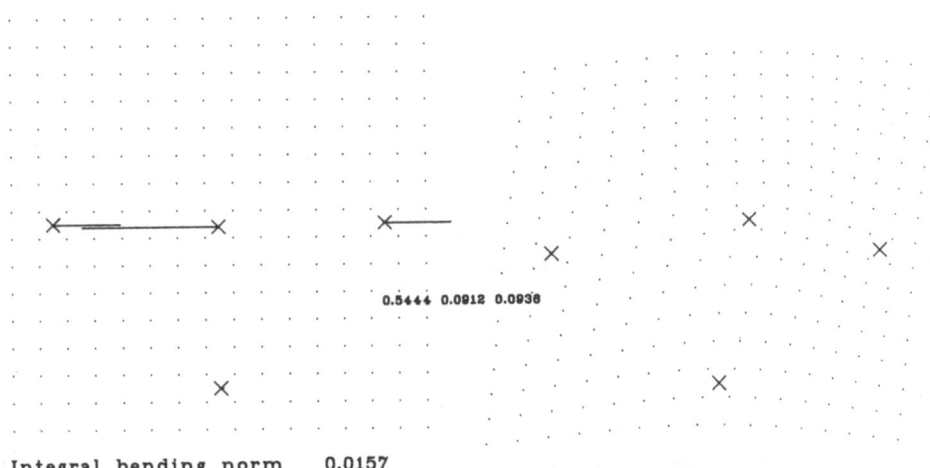

Integral bending norm    0.0157

Figure 6

31

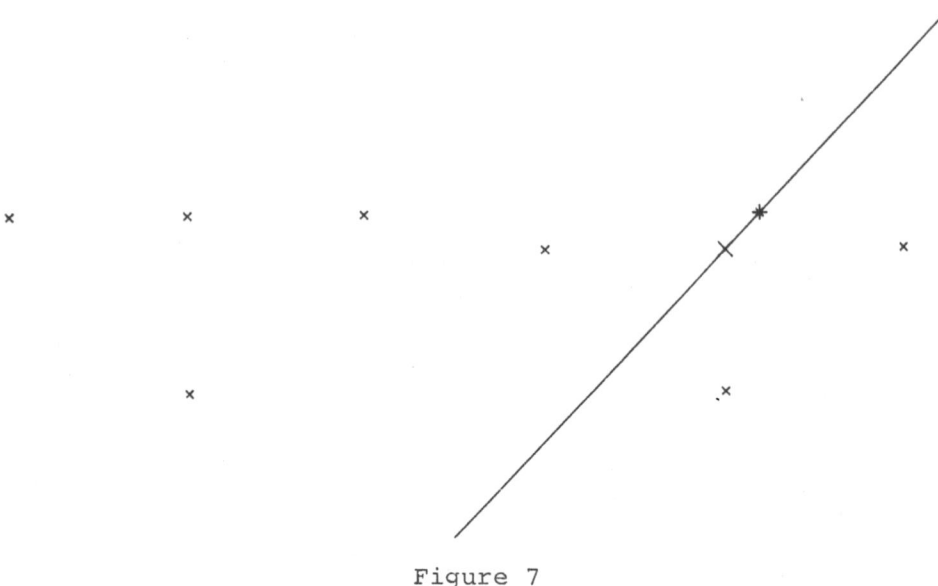

Figure 7

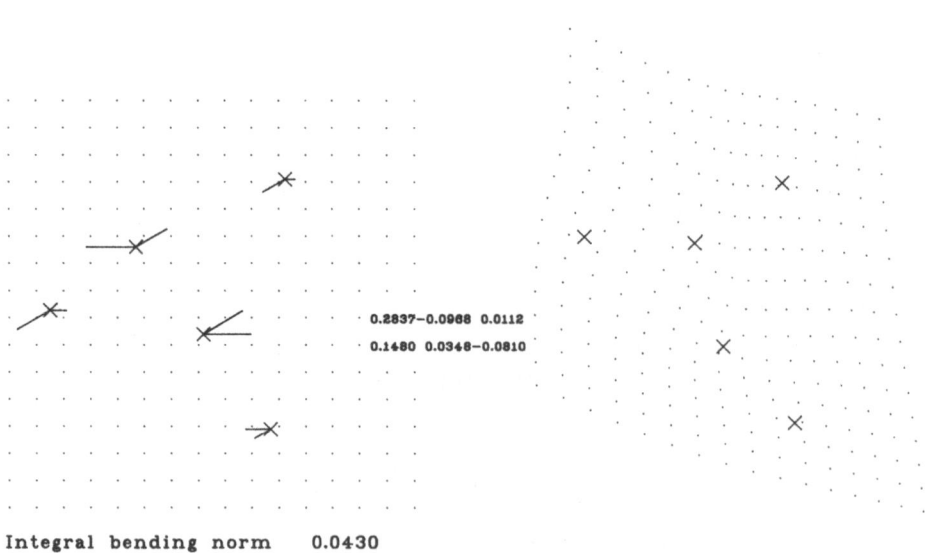

0.2837−0.0968 0.0112
0.1480 0.0348−0.0810

Integral bending norm    0.0430

Figure 8

position of the homologue of the lowest landmark may now be anywhere in the plane without affecting the computed bending $I_f$ of the transform; consequently, this point has no loading upon the nontrivial eigenvector—it does not contribute to our measure of inhomogeneity in any way. When we relax the position of the landmark near the middle of the baseline, for instance (Figure 7), we send it in the direction of the point for which the transformation is linear along that line alone.

Local features begin to emerge from this analysis when five or more landmarks are involved. Figure 8, for instance, shows the two eigenvectors of non-zero eigenvalue for the form $I_f$ corresponding to a deformation discussed later in connection with Figure 12. The last non-zero eigenvalue, plotted at 30° to the horizontal, is equivalent to the global nonhomogeneous term of the previous discussion: it represents a pattern of reversals of displacement between each pair of adjacent landmarks in the design, and bears no local information. But the eigenvector of largest eigenvalue—in general, any eigenvector after the lowest—does bear local information. Discrepancies between the two points most central in this configuration (that at the cross of the "T" and that at the center of the figure) represent a greater modulus of nonlinearity per mm displacement—a greater "bending energy"—than discrepancies between other landmark pairs. Of these two terms for inhomogeneity, all there are for five landmarks, this first, drawn with horizontal dashes in the figure, is thus considerably more localized than the second.

The eigenvectors of $I_f$ depend on the landmarks $(x_i, y_i)$ of the left-hand form only, but the projections of $f$ upon those eigenvectors involve the homologous locations $(x_i', y_i')$ as well. These projections are listed following the eigenvalues in the central table of the figure: first, the projections of the $x$-coordinate of $f$, then those of the $y$-coordinate. In the actual deformation shown, the loading for the largest eigenvector is largest in the $x$-direction (.0968), by virtue of the notable decrease of the horizontal separation between the two landmarks at the center. (But any metaphor of material compression of a segment is misleading. One landmark may move to lie atop another, or jump right across it and continue; the thin-plate spline mapping, not constrained to positive Jacobian, remains perfectly well-defined.) The other eigenvector, the more "global" inhomogeneity, emphasizes the $y$-coordinate (loadings of .0810 vs. .0348) of the deformation under study here; it corresponds to the apparent vertical descent of both "interior" landmarks with respect to the triangle of the three outermost.

Figure 9 augments Figure 8 by two more landmarks, the same two to be added in connection with the transition from Figure 12 to Figure 13. Once again the eigenvector of lowest eigenvalue (now plotted in vertical dashes out of the landmarks, as it is fourth-largest) is a contrast of one "diagonal" of the configuration against the other; it is the most global inhomogeneous term. At the other extreme of eigenvalues is the contrast of shift at the central landmark and that farthest left vis-a-vis the two landmarks in-between them. This term thus corresponds to the "global" inhomogeneity term for a subset of the landmarks, the smallest quadrilateral that can be formed from the original four. In this particular deformation, inhomogeneity of strain seems evenly distributed over all four features except for one of the bending modes of the central "T," already reviewed in connection with the preceding figure: the considerable $x$-shift of the central landmark. Notice that the landmark most centrally located loads almost equally on all four of these eigenvectors, as the configuration is not far from a regular hexagon.

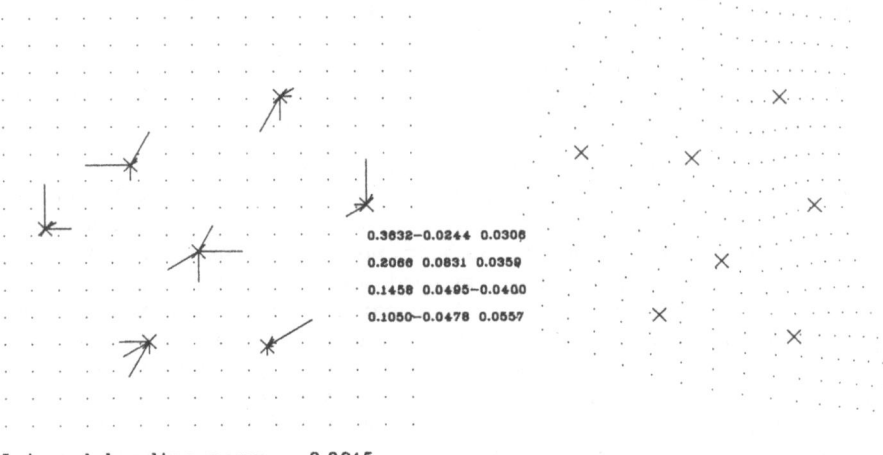

0.3632-0.0244 0.0306
0.2066 0.0831 0.0359
0.1456 0.0495-0.0400
0.1050-0.0476 0.0557

Integral bending norm    0.0615

Figure 9

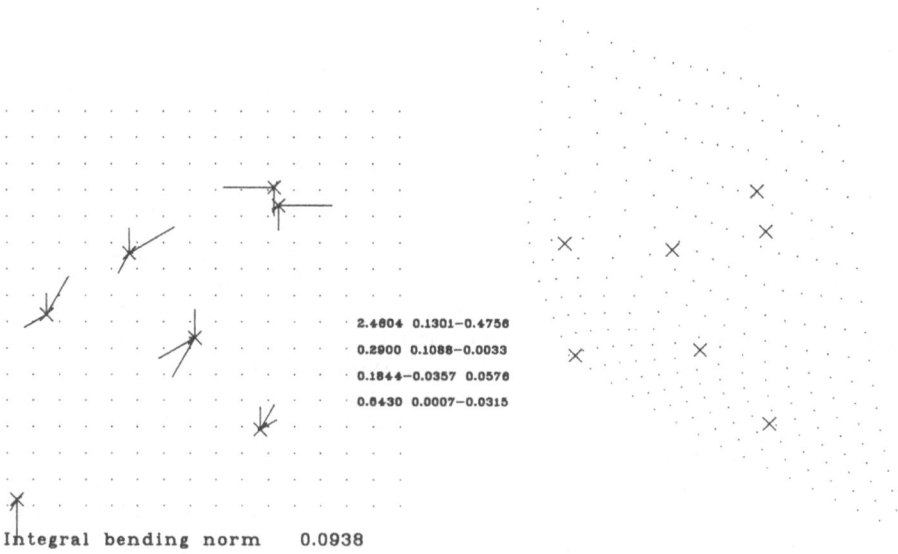

2.4604 0.1301-0.4756
0.2900 0.1086-0.0033
0.1844-0.0357 0.0576
0.6430 0.0007-0.0315

Integral bending norm    0.0938

Figure 10

Other geometries of landmarks yield feature spaces—eigenanalyses of the matrix $L_n^{-1}KL_n^{-1}$—which combine aspects of each of these examples. For instance, Figure 10 arises from the augmentation of Figure 8 by a different pair of points taken with some care to demonstrate the following points. There is an eigenvector of very large eigenvalue—very large bending cost per millimeter of displacement—which, naturally, contrasts displacements at the two landmarks at upper right, those closest together. It thus represents a purely local feature of any deformation based on these points. At the other extreme of stiffness is the eigenvector contrasting joint displacement of the northeast and southwest landmarks with the displacement of all the landmarks along the other diagonal—the same most-global inhomogeneity we have noted three times before. Between these two extremes lie two other eigenvectors whose eigenvalues happen to be nearly equal. Both refer to the set of four landmarks nearest the center of the figure: one involves compression of the "baseline" (the segment along the upper left margin) together with bending of the spur toward the lower right, the other involves extension of that baseline together with the same bending.

## INTERACTIVE FEATURE EXTRACTION

This numerical software for exploiting the bending integral $I_f$ and the quadratic form it represents may be augmented by interactive graphical aids into a little package for determining a "best" description of the relation between two images. I will demonstrate this application using the pair of images in Figure 11, presumed extracted by appropriate processing from a pair of corresponding grey-valued images. The size of the little $x$'s is intended to represent a local measure of lack of edge definition. As these analyses were computed on Mother's Day, it might help to think of the figures as a pair of flowers, each including a stem, two petals, and two seeds.

At the outset we might imagine a suitable homology mapping to be that given by the five obvious landmarks in the image. There results the mapping shown in Figure 12, which has a bending norm of 0.0430 (to arbitrary units). We studied its "features" (shift of the lower "seed" horizontally, shift of both "seeds" vertically) in connection with Figure 8 above. The dots represent a square grid superimposed over the left-hand form and its deformation on the right according to the computed thin-plate spline $f$. (This grid has nothing to do with the computation of $f$; it is a mere visual convenience.) There are three classes of $X$'s in this figure. The largest indicate the landmarks chosen to correspond exactly between the images: the discrete pairs $(x_i, y_i)$ and $(x_i', y_i')$ corresponding under this thin-plate spline. The middle-sized $X$'s are copies of the original data, the outlines of Figure 11. And the smallest $X$'s on the right are the images of the original data from the left according to the mapping function $f$ specified by the landmark correspondence of large $X$'s shown. From the failure of the little $X$'s to overlie the middle-sized $X$'s in Figure 12, we see that these "features"—scores on the eigenvectors of $I_f$ for the current spline basis—are not an adequate representation of the deformation, as this $f$ substantially fails to apprehend the changes of curving form around the "petals" of these two "flowers."

In Figure 13 we have added the sixth and seventh corresponding points, one along each "petal." There results the analysis already reviewed in connection with Figure 9. Only one "feature" is larger than the others, that corresponding to the $x$-component of the second-stiffest eigenvector. Although we have added considerable

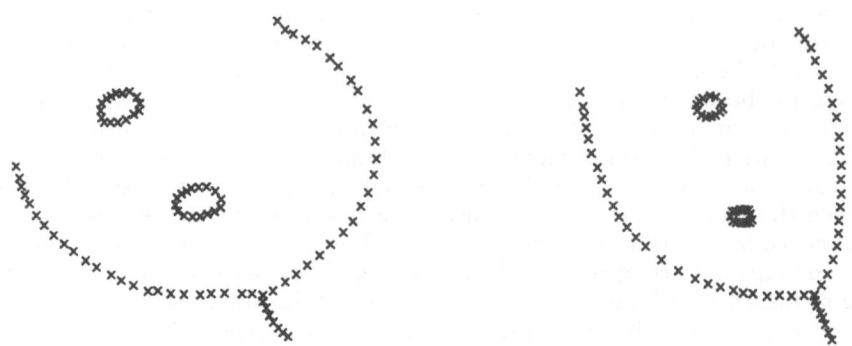

Figure 11

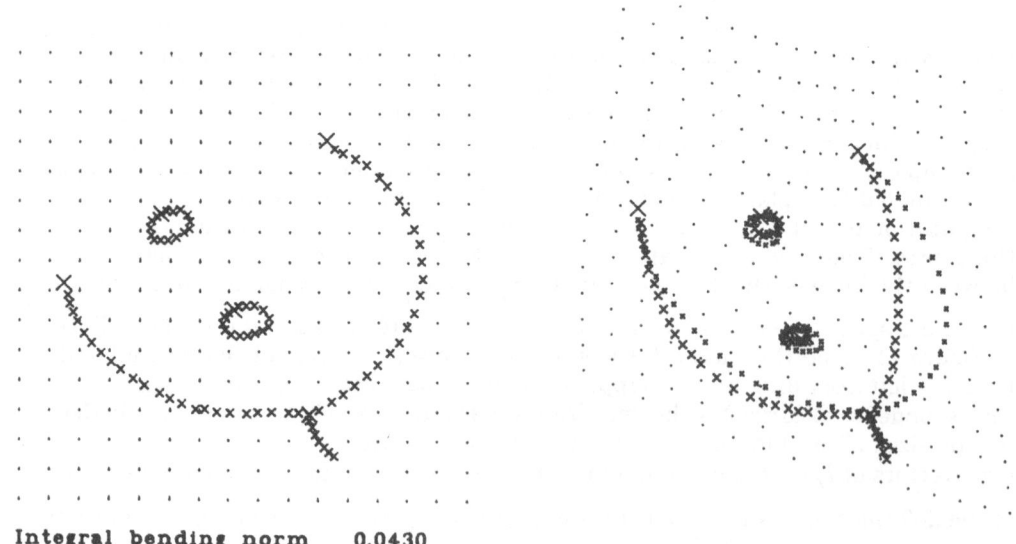

Integral bending norm    0.0430

Figure 12

36

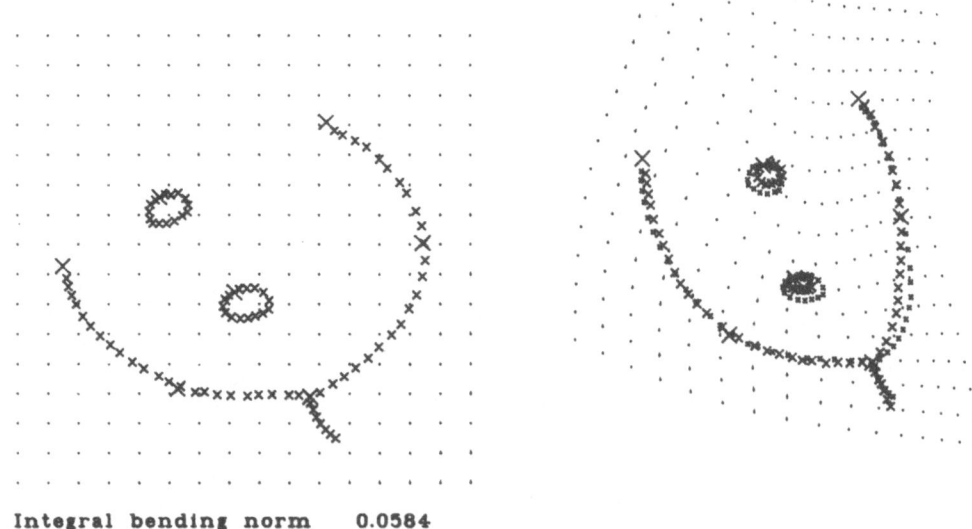

Integral bending norm    0.0584

Figure 13

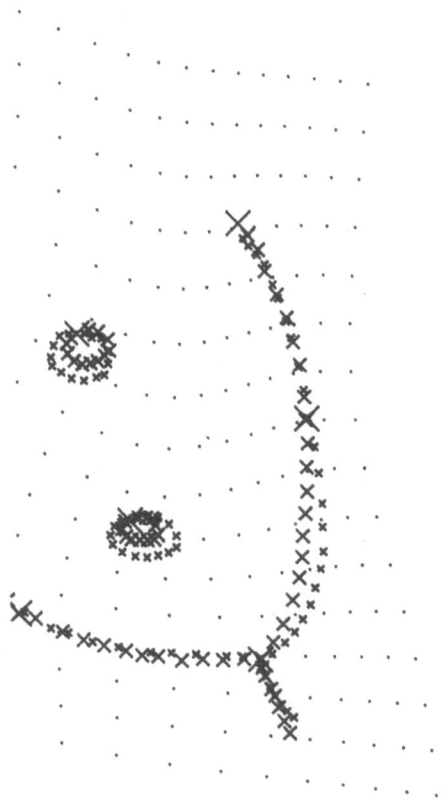

Figure 14

37

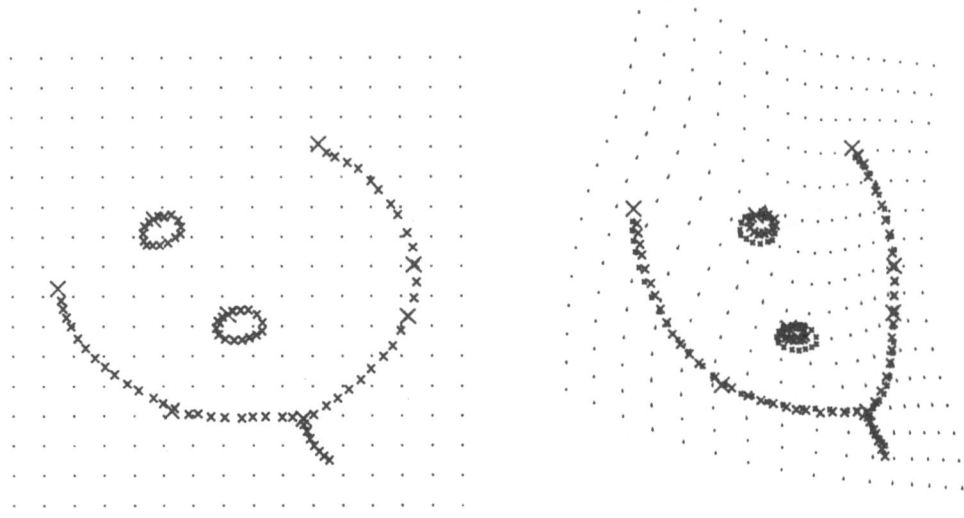

Integral bending norm    0.0622

Figure 15

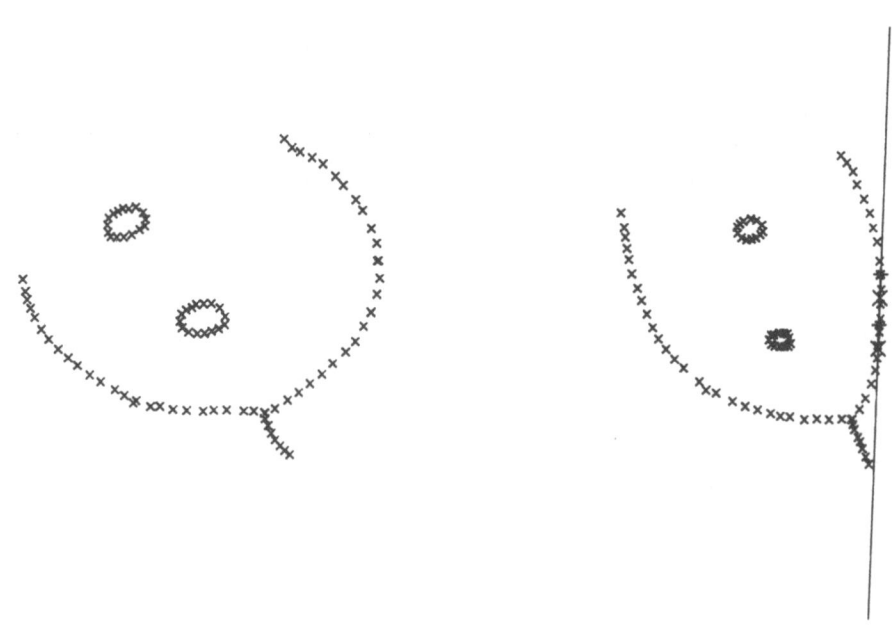

Figure 16

deformation in connection with the considerable displacement of the landmark at center right from its previous location (reduction of the "bulge" of the right-hand petal from left to right), the displacements of this most lateral point (see Figure 9) load most heavily on the <u>last</u> component, the global inhomogeneity of this transformation. The effect of reducing the bulge is, in effect, to "rotate" the axis of this net inhomogeneity from the vertical position it occupied earlier, but not to change more local aspects of the description to any extent.

In the resulting superposition of warped left-hand image over original right-hand image, Figure 14, we see that there is still a systematic failure-of-fit near the base of the right-hand petal. The curve between pseudolandmark and stem diverges between the images. That is, the direction that the spline $f$ assigns to the tangent to the pseudolandmark on the left is not the direction appropriate for the actually corresponding tangent in the scene on the right. We may remedy this discrepancy by requiring the spline to cope with another pseudolandmark on the right-hand arc, below the first and close to it. There results the map of Figure 15, in which the arcs are superimposed correctly. But there is less here than meets the eye: both pseudolandmarks at the right are arbitrary choices from the curve upon which they lie. We may allow the pair to slide up and down as a unit (so as to preserve that tangent direction), Figure 16—the plus signs mark the original positions of these $(x_i', y_i')$, the large $X$'s their new positions—and then free the lower point to slide independently, Figure 17 (so as to relax the implied constraint upon the directional derivative). These represent separate computations minimizing integrals $I_f(t_1, t_2)$ and $I_f(t_1)$, respectively. The net effect of the pair of relaxations is to have specified one aspect only of the affine derivative in this region: that it map the left-hand petal direction onto the right-hand petal direction. The magnitude of the derivative in that direction is constrained to yield the lowest net $I_f$ for the mapping as a whole: to be "least informative" of deviations from homogeneity. (A similar sliding of the landmark on the left-hand petal is null: we guessed well about the position of smoothest correspondence.)

While we are tinkering with such details of the picture, we may add two explicitly local features: the correct rescaling of the two inclusions at the center. These are managed by specifying that differentials (here taken as small finite separations) in two directions preserve both their ratio and their angle between the scenes: the sides of the little isosceles right triangles in Figure 18. (The right-hand triangles should have been freed to rotate within their image, but I couldn't get the software to work in time for the deadline for this manuscript.) There results the overlay of Figure 19, which uses twelve landmarks to map the scene. Now the images at the right fail to overlay only in the region of the trifurcation (Figure 20). Once this is corrected by the addition of two more landmarks, each permitted to slide freely (Figure 21), our editing session is finished (Figure 22).

It is clear that all manipulations subsequent to Figure 14 have dealt with relatively local features. The passage from Figure 18 to Figure 20, for instance, comprises merely a specification of two degrees of freedom of the affine derivative at the stem; the little triangles of crosses at the "seeds" merely specify relative scales of the transformation at those points, and so forth. These features are very nearly $I_f$-orthogonal to those in the eigenvectors of lower eigenvalue, which deal with regional, then global features of the mapping between the images.

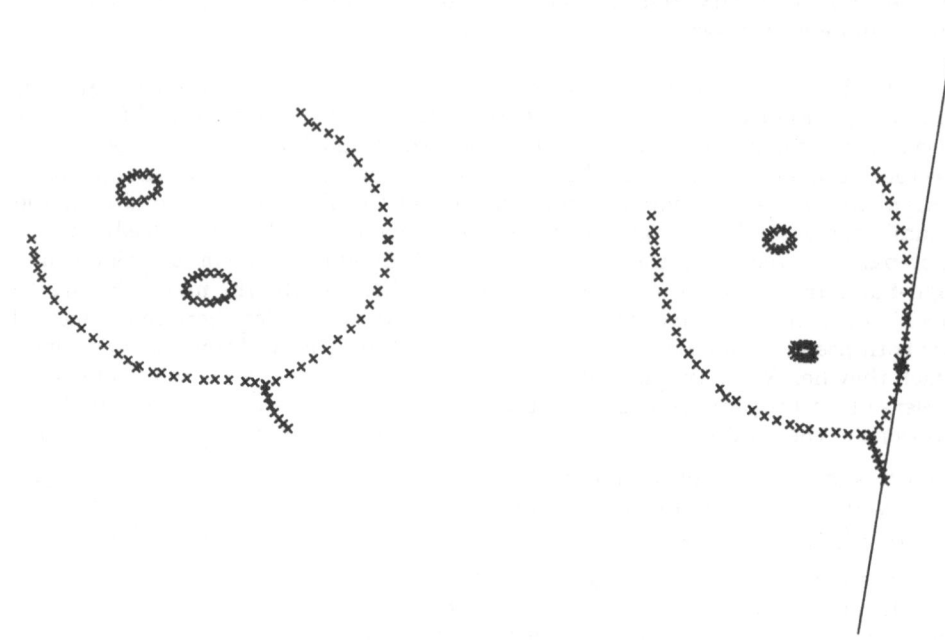

Figure 17

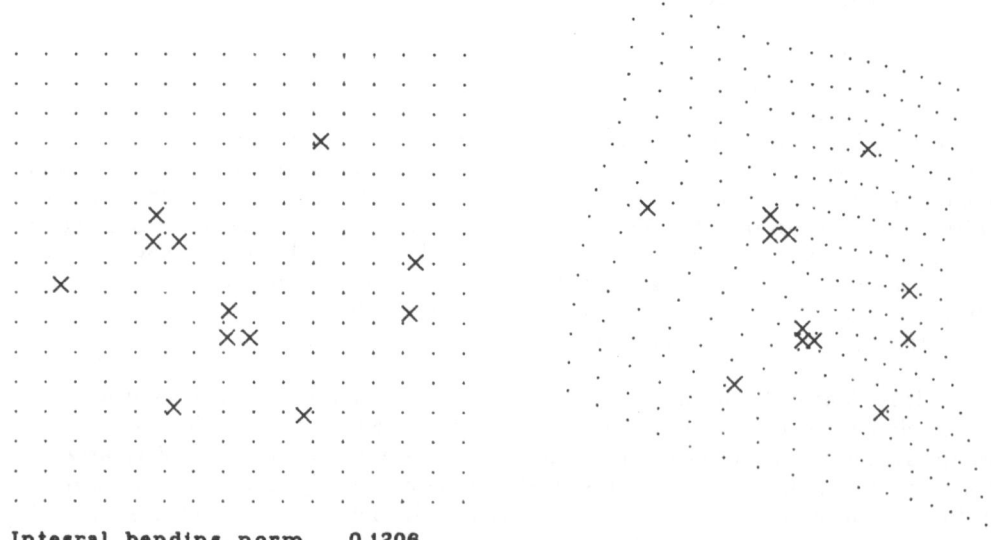

Integral bending norm    0.1206

Figure 18

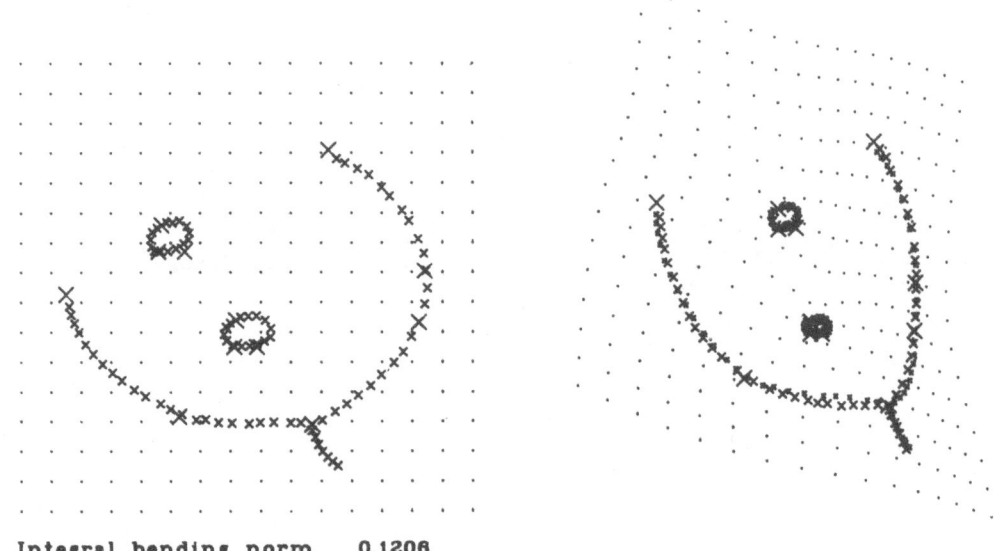

Integral bending norm    0.1206

Figure 19

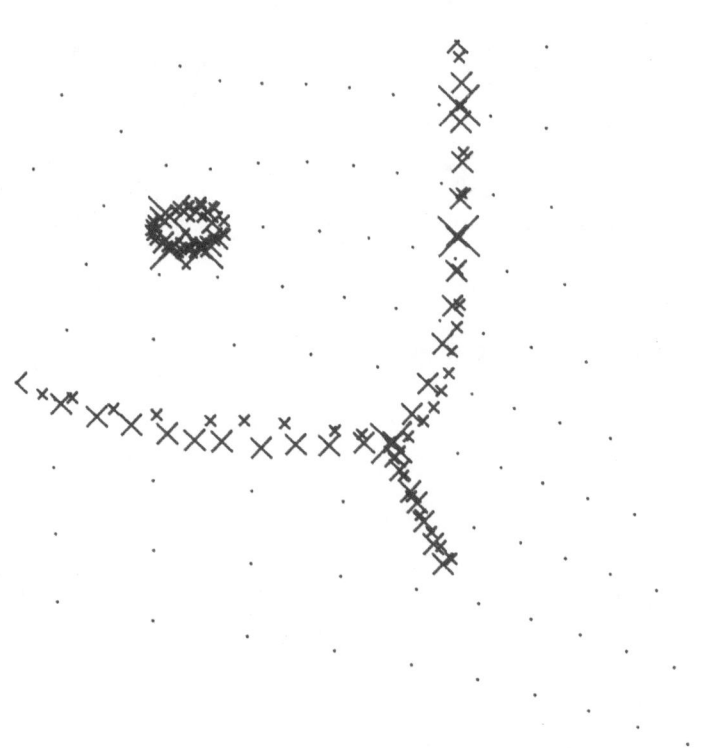

Figure 20

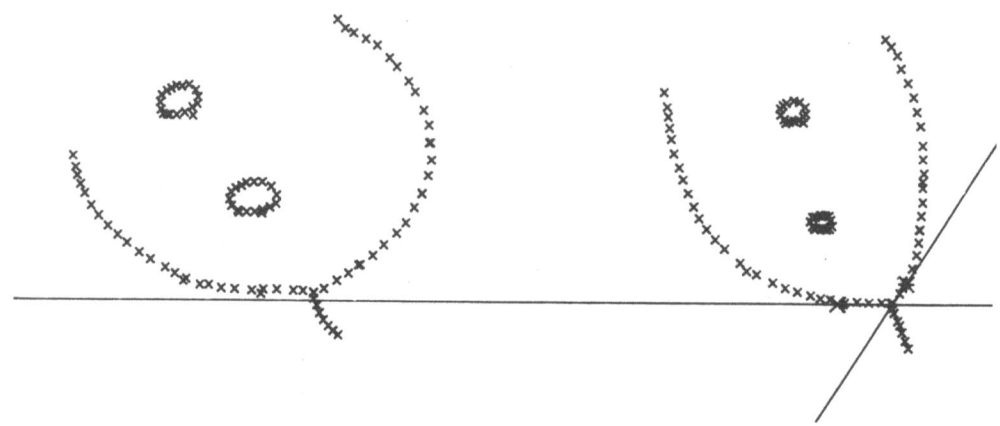

Figure 21

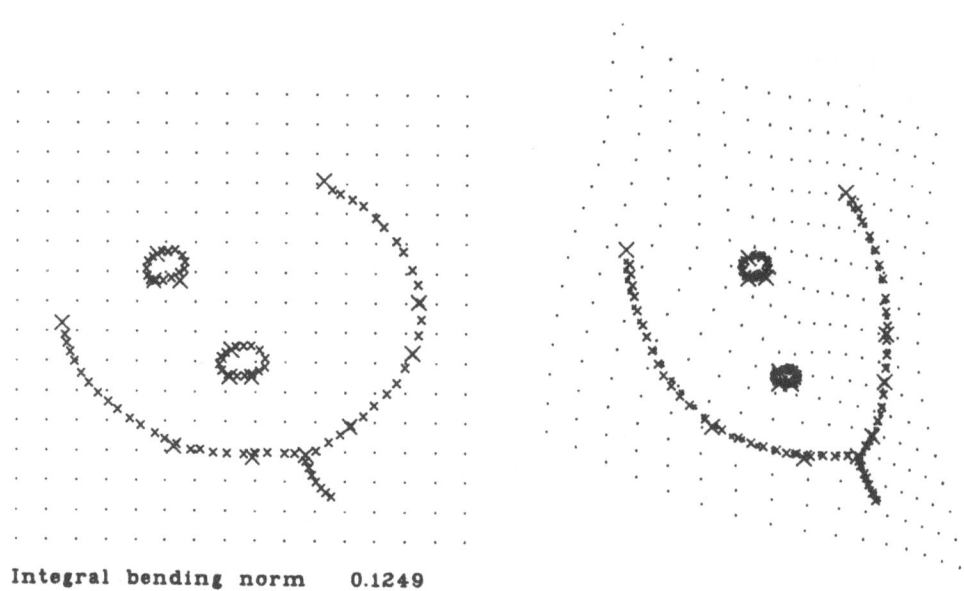

**Integral bending norm    0.1249**

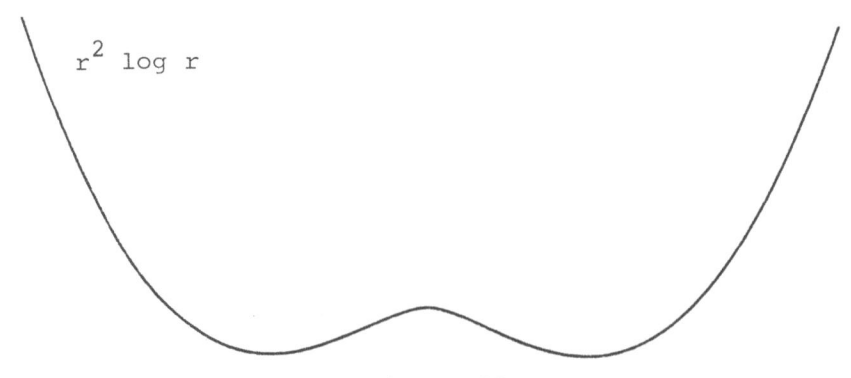

$r^2 \log r$

Figure 22

42

# CONCLUDING REMARKS

The software just demonstrated is based on the identification of local "features" of shape change with eigenvectors of $I_f$ having high eigenvalue, and so with the specification of aspects of the affine derivatives of mappings: local scale, local scale-plus-rotation (not demonstrated here), orientation of a directional derivative, magnitude of such a derivative (not demonstrated), or orientation-plus-magnitude of such a derivative. These are local features both on the screen and in the eigenanalysis (where they arise as high-order eigenvectors expressing the close adjacency of certain landmark pairs). Other features, global features, express fundamental "bending modes" of the configuration of landmarks as a whole: as we have seen, the highest-order such feature, the global inhomogeneity component, is more-or-less common to all sets of four or more landmarks. In offering us a descriptive system for which the effects of specifying displacements and of specifying differentials are expressed in common units, this system of variously scaled features for describing important aspects of image-matching exploits the origin of the thin-plate spline in a problem of real physics. Thin metal plates under a combination of point constraints and clamps "know" what forms to take, and so, apparently, does our software.

In my view these maneuvers have brought us perhaps halfway toward a flexible technology of feature extraction for mappings. There remains the problem of using these features as features: the quantitative summary and comparison of eigenanalyses on starting configurations of somewhat diverse aspect. We have seen that the eigenvectors of lower eigenvalue are robust against small-to-moderate changes in these configurations, while those of higher eigenvalue express mostly the presence of pseudolandmarks at close spacing, those used for the specification of differential structures in the correspondence of the pair of images: information which is, so to speak, "purely local" to begin with. In the resulting feature space, differential structure is expressed as "features" only to the extent that it differs from that induced by the highest-scale aspects of bending. In the final analysis of our pair of flowers, Figure 20, there is barely one "feature" upon the left-hand petal, but a considerable number upon that at the right.

If by "information" we mean geometric localization of features of form suited for comparison between organisms, then medical images contain much less usable information than meets the eye (Bookstein, 1986a). If such information is to be extracted pure, in a form suited to the usual maneuvers of quantitative biology—averaging, diagnosing, discriminating, and predicting, then attention must be paid to the geometric design of the feature space in which these operations are to take place. In this essay I have sketched one such feature space, having a different count of features for each comparison, but with a common geometric language for the expression of those features: the inhomogeneities of transformation.

Acknowledgements. The tentative match of problem with solution set forth here owes mainly to an extended conversation with David Ragozin, University of Washington at Seattle, during the course of my appointment as Visiting Professor of Statistics in 1985. I have also benefitted greatly from conversations with Paul Sampson, University of Washington, and with Stephen Pizer, University of North Carolina at Chapel Hill. Programming of the thin-plate spline and preparation of these comments was supported in part by N.I.H. grant GM-37251 to Fred L. Bookstein.

Bookstein, F. L. (1986a). From medical imaging to the biometrics of form. Pp. 1–18 in Proceedings of the 9th International Conference on Information Processing in Medical Imaging, S. L. Bacharach, ed., Martinus Nijhoff, The Hague, Netherlands.

Bookstein, F. L. (1986b). Size and shape spaces for landmark data in two dimensions, Statistical Science. 1, 181–242.

Bookstein, F. L. (1987a). Morphometrics for functional imaging studies. In J. C. Mazziotta and S. H. Koslow, Assessment of Goals and Obstacles in Data Acquisition and Analysis from Emission Tomography, Journal of Cerebral Blood Flow and Metabolism, 7, S23-S27.

Bookstein, F. L. (1987b). Software requirements for morphometric analysis. To appear in Proceedings of the XIX Conference on the Interface between Computer Science and Statistics, American Statistical Association.

Bookstein, F. L. (1987c). Describing a craniofacial anomaly: Finite elements and the biometrics of landmark location, American Journal of Physical Anthropology, accepted for publication.

Bookstein, F. L., Chernoff, B., Elder, R., Humphries, J., Smith, G., and Strauss, R. (1985), Morphometrics in Evolutionary Biology: The Geometry of Size and Shape Change, with Examples from Fishes, Academy of Natural Sciences of Philadelphia.

Franke, R. (1982). Scattered data interpolation: Tests of some methods, Mathematics of Computation, 38, 181–200.

Meinguet, J. (1979a). Multivariate interpolation at arbitrary points made simple, Zeitschrift für Angewandte Mathematik und Physik (ZAMP), 30, 292–304.

Meinguet, J. (1979b). An intrinsic approach to multivariate spline interpolation at arbitrary points. Pp. 163–190 in Polynomial and Spline Approximation, B. Sahney, ed., D. Reidel Publishing Co., Dordrecht, Netherlands.

Meinguet, J. (1984). Surface spline interpolation: Basic theory and computational aspects. Pp. 127–142 in Approximation Theory and Spline Functions, S. P. Singh et al., eds., D. Reidel Publishing Co., Dordrecht, Netherlands.

Silverman, B. W. (1985). Some aspects of the spline smoothing approach to non-parametric regression curve fitting, Journal of the Royal Statistical Society, B47, 1–52.

Wahba, G., and Wendelberger, J. (1980). Some new mathematical methods for variational objective analysis using splines and cross-validation, Monthly Weather Review, 108, 36–57.

# A META-MODEL FOR SEGMENTATION PROBLEMS

# IN MATHEMATICAL MORPHOLOGY

Isabelle Bloch[*], Françoise Preteux[*], Frédéric Boulanger[*], and
Françoise Soussaline[**]

\* Ecole des Mines de Paris, Centre de Morphologie Mathématique
   35 rue St Honoré, 77300 FONTAINEBLEAU, FRANCE.
\*\* IMSTAR, 60 rue Notre Dame des Champs, 75006 PARIS, FRANCE.

## INTRODUCTION

In Image Analysis, segmentation is a concept widely in use, being a
basic transformation in most studies. As a general rule, the word
segmentation is intended for "partition", or "division" of an image into
regions that are uniform according to given criteria. However, we shall use
it in a more restricted sense, i.e. the extraction of an object in a complex
image, a meaning which is closer to that used in pattern recognition.

In medical imaging, segmentation is a particularly critical problem
owing to the complexity of the images. To deal with such a difficulty,
multiplying ad hoc algorithms, we propose, within the context of
Mathematical Morphology, a general method independant of the problem under
study. This method consists of a series of rules, a procedure to follow, in
order to design a specific algorithm, for a given problem, based on an a
priori knowledge of the object to be segmented.

In the first part, the basic principles of mathematical morphology are
introduced.

In the second part, the three essential steps of the method are
presented.

In the third part, the results are discussed when the method is applied
to medical images obtained by different modalities (C.T. scanner, Digital
Angiography, Positron Emission Tomography, Magnetic Resonance Imaging).

As a conclusion, the enlarged prospects provided by the method, as well
as it possible developments are evoked.

## MATHEMATICAL MORPHOLOGY

Mathematical Morphology (Matheron, 1975 ; Serra, 1982 ; Coster and
Chermant, 1985) was born more than twenty years ago, through the impetus
given by G. Matheron, at the Centre de Géostatistique et de Morphologie
Mathématique (Ecole des Mines de Paris).

What is it about ? Strictly speaking, it designates the study of shapes and structures, by means of mathematics and expressed by mathematics. Beyond words, it is actually much more than a mere analysis of shapes, it is a way of thinking image analysis. A School was formed, which has been enriching and diversifying ever since, imposing, step by step, not only its terminology and notations, which are now generally acknowledged, but also its original approach, where "the concept precedes the measure".

What are the foundations, principles and concepts of mathematical morphology ?


## Fundamental concepts

The concept of shape, which may be considered as being at the origin of mathematical morphology, assimilated to the notion of structure in the mathematical sense, was defined by the knowledge of a family $\mathcal{R}$ of relations considered as possible and a given family $\mathcal{B}$ of geometrical sets, arbitrary yet explicit, called structuring elements.

From a deterministic point of view, characterizing the shape of an object is to know whether or not, for each structuring element, the possible relation is satisfied. Now, if we stick to this general principle we face infinite possibilities.

By emphasizing the relations of the boolean logic and the context of the lattices, mathematical morphology was confered a set foundation, which makes it different from other methods of image processing, mostly based on relations of linear algebra. In fact, mathematical morphology inherits all the properties resulting from this choice : increasing and anti-extensivity with respect to order relationship, convergence via idempotence, algebraic opening and closing...

The second concept that had to be defined concerned the topological nature of the objects to analyse. Indeed, if we take the example of a porous medium with two components : the set A of the grains and the complementary set, the set of pores. Does a point situated on the border of A belongs to the grains or to the pores ? In other words, what is the topological status of A : open or closed ? If the structuring element B is a compact set or an open set relatively compact, we cannot distinguish between two porous media if they have the same interior and the same adherence.

This remark, suggested by experimental constraints, lead G. Matheron to define a topology, the "Hit or Miss topology", not on all the parts of a set, but on a subset which is that of the closed sets, and to restrict the class $\mathcal{B}$ of the structuring elements to the compact sets. There again, the consequences of this choice are essential, since they induce the continuity or the semi-continuities (upper or lower) of the transformations and operations.

The next conceptual step consisted in using the probabilities theory. G. Matheron's Random Set Theory established that logical propositions such as "B is included in A" or "B is not disjoined from A", were events of a certain $\sigma$-algebra and that they could be assigned a probability. In other words, the studied object can be assimilated to a random set realization. The probabilities of the preceding events are, in a way, the moments of a spatial distribution, with this fundamental restriction, that they can, in particular, involve a neighbourhood, in the topological sense, and thus, involve an uncountable infinity of points.

## Evolution and development

Thanks to these general mathematical foundations, the method, initially developed for binary images only, could evolve when they gave place to grey-levels images, assimilated then to functions. The theory was adapted to this new context, richer and more complex :

- either by means of a mere transposition of certain set of operations,
- or by a different interpretation of other operations,
- or by new developments.

Grey-levels images with their intrinsic imperfections (noise, artifacts...), lead to original studies on filtering (Matheron, 1983 ; Sternberg, 1980 ; Serra, 1982) which resulted in a theory of morphological filtering (Serra 1982), totally different from the theory of the filtering based on convolution.

Along with the developments on the set, topological and probabilistic, a technological evolution gave birth to texture analysers designed for the study of binary images, and, further, to grey-levels image analysers (Klein, 1976 ; Beucher and Meyer, 1977).

These considerations show that mathematical morphology does not constitute a doctrinal body delimited in space and time, but, more accurately, a way of dealing with image analysis problems, that is capable of evolution and flexibility in order to fit the nature of the images and the needs of the users.

An attempt at a definition can only be a review, at a given moment, of the state of the art of the theory, the technology and the involved fields of applications.

Thus, when we propose a method for segmentation and examples of problems that been solved, it only indicates the philosophy of the method, which is to simplify, transform, characterize, quantify and interpret thanks to "primitives" integrating the a priori knowledge of the images to analyse (Prêteux, 1986).

## A consistent and evolutive body

One of the original features of mathematical morphology is that it provides not only a collection of primitives, but also a true construction, ordered according to the actions and effects of the transformations. Thus it answers to the actual needs of practical image analysis.

To describe the original generation of the mathematical morphology primitives, we represent them as a pyramid of variable geometry built on its summit. Indeed, we have here a mathematical design made up of primitives of higher order that become more and more complex, specific and efficient as we go up the pyramid.

Still, all of them can be written from a single basic morphological primititive, by using numerical primitives of "sup" and "inf", and the principle of duality.

Thus, the effects of higher order primitives are in close relationship with the mathematical structures and properties from which their are composed and with the a priori knowledge they integrate and convey.

This explains why, at every step of image analysis, for every problem, one must choose either a primitive that already exists, or create one or more primitives able to solve the problem or aim to a solution by a necessary step, a sub-goal. These are the primitives which will be subsequently used in automatic programming systems, as well as in our problem solving method. This gives an inkling of the forecoming shift from image analysis to artificial intelligence.

## THE METHOD

The basic principle is to translate the properties of images and objects submitted to segmentation, into terms of image analysis, and, more precisely, into primitives of mathematical morphology.

These properties involve the shape, the size, the neighbourhood relationships existing between the object of interest and the image as a whole, and also the "colour". Here, the colour is meant for intensity of grey levels being real colour for natural images, texture density in C.T. imaging, radioactivity in nuclear medicine, relaxation time in MRI, artificial staining in microscopy.

The first step consists in listing the properties of the images, related to imaging modality, and the properties of the object to be analysed. It is then possible to evaluate their influence on the analysis methods, and, in particular, to eliminate the methods for which these properties do not satisfy the conditions of application. For instance, high noise prevents the direct use of a gradient.

Secondly, the access to these properties and their translation into useful information is performed by means of the primitives of mathematical morphology, which associate a structuring element with an imposed relationship between this structuring element and the analysed image. In summary, the structuring element enables the access to information concerning size and shape, and a set relationship gives information on the neighborhood, whereas a functional relationship informs on "colour". In order to achieve this translation, we have to define at each step of the analysis the criteria according to which the necessary choices of image analysis will be made. In the case of mathematical morphology, these choices are :

- the structuring element,
- the relationship,
- the interpretation of the image, as a function or a set,
- the model to be used in order to analyse a texture, or estimate various parameters.

The choice involves a highly complicated process, without any true hierarchical structure. However, there are some relationships between certain choices, either bilateral relationships (equivalence, incompatibility) or unilateral relationships (conditioning, implication), that should be taken into account.

In order to face the complexity of the choice process, the translation of the properties of the images and objects to be segmented into primitives of image analysis, is actually performed by means of a double movement from the image to mathematical morphology, and vice versa, according to the following :

Properties → Methods → Hypotheses to satisfy → New Properties

This approach allows to associate a method with a set of properties on the one hand, and to determine the necessary properties for a satisfactory application of the method (ability to deal with noise, etc...) on the other hand. Let us take a typical situation. Let us assume that the object to be segmented highly contrasts with its surrounding. This property suggests to use a gradient. But, as we have seen, the presence of noise in the image prevents from using the gradient directly. This noise information has to be taken into account by a filtering, in order to increase the gradient robustness.

It can be noticed about the second step (fig.1), that it starts from the set of properties which is obtained at the end of the first step. But this set varies during the translation : the properties deduced from the performed transformations are added to it (e.g., the fact that we have a binary image after a thresholding, or that we have a marker of the object, etc...). The deduced properties are taken into account in the same way as are the initial properties for determining the following transformations.

The translation of a property may suggest several algorithms. We introduce here a classification of the primitives of mathematical morphology according to their complexity, i.e. the primitives of higher order belong to classes of higher complexity.

Among several suitable algorithms, we shall always choose first the one which belongs to the class of least complexity. If the algorithm is unconvenient, we shall move to a class of higher complexity.

There are many possible reasons why the algorithm may not be convenient : e.g. the translated properties are not characteristic of the object, or the conditions of application of the algorithm are not satisfied, or the deduced properties are incompatible with the other ones, or the algorithm simply leads to nowhere (idempotence, convergence problems).

It is our bivocal approach based on a non monotonous logic which allows to go back over the choices made at each step and thus answer to the different causes of failure.

These remarks shows the complexity of the second step, the numerous problems involved and the difficulty to establish the translation rules between the language describing images and the language of mathematical morphology. In particular, dealing with "synonyms" requires to consider the whole context.

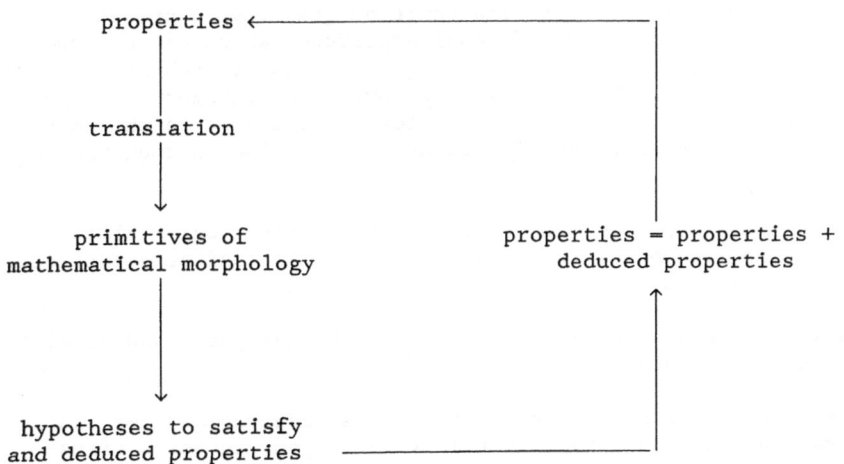

Fig.1 : Diagram symbolizing the second step

The last choices to be made concern the precise value of the different parameters involved (size of filtering, size of structuring element, number of iterations of a procedure,...). Therefore, the purpose of the third step is to define the characteristic criteria of the object to be segmented, and, thus, to allow the setting of the parameters values and, finally, to determine the exact algorithm which is required.

At this stage, thanks to the very principle of this approach, we notice that all the imperfections difficult to eliminate (such as under- or over-segmentation) which usually result from classical methods have disappeared. Most often, only a few artifacts remain and we can easily obtain the exact contour (a simple pruning is generally sufficient).

## APPLICATIONS IN MEDICAL IMAGING

In order to illustrate our approach step by step, we chose four examples amongst studies performed at the Centre de Morphologie Mathématique, Ecole des Mines de Paris.

### The lung in C.T. imaging

Our first example deals with the segmentation of lung lobes from C.T. scanner. In this study, carried out jointly with the Service of Radiology of the Hospital Beaujon, Pr. Grenier, (Paris, France), we wanted to calculate the lung volumes, distinguishing the healthy parts from the ones affected with vesicular emphysema (Prêteux et al., 1985 ; Merlet, 1987). The first indispensable step was to segment lungs and trachea in each slice. It is described in the following.

The segmentation algorithm is based on the exploitation of two properties of lung C.T. images :

- they display four zones of different intensity : a low signal zone (ranging between 0 and 1000), corresponding to the image background, the lungs, the trachea and to some noise pixels, a high signal zone corresponding to bony parts, and two intermediary zones corresponding to tissues of mean density ;

- lungs and surrounding tissues are clearly contrasted.

The first property is translated into a thresholding suited to each image, in an automatic manner. The range of grey levels present on the image is divided into four domains of equal amplitude, which correspond to the four zones described above. Next, the grey levels of each area are reduced to the lower level of the area. We thus obtain a transformed image encoded on four grey levels, where the lowest level correspond to the lungs, the trachea and image background. The thresholding value is then the lower level.

At this stage, we go back to the initial image, which allows, according to our "to and fro" model, to eliminate the background as a particle touching the image border.

As to the second property, it insures the sharpness and precision of the resulting segments.

Here, the third step just consists in an opening of size two to eliminate the small particles that only correspond to noise (first property).

In this example, the properties order conveys their importance. Respecting this order allows to determine a simpler and more performing algorithm. Indeed, the sole second property would be translated under the form of a gradient. But this transformation is more complex than a thresholding and requires a certain processing in order to obtain a binary image, which is difficult since this property is not characteristic of the lung.

## Left ventricle mask in digital angiography

The automatic detection of a left ventricle mask in digital angiography is a necessary step for the automatical quantification of the left ventricle volume from densitometric measurements (Lavayssière and Prêteux, 1987).

At the first stage of the method, three types of properties are identified. The first type consists of the images properties related to the imaging technique, i.e. direct X imaging with logarithmic subtraction :

1) the information contained in the subtracted image is "relative", as opposed to the information obtained with C.T. images,

2) a background noise remains after the logarithmic subtraction interfering with the actual information, especially in zones which are not very thick (apex, myocardium pillars),

3) a collimation (with an elliptic geometry by passing to a hexagonal grid) of the image is realistic, owing to the presence of luminance amplificators.

The second type involves the properties due to the medical examination procedure :

4) continuity of grey-level functions (i.e. absence of strong gradients) due to the intravenous injection mode in which the contrast agent is diluted in its course from "injection site to left ventricle",

5) the orientation of the left ventricle is invariable, due to the invariance of the acquisition incidence,

6) the lowest densities correspond to the pixels made opaque, since the contrast agent is located in cardiac cavities (ventricles, auricles) and afferent and efferent vessels on the one hand , and, to isolated pixels due to artifacts (patient's movement, defects in X-rays emission) on the other hand.

7) Lastly, the third type is constituted of a property due to anatomic variabilities among patients, which induces some variations in the injected dose and the injection site (property 7).

At the second step,of the reasoning, properties 1, 2, 4, and 7 forbid all methods based on thresholding and/or gradient.

The translation of the third property, that we will not describe here in details, provides spatial and temporal criteria allowing the detection of an ellipse of collimation and thus the reduction of the field of analysis (fig.2).

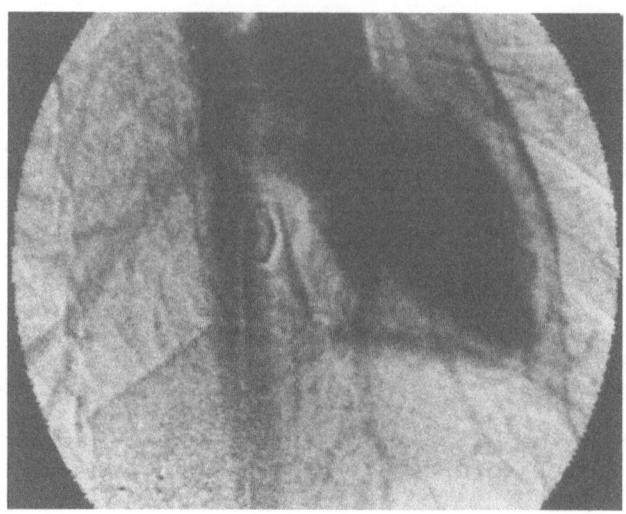

Fig.2 : Left ventricle in digital angiography :
initial image after reduction

The sixth property suggests to search for regional minima of the grey-tone function associated with the image (the valleys), in order to obtain a left ventricle marker, which is then dilated until the required mask is obtained. To know where to stop the dilation, we have to know the pixels or regions which are certainly outside the ventricle. According to the same property 6, the regional maxima (Meyer, 1986) of the grey function are actually such regions.

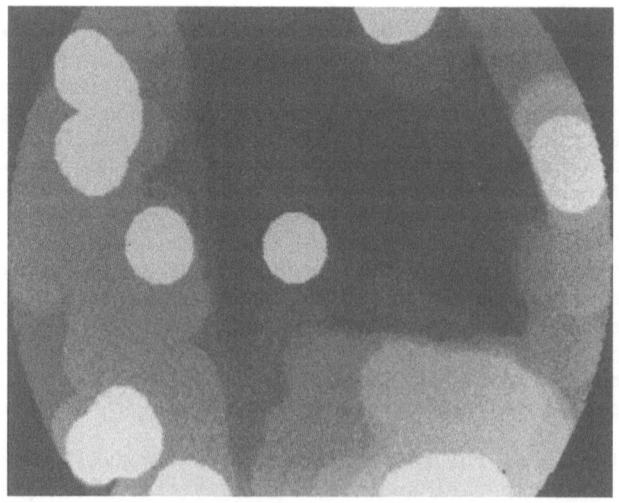

Fig.3 : Large size opening and regional maxima

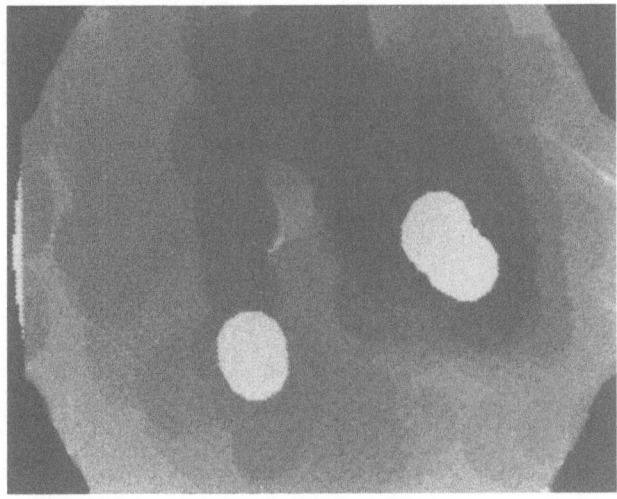

Fig.4 : Large size closing and regional minima

The search for regional minima and maxima leads to a cluster of points which cannot be exploited. Then, it is necessary to go back over the second property (background noise) and take it into account under the form of a filtering. The simplest morphological filterings are the grey-level openings and closings. By assimilating the numerical function to a relief where the altitude corresponds to grey levels, morphological closings partially fills the valleys of this relief, while preserving peaks, whereas morphological openings cut the crests of peaks while preserving valleys. On an opened image, regional maxima have at least the same size as the structuring element used for the opening.

Thus, we have performed a large size opening and searched for regional maxima in order to locate the non opaque regions (fig.3), and, on the other hand, we have performed a large size closing and searched for regional minima so as to obtain a partition of the regions that have become very opaque and the residual artifacts (fig.4).

Therefore, it is necessary to eliminate the parasitic valleys to retain only those marking the left ventricle. To do so we just have to exploit the property 5, according to which the ventricular axis is oriented at about $-30^0$, whereas the vessels that come from it (aorta) are oriented at $120^0$, $150^0$ to the left of the ventricle. The ventricular valley is then the first encountered in a linear dilation ($0^0$) of the righthand border of the image (fig.5).

We have now a marker of the left ventricle as well as numerous particles marking the exterior of the ventricle (plateaux) (fig.6). It is finally possible to perform a dilation of the ventricle marker, conditionally to the plateaux and giving greater importance to the direction $-30^0$ (property 5), so as to obtain the minimal ventricular mask (fig.7).

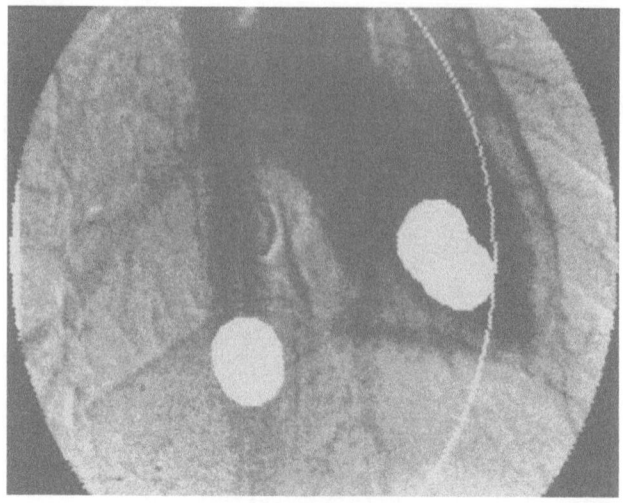

Fig.5 : Selection of the minimum marking the left ventricle

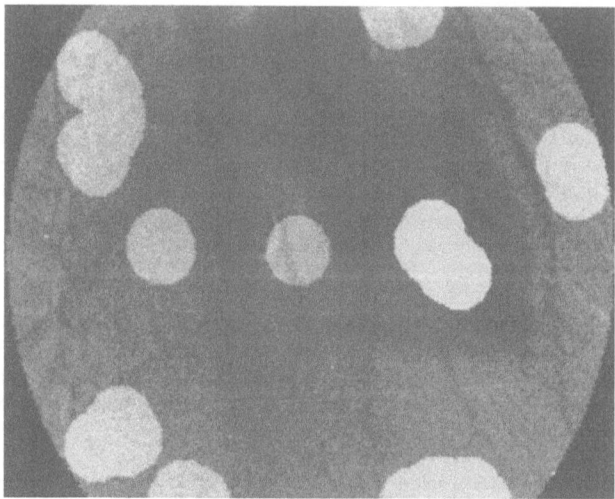

Fig.6 : Marker of the left ventricle and numerous partcles marking the
exterior of the ventricle

The third step consists in determining the sizes of the opening and
closing used in the filtering. They have been respectively set to 12 and 14,
considering the relative sizes of the left ventricle and the other
structures. Moreover, to take into account the ventricle shape, it was
necessary to use dodecagonal structuring elements, which are the best
approximate circles on a hexagonal grid.

In this application, the approach we propose allows to obtain an
automatic, simple and very robust algorithm (we elaborated it from images
with particularly high parasitic noise) thanks to the optimal exploitation
of numerical information. This feature sets it apart from classical
algorithms, which immediately perform a binarization and therefore ignore
many interesting properties.

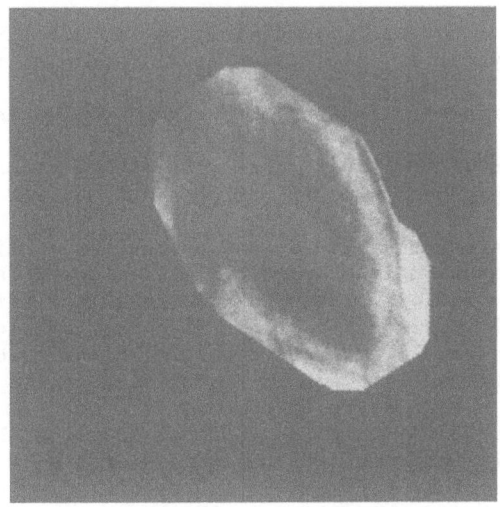

Fig.7 : Minimal ventricular mask

## The myocardium in Positons Emission Tomography (P.E.T.)

The goal of this study undertaken at the SHFJ laboratory of Orsay, CEA, France (Pr A. SYROTA) was to analyse the radioactive distribution in the functional myocardium (Boulanger et al., 1987), using a positron emettor 11C labelling a specific muscarinic receptorspharmaceutical (MQNB). We shall only present here the segmentation stage. We had a collection of 525 images of myocardium obtained by P.E.T., with the following characteristics (Syrota et al., 1985) : (fig.8)

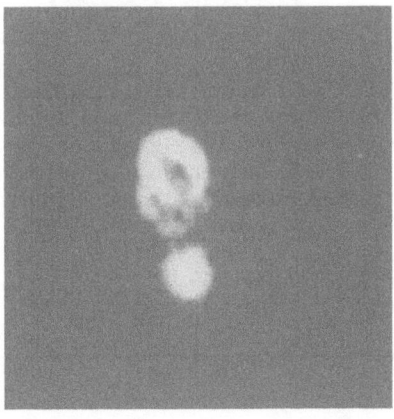

Fig.8 : Myocardium in PET : initial image

1) low signal/noise ratio varying from 1.3 to 3,

2) three main grey levels of radioactive distribution, corresponding approximately to :
   - the muscarinic receptors (myocardium) and to the liver (higher level),
   - to the right myocardium wall (mean level) and also to the hypoactive areas,
   - to the lung parenchyma and to the background (low level).

3) constant position of the liver relatively to the myocardium (at the bottom on the right-hand side in the conventional PET representation).

Properties 2 and 3 are translated by an automatic reduction of the image to a minimal window containing the heart. This is a simple step which needs not to be detailed here. The high activity areas are then defined biunivocally by a high grey level and a high contrast (fig.9a). None of these two properties taken separately is characteristic of the myocardium. Only their combination is so, taking into account both the absolute information of the high grey level and the relative information of the high contrast. Thus, we developed a new algorithm : the h-conditional gradient (Boulanger et al., 1987), where the relative information is translated by a morphological gradient, and the absolute information is translated by coding the image with the purpose of reinforcing interesting areas. The two are combined by means of a multiplication.

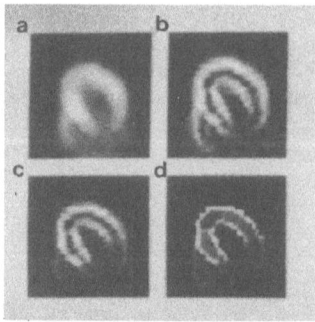

Fig.9 : h-conditional gradient
9a- reduced filtered image
9b- classical gradient
9c- h-conditional gradient
9d- numerical thinning on
    the h-conditional gradient

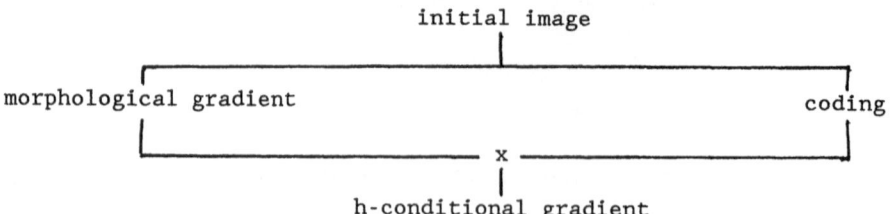

Figure 10 : h-conditional gradient diagram

The coding step aims at amplifying the grey tone values of the morphological gradient corresponding to the appropriate contours and can be described as follows :

1) the initial image IM1 is transformed by a continuous function $\psi$ such that all pixels being at h level (mean grey level of the zone to be contoured) bears a maximal value in a new image IM2 (e.g. $\psi(x) = \sup(h,M-h) - |h-x|$ where M is the maximal grey level in IM1) ;

2) the image IM2 is dilated (i.e. the propagation of the IM2 maxima on a unity neighbourhood) to take account of the fact that the numerical contours of the morphological gradient correspond to the exterior contours of the regions of high intensity ;

3) the dilated image IM3 is coded on N areas of amplitude a(i) ($i\epsilon[1,\ldots,N]$) and of grey level b(i) into the coded image IM4 .

The 2N coefficients a(i) and b(i) satisfy :

$$* \; b(1) = 0 \text{ and } b(2) = \frac{\alpha(2)}{2\alpha}$$

$$* \; b(i) - b(i - 1) = \frac{\alpha(i) + \alpha(i-1)}{2\alpha}$$

$$* \; b(N) - b(N-1) = 1$$

where $\alpha = \inf (\alpha(i), i\epsilon[2,\ldots,N-1])$.

The coded image is then defined by function g :

$$g(x) = b(i) \text{ if x belongs to the area i in IM3.}$$

The h-conditional gradient (fig.9c) is finally obtained by multiplying the coded image by the morphological gradient. A unity thickness gradient is obtained after a numerical thinning (fig.9d). The required contours now appear with a high grey level.

The coding form insures the flexibility of the h-conditional gradient. Indeed, it allows to take into account not only the number of the components contained in the image, thanks to the choice of N, but also the "degree" of the contour's fuzzyness by adding transitional areas between the different components. The expression of b(i) enables to obtain slight variations of grey on the coded image between transitional areas. Area 1, which corresponds to low levels, is not involved in the calculation of b(i) which allows to determine the form of b(1) and b(2). The expression of b(N) enables to obtain slight variations of grey levels on the coded image in the contour neighbourhood.

However, because of the first property, the h level is not very well defined. In order to use the algorithm under proper conditions, it is necessary to first filter the noise. The great variability of grey levels on the numerical contour prevents the use of a thresholding to obtain the binary contour of the myocardium. We have then to exploit the delineation properties at the neighbourhood of the required contour by means of a crest line tracking algorithm (fig.11).

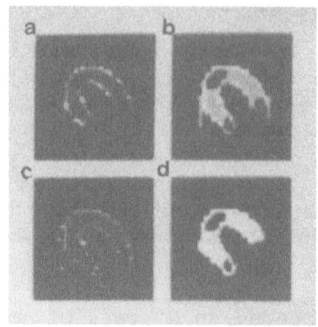

Fig.11 : Crest line tracking
11a- markers
11b- propagation
11c- extreme points
11d- closed contour


The second properties of the images allowed us to perform the last step of the method, i.e. set the h-conditional gradient parameters. Thus, h is the maximal value of the grey levels in the image, there are 3 areas, and the corresponding coefficients $\alpha(i)$ are 1/3. Since the contours are clear enough, it is not necessary to introduce transitional areas.

The resulting contour is that of the high activity regions of the myocardium (fig.12). It is superimposed on the functional myocardium only in healthy patients (fig.12a) and never in pathological patients (fig.12b,c), since the choice of the criteria and the adjusting of these parameters are only characteristic of the areas of high activity (fig.12a',b',c').

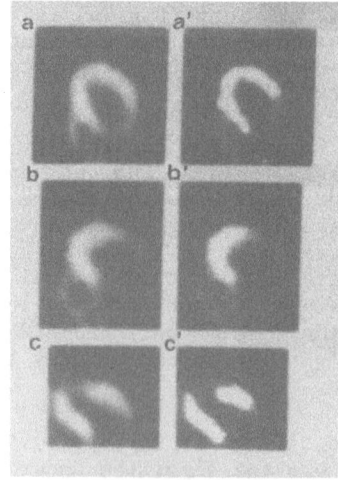

Fig.12 : Areas of high activity
12a,b,c- reduced initial images in 3 cases
12a',b',c'- areas of high activity superimposed
on the initial imges

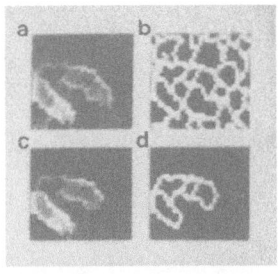

Fig.13 : Detection of hypoactive areas
  13a- gradient
  13b- watersheds : sursegmentation
  13c- region containing hypoactive areas
  13d- watersheds in this region : contour

Here, we have a deduced property which is defined by the contour of high activity areas. This property is associated with the grey levels properties and so enables the detection of a region containing hypoactive areas. In the end, it is the contrast property which allows to characterize hypoactive area and thus extract the exact contours from them and, consequently, those of the functional myocardium (fig.13).

The approach proposed in the TEP example, making use of a priori knowledge, enabled us to overcome the problems related to the poor definition of the images, to the presence of noise and hypoactive areas. It is then possible to determine on the result an absolute reference mark of the heart, defining $30^{\circ}$ sectors. The physician can now obtain temporal distribution curves of radioactivity in a given sector and spatial distribution curves of activity at a given time. These two classes of curves enable a quantitative diagnosis.

Comparing the results with those obtained by a classical method of a statistical type and based on the geometric modelization of the muscarinic receptor (Travère et al., 1986) proved the good performance of the algorithm resulting from our approach. If the same absolute reference (up to 3%) was obtained by the two methods, ours is, up to now, the only one that is capable of detecting automatically pathological zones. Moreover it allows the study of the transitional stage (corresponding to the uptake of radiopharmaceutical on the receptors sites) ; and, finally, the result is independent of the operator, as opposed to the classical method.

This example shows how the proposed method allows the design of primitives of higher order (as the h-conditional gradient, for instance) by highlighting the requirements and components that have to be taken into account in the solution of a segmentation problem, justifying the development of such primitives.

## Brain lesions in Magnetic Resonance Imaging (M.R.I.)

The last example (fig.14) deals with the segmentation of brain lesions in MRI (Bloch et al., 1986). This study was carried out in collaboration

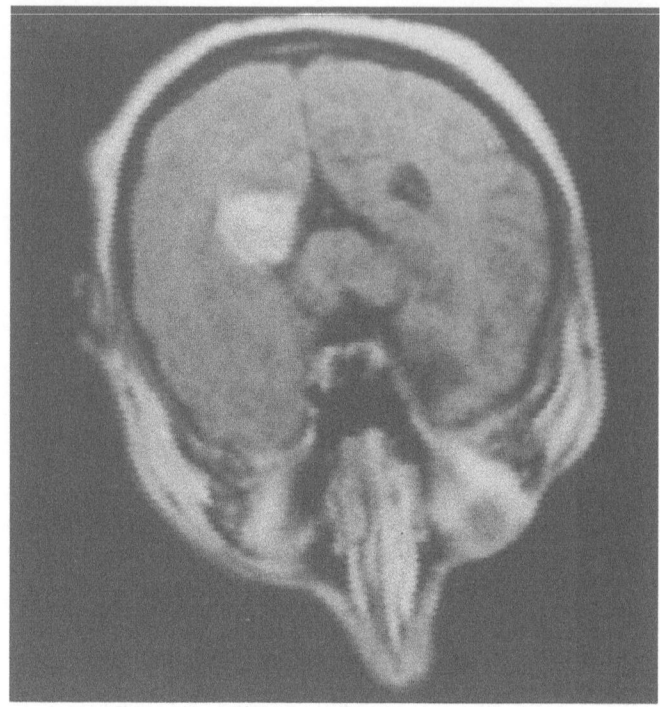

Fig.14 : Brain by NMR : initial image

with the Centre National Ophtalmologique des XV-XX, Paris, France
(Neuroradiology Service, Pr Cabanis).

The properties of the images (noise, absence of absolute reference of
the signal due to a systematic normalization on 12 bits) are related to the
M.R.I. acquisition mode. As to the lesions characteristics, they can be
divided into two categories :

- their intensity is generally high, and they clearly contrast with the
  brain, due to the injection of a paramagnetic contrast agent
  (Gadolinium-DTPA),

- their round shape (simple or polylobe), their heterogeneity, their
  variable location and size, are purely anatomical.

The images properties immediately ruled out all the classical methods
based on thresholding, gradient or region growing.

The second step, consisting of the translation of these characteristics
under the form of primitives of mathematical morphology, lead, successively,
to the search for the regional maxima (fig.16) of the numerical function
associated with the image, to the selection of the maxima actually
corresponding to the lesion (fig.17) by means of an r,h maxima algorithm
(Prêteux and Schmitt, 1986) (if an image shows a regional maximum at the
altitude $h_{max}$ , the set of points at an altitude higher than $h_{max}$ - h around
this maximum is kept provided that this zone is preserved by an erosion of r
size), and next, by means of the extraction of concavity primitives by
performing a closing with a three-dimensional structuring element
(rhombododecahedron) (Serra, 1987).

Here, is another example of the "to-ings and fro-ings" between the image and mathematical morphology, especially through the criterion of high intensity signal, whose mathematical translation corresponds to the notion of regional maxima. Indeed, exploiting this sole criterion does not a priori require to start with a filtering of the image. But, in practice, the search for the maxima must be performed on a filtered image, in order to be able to

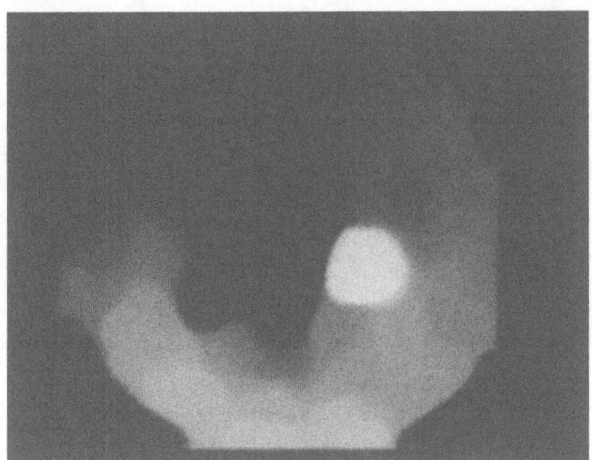

Fig.15 : Morphological filtering

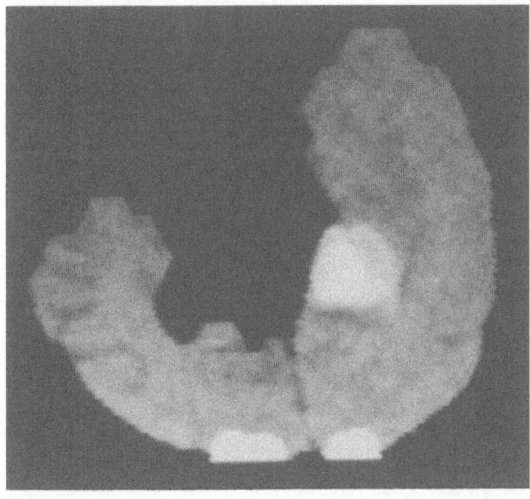

Fig. 16 : Regional maxima

deal with noise and heterogeneity of the intralesional signal. For this reason, we adopted an alternate sequential filtering (Sternberg 1980, Serra 1982). Besides, to preserve the roundness of lesional contours, this filtering has to be performed with dodecagonal structuring elements (fig.15).

The last step of the method corresponds to the adjustment of the parameters values. The maximal size of the structuring element used in the filtering corresponds to the minimal size of the lesions to be detected. The parameters r and h were set experimentally (r = 8 and h = 70). These values allowed, in particular, the distinction between ocular globes lesions,

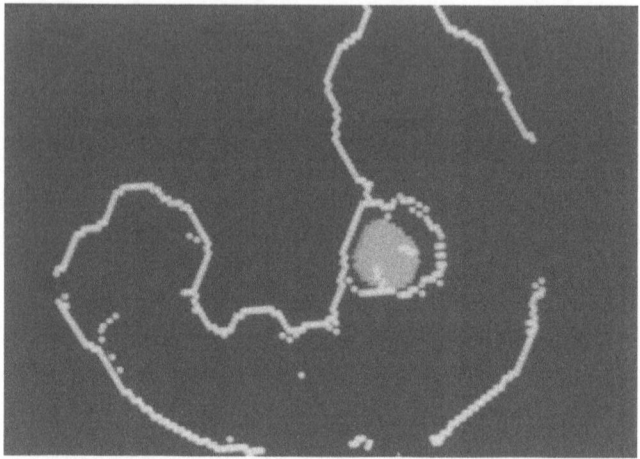

Fig.17 : Oversegmented contours (in white)
Marker of the lesion (in grey)

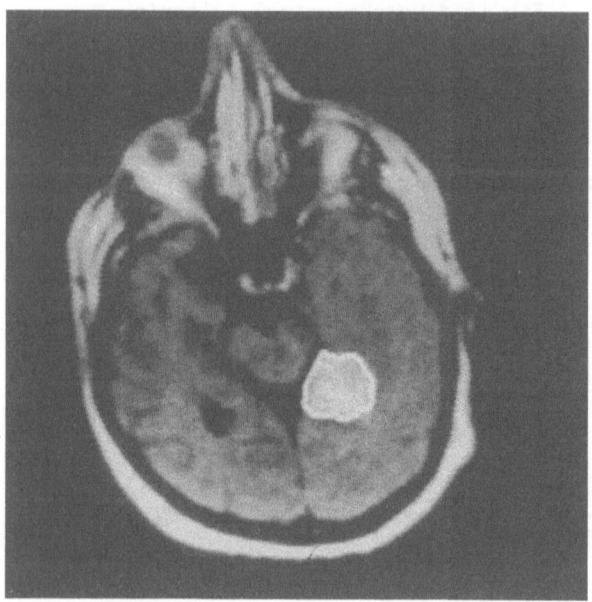

Fig. 18 : Result superimposed on the initial image

though the intensity of their signal was the same on the initial image. Note that the set values for r and h can bear variations up to 15%, which emphasizes the robustness of the r,h maxima algorithm and its capacity to take appropriate account of the anatomical diversity of the lesions. At this stage, the lesions are located by the "markers" constituted by the selected maxima.

The last implemented algorithm (extraction of concavity primitives) provides, in this case, oversegmented contours (fig.17), imposing to perform a simple transformation between these two images (reconstruction after pruning), in order to obtain the appropriate contours (fig.18).

The adopted approach, using anatomical, morphological and two- or three- dimensional geometrical criteria, has allowed the establishment of an automatic algorithm for the segmentation of brain lesions and thus gives access to studies of contour regularity and texture homogeneity, with the aim of lesions classification. Therefore, this approach constitutes a good starting point for an aid to diagnosis.

## CONCLUSION

The approach proposed here is very general as to its principle. Since it is based on the a priori knowledge we have of the images and the objects to be segmented in terms of image analysis, this approach can be applied under any circumstances and provides an answer under the form of an appropriate algorithm for every particular problem. The resulting algorithm, specific to the problem, is most of the time automatic (i.e. is applied without modification for all the images concerning the problem).

The method is especially well suited to segmentation problems in medical imaging. Indeed, the images to be processed are complex (e.g. the distinction between two anatomical segments may be difficult to see for a non experienced observer). On the other hand, segmentation is rarely a self-sufficient goal, and therefore must be of a quality good enough to enable the proceeding of the study.

The approach, proposed here, is very close to an expert system (Prêteux and Laval-Jeantet, 1986 ; Haton, 1987). Indeed, the associating rules between the properties of the image and of the objects to be segmented and the primitives of mathematical morphology correspond to the basis of knowledge. The description of the images and objects through their properties corresponds to the basis of facts. The bivocal approach may be seen as an inference engine working in a mixed chaining : the association of a method with a set of properties constitutes a forward chaining and the determination of the properties required for the proper application of an algorithm constitutes a backward chaining.

This similarity enhances powerful perspectives offered by this method. Obviously, it can be considered as the first step of a true segmentation expert system in mathematical morphology.

REFERENCES :

Beucher, S., and Meyer, F. (1977). Méthodes d'analyse de contraste à l'analyseur de textures, N-536, C.M.M, Fontainebleau.

Bloch, I., Prêteux, F., Cabanis, E.A., Iba-Zizen, M.T., Bourgoin, C., and Tamraz, J. (1986). Mathematical morphology for automatic detection of MR brain lesions : primary results, XIII symposium neuroradiologicum, Stockholm.

Boulanger, F., Soussaline, F., and Prêteux, F. (1987). A new segmentation algorithm in mathematical morphology, MARI87, La Villette, France, 342-349.

Coster, M., and Chermant, J.L. (1975). Précis d'Analyse d'Images, éd. CNRS.

Haton, J.P. (1987). Knowledge-based systems for pattern recognition and interpretation, MARI87, La Villette, France, 73-80.

Klein, J.C. (1976). Conception et réalisation d'une unité logique pour l'analyse quantitative d'images, Thèse de doctorat, Université de Nancy.

Lavayssière, B., and Prêteux, F. (1987). Repérage automatique du ventricule gauche en angioradiographie numérique par la morphologie mathématique, 11ème colloque GRETSI, Nice, France.

Matheron, G. (1975). Random Sets and Integral Geometry, Wiley and S., New York.

Matheron, G. (1983). Filters and Lattices, N-851, C.G.M.M., Fontainebleau.

Merlet, N. (1987). Détermination du volume pulmonaire dans le cadre du traitement de l'emphysème bulleux, C.M.M., Fontainebleau.

Meyer, F. (1986). Erodés ultimes, maxima régionaux : algorithmes rapides, N-5/86/MM, C.M.M, Fontainebleau.

Prêteux, F., Laval-Jeantet, A.M., Roger, B., and Laval-Jeantet, M. (1985). New Prospects in CT Image Processing via Mathematical Morphology, Europ. J. Radiol. 5, 313-317.

Prêteux, F. (1986). Primitive Extraction and Mathematical Morphology, Second Image Symposium GRETSI-CESTA, Nice, France, 719-725.

Prêteux, F., and Schmitt, M. (1986). A new mathematical morphological algorithm : r,h maxima, r,h minima ; applications to X-rays tomographs, N.M.R., Angiography, Second Image Symposium GRETSI-CESTA, Nice, France, 469-475.

Prêteux, F., and Laval-Jeantet, M. (1986). Les systèmes experts en radiologie, réponse à l'inflation et à la complexité des images, 3ème Forum des Jeunes Chercheurs GBM, Paris, France.

Serra, J. (1982). Image Analysis and Mathematical Morphology, Academic Press, London.

Serra, J. (1982). Les filtres morphologiques, N-744, C.M.M., Fontainebleau.

Serra, J. editor (1987). Advances in Mathematical Morphology (to be published in Academic Press).

Sternberg, .R. (1980). Cellular Computers and Biomedical Image Processing, U.S. France Seminar on Biomedical Image Processing, Grenoble, France, 294-319.

Syrota, A., and Comar, D. (1985). Muscarinic cholinergic receptor in the human heart under physiological conditions by positron emission tomography, Proc. Nat. 1 Acad. Sci., USA.

Travère, J.M., Lailler, P., Plancoulaine, B., Bloyet, D., Syrota, A., and Charbonneau, P. (1986). Automatic analysis and graphic image modeling for muscarinic receptors study by time of flight positron emission tomography, Second Image Symposium GRETSI-CESTA, Nice, France, 497-503.

# OPTIC FLOW ESTIMATION BY ADAPTIVE AFFINE TRANSFORM

A. Toet[+], P. Werkhoven[+], B. Nienhuis[+], J.J. Koenderink[+],
and O Ying Lie[#]

[+]University of Utrecht, Physics Laboratory
P.O. Box 80000, 3584 CC Utrecht, The Netherlands

[#]University Hospital Utrecht, Dept. of Nuclear Medicine
Catharijnesingel 101, 3511 GV Utrecht, The Netherlands

## INTRODUCTION

Optic flow is the velocity field in the image plane that arises due to the projection of moving points in the scene onto the image plane. The motion of points in the image plane may be due to the motion of the observer, the motion of objects in the scene, or both. Optic flow also represents the apparent motion due to the temporal rate of change of gray value structures. Figure 1 illustrates the distinction between real (fig. 1a) and apparent (fig. 1b) motion.

Currently, there has been much interest in the computation and description of optical flow in time varying imagery. Several reasons for this can be identified. Firstly, optic flow provides information relating to the depth, shape and orientation of visible surfaces in a scene (Prazdny, 1983). Secondly, knowledge of motion in the scene can lead to a more compact transmission or storage of image sequences. Thirdly, it faciliates the segmentation of a scene.

## FORMULATION OF THE PROBLEM

Optic flow induces a relative displacement between the same identifiable features in two images in a time varying sequence. The image velocity field can therefore be estimated by computing a mapping between two consecutive images. This mapping will be called the *displacement vector field*. It can be obtained by finding the correspondence between features in two images (e.g. Prager and Arbib, 1983). An alternative approach is to assume that all changes in image irradiance in a time sequence of images are attributable to optic flow. Under the assumption that the intensity of an object's surface element will not change during motion (uniform constant illumination and neglegable shading effects) Horn and Schunck (1981) derived an equation which relates the change in gray value $g(r;t)$ at a point $r(x,y)$ in the image plane due to the displacement dr of the corresponding local intensity pattern to the temporal change of the intensity at r:

$$dg(r;t)/dt = 0 \qquad\qquad\qquad (1)$$

This is the so-called *motion constraint equation* . Assume that g may be approximated by a first order Taylor series with respect to t. Equation (1) can then be written as

$$\delta g(r;t)/\delta t + \delta g(r;t)/\delta r \; dr/dt = 0 \qquad\qquad (2)$$

or, for the sake of brevity, as

$$g_t(r) + \nabla g(r) \; v(r) = 0 \qquad\qquad\qquad (3)$$

where $\nabla$  denotes the gradient operator,
 and  v(r) denotes the local image velocity
(e.g. Horn and Schunk, 1981).

The motion constraint equation can only be solved if v(r) is uniform across the image plane and there exist at least two linear independent gray value gradients in the image. However, v(r) is generally not uniform and a first order Taylor series may not be sufficient to take into account second order characteristic gray value variations at locations where the gray value gradient vanishes (e.g. extrema).

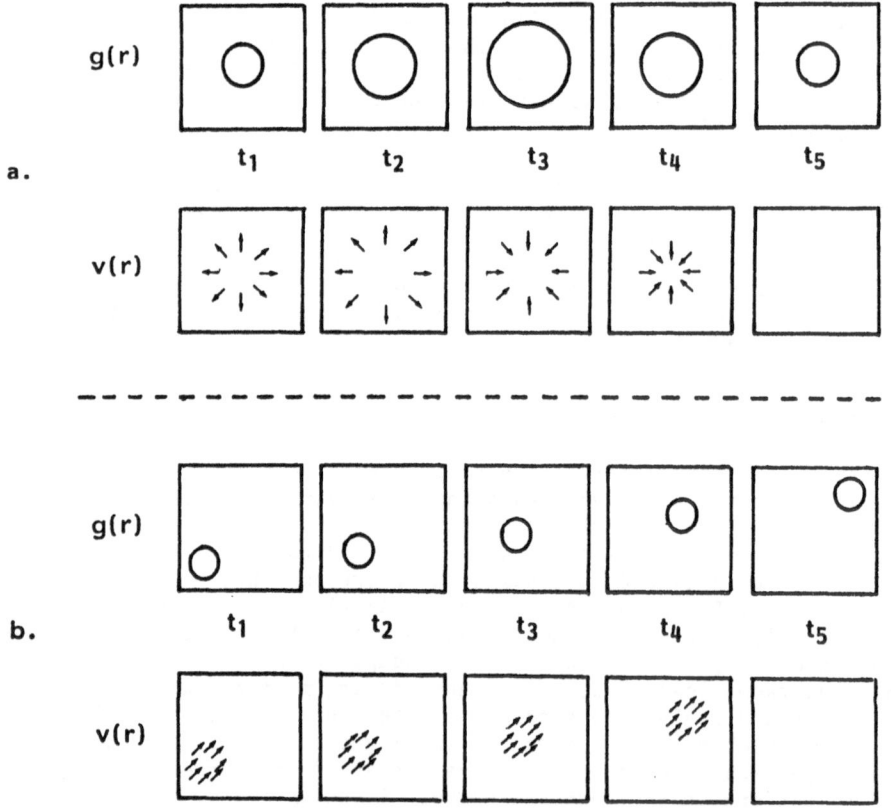

Figure 1. (a) Real motion and (b) apparent motion.

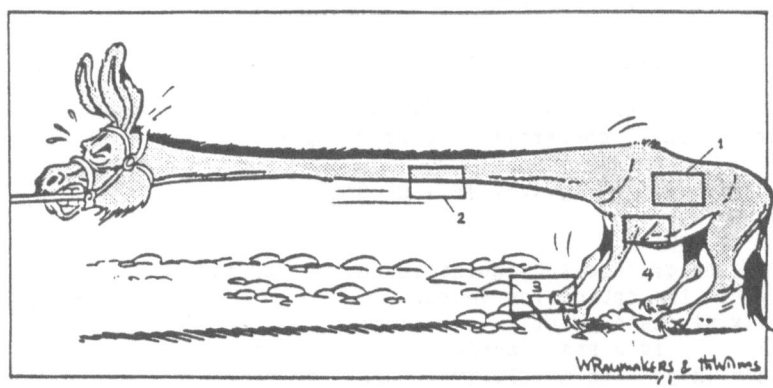

Figure 2. The different effects of object motion on gray
value changes.


In the sequel we will denote the points of local maximum curvature in a
zero-crossing contour (i.e. in the locus curve of the steepest gray value
slope) as *gray value corners*. Corner points exhibit a local unique curvature
in two perpendicular directions. This enables the determination of both
components of the flow vector at these points.
At *edges* (the gray values vary only in one direction), only the component of
the flow vector along the direction of the gradient can be computed. In
homogeneous regions, no unique flow vector estimates can be obtained.

In most situations, the mere gray value variations do not provide
sufficient information to obtain a unique solution (displacement vector
field) for the motion constraint equation. Figure 2 illustrates that the
changes of the gray value structures in the image that result from the
relative motion of objects in the scene are strongly context dependent
(assuming the attempts to move the stubborn animal are successful in the
first place). Small displacements of homogeneous surface areas (fig. 2;
window 1) leave the gray value structure in the image essentially the same.
Therefore, no unique estimate for the displacement vectors can be determined
in these areas. On gray value edges (fig. 2; window 2) only a single
component of the displacement vector can be estimated. In occlusion
situations (fig. 2; window 3) parts of surfaces may appear and disappear. No
displacement vector estimates can be obtained without additional knowledge
of the context of these occluded parts. As illustrated in figure 3,
occlusion may even introduce false features.

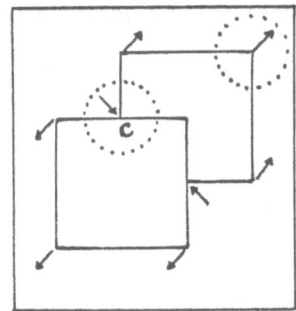
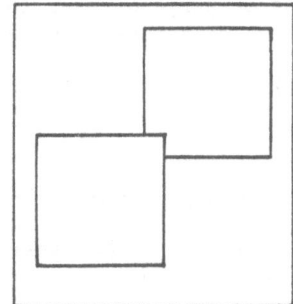

Figure 3. An occlusion situation in which a false feature
(corner C) can induce unrealistic motion estimates.

# LOCAL CONSTRAINT AND ORIENTED SMOOTHNESS

## A constrained least-squares formulation

As noted before, equation (2) is ill-posed (e.g. in homogeneous areas). Therefore, a local constrained least-squares approximation is formulated:

$$\text{Min}_{v} \sum_{z \varepsilon P} \{g_2(z) - g_1(z-v)\}^2 + \alpha^2 \, S(z) \qquad (4)$$

where $g_1$ and $g_2$ are subsequent images at $t_1$ and $t_2$,
$v$ is the optic flow vector,
$r(x,y)$ is a point in the image,
$P$ is a small surface patch around $r$,
$z = [x \; y]^\top$ is a relative coordinate vector w.r.t. $r$,
$\alpha^2$ is the stabilizing factor,
and $S(z)$ is the stabilizing functional.

Note that it is possible to introduce a weight function $w(z)$ with weight factors that depend on the relative distance $|z|$ into this procedure.

## The stabilizing funtional

Nagel (1986) suggested to restrict variations of the displacement vector field over the image plane in directions with small or no variation of gray values. The rationale for the choice of this particular constraint is the fact that there is not sufficient information to estimate a unique mapping between consecutive time slices at locations where the gray value distribution does not exhibit any sizable discontinuity (i.e. where there are no distinct features).

The oriented smoothness constraint can be formulated as follows:

(i) The variation of the flow vector in the direction perpendicular to the gradient should become as small as possible. The variation is captured by

$$\nabla g^+ \; \nabla v \qquad (5)$$

where $\nabla$ denotes the gradient operator,
and $+$ denotes the normal to a vector.

(ii) The variation of the flow vector should be as small as possible in the direction perpendicular to the principal curvature direction associated with a large curvature. The variation is given by

$$(\nabla \nabla g)^+ \; \nabla v \qquad (6)$$

The stabilizing functional can then be written as

$$S = \sum_{z \varepsilon P} \{(\nabla g^+)^2 + b^2 \, (\nabla \nabla g^+)^2\} \, \nabla v^2 \qquad (7)$$

The spatial range of the smoothing process induced by the stabilizing functional S can be adjusted by setting the parameter $\alpha$.

## Solution method

Estimates of the solution of equation (4) can be obtained from an iterative process

$$v(r) = v_0 + dv_1 + dv_2 \tag{8}$$

where $v_0$ is the precomputed value.
The term $dv_1$ results from the least-squares term in equation (4);
the term $dv_2$ results from the stabilizing functional.

Consider the least-squares term in equation (4):

$$\min_{v} \sum_{z \varepsilon P} \{g_2(z) - g_1(z-v)\}^2 \tag{9}$$

The Euler-Lagrange equation for this problem is

$$\sum_{z \varepsilon P} \{g_2(z) - g_1(z-v)\} \, \delta g_1(z-v)/\delta v = 0 \tag{10}$$

A first order Taylor series expansion w.r.t. $v$ yields

$$\sum_{z \varepsilon P} \{g_2(z) - g_1(z-v_0) + \nabla g_1(z-v_0) \, dv\} \, \nabla g_1(z-v_0) = 0 \tag{11}$$

In matrix notation:

$$(G_2 - G_1 + \nabla G_1 \, DV)^T \, \nabla G_1 = 0 \tag{12}$$

or, equivalently

$$(G_2 - G_1) \, \nabla G_1^T + \nabla G_1 \, DV \, \nabla G_1^T = 0 \tag{13}$$

The matrix $\nabla G_1 \, \nabla G_1^T$ is ill-posed. By the use of a second order Taylor series expansion it can be approximated by

$$C = \nabla G_1 \, \nabla G_1^T + dz^2 \, \nabla \nabla G_1 \, \nabla \nabla G_1^T \approx \nabla G_1 \, \nabla G_1^T \tag{14}$$

The solution of equation (9) can then be obtained from the iterative process

$$V = V_0 + DV$$

with $\tag{15}$

$$DV = - \, C^{-1} \, (G_2 - G_1) \, \nabla G_1^T$$

C represents a combination of gray value gradients and principle curvatures of the local gray value structure of g. The eigenvalues of C will be denoted as the "main curvatures". At extrema C represents the principle curvatures and at linear gray value distributions C represents the gray value gradients.

Because corner points exhibit a local unique curvature in two perpendicular directions, the matrix C is regular at corner points. Therefore, both components of the flow vector can be determined. At edges, only the component of the flow vector along the direction of the gradient can be computed. In homogeneous regions, no unique flow vector estimates can be obtained.

Now, the second term of equation (4) will be incorporated into the iteration process:

$$S = \sum_{z \varepsilon P} \{(\nabla g_1{}^+)^2 + b^2 (\nabla\nabla g_1{}^+)^2\} \nabla v^2 \tag{16}$$

or, in matrix notation

$$S = \text{trace}(\ \nabla V^T\ (\nabla G_1{}^+\ \nabla G_1{}^{+T} + b^2\ \nabla\nabla G_1{}^+\ \nabla\nabla G_1{}^{+T})\ \nabla V\ ) \tag{17}$$

By choosing $b^2 = dz^2$ we get

$$S = \text{trace}(\ \nabla V^T\ C^{-1}\ \nabla V\ ) \tag{18}$$

Combining the two terms as in equation (4) yields

$$\underset{V}{\text{Min}}\quad (G_2-G_1)^T(G_2-G_1) + \alpha^2 \cdot \text{trace}(\nabla V^T\ C^{-1}\ \nabla V) \tag{19}$$

Assume that the coordinate system is aligned with the eigenvector directions of C at the image location of interest. This results in a diagonal matrix of eigenvalues of $C^{-1}$. If these eigenvalues are small, the contribution of the stabilizing functional S is small compared to the first term in equation (4).

To simplify the solution of this equation, Nagel (1986) assumes that the components of C vary slowly over the image plane. In this case, the derivatives of C can be neglected and the iterate is given by

$$DV = -\ C^{-1}\ (G_2-G_1)\ \nabla G_1{}^T + \alpha^2\ C^{-1}\ \left(\begin{array}{c}\text{trace}([C^{-1}\ O]\ \nabla\nabla V_0)\\[4pt]\text{trace}([O\ C^{-1}]\ \nabla\nabla V_0)\end{array}\right) \tag{20}$$

$$=\qquad DV_1\qquad +\qquad DV_2$$

where  O  denotes the zero matrix,
  and  [] denotes a matrix that contains two submatrices.


## The interpretation of oriented smoothness

In this section we will show that Nagel's (1986) oriented smoothness constraint derived in the previous section is equivalent to a local weighted averaging of the solution of the least-squares equation (9), given by the iteration process (15). Moreover, we will show that the weight functions used for both components of $DV_2$ in the averaging process adapt in form and orientation to the local gray value structure of the image.

C is positive symmetric, hence

$$L = P^T\ C\ P\quad \text{or}\quad L^{-1} = P\ C^{-1} P^T \tag{21}$$

where  P  is the matrix of eigenvectors of C,
  and  L  is the diagonal matrix of eigenvalues of C:

$$L^{-1} = \left(\begin{array}{cc}1 & 0\\0 & m\end{array}\right)$$

Hence, by alignment of the axes with the eigenvectors of C

$$DV_2 = \alpha^2 \; L^{-1} \; \binom{\text{trace}([L^{-1}\; O] \; \nabla\nabla V_0)}{\text{trace}([O \; L^{-1}] \; \nabla\nabla V_0)} \qquad (22)$$

Consider a symmetric patch P and window W such that

$$\sum_{z \varepsilon P} w(z) \; z = 0 \qquad (23)$$

A second order Taylor series expansion of V w.r.t. z within the patch P yields

$$\sum_{z \varepsilon P} w(z) \; v(z) = v_0 + \sum_{z \varepsilon P} w(z) \; z \; \nabla v_0 + 1/2 \sum_{z \varepsilon P} w(z) \; z^2 \; \nabla\nabla v_0 \qquad (24)$$

and thus

$$DV_2 = 1/2 \; \binom{\text{trace}([W \; O] \; \nabla\nabla V_0)}{\text{trace}([O \; W] \; \nabla\nabla V_0)} \qquad (25)$$

where W is a diagonal matrix with elements $\sum_{x \varepsilon P} w(x) \; x^2$ , $\sum_{y \varepsilon P} w(y) \; y^2$ .

As a result, equation (22) equals equation (25) by taking

$$\alpha^2 l^2 = 1/2 \sum_{x \varepsilon P_1} w_1(x) \; x^2 \quad \text{and} \quad \alpha^2 lm = 1/2 \sum_{y \varepsilon P_1} w_1(y) \; y^2$$

and

$$\alpha^2 lm = 1/2 \sum_{x \varepsilon P_2} w_2(x) \; x^2 \quad \text{and} \quad \alpha^2 m^2 = 1/2 \sum_{y \varepsilon P_2} w_2(y) \; y^2 \qquad (26)$$

where $P_1$ and $P_2$ are patches,
and $w_1$ and $w_2$ are window functions.

As a result, the elaborate computation of the expression for $DV_2$ in equation (20) can now be replaced by a local weighted averaging.

The x and y components of $DV_2$ are computed by weighted averaging over respectively the windows $W_1$ and $W_2$. Adaptation of these windows to the density of the flow vector field can be realized by adopting two bivariate Gaussian functions $w_1$ and $w_2$:

$$w_i(x,y) = \exp \; -(x^2/\sigma^2_{xi} + y^2/\sigma^2_{yi}) \qquad (i=1,2) \qquad (27)$$

The two standard deviations of each Gaussian function are related to the eigenvalues l and m of $C^{-1}$ as follows:

$$\sigma_{y1}/\sigma_{x1} = \sigma_{y2}/\sigma_{x2} = \sigma_{x2}/\sigma_{x1} = 1/m \qquad (28)$$

The proportions of the length and width of the windows are determined by the magnitude of the eigenvalues of $C^{-1}$. The window $W_2$ used to compute the y component of the flow vector is congruent to the window $W_1$ used to compute the x component and scaled by a factor $1/m$. The standard deviations of the weight functions are chosen in the order of a few times the spatial *sampling* interval of the image plane.

71

The spatial range of the averaging process can be adjusted by setting the parameter $\alpha$. Nagel (1986) used a heuristic criterium to increase $\alpha$ during the iteration process. It is preferable to adapt $\alpha$ to the local "feature" density in the image. In the absence of corners or edges ("features") in the direct neighbourhood of r (no characteristic curvatures) the window over which the unknown components of V are computed should be large. When the local gray value structure varies heavily a small window suffices.

## ADAPTIVE AFFINE TRANSFORM

A small deformation of the gray level structure in a patch can be approximated by a linear (affine) transform. The deformation can be made arbitrarily small if the size of the patch P or the timespan dt in which the patch is subjected to the flow are chosen small enough. An affine transform can be described by 6 parameters, representing respectively the effects of rotation (1 parameter), dilatation (3 parameters) and translation (2 parameters).

First, a solution for equation (9) is estimated at corner points and at gray value edges. Thereafter, these estimates are used to compute the local affine transform. The parameters of this transform are computed over a patch P weighted by a bivariate Gaussian function $w(x,y)$ as given by expression (27).

Consider an image point at $r(x,y)$. The flow vector v at r can be approximated by

$$v(r) = T\ r \tag{29}$$

where T denotes the affine transform.

The parameters of T can then be obtained by minimizing the weighted least-squares function

$$\text{Min} \quad \Sigma\ w(z_c)\ \{v_c - Tz_c\}^2 + \Sigma\ w(z_e)\ \{(v_e - Tz_e\ e_e)\ e_e\}^2 \tag{30}$$
$$T \quad z_c\ \varepsilon P \qquad\qquad z_e\ \varepsilon P$$

where $w(z)$ is the window function of r w.r.t. z given by (27),
   $z_c$ are the corner points in P,
   $v_c$ are the flow vector estimates resulting from the iterative
      approximation of (9) at corner points $z_c$,
   $z_e$ are the edge points in P,
   $v_e$ are the flow vector estimates resulting from the iterative
      approximation of (9) at edges $z_e$,
   $e_e$ are the normalized eigenvectors of $C^{-1}$ at edges $z_e$ with the
      largest eigenvalues.

As noted before, the solution of equation (9) only provides estimates of the flow vector components perpendicular to gray value transitions. Thus, for edge points only the component perpendicular to the edge can be used in the assessment of the local affine tranform. This is the reason why only the projections of the flow vectors on the gray value gradient enter the minimalization process of equation (30) at edge points.

Once the affine transform T is known within a patch P a flow vector T r can be assigned to the centre of P. Because the window size is adaptive to the local gray value structure (feature density), there is no need to propagate information by means of an iterative process. Instead, after completing the iterative solution of equation (9), the adaptive affine reconstruction (30) can be carried out in a single step. The flow vector estimates obtained at corner points are preserved in the affine reconstruction process.

Consider for instance the interior of a homogeneous gray value segment. An adaptive oriented smoothing process needs many iteration steps to propagate flow vector estimates determined for corner and edge points into the interior (were no initial flow vector estimates are available). On the other hand, the adaptive affine transform can reconstruct the entire flow field in a single step. Therefore, this method is more efficient than the oriented smoothness approach. The latter also requires the calculation of second order partial derivatives of the flow vector components at each point on every iteration step. Moreover, a local affine transform tolerates sharp discontinuities in the flowvector field. The results are therefore more realistic than the ones obtained from an oriented smoothing process.

## NUMERICAL IMPLEMENTATION

### Corner detection

We used the Zuniga-Haralick (1983) operator to detect gray value corners. For an n x n neighbourhood around each pixel a least squares fit of a bicubic polynomial to the gray level function is computed. This fit yields estimates for the first and second derivatives of the gray value function.

A pixel is declared an edge point if the norm of the gradient is large and the derivative of this norm in the direction of the gradient is small:

$$|\nabla g| \geq M_1 \quad \text{and} \quad |(\nabla |\nabla g| \ \nabla g) / (|\nabla g|)| \leq \varepsilon$$

where $|.|$ denotes the Euclidean norm,
and $M_1$ and $\varepsilon$ are threshold parameters.

A corner is defined by its "cornerness", that is the derivative of the orientation angle of the normal to the gradient. Thus, a pixel is declared a corner if it is an edge point and the "cornerness" is large:

$$(\nabla g^{+T} \ \nabla \nabla g \ \nabla g^{+}) / (|\nabla g|^3) \geq M_2$$

where $M_2$ is a threshold parameter.

Because of the condition that a corner point should also be an edge point, the Zuniga-Haralick corner detector eliminates all false corners in the background which might appear due to noise. Moreover, this detector is insensitive to the effects of image blur (Shah and Jain, 1984).

The faithfulness of the bicubic polynomial approximation to the local gray value structure is limited by the spatial frequency content of the image. To prevent the occurence of unrealistic values for the derivatives we reduced the high spatial frequency content of the input images by convolving these images with a Gaussian kernel.

### Algorithms

Algorithm 1: Adaptive smoothing.

Step 1: Convolution of $g_1$ with a Gaussian kernel to smooth the image before making a bicubic polynomial approximation.

Step 2: Calculation of the derivatives of $g_1$.

Step 3: Corner detection in $g_1$.

Step 4: Iteration for corners without smoothness constraint using formula (15).

Step 5: Iteration for other pixels using formula (15) followed by averaging within adaptive window functions as specified in expression (27).

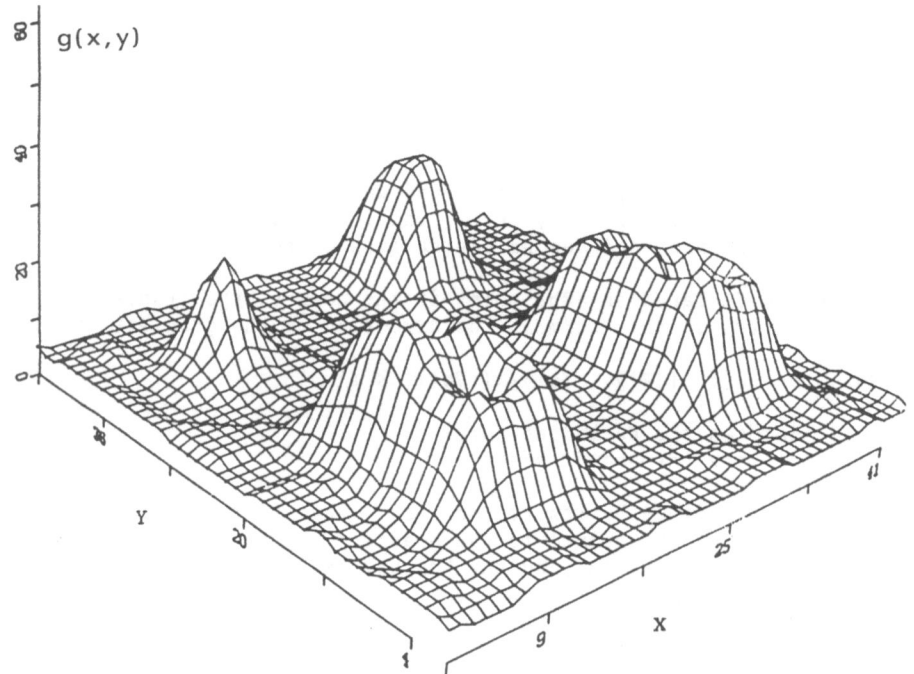

Figure 4. An artificial test image.

Algorithm 2: Adaptive affine transform.

Step 1 to 3: as in Algorithm 1.

Step 4: Iteration for corners and edges without smoothness constraint using formula (15).

Step 5: Solution for other pixels by means of adaptive affine transform represented by equation (29).

74

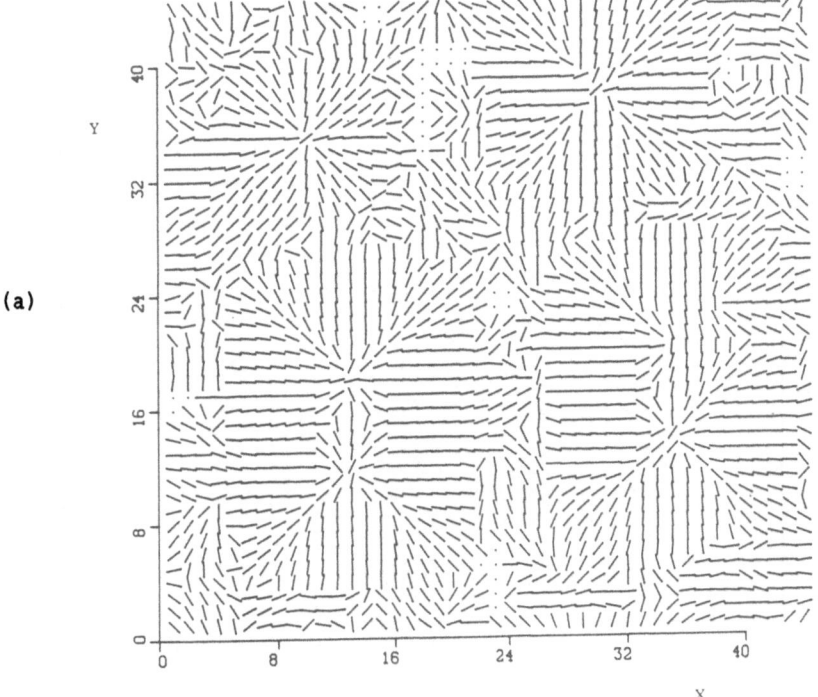

(a)

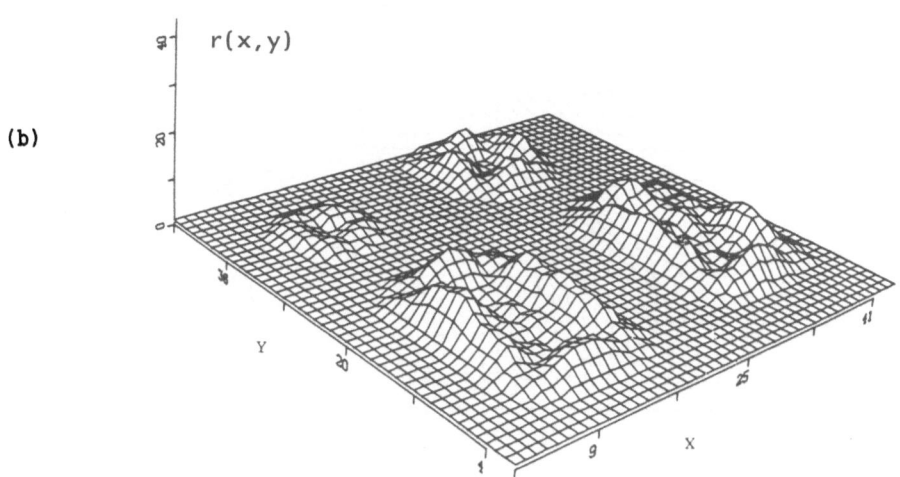

(b)

Figure 5. (a) The direction of the eigenvector of
matrix C with the largest eigenvalue.
(b) The ratio of the eigenvalues corresponding with the eigenvectors of C.

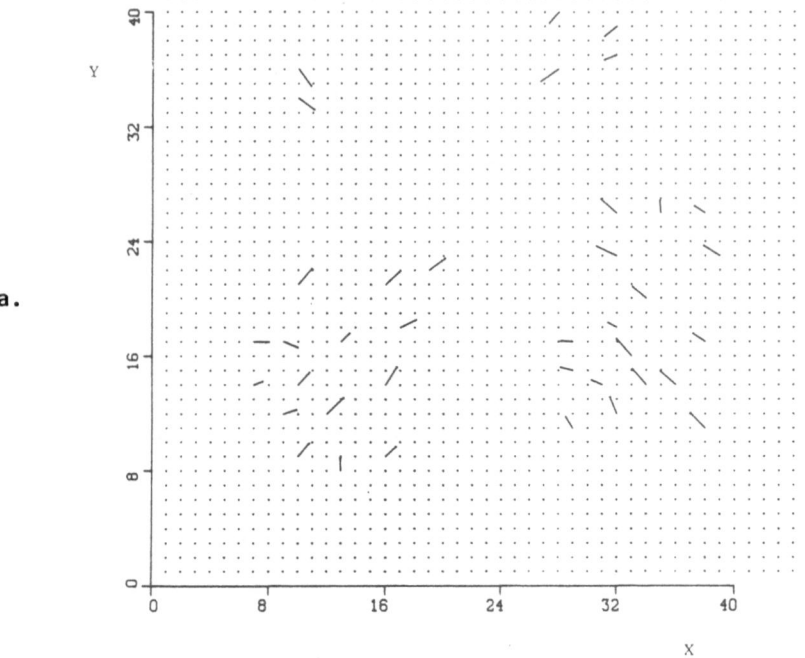

a.

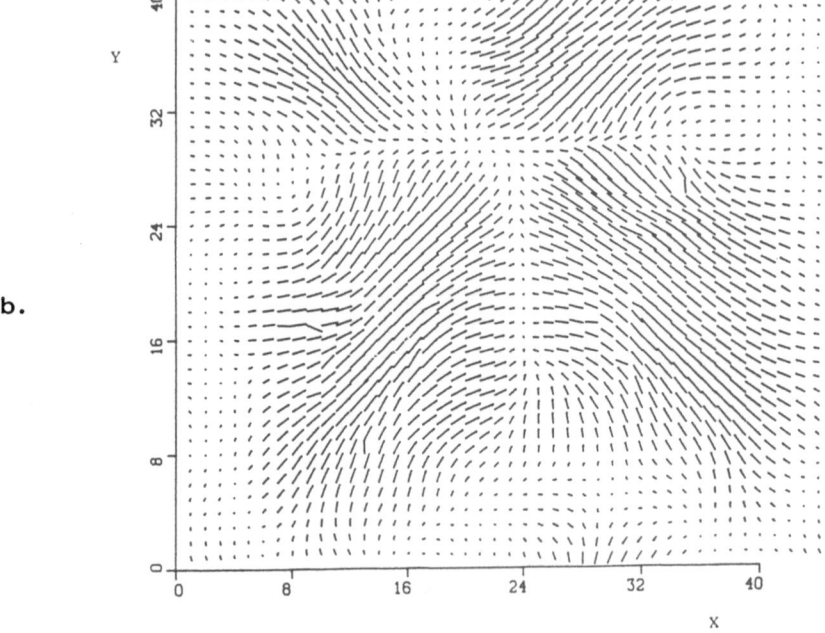

b.

Figure 6. The result of Algorithm 1.
       (a) Estimates for the displacement vectors
           at gray value corners.
       (b) The final displacement vector field.

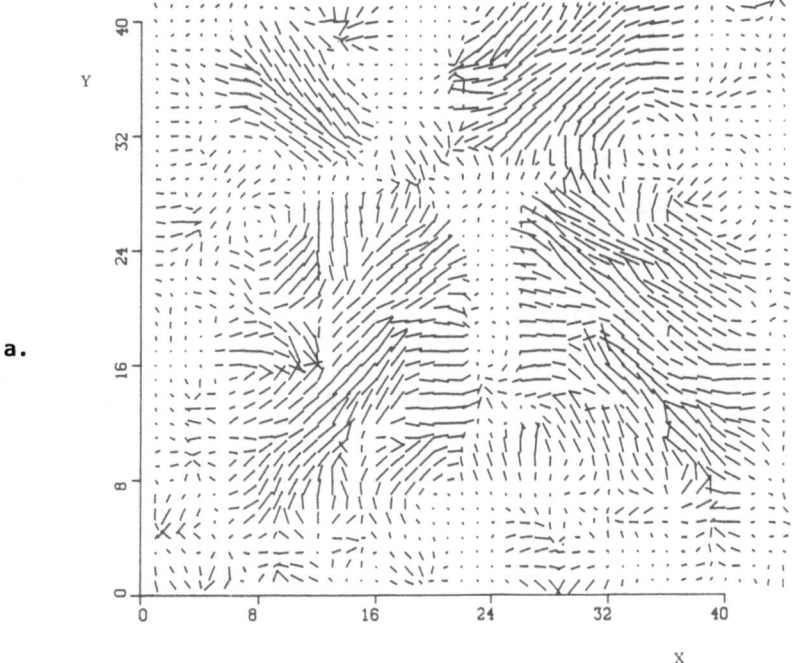

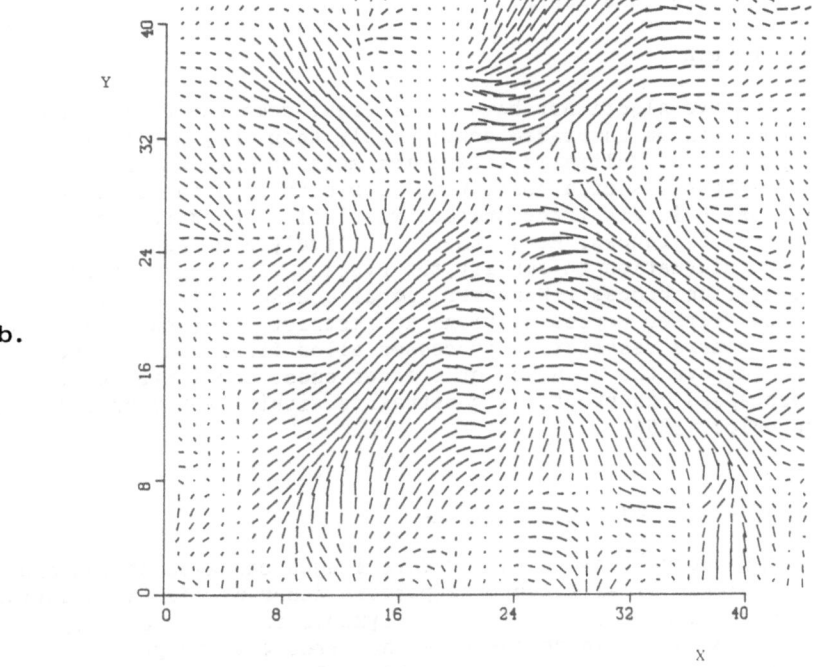

Figure 7. The result of Algorithm 2.
(a) Estimates for the displacement vectors
on corners and on gray value edges.
(b) The final displacement vector field.

77

RESULTS

Both algorithms have been implemented and applied to synthetic image sequences. To simulate a realistic situation, we corrupted our artificial images with poissonian noise (12 dB signal/noise ratio). The spatial frequency bandwidth of the noise-corrupted images was reduced by convolving them with a Gaussian kernel (low-pass filtering). As a result the spatial cut-off frequency of the images was 0.32 cycles per pixeldistance. Figure 4 shows the image that was used to obtain the results that will be presented in the rest of this section. It contains the numbers 6 and 8 and two different squares.

The form and orientation of the adaptive windows applied in both algorithms is determined by the eigenvectors and corresponding eigenvalues of the matrix C. Figure 5 shows for each point in the image from Figure 4 the direction of the eigenvector with the largest eigenvalue (5a) and the ratio of the two eigenvalues (5b).

Both algorithms first produce sparse displacement vector fields. Algorithm 1 first yields estimates for the displacement vectors at gray value corners (Figure 6a). Algorithm 2 first produces estimates for displacement vectors on corners and on edge points (Figure 7a). The final displacement vector fields produced by both algorithms are shown in respectively figures 6b and 7b.

Only minor differences can be noted between the flow vector fields produced by both algorithms. The displacement vector field is filled in correctly in most structureless gray value regions.


DISCUSSION AND SUGGESTIONS FOR FURTHER RESEARCH

A multigrid approach

Local iterative algorithms have an inherent computational sluggishness. Their efficiency can be increased considerably when they are implemented in a multigrid structure. Multigrid relaxation methods take advantage of multiple discretizations of a continuous problem over a range of resolution levels. The coarser levels trade spatial resolution for direct communication paths over larger distances. Hence they effectively accelerate the global propagation of information to amplify the overall efficiency of the iterative relaxation process. Moreover, local coarse-to-fine intralevel processes allow coarser representations to restrict finer ones and, vice versa, fine-to-coarse restriction processes allow finer representations to constrain and improve the accuracy of coarser ones. Local iterative relaxation processes can propagate constraints within each representational level (Terzopoulos, 1986).


Matching hierarchical image descriptions

The correspondence between two or more images can also be found by matching their hierarchical structural pattern descriptions. An additional advantage of such an approach is that the symbols in such a description can also be matched to models which describe the structural properties of pattern classes (Crowley and Sanderson, 1987). As a result, the matching process may become relatively insensitive to intensity changes, rotations, deformations, changes of spatial scale and even occlusions. The stack-based image segmentation tree introduced by Pizer (1986) seems very suited for this approach. Initial results show that the method is indeed very robust.

## Integrating segmentation and optic flow calculation.

Optic flow is useful as a cue for scene segmentation. Motion information may be used to link adjacent but visually dissimilar surfaces or to split surfaces not easily separable by static criteria alone. Often object boundaries that are ambiguous in a single image frame are easily resolved when dynamic effects are evaluated based on a sequence of frames. On the other hand, a priori knowledge of the scene segmentation may be used to estimate flow vectors for regions that have no characteristic or resolvable features within their boundaries (e.g. homogeneous regions or regions with fine texture).

The use of motion as a basis for segmentation velocity estimation must be independent of extensive analysis of static boundaries. The optic flow calculation procedures described in this paper operate on local gray value properties rather than on coherent/ closed contours. Because these local area velocity estimation techniques require no prior image partitioning, the resulting displacement map may be used as a primary source of data for motion-based segmentation. The parameters provided by the local adaptive affine transform reconstruction method can be a valuable source of information for scene segmentation.

## REFERENCES

Crowley, J.L. and Sanderson, C. (1987). Multiple resolution representation and probabilistic matching of 2-D gray-scale shape, IEEE Tr. Patt. An. and Mach. Int., 9, 113-121.

Horn, B.K.P. and Schunck, B.G. (1981). Determining optical flow, Artificial Intell., 17, 185-203.

Nagel, H.H. and Enkelmann, W. (1986). An investigation of smoothness constraints for the estimation of displacement vector fields from image sequences, IEEE Tr. Patt. An. and Mach. Int., 8, 565-593.

Pizer, S.M., Koenderink, J.J., Lifshitz, L.M., Helmink, L. and Kaasjager, A.D.J. (1986). An image description for object definition, based on extremal regions in the stack, in: "Information Processing in Medical Imaging, Proc. of the 9th Conference", 24-37. S.L. Bacharach, ed., Martinus Nijhoff, Den Haag.

Prager, J.M. and Arbib, M.A. (1983). Computing the optical flow: The MATCH algorithm and prediction, Comp. Vision, Graphics and Image Processing, 24, 271-304.

Prazdny, K. (1983). On the information in optical flows, Comp. Vision, Graphics and Image Processing, 22, 239-259.

Shah, M.A. and Jain, R. (1984). Detecting time-varying corners, Computer Vision, Graphics and Image Processing, 28, 345-355.

Terzopoulos, D., (1986). Image analysis using multigrid relaxation methods, IEEE Tr. Patt. An. and Mach. Int., 8, 129-139.

Zuniga, A. and Haralick, R.M. (1983). Corner detection using the facet model, in: Proc. IEEE Conf. Comp. Vision and Patt. Rec., 30-37.

# IMAGE REGISTRATION : A REVIEW AND A STRATEGY FOR MEDICAL APPLICATIONS

Pascale GERLOT [*] and Yves BIZAIS [+]

\* : LAN, UA CNRS 823, ENSM
    NANTES, FRANCE

\+ : Projet DIMI, HGRL, CHRN
    NANTES, FRANCE

## INTRODUCTION

Similarity measurements of biomedical images are of interest when a diagnosis is derived from comparing images produced by various modalities and/or in various patients.

Information in images depends on various features (Bookstein, 1986) and different types of information can be distinguished (Kropatsch, 1983). Therefore image comparison can be considered as a two-stage process. The first step consists in registering images in order to discard information relative to displacements and to the patient without diagnosis meaning, such that only relevant information is kept. Components pertaining relevant information - information relative to the image formation and recording process and to the patient with potential diagnosis meaning - are used in the second stage in order to lead to one or several combined images allowing improved diagnosis.

In this paper, we focus on the first stage named registration thereafter. A general approach for registration is (i) to extract features common to the image pair (preprocessing stage), (ii) to match common features in the first image with common features in the second one and (iii) to compute the transformation which maps one image into the other. The preprocessing stage depends on images operated on so that a priori information (such as information relative to the patient without diagnosis meaning) may be involved.

Many different kinds of medical images exist ; therefore we present a review of image registration methods in order to define appropriate preprocessing and matching techniques for the various biomedical applications.

The registration problem is presented in the first section ; control-point based registration methods in the second one ; moment-based normalization techniques in the third section ; edge-based registration methods in the fourth one and the optimization of a similarity measurement as a registration method in the fith one are reviewed. Application of the above methods to biomedical images registration is considered in the sixth section.

## DEFINITION OF THE REGISTRATION PROBLEM

The following definition has been proposed by Henderson et al. (1985) :
let $f(x,y)$ and $g(x,y)$ be two digital images ;
let $C = \{(x,y,u,v) \mid (x,y) \text{ in } f \text{ corresponds to } (u,v) \text{ in } g\}$ ;

In order to register f with respect to g,
f'(u,v) = f ( T(u,v) ) where T is a registration function defined by :
    T(u,v) = (x,y) for any (x,y,u,v) belonging to C
must be computed.
    The registration problem can be defined as :
1) determining C : selecting control-points in f and assigning them to
control-points in g (correspondence of control-points),
2) determining the registration transform T,
3) computing f' : resampling of f because T(u,v) is often a real coordinate
for which no f value exists.
    This definition, despite the many existing resolution methods is gene-
ral ; differences between approaches lie on the way used to perform the three
steps described above. For example, when a criterion is optimized (cf : optimization of a similarity measurement as a registration method)
1) determining C corresponds to :
    choosing a region of interest in g, and a registration parameter model
(translation, rotation...)
    minimizing a similarity criterion in this region of interest with res-
pect to registration parameters. This operation matches control-points in f
with control-points in g ;
2) determining T using registration parameter values ;
3) computing f'.

CONTROL-POINT BASED REGISTRATION METHODS

Defining control-points

    Determining C (preprocessing stage) consists in choosing some peculiar
points in images named control-points, defined by :
    - their features are unique in order to reliably identify control-points
in the various images ;
    - their geometric properties must lead to an accurate description of the
image transformation.
    They can be obtained manually (Merickel and Mc Carthy, 1985) by choosing
particular points such as edge intersections or points having specific locations. They can be provided by the imaging process itself such as point sources attached to the patient (Fleming 1984) and fiducial markers in stereotactic studies (Kall et al., 1985). In these methods control-points are
provided by the user and choosing them is often cumbersome and not always accurate. In order to overcome this latter problem, Frei et al. (1980), Singh
et al. (1979) have proposed a method consisting in roughly identifying the
control-points visually, estimating their relative location and correcting
the estimates using a cross-correlation coefficient. Alternatively, control-
points can be computed automatically (Merickel and Mc Carthy, 1985 ; Mitiche
and Aggarwal, 1983 ; Yam and Davis, 1985) using centroid, radius weighted
mean point...

Registration step

    Registration is an easy operation consisting in estimating coefficients
of the transformation which maps the control-points of the first image into
the ones in the second image (i.e. using mse minimization : Frei et al.,
1980 ; Singh et al., 1979).

Potential use in medical imaging

    The difficult operation to be done using control-points is preproces-
sing.
    User-provided control-points lead to satisfactory and fast registration;
a priori information being given by the user's knowledge is straightforwardly
introduced in the process. However generality is lost since a priori informa-

tion is defined narrowly (application and user dependence).

Computer generation of control-points is not well suited for complex images such as medical ones because erroneous location of control-points induced by noise may lead to misregistration and produce severe artifacts.

However this approach can be efficient in some particular cases when control-points are provided by the imaging process itself.

## MOMENT-BASED REGISTRATION

### Description

The basic idea used here is to extract common information in images without user participation.

Gray-level and geometric properties of images are characterized by complex moments as defined in Abu-Mostafa and Psaltis (1985), (1984), Hu (1962) and Maitra (1979), and parameters (translation, rotation, scaling...) of the transform leading to "standard" images are computed by normalizing moments in each image, normalized moments being invariant features of images (Goshtasby, 1985).

Noise tolerance is rather weak since noise can lead to imperfect moment estimates and large errors in parameter determination (Abu-Mostafa and Psaltis, 1985).

### Potential use in medical imaging

For complex images, misregistration may occur because :
1) the normalization criterion based upon moments is a general feature of an image characterizing shape and location which can vary significantly without significant differences in images because of noise dependence ;
2) moments do not involve enough knowledge about a priori information which is present only through the registration model. It is clearly insufficient to permit robust registration.

Field of use is restricted to the matching of simple objects in image pairs.

## EDGE-BASED REGISTRATION METHODS

This class of methods has been usually performed to register images where neat contours exist. Preprocessing stage consists in discarding all information except edges in each image.

### Extracting edges

The edge extraction step can be solved in many different ways : template matching, zero-crossing... (Medioni and Nevatia, 1984 ; Mokhtarian and Mackworth, 1986 1-2 ; Moring and Hakalahti, 1985 ; Rosenfeld, 1981 ; Svedlow et al. 1978 ; Wong and Hall, 1979 ; Wong, 1978 ; Yam and Davis, 1981). Nevertheless contours are not easily extracted from noisy images and resulting contours must be characterized properly for the associated matching algorithm to be run, such that it may be difficult to provide a robust input to it.

### Maching edges

This operation can be performed by comparing intensity values of edge pixels (Andrus et al., 1985 ; Svedlow et al., 1978) ; available information about edges is incompletely used since only appearance of edges is involved in this method (Henderson et al., 1985) and the optimization criterion often presents a very sharp minimum which can be missed during optimization. Fig. 1 demonstrates a type of error which may occur with the comparison of contours. Contours in the original image are shown in the upper left quadrant and con-

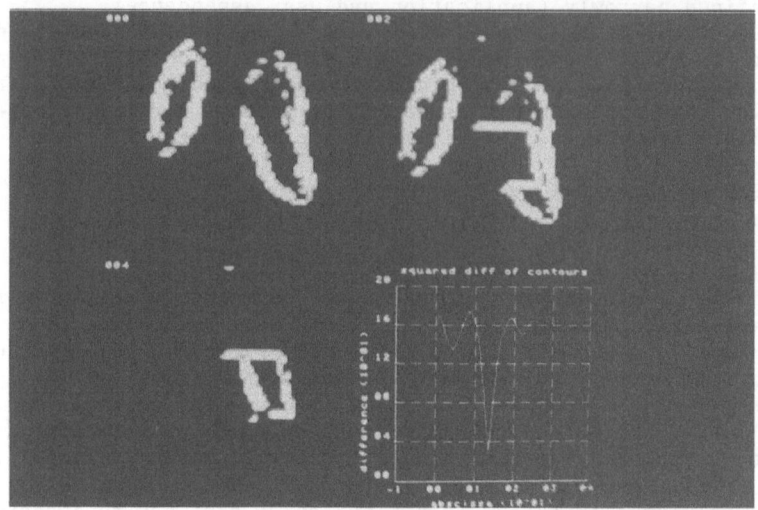

Fig. 1. Edge-based methods. Upper left : contours of the
original image ; upper right : contours of the
image translated and modified ; lower left : difference image for translation value giving the
minimum criterion ; lower right : sum of squared
values in the difference image versus translation
value.

tours in the same image after translation and modification, in the upper
right quadrant. The distance between the two contours as defined by the sum
of squared values in the difference image has been plotted for several translation values in the lower right quadrant. Because either the two contours
are superimposed and the criterion is small, or the two contours are not
superimposed and the criterion is high, the graph exhibits a very sharp
minimum. And because of noise in contour images, this minimum can be missed
and a local minimum selected instead, leading to a totally meaningless registration. In order to overcome this failure, and to ensure high reliability,
contour-based methods must involve systematic search, symbolic representation
or global optimization techniques.

Such comparisons of edges at a symbolic level can be implemented through
the use of segments (Bhanu and Faugeras, 1984 ; Price and Reddy, 1979) ;
scale-based description (Mackworth and Mokhtarian, 1984 ; Mokhtarian and
Mackworth, 1986 2) ; Fourier descriptors (Kuhl and Giardina, 1982), or the
Hough transform (Aggarwal et al., 1981 ; Davis, 1982 ; Henderson et al.,
1985 ; Moring and Hakalahti, 1985 ; O'Rouke, 1981 ; Yam and Davis, 1981) ;
dynamic programming has been used as well (Wu and Maitre, 1986, 1985) in the
context of image/map registration.

The use of segments requires edges well modelled by long segments
(Medioni and Nevatia, 1984) ; the use of the Hough transform is computationally simple but requires huge computer ressources (Mackworth and Mokhtarian,
1984 ; Mokhtarian and Mackworth, 1986 2 ; Wu and Maitre, 1986, 1985) ; dynamic programming requires an edge representation in an ordered sequence which
cannot be provided in the context of image/image registration.

## Potential use in medical imaging

The above methods are particularly well suited when images obtained from
different modalities are compared, because in most instances edge information
is the only common feature found in each image of the set (no common elements
in textural information).

OPTIMIZATION OF A SIMILARITY MEASUREMENT AS A REGISTRATION METHOD

The methodology involved here is not the extraction of features but rather transforming one of the images and measuring the similarity between images until the best fit is achieved.

## Description

Registration is usually performed by optimizing a similarity criterion such as a correlation coefficient, a correlation function, a sum of absolute differences (Appeldorn et al., 1980 ; Barnea and Silverman, 1972 ; Lillestrand, 1972 ; Pratt, 1974 ; Ros et al., 1984 ; Rosenfeld, 1981 ; Svedlow et al., 1978).

Using these similarity measurements for the registration of images may lead to misregistration (Venot et al., 1984 2), because criterion values take into account differences in pixel values due to processes which cannot be explained by statistical fluctuations or by the registration parameter model, such as variations in the amount of contrast medium during angiography, presence of a tumor in only one image... These pixels can be considered as outliers. This is demonstrated by fig. 2 where the original image is shown in the upper left quadrant and the same image, translated and modified in the upper right quadrant. Modification consists in creating a region of mismatch made up of outlier pixels. The minimum value of the sum of squared values in the difference image is not reached for the correct translation values. This can be understood by looking at the difference image (in the lower left quadrant) giving the minimum criterion value. The region of mismatch "pulls" the translation values to the right, the average intensity in the difference image being spread out in regions of mismatch as well as in matching regions. A reliable registration method using a similarity criterion can be obtained by maximizing the number of points for which regions match.

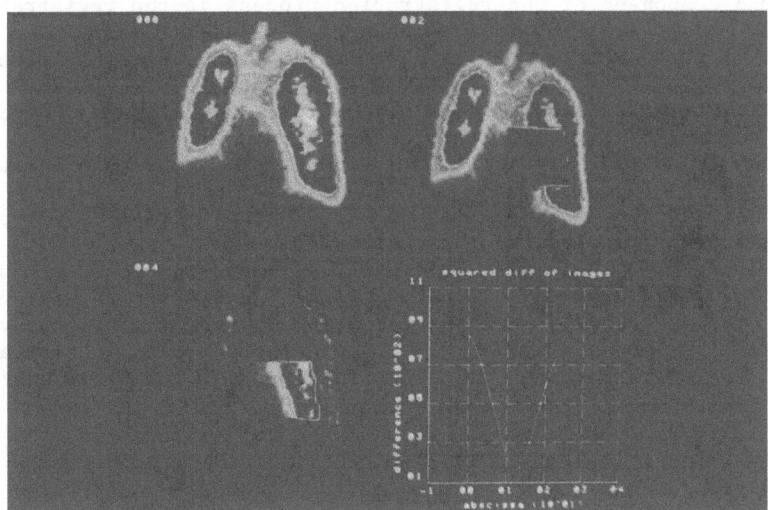

Fig. 2. Similarity criterion based method. Upper left : original image ; upper right : original image translated and modified ; lower left : difference image for translation value giving the minimum criterion ; lower right : sum of squared values in the difference image versus translation value.

Therefore Venot et al. (1986 1-2-3, 1984 1-2-3, 1983), Liehn et al. (1985), Pronzato et al. (1984) have developped a new class of similarity criteria insensitive to the presence of outliers, the optimization of which permits robust registration procedures.

In order to register two noisy images f and g, several registration vectors are tried successively and the difference image dv is computed. dv is defined by :
dv (x,y) = f (Tv (x,y)) - g (x,y) where Tv is a registration function.
Then the number of sign changes is computed by scanning dv row by row : this number is called the SSC (stochastic sign change) criterion. When the two corresponding regions in f ang g match, the number of sign changes is high, while when the two regions do not match, no sign change occurs. Maximization of the SSC criterion with respect to registration parameters leads to the estimation of parameter values.

## Potential use in medical imaging

This class of methods does not necessarily involve a preprocessing stage, all the information being used in order to correlate the image pair.

The use of classical similarity measurements may induce misregistration: the used criterion operates in the same way on local and global differences.

The sign change criterion leads to robust registration : computing the number of sign changes is equivalent to preprocess images in order to extract relevant information (as in the extraction stage of edge-based methods). However this method may fail when comparing very different images or images with different textural information.

## APPLICATION TO REGISTRATION OF BIOMEDICAL IMAGES

Comparison of biomedical images may involve images produced by :
1) the same modality for the same patient,
2) different modalities for the same patient,
3) the same modality for different patients.

A second component of the registration process is the registration parameter model. Usual parameters are translation, rotation, gray-scale and spatial scaling ; in some cases, it is necessary to include more parameters such as shear (Barber, 1982). A compromise as to be found :
- a too rudimentary model cannot describe actual displacements correctly but constrains parameter estimates drastically ;
- a too elaborate model potentially describes any complex displacements, but constraints are too weak.
A priori information plays an essential role in the model elaboration.

A last element involved in the choice of a robust registration method is the existence or absence of contours. For images such as CT scans or DSA images, well described by almost uniform regions separated by neat contours, edge-based or control-point based registration methods are obviously well suited, while they are not appropriate in other cases such as Nuclear Medecine images where moment-based registration or similarity measurement methods can be applied succesfully.

In case 1 (same modality, same patient)
- edge-based registration is a more general approach than control-point based registration and should be preferred if contours exist ;
- if contours do not exist, the sign change criterion leads to a more robust registration than moment-based methods ;
- the registration parameter model is simple and not a limitation for good registration.

In case 2 (different modalities, same patient)
- since common information is very difficult to extract, the more important step here is preprocessing, a priori information being essential ;

- either preprocessing produces control-points or edges and robust registration can be achieved using corresponding methods ; or highly specific preprocessing is necessary before applying similarity measurement or moment-based methods ;
- the registration model is not a limitation for good registration.

In case 3 (same modality, different patients)
- the choice of a registration method depends on the existence of contours,
- patients are different so the registration model has to be representative of actual displacements for the registration to be robust.

The above methods are being implemented on our image processing system and tested on a set of medical images (X-rays, Radionuclide, CT scans, Ultrasounds, MRI).

## CONCLUSION

The image registration problem has been reviewed, four general approaches (control-point based registration, moment-based registration, edge-based registration, optimization of a similarity measurement) are described and use of each method in the context of medical imaging is considered which can be summarized by the following remarks :
- a priori information has to be used in almost any instances to extract information relevant to registration ; only in simple cases for which images are very similar, preprocessing is of little importance.
- as for registration methods themselves, contour or similarity criterion based methods are best suited, even though control point based methods have been used extensively. Use of one method or the other depends on the existence of features such as neat contours.
- more precisely, recent contour based methods make use of symbolic representation, systematic search or global optimization which ensures high reliability. On the other hand, the sign change criterion is much more robust than previously used criteria because its takes into account non stationnarity in images.

## REFERENCES

Abu-Mostafa, Y. S., and Psaltis, D. (1985). Image normalization by complex moments, IEEE Trans. Pattern Anal. Mach. Intel., 7, 46-55.

Abu-Mostafa, Y. S., and Psaltis, D. (1984). Recognitive aspects of moment invariants, IEEE Trans. Pattern Anal. Mach. Intel., 6, 698-706.

Aggarwal, J. K., Davis, L. S., and Martin, W. N. (1981). Correspondence processes in dynamic scene analysis, Proc. IEEE, 69, 562-572.

Appeldorn, C. R., Oppenheim, B. E., and Wellman, H. N. (1980). An automated method for the alignment of image pairs, J. Nucl. Med., 21, 165-167.

Andrus, J., Campbell, C., and Jayroe, R. (1975). Digital image registration method using boundary maps, IEEE Trans. Comput., 19, 935-940.

Barber, D. C. (1982). Automatic alignment of radionuclide images, Phys. Med. Biol., 27, 387-396.

Barnea, D. I., and Silverman, H. F. (1972). A class of algorithms for fast digital image registration, IEEE Trans. Comput., 21, 179-186.

Bhanu, B., and Faugeras, O. (1984). Shape matching of two dimensional objects, IEEE Trans. Pattern Anal. Mach. intel., 6, 137-155.

Bookstein, F. L. (1986). From medical images to biometrics of form, in : Proc. 9th IPMI Conference, Washington/DC, S. L. Bacharach, ed., Martinus Nijhoff, The Hague, 1-18.

Davis, L. S. (1982). Hierarchical generalized Hough Transform and line-segment based generalized Hough transforms, Pattern Regognition (GB), 15, 277-285.

Fleming, J. S. (1984). A technique for motion correction in dynamic scintigraphy, Eur. J. Nucl. Med., 9, 397-402.

Frei, W., Singh, M., and Shibata, T. (1980). Digital image change detection, Optical Engineering, 19, 331-338.

Goshtasby, A. (1985). Template matching in rotated images, IEEE Trans. Pattern Anal. Mach. Intel., 7, 338-344.

Henderson, T. C., Triendl, E. E., and Winter, R. (1985). Edge and shape based geometric registration, IEEE Trans. Geosci. and Remote Sensing, 23, 334-342.

Hu, M. K. (1962). Visual pattern recognition by moment invariants, IRE Trans. on information theory, 8, 179-187.

Kall, B. A., Kelly, P. J., Goerss, S. J., and Earnest, F. (1985). Cross registration of points and lesion volumes from MR and CT, IEEE 7th annual conference of the engineering in medecine and biology society, 939-942.

Kropatsch, W. (1983). Segmentation of digital images using a priori information about the expected image contents, in : Proc. NATO ASI on Pictorial Data Analysis, R. M. Haralick, ed., Springer-Verlag Berlin Heidelberg, F4, 107-132.

Kuhl, F. P., and Giardina, C. R. (1982). Elliptic Fourier features of a closed contour, Comput. Graphics and Image Process., 18, 236-258.

Liehn, J. C., Venot, A., and Lebruchec, J. F. (1985). A new approach to double tracer studies, in : Proc. 9th IPMI conference, Washington/DC, S. L. Bacharach, ed., Martinus Nijhoff, The Hague, 280-287.

Lillestrand, R. L. (1972). Techniques for change detection, IEEE Trans. Comput., 21, 654-659.

Mackworth, A. K., and Mokhtarian, F. (1984). Scaled-based description of planar curves, Proc. 5th Canadian Soc. Computational studies of Intell., London. Ont. Canada, 114-119.

Maitra, S. (1979). Moment invariants, Proc. IEEE, 67, 697-699.

Medioni, G., and Nevatia, R. (1984). Matching images using linear features, IEEE Trans. Pattern Anal. Mach. Intel., 6, 675-685.

Merickel, M., and Mc Carthy, M. (1985). Registration of contours for 3-D reconstruction, IEEE 7th annual conference of the engineering in medecine and biology society, 616-620.

Mitiche, A., and Aggarwal, J. K. (1983). Contour registration by shape-specific points for shape matching, Comput. Vision, Graphics and Image Process., 22, 396-408.

Mokhtarian, F., and Mackworth, A. (1986) (1). Authors'reply, IEEE Trans. Pattern Anal. Mach. Intel., 8, 675.

Mokhtarian, F., and Mackworth, A. (1986) (2). Scale-based description and recognition of planar curves and two-dimensional shapes, IEEE Trans. Pattern Anal. Mach. Intel., 8, 34-43.

Moring, I., and Hakalahti, H. (1985). Scale independent method for object recognition, Proc. 4th Scandinavian Conference on Image Analysis, Trondhein, 881-889.

O'Rouke, J. (1981). Motion detection using Hough techniques, IEEE Conference on Pattern Recognition and image Processing, Dallas/TX, 82-87.

Pratt, W. K. (1974). Correlation techniques of image registration, IEEE Trans. Aerosp. Electron. Sys., 10, 353-358.

Price, K., and Reddy, R. (1979). Matching segments of images, IEEE Trans. Pattern Anal. Mach. Intel., 1, 110-116

Pronzato, L., Walter, E., Venot, A., and Lebruchec, J. F. (1984). A general purpose global optimizer : implementation and applications, Math. Comput. Simul., 26, 412-422.

Ros, D., Juvells, I., Vallmitjana, S., and R. De F. Moeno, J. (1984). A simplified method for the automatic alignment of images affected by random noise, Opt. Acta, 31, 1151-1159.

Rosenfeld, A. (1981). Image pattern recognition, Proc. IEEE, 69, 596-605.

Singh, M., Frei, W., Shibata, T., and Huth, G.C. (1979). A digital technique for accurate change detection in nuclear medical images with application to myocardial perfusion studies using Thallium-201, IEEE Trans. Nucl. Sci., 26, 565-575.

Svedlow, M., Gillem, C.D., and Anuta, P. E. (1978). Image registration : similarity measure and preprocessing method comparisons, IEEE Trans. Aerosp. Electron. Syst., 14, 141-149.

Venot, A., Pronzato, L., Walter, E., and Lebruchec, J. F. (1986) (1). A distribution-free criterion for robust identification with applications in system modelling and image processing, Automatica (in press).

Venot, A. (1986) (2). Nouvelles méthodes de comparaison d'images numériques, Thèse de doctorat d'état es sciences mathématiques, Université Pierre et Marie Curie Paris VI.

Venot, A., Liehn, J. C., Lebruchec, J. F. and Roucayrol, J. C. (1986) (3). The automated comparison of scintigraphic images, J. Nucl. Med. (in press).

Venot, A., Golmard, J. L., Lebruchec, J. F., Pronzato, L., Walter, E., Frija, G., and Roucayrol, J. C. (1984) (1). Digital methods for change detection in medical images, in : Proc. 8th IPMI Conference, Brussels, F., Deconinck, ed., Martinus Nijhoff, The Hague, 1-16.

Venot, A., Lebruchec, J. F., and Roucayrol, J. C. (1984) (2). A new class of similarity measures for robust image registration, Comput. Vision, Graphics and Image Process., 28, 176-184.

Venot, A., and Leclerc, V. (1984) (3). Automated correction of patient motion and gray values prior to subtraction in digitized angiography, IEEE Trans. Med. Imaging, 3, 179-186.

Venot, A., Lebruchec, J. F., Golmard, J. L., and Roucayrol, J. C. (1983). An automated method for the normalization of scintigraphic images, J. Nucl. Med., 24, 529-531.

Wong, R. , and Hall, E. (1979). Performance of scene matching techniques, IEEE Trans. Pattern Anal. Mach. Intel., 1, 325-330.

Wong, R. (1978). Sequential scene matching using edges, IEEE Trans. Aerosp. Electron. Sys., 14, 128-140.

Wu, Y. F., and Maitre, H. (1986). Registration of rotated picture with hidden parts using dynamic programming, Proc. 8th international conference on pattern recognition (IAPR-AFCET), Paris France, 792-794.

Wu, Y. F., and Maitre, H. (1985). Utilisation de la programmation dynamique au recalage carte-image, problèmes théoriques, Proc. 5ième Congrès reconnaissance des formes et intelligence artificielle (AFCET), Grenoble France, 641-648.

Yam, S., and Davis, L. S. (1981). Image registration using generalized Hough transform, IEEE conference on pattern recognition and image processing, Dallas/TX, 526-533.

# SEGMENTATION OF MAGNETIC RESONANCE IMAGES USING FUZZY CLUSTERING

Douglas A. Ortendahl and Joseph W. Carlson

Radiologic Imaging Laboratory
University of California
San Francisco, California

## INTRODUCTION

Magnetic Resonance Imaging (MRI) is unique among imaging modalities in that image contrast can be varied over a wide range by manipulation of the acquisition parameters. The signal intensity depends indirectly on particular physical and chemical characteristics of the tissues being imaged. These tissue properties influence the behavior of the nuclei undergoing resonance, and their behavior is what directly affects the MRI signal. The parameters of interest that describe this behavior are the relaxation times T1 and T2, the spin density (for hydrogen, N(H)), and the microscopic (diffusion) and macroscopic (flow, motion) motional states of the nuclei. These parameters exist, in turn, because of certain properties of the tissues: water content, fat content, macromolecules, paramagnetic ions and flow being among the significant variables.

This work is grounded in the conviction that maximum information content can only be obtained by proper integration of the data available from these multiple images. Recently there has been an application of multispectral techniques using LANDSAT technology to analysis of breast images (Gohagan et al., 1987). The goal in our present work is the segmentation of images, that is the grouping of the pixels into classes with similar properties. These properties are intensity, T1, T2 etc. Spatial location is also an important consideration as is the proximity to other segments with similar properties. The two segmentation extremes are the original image (1 pixel per segment) and the image mean where 1 value represents the whole image. Obviously we are interested in an intermediate position, but the number of segments we ultimately desire has an important influence on our approach. Our ultimate goal is to expedite the analysis of tissue properties, which requires facilitating the identification and specification of areas of such tissue. Ideally, we would want one segment associated with each tissue type, but for reasons that will become more apparent,this will be unrealizable in many cases. But in any event minimizing the number of segments is important for reducing the complexity of the analysis. The caveat is of course that we must always be alert to the possibility of losing significant differences between tissue in our zeal to simplify the image.

Several approaches to this segmentation problem suggest themselves. One is template matching (Ortendahl et al., 1984). Define the MR characteristics of the various tissues and use this definition to label the pixels within the image. There are several problems with this method. First, while the sensitivity of MR is very high the specificity has not been as impressive. Reliable tissue signatures are not available except for a limited number of tissues. Second, nature does not oblige us by placing pure tissue in each voxel; partial volume averaging is a significant problem. Our visual system, allows us to disregard the partial volume problem in many cases by using context to make these areas appear as junctional regions between tissues. One of the methods used is simultaneous analysis of the scene at multiple levels of resolution. This motivates hierarchical processing as a means of segmentation (Ortendahl and Hylton, 1986). The segmentation is done over a local area which becomes larger as we move up vertically. In previous work, we have applied the use of the pyramid to MRI. However, for our purposes to obtain a small enough set of segments directly required too great a loss of spatial resolution by down projecting from high in the pyramid. Rising too high in the hierarchy also significantly increases the problem with partial volume effects. If we start from lower level of segmentation from the pyramid or stack, we are faced with finding other methods of merging these segments together. In this paper we discuss another alternative, the direct segmentation of the data set into clusters of pixels with similar properties. We will see that with this algorithm we can directly obtain a manageable number of clusters per tissue. Tools are described which aid in further merging of these clusters into single segments associated with a tissue type.

SEGMENTATION ALGORITHM

Fuzzy Clustering

While there are a variety of clustering algorithms in the literature such as maximum likelihood, recently there has been increased interest in a class of algorithms called fuzzy c-means (FCM) (Cannon et al., 1986). It has been shown that this algorithm may be applied to the segmentation of MR images (Delapaz et al., 1986). FCM is based on the branch of mathematics known as fuzzy set theory.

Let R be the set of reals and $R^p$ be the set of p tuples of reals. $R^p$ is the feature space and elements x of $R^p$ are the feature vectors where x = $(x_1, x_2, \ldots, x_p)$. Let X be a subset of $R^p$. Let us consider the set of functions u defined over X which satisfy the constraint, u:X → [0,1]. Each such function is said to assign to each subelement, x its grade of membership in the fuzzy set u. The function u is a fuzzy subset of X. There are of course an infinite number of such fuzzy sets associated with X. We can further limit the number of fuzzy sets which need be considered by defining a partition of X which is a group of fuzzy sets with the constraint that for every x the sum of the fuzzy memberships of x in the fuzzy subsets is one. Those who are uncomfortable with the concepts of fuzzy set theory will recognize that this last statement is equivalent to the statement that the probability that each element will be a member of one of the subsets is one.

Now let X be a finite set with n elements and c be an integer, $2 \leq c \leq n$. A fuzzy c partition of X can be represented by a c x n matrix U. Row i of U, $U_i = (u_{i1}, u_{i2}, \ldots, u_{in})$ is the ith membership or fuzzy subset of X. Column j of U, $U^j = (u_{1j}, u_{2j}, \ldots u_{cj})$ gives the values of the c different membership functions for the jth data point in X. For each j, $\Sigma_i u_{ij} = 1$. The task is to choose the partition that is in some sense optimal. For this purpose we introduce a set of vectors, v consisting of c elements from the set X. This relates each fuzzy set to a location in the feature space. The fuzzy c-means functional $J_m$ is defined as

$$J_m(U,v) = \sum_{k=1}^{n} \sum_{i=1}^{c} (u_{ik})^m (d_{ik})^2 \tag{1}$$

$d_{ik} = || x_k - v_i ||$ where this is any norm metric and m must be larger than 1. Note that with this definition the squared distance is weighted by the mth power of the membership function. Thus minimization of $J_m$ will produce a set of fuzzy clusters which are optimal in a generalized least squares sense. The vectors $v_i$ are the centers for the cluster or fuzzy subset i.

Implementation of the algorithm requires the selection of a value for m and choice of the number of clusters c. A norm metric for d must also be provided. A set of c cluster centers, v, is chosen. This could be from some a priori knowledge, but in our implementation these are selected randomly. At this point iteration begins.

1. Compute a new set of membership functions, $u_{ik}$. For each cluster i check if $d_{ik} = 0$ for any of the n data vectors. If this is satisfied then $u_{ik} = 0$ for all but the k for which the distance is 0 and then $u_{ik} = 1$. This of course makes sense because if a cluster center falls on top of a data point then its membership should be 1 and all others 0. Otherwise we define the membership function by

$$u_{ik} = \{ \sum_{j=1}^{c} [ d_{ik} / d_{jk} ]^{2/(m-1)} \}^{-1} \tag{2}$$

2. We then recalculate the cluster centers using these new membership functions

$$v_i = \{ \sum_{k=1}^{n} u_{ik} x_k \} / \{ \sum_{k=1}^{n} u_{ik} \} \tag{3}$$

3. The convergence criteria is checked and if convergence is not reached return to step 1.

In our implementation we use the movement of cluster centers as a test of convergence. Convergence is declared when from one iteration to the next no cluster moves more than a fixed amount. For this study this distance was usually 2 intensity units. As a point of reference mean brain intensity is typically 3000-4000. This is probably more conservative than necessary, but computational speed was not the prime concern. This differs from the criterion used by (Cannon et al., 1986) which is that the change in the membership function be less than a specified amount. The difference should only be important when it is desired to obtain the last bit of speed from the algorithm. Each data point is assigned to the fuzzy set or cluster for which the membership function is the largest. For the work described here we chose m = 2 which makes the calculations easier by making 2/(m-1) = 2. There is no theoretical basis for choosing m and values from 1.1 to 5 have been typically reported as being useful (Cannon et al., 1986). Application of fuzzy c-means to LANDSAT data of corn and soybeans found best results for m between 1.3 and 1.8 (Cannon et al., 1986a). The distance norm we choose is simple Euclidean distance in feature space with equal weights for each component.

One of the complaints about fuzzy c-means that one finds in the literature is that it is slow, even though FCM is several orders of magnitude faster than maximum likelihood iteration (Bezdek et al., 1984).

For this reason an approximate version AFCM was developed which uses lookup tables for most of the intensive calculations and gains a factor of 6 in speed. We have implemented the exact version of FCM on a VAX 11-730 and on a CSPI Mini-Map array processor. Memory constraints on the use of lookup tables prevented us from using the AFCM.

The data used for the cluster determination can come from a single or section or multiple sections. A selection mask is constructed to determine which pixels should be clustered. This mask can either pass every pixel or be dependent on a region of interest or a threshold. It is also possible to recluster segments into finer divisions. This is faster than clustering the whole image into a large number of clusters. An effective way to avoid the necessity of choosing a threshold is to cluster the whole image into 3 clusters and then discard the cluster with lowest mean value as noise and do a finer division of the two main clusters. However, for simplicity most of the work described here was performed with a threshold which was typically 10% of the maximum value in the long TR image. The maximum array size in the array processor limits the number of vectors which can be clustered at one time. This will often be smaller than the total number of data points selected. For 16 clusters the limit is 12287 data points. In this case a randomly selected subset is run through FCM and cluster centers are determined. For the remaining points, we use the calculated cluster centers to recalculate membership functions and make cluster assignments.

Color assignment is an important issue. Ideally since we are discussing segmentation we would want color to be indicative of some intrinsic property of the tissue beyond merely intensity or relaxation time. We leave this for future work and instead rely on a simple expedient. At the output of the FCM algorithm the clusters are ranked in random order, a very unpleasing display. We resort them according to hydrogen density and then divide the color scale equally. The choice of hydrogen is somewhat arbitrary, but it is reasonably effective. If the number of clusters chosen is not too large then the differences between segments is apparent using equally spaced levels.

The number of clusters to use is another parameter which we must set. A priori we do not know the number of tissues and this is further complicated from problems with partial volume effects. One way to handle this dilemma is to use more clusters than one expects to need and then merge them later using a similarity measure. One construct which has been used effectively in the analysis of LANDSAT images is the minimum spanning tree (MST) (Cannon et al., 1986a). This is a projection onto a "hyperplane" of the feature space which shows the relationship between the clusters. It should not be taken too literally since it is not to scale, but it does provide a minimum path through which all the clusters link together using the same distance metric as for FCM. By using more clusters than needed, it is more likely that small features with unique characteristics will be preserved.

## Basis Image Selection

For the choice of basis images, the fundamental images T1, T2 and N(H) come to mind. The problem with using these images is the very different scale of the image values which makes the definition of a distance metric difficult. The other choice is acquired intensity images which for our purposes consist usually of three: a short TR = 0.5 sec with TE of 30-50ms, and long TR = 2.0 sec with a first echo at the same TE as the short TR and a second at twice that value. The electronic noise is the same in each image, but it is not electronic noise that is our main adversary in segmentation, rather it is biologic variability and partial volumes.

A well known feature of the acquired images is that they are highly correlated. The classical principal component analysis (PCA) (also known as the Karhunen-Loeve transform) has traditionally been used in multivariate analysis to remove this correlation and in the process reduce dimensionality by providing the bulk of the information in the first few principal components (Mardia et al., 1978). This approach has been used successfully in satellite imagery where images are typically obtained over multiple bands in the optical spectrum and false color displays limited to the three primary colors are often used (Ready and Wintz, 1973; Dave et al., 1982). PCA allows these colors to be used to present the maximum information by driving each of the primary color guns with the three most important components. We have recently applied PCA to the analysis of MRI data (Ortendahl, 1986; Schmiedl et al., 1986). Principal component analysis starts with the covariance matrix of the initial images. If N input images are used then the covariance matrix S will be size NxN and defined by:

$$S_{ij} = (1/M) \sum_k (x_{ik} - \mu_i)(x_{jk} - \mu_j) \tag{4}$$

where $x_{ik}$ is the intensity of the kth pixel in the ith image and $\mu_i$ is the mean intensity value of the ith image. The sum is over all desired pixels in the image, this may be the whole image, a small region or all pixels whose intensity is above some specified threshold. M is the total number of contributing pixels. The diagonal elements are just the variances of the input images. By definition S is real and symmetric and thus may be diagonalized. The principal component transformation is defined by $y = \Gamma^t x$ where $\Gamma$ is the NxN unitary matrix which diagonalizes S such that:

$$\Gamma S \Gamma^t = \Lambda \tag{5}$$

where $\Lambda$ is a diagonal matrix where the diagonal elements of $\Lambda$, $\lambda_1$, $\lambda_2$, $\cdots$ $\lambda_N$ are the eigenvalues and variances of the principal components. In the above definition, x is a vector of spectral intensities associated with each pixel. The vectors $y_i$ are principal components or eigenvectors of S such that $Sy_i = \lambda_i y_i$. One of the most important features of PCA is that these principal components will be orthogonal and uncorrelated, but since it is simply a rotation, scale is preserved. Once we have diagonalized the covariance matrix we can define the Mahalanobis transformation (Mardia et al., 1978) as:

$$z = S^{-1/2} x \tag{6}$$

$$S^{-1/2} = \Gamma^t \Lambda^{-1/2} \Gamma \tag{7}$$

where $\Lambda^{-1/2} = \text{diag}(\lambda_i^{-1/2})$. This transformation eliminates the correlation between the images and equalizes the variances.

## Introduction of Spatial Relationships

In the above discussion, the data elements are treated as independent voxels. The results would be the same if the voxel locations were completely scrambled. But experience in previous work and this current project shows the necessity of spatial information and relationships for both supervised and unsupervised segmentation. Several different pieces of information are used in this study. First is the adjacent cluster matrix (ACM). The ACM is c x c and ACM(i,j) is the number of pixels of cluster i which are found to be adjacent to a member of cluster j. An ACM is computed for each section, this only takes into account information within the plane. While the the ACM is being computed we also compute the perimeter/area ratio (PAR) for each cluster which is the number of pixels which are on a cluster boundary compared to the total mass of the cluster. The combined ratio matrix (CRM) is defined such that CRM(i,j) is the perimeter/area ratio which would result if the ith and jth clusters where to be combined into a single one. The perimeter/area ratio is a measure of the compactness of a segment. In general we think of tissues as being relatively compact. Some caution is in order since there are some exceptions such as a ring of edema surrounding a tumor. If the PAR decreases when 2 clusters are combined, then this may be evidence to justify the merging of the two. This can of course be carried to a logical extreme, since the best PAR would be obtained by combining the entire image into 1 cluster. Another statistic is the adjacent section matrix ASM where ASM(i,j) is the number of pixels in cluster j found in the adjacent section at the same location as the cluster i. This is computed for each section.

Hierarchical processing can also be of assistance in incorporating spatial relationships. The structure we use here is the pyramid which is discussed extensively in (deGraaf et al., 1984). Briefly the pyramid is a linked structure which allows the simultaneous analysis of images at multiple levels of spatial resolution. Segmentation is obtained by down-projecting the values of the elements in a particular level within the pyramid. In forming this pyramid we use the method described in (Ortendahl and Hylton, 1986) where a single pyramid is constructed from the multispectral information using the same distance metric for determining the links as was used for FCM. We considered using FCM to cluster at different levels of resolution. This was rejected since partial volume averaging was expected to increase. Instead, the cluster centers determined at the highest resolution were used to compute membership functions and cluster assignments at each level within the pyramid. This provides some smoothing of the clustered image and tends to remove isolated clusters which have no similar clusters in the vicinity.

## Partial Volume Model

A simple model for partial volume averaging can also be useful in analyzing the relationships between clusters. Let $I_{ij}$ be the intensity of the ith cluster in the jth basis image. Then if a voxel contains a mixture of tissue i and tissue k then naively we might assume that the intensity for the jth image would be

$$I_j = rI_{ij} + (1-r)I_{kj} \qquad (8)$$

Where r is the fraction of tissue i within the voxel. With this construct we can now ask whether a cluster can be considered to be a mixture of two others by doing a chisquare fit to find the best value of r. The model is not meant to be taken too seriously, since it is not designed to account for the molecular interactions and changes in relaxation time that occur at that level when different substances combine. There is also the very real possibility of clusters lining up by chance. Thus this must be applied with some caution, but it can provide useful information by suggesting some clusters as potential partial volume mixture of others.

## RESULTS

The FCM algorithm has been coded in Fortran for the VAX 11-730 and for the CSPI Mini-Map array processor. While speed of computation is not or primary concern here, the VAX alone implementation was hopelessly slow and consumed an unacceptable fraction of the CPU on a multiuser system. The array processor provides a factor of 60 improvement in speed while requiring minimal host interaction. Clustering a 256x256 image into 10 clusters takes approximately 3 minutes real time which includes about 50

Table I. Cluster centers and parameter values for the 15 clusters found for the patient of Figure 1. Tissue type is not given for the tissues found only outside the brain in scalp and skull.

| Color | I1 | I2 | I2 | T1 | T2 | H | Tissue |
|---|---|---|---|---|---|---|---|
| 3 | 370 | 724 | 398 | 729 | 50 | 1416 | |
| 4 | 595 | 1066 | 601 | 616 | 52 | 1976 | |
| 5 | 786 | 1443 | 873 | 645 | 60 | 2509 | |
| 6 | 1066 | 2262 | 1535 | 857 | 77 | 3723 | |
| 7 | 1175 | 1814 | 871 | 463 | 41 | 3838 | |
| 8 | 2006 | 2393 | 1314 | 259 | 50 | 4359 | |
| 9 | 1379 | 3142 | 2251 | 997 | 90 | 5118 | CSF |
| 10 | 2055 | 3151 | 1930 | 457 | 61 | 5220 | white |
| 11 | 2131 | 3342 | 2038 | 477 | 61 | 5578 | white |
| 12 | 2034 | 3502 | 2169 | 571 | 63 | 5847 | white |
| 13 | 1960 | 3706 | 2329 | 682 | 65 | 6261 | gray |
| 14 | 1670 | 3691 | 2446 | 933 | 73 | 6367 | gray |
| 15 | 1851 | 3878 | 2496 | 835 | 68 | 6680 | gray |
| 16 | 1958 | 4087 | 2592 | 829 | 66 | 7133 | gray |
| 17 | 3498 | 4391 | 2599 | 297 | 57 | 7428 | fat |

iterations. The number of iterations required was quite variable and could vary as much as a factor of two for repeat runs over the same data. The only difference between the runs is that the random selection of starting cluster values is different. Since the available minimap memory limits us to cluster only a fraction of the data points in the sample, the computation time is not very dependent on sample size. Almost any study of interest will exceed the capacity of the processor. The calculation of cluster membership for the remaining data points is a small fraction of the overall time.

In Figure 1 we show three acquired images for a patient with multiple

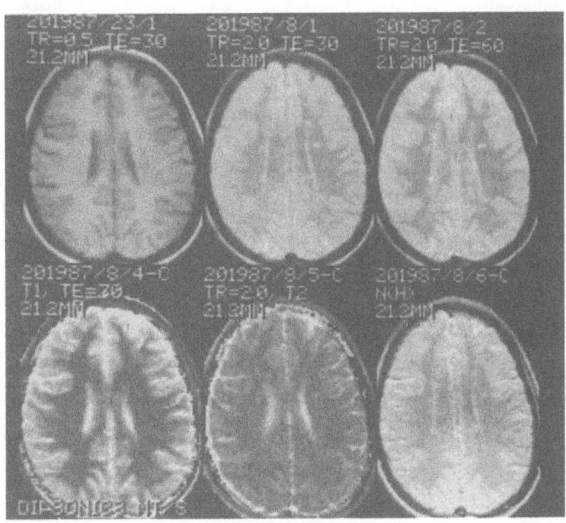

Figure 1. For a patient with multiple sclerosis we show the basis set of acquired images (TR=0.5s, TE=30ms; TR=2.0s, TE=30ms; TR=2.0s, TE=60ms). Also shown are the calculated relaxation time and N(H) image. The section thickness is 1.0 cm, the pixel resolution is 0.9mm x 0.9mm.

sclerosis along with the calculated relaxation time and density images. This single section was analyzed with FCM using 15 clusters with the acquired images as the basis set. The cluster centers are shown in Table I. The clusters have been sorted by the hydrogen density and equally spaced colors or gray values are assigned to each cluster. Throughout this paper clusters will be identified by their color. We start the coloring with value 3 in order to be distinct from the background. In Figure 2 we show the cluster map. The white and gray matter are well delineated although at this point we have not identified which clusters are associated with which lesion. Also shown is a the result of segmenting the image from the second level of the pyramid using the acquired images as input. New membership functions were calculated using the same cluster centers and cluster assignments were made. This segmentation is somewhat smoother by removing some of the isolated pixels which are not supported by their neighbors.

The minimum spanning tree is shown in Figure 3. This diagram is only meant to be a schematic representation of the minimum path through feature space. It is not to scale and the distance between clusters is shown in parentheses. For simplicity we have not included the colors below 8 which are found only in the skull and scalp, are of lower intensity and far away from brain tissue in feature space. The MST can be used as a guide for the merging of the segments. A brief example of this is given. The clusters closest together are 11 and 12. Examination of the spatial relationships finds support for this assignment. Looking at the 4511 pixels which are adjacent to segment 11, 33% are segment 12, 33% segment 10 with the next highest being segment 13 with 10%. For the 5041 pixels adjacent to cluster 12 we have 13: 32%, 11: 32% and 10: 13%. The

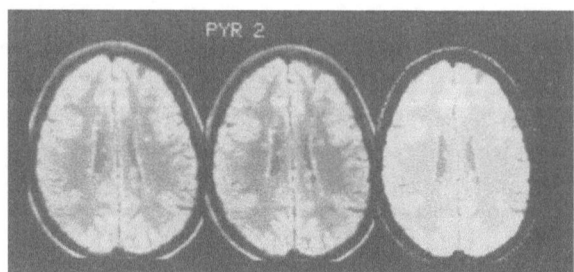

Figure 2. For the patient of Figure 1 we show the 15 segment cluster map(left). In the middle is a segmented image using the same 15 clusters, but with a level 2 pyramid segmentation to obtain a small amount of smoothing. On the right the clusters are merged into the 3 major tissues: white matter, gray matter and CSF.

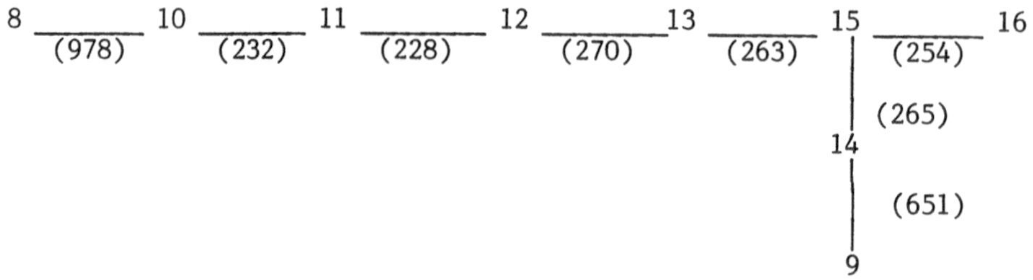

```
8 _____ 10 _____ 11 _____ 12 _____ 13 _____ 15 _____ 16
  (978)     (232)     (228)     (270)     (263)  |   (254)
                                                 |
                                                 |  (265)
                                                 |
                                                14
                                                 |
                                                 |  (651)
                                                 |
                                                 9
```

Figure 3. The minimum spanning tree (MST) for the patient of Figure 1. For simplicity only the clusters found within the brain are shown.

perimeter to area (PAR) for 11 and 12 is 0.93 and 0.96 respectively. Merging the two segments gives PAR = 0.75, a significant improvement. A similar analysis suggests that 10 and 11 be combined. Examination of the cluster image shows that 10, 11 and 12 are located within what appears to be the white matter. Continuing the analysis we can combine and make the assignment shown in Table I. One might be tempted to combine segments 12 and 13 since the distance is only 270, but this would cause all the white and gray matter to combine. This is where the operator's expert judgment is required to intervene. One of the considerations is that the T1 of 571 ms is more consistent with what we attribute to white matter.

The significant lesion found isolated in the white matter on the left side of the brain is found to be composed of a central core containing 3 pixels of cluster 15, 1 of 16, surrounded by 10 pixels of cluster 13 and all of this within a sea of cluster 10. Cluster 15 and 16 make up much of the presumably normal gray matter. Thus on the basis of parameter values alone, we can not distinguish MS lesions from normal gray matter. We had similar experience in previous work (Ortendahl and Hylton, 1986). MR is so effective for the detection of MS because the lesions are normally seen in or adjacent to the white matter. The lesion is surrounded by cluster 13. It is interesting to use our partial volume model to fit 13 as a mixture of two other clusters. We get a good fit by mixing 35% cluster 11 with cluster 15. The distance between the cluster 13 and its expected position by the model is only 19 units. This is consistent with the MST and the fact that cluster 13 in the image appears to be a transition zone between the white and gray matter.

In Figure 4 we show the acquired and calculated images for a patient with a glioma in the brain. Figure 5 shows the effect of varying the number of clusters. The major differentiation between the white and gray matter is seen with as few as 3 clusters. The border between the glioma and the surrounding tissue is seen with as few as 8 clusters. However, with only 8 clusters, a larger section of the gray matter appears to have the same properties as the tumor. Increasing the number clusters improves

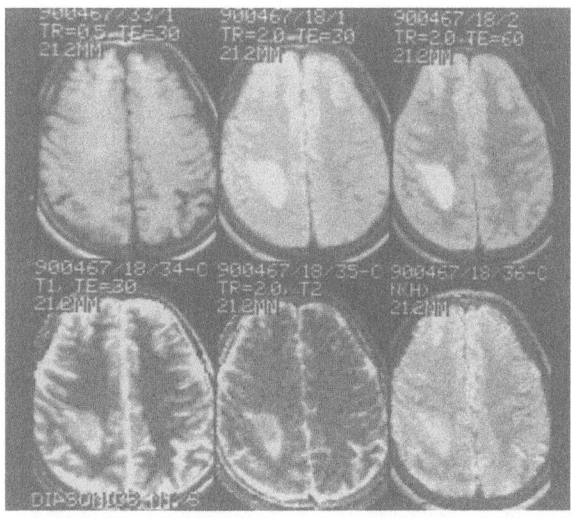

Figure 4. For a patient with a glioma we show the basis set of acquired images (TR=0.5s, TE=30ms; TR=2.0s, TE=30ms; TR=2.0s, TE=60ms). Also shown are the calculated relaxation time and N(H) image. The section thickness is 1.0 cm, the pixel resolution is 0.9mm x 0.9mm.

Table II.  Cluster centers and parameter values for the 15 clusters found for the patient of Figure 4.  Tissue type is not given for the tissues found only outside the brain in scalp and skull.

| Color | I1 | I2 | I2 | T1 | T2 | H | Tissue |
|---|---|---|---|---|---|---|---|
| 3 | 342 | 598 | 295 | 587 | 42 | 1261 | |
| 4 | 597 | 896 | 477 | 438 | 48 | 1702 | |
| 5 | 754 | 1242 | 712 | 526 | 54 | 2224 | |
| 6 | 1045 | 1545 | 813 | 425 | 47 | 2968 | |
| 7 | 807 | 1767 | 1178 | 914 | 74 | 3011 | |
| 8 | 1287 | 2032 | 1069 | 484 | 47 | 3934 | |
| 9 | 1711 | 2633 | 1523 | 460 | 55 | 4622 | white |
| 10 | 1764 | 2794 | 1635 | 487 | 56 | 4865 | white |
| 11 | 1154 | 2803 | 1970 | 1151 | 85 | 4896 | CSF |
| 12 | 1729 | 2940 | 1741 | 558 | 57 | 5122 | white |
| 13 | 1399 | 3070 | 2003 | 919 | 70 | 5353 | gray |
| 14 | 1671 | 3092 | 1872 | 654 | 60 | 5384 | gray |
| 15 | 763 | 2394 | 1875 | 2458 | 123 | 5601 | CSF |
| 16 | 1637 | 3274 | 2020 | 761 | 62 | 5753 | gray |
| 17 | 1656 | 3470 | 2196 | 835 | 66 | 6078 | tumor |

the separation between tumor and gray matter, although there are still sections of the gray matter which share the same cluster as the tumor. These images were acquired as part of a multisection acquisition, and in Figure 6 we show the results of simultaneously segmenting 5 sections into 15 clusters.  It is gratifying that the tumor is still relatively distinct even when a larger data volume is analyzed.  The cluster values are given in Table II.  The MST is shown in Figure 7.  The MST along with the statistics on spatial relationships is used to aid the operator in the further merging of the clusters.  For example segments 9 and 10 have a PAR of 0.82 and 0.96 which reduces to 0.62 when they are combined.  It is also interesting to note that even though the tumor, cluster 17, is close in feature space to cluster 16, it is an outrigger in the sense that application of the partial volume model shows that it does not come anywhere near a line between any of the other clusters.  The assignments

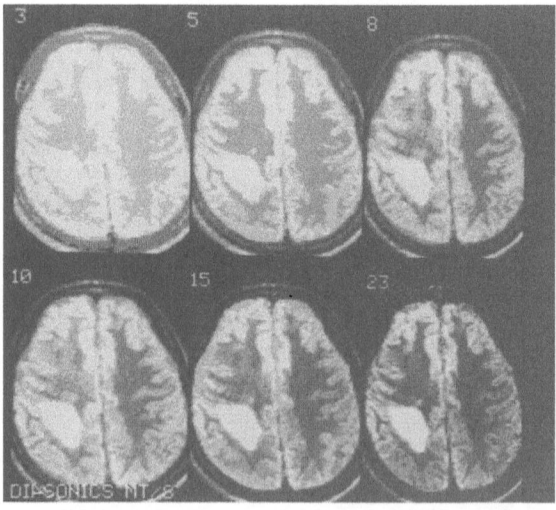

Figure 5.  The images of Figure 4 are segmented with 6 different values for the cluster number.

of tissues within the brain is given in Table II. The final tissue maps
showing the white and gray matter, CSF and tumor are shown in Figure 8.
Excellent delineation is seen for the white, gray matter, CSF and the
tumor.

The reproducibility of the algorithm was tested by taking a subset of
the data in Figure 4 which was small enough that all the data could fit in
one array processor load. This was to guarantee that exactly the same
data would be analyzed each time instead of a randomly selected subset.
Two simultaneous runs were done with randomly selected starting centers.
The differences between them where small with an RMS deviation of
25 intensity units. We also investigated the choice of basis images. A
principal component transformation was performed on the 3 acquired images
of figure 4. These are shown in Figure 9. As is typical of our previous
experience with PCA (Ortendahl, 1986; Schmiedl et al., 1986), the first
principal component is a weighted (positive) average of the 3 input
images. The second enhances differences between image 1 and 2 while the
third appears to contain little information. The three PCA images were
segmented into 15 clusters. The cluster numbers were rearranged to agree
with the assignments used in Figure 5, and the absolute difference was

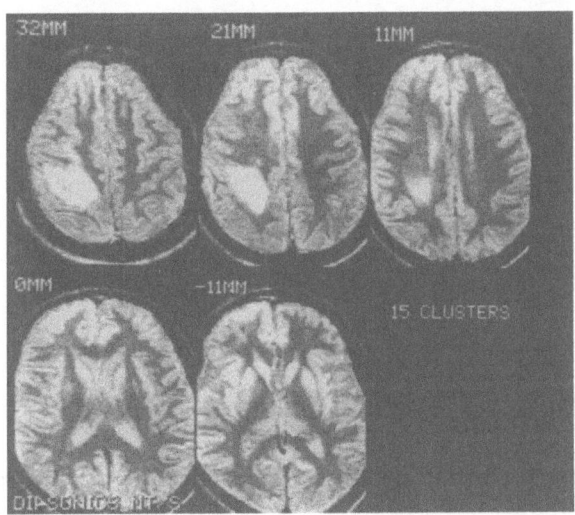

Figure 6. For the patient of Figure 4 we segment 5 contiguous sections
simultaneously into 15 clusters. The lesion is well delineated in the
first three sections.

```
8 _____ 9 _____ 10 _____ 12 _____ 14 _____ 13 _____ 11
 (864)     (204)      (183)      (208)   |  (303)       (364)   |
                                         |                      |
                                         |  (238)       (574)   |
                                        16                     15
                                         |
                                         |  (264
                                         |
                                        17
```

Figure 7. The minimum spanning tree (MST) for the patient of Figure 4.
For simplicity only the clusters found within the brain are shown. This
is the result of segmenting 5 sections at once.

taken between the segmented PCA image and the 15 segment image of Figure 5. Pixels which differ in cluster number are assigned maximum gray and pixels which are the same are given a value of 0. This image is overlayed on a TR=2.0, TE=30ms image and displayed in Figure 10. We see that the number of pixels in disagreement is small with no apparent pattern. Of the 27349 pixels in the image 5% change value. If we combine the segments into the major tissue groups and ignore the clusters which have no members within the brain cavity, the differences between this clustering and the one in Figure 5 is a smaller 2%, and the differences are mainly along tissue boundaries. We also considered reducing the number of basis images by clustering with only the first two principal components. This image was again merged into the major tissue groups within the brain and the difference with that obtained with 3 basis images was produced. This is also shown in Figure 9. The difference is more substantial with 10% of the pixels changing cluster value. We can see that there are sections of gray matter which are misclassified if only 2 images are used. This is despite the fact that the third PCA image

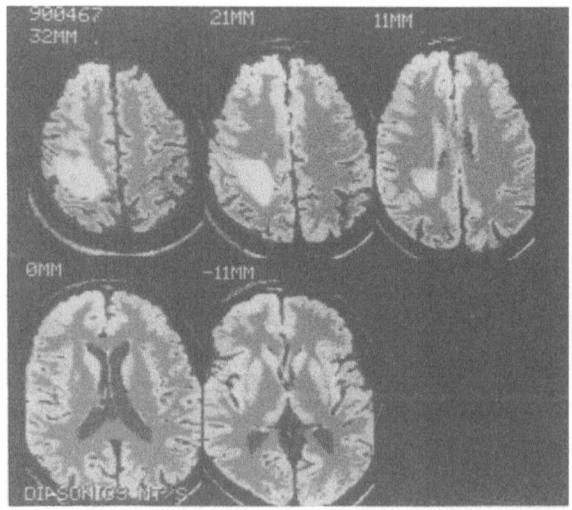

Figure 8. The segmented shown in Figure 6 are merged into four types of tissue: gray matter, white matter, CSF and the tumor. Excellent delineation is observed.

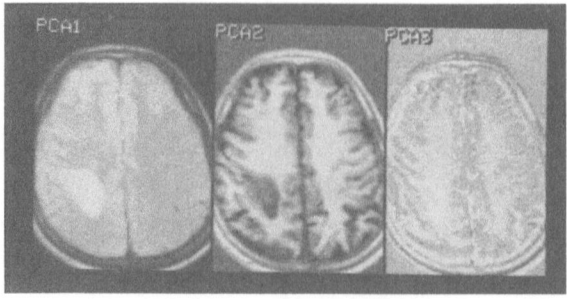

Figure 9. A principal component transformation is performed on the basis images of Figure 4. Most of the information content is found in the first two components.

appears to contain little information. When 3 PCA images are used, we would expect that the results would be same as with the original basis set, since PCA is simply a rotation which preserves distances in feature space. We found that if 3 Mahalanobis transformed images were used that the results were not satisfactory. For example, in the white matter where we find 3 different clusters for this case using the standard basis, we found 5 clusters with the Mahalanobis transformation. This transform was not considered further.

As a final example we show a patient with a hemorrhagic infarct in Figure 11. Eight sections were analyzed to produce 15 clusters. Six of the clustered images are shown in Figure 12. As in the previous examples, the clusters were merged with the tissue assignments for the clusters within the brain given in the table and the results of this merging is shown if Figure 13. Note in particular the resolution which allows us to find clusters of apparent gray matter in the eye corresponding to the optic nerve.

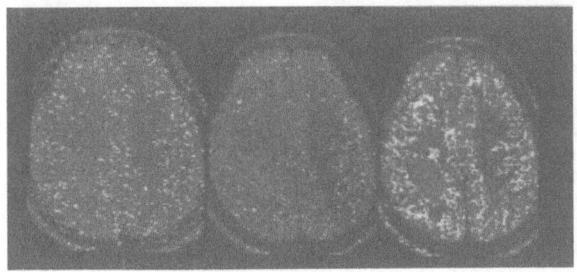

Figure 10. On the left is the difference between a segmentation by the acquired images and one using the PCA images. Differences are shown as white dots overlayed on a TR=2.0 sec intensity images. In the middle is the difference after clusters are merged into tissue types. On the right is the difference when only 2 PCA images are used after merging into tissue types.

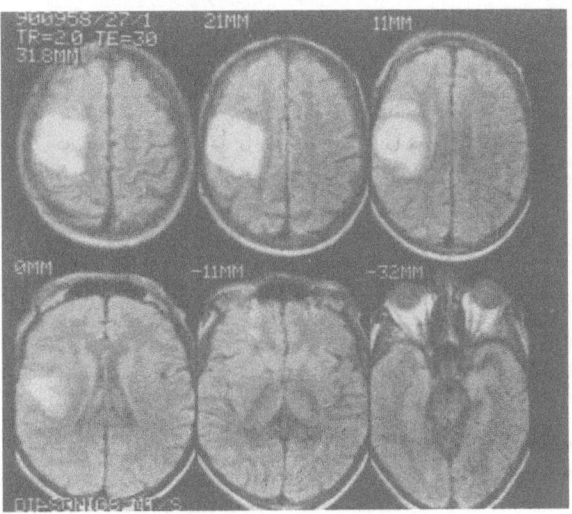

Figure 11. Six TR=2.0s, TE=30 ms images from an eight section data set of a patient with an infarct.

103

DISCUSSION

Fuzzy set clustering provides an effective method of segmenting MR images. With the use of an array processor, the throughput is within practical limits. Even if more data memory is available than we currently are using, it would appear that there is a computational advantage to limiting the clustered data set to some reasonable fraction of the data of

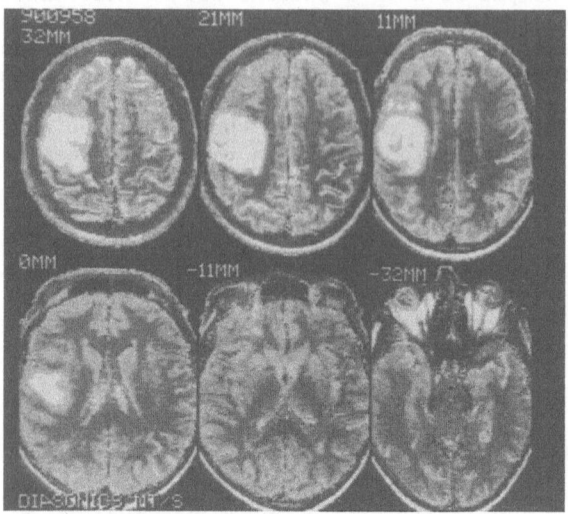

Figure 12. Eight sections for the patient of Figure 12 are are segmented into 15 clusters. Six sections are displayed.

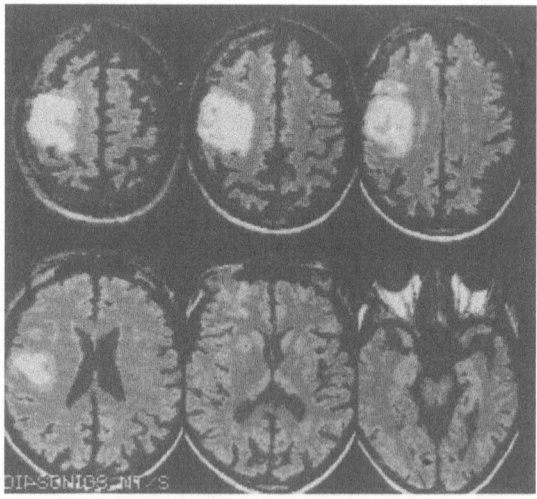

Figure 13. The segments of Figure 13 are merged into five tissue types: white matter, gray matter, CSF, lesion and fat. Note the resolution of the optic nerve. Fat is observed surrounding eye. The vitreous in the eye is in the same cluster as the CSF.

interest and using these cluster centers to assign fuzzy memberships to the rest of the data. Our experience is that the reproducibility is more than adequate. As discussed by others (Cannon et al., 1986) there is no guarantee that FCM will converge to the absolute minimum. Our experience suggests that if the segmentation does sometimes converge to saddle points, these are not significantly different from either the minimum or other saddle points. Numerous repeat runs with different starting cluster centers did not reveal any noticeable discrepancies. We also did not investigate the possibility of using a set of cluster centers from one patient as an initial guess for another. This could reduce the number of iterations required, but might it lead to false minima?

Of more concern is the choice of the number of clusters. The ideal number is task and patient specific. For a patient with a tumor we want enough clusters to separate the pathology from the normal tissue, but not so many that we are overwhelmed with segments. Yet if the goal is automated analysis, specific rules must be provided. For the normal tissue, the number of clusters (such as 3 to describe the white matter) is adequate. Doubling the number could be handled, but increasing much beyond that will make the necessary cluster merging more difficult. The number of clusters which are borderline between two major tissue groups will increase. Automating this decision making is a formidable task. The minimum spanning tree is clearly not enough. The statistical information about the spatial relationships was helpful, but we were not able to find an algorithm which would could be relied on to merge clusters automatically. Some cases are often easy, for example combing two clusters which are in the white matter and heavily mixed so that the PAR is substantially improved by combining them. But we find many cases of subtle differences at the boundary of the white and gray matter where some supervision is required which is certainly to be true in other tissues. Improved pattern recognition capability is required.

It may also be that it is unnecessary to perform a lot of segment merging. The current segmentation could be used as input to a data base which may reveal statistical pattern in the occurrence of pathology as suggested by (Gohagan et al., 1987). Also with the current implementation the operator can readily identify the clusters associated with the pathology and ask for further segmentation of them to elucidate lesion structure that may not be readily apparent in the acquired images.

## ACKNOWLEDGEMENTS

This work is supported in part by USPHS Research Career Development Award GM00493 from the NIGMS(DHHS); USPHS Grant CA 32850 from the NCI; and by Diasonics (MRI), Inc.

## REFERENCES

Bezdek JC, Hathaway R and Huggins V, 1984, Parametric estimation for normal mixtures, Pattern Recognition Letters, 3:79.

Cannon RL, Dave JV, and Bezdek JC, 1986, Efficient implementation of the fuzzy c-means clustering algorithms, IEEE Trans Pattern Anal. Machine Intell, PAMI-8:248.

Cannon RL, Dave JV, Bezdek JC and Trivedi MM, 1986a, Segmentation of a thematic image using the fuzzy c-means clustering algorithm, IEEE Trans on Geoscience and Remote Sensing, GE-24:400.

Dave JV, Bernstein R and Kolsky HG, 1982, Importance of higher-order components to multispectral classification, IBM J Res Develop, 26:715.

deGraaf CN, Toet A, Koenderink JJ et al., 1984, Some applications of

hierarchical image processing algorithms, Proceedings of the 8th
International Conference on Information Processing in Medical Imaging,
Martinus Nijhoff Publishers, The Hague, 343.

Delapaz RL, Bernstein R, Dave JV and Chang PJ, 1986, Tissue
characterization with MRI using advanced digital processing techniques
("fuzzy clustering"), Fifth Annual Meeting Society of Magnetic
Resonance in Medicine, Montreal.

Gohagan JK et al., 1987, Multispectral analysis of MR images of the
breast, Radiology, 163:703.

Mardia KV, Kent JT and Bibby JM, 1978, "Multivariate Analysis," Academic
Press, London.

Ortendahl DA, Hylton NM, Kaufman L and Crooks LE, 1984, Automated tissue
characterization with NMR imaging, Proceedings of the 8th
International Conference on Information Processing in Medical Imaging,
Martinus Nijhoff Publishers, The Hague, 392.

Ortendahl DA, 1986, The application of principal component analysis to
multivariate MRI data, Proceedings of the 8th Annual Meeting of the
IEEE Engineering in Medicine and Biology Society, Fort Worth, Texas,
1065.

Ortendahl DA and Hylton NM, 1986, Tissue type identification by MRI using
pyramidal segmentation and intrinsic parameters, Proceedings of the
9th International Conference on Information Processing in Medical
Imaging, Washington, D.C., 62.

Ready PJ and Wintz PA, 1973, Information extraction, SNR improvement, and
data compression in multispectral imagery, IEEE Trans on Commun, COM-
21:1123.

Schmiedl U, Ortendahl DA et al., 1986, The utility of principal component
analysis for the image display of brain lesions: a preliminary
comparative study, Magnetic Resonance in Medicine, 4:471.

# A MULTIRESOLUTION HIERARCHICAL APPROACH TO IMAGE SEGMENTATION BASED ON INTENSITY EXTREMA

Lawrence M. Lifshitz[*][+] and Stephen M. Pizer [*][‡]

Departments of Computer Science[*] and Radiology[‡]
University of North Carolina
Chapel Hill, N.C., U.S.A.

## SECTION 1 - BACKGROUND ON SEGMENTATION

### Segmentation as a Step towards Interpretation

An image as it is stored by a computer is just a multi-dimensional array of pixel values. Although we as humans may look at the displayed image and recognize it as meaningful, the computer must algorithmically analyze the array of pixel values before it can reach any conclusions about the content of the image.

A computer must deal with objects in an image, as objects and not just as unrelated pixels, for many reasons:
1. computer vision (e.g., robotics)
2. computer analysis of quantitative properties of objects
3. computer manipulation of objects for image display via man-machine interactions
4. object-based nonstationary image restoration.

Before any of the above mentioned object-related actions can be taken, one or two conditions must be met:
1. The object must be recognized as an entity distinct from other objects in the image (i.e., pixels belonging to the object must be understood to be related in some way).
2. The entity must be labeled. It must be understood that it is, in fact, the specific object that is being searched for.

Most image processing techniques perform step # 1 first and independently of step # 2. Step # 1 is commonly called the image segmentation step.

### The Stack

There exists a large number of image segmentation techniques. Most techniques, however, fall into one of three broad categories: region growing, boundary detection, or multiresolution. Multiresolution techniques attempt to gain a global view of an image by examining it at many different resolution levels. The lower resolution provides a global view of the image, and the higher resolution provides the detail.

The stack approach initially proposed by Koenderink (1984) is a multiresolution image description and segmentation technique. The stack calculates image segments and an image

---

+ Present address: Biomedical Imaging Group, University of Massachusetts Medical School, Worcester, Massachusetts, U.S.A.

description tree by associating every pixel in an image with a local intensity extremum (Pizer et al., 1986). The approach focuses on decomposing the image into light and dark spots, each, except for the spot representing the whole image, contained in others. Thus a face might be described as a light spot containing a light spot (a reflection from the forehead) and three dark spots (the mouth and the regions of the two eyes). In turn the eye regions would be described as containing a dark spot (the eyebrow), a light spot (the eyelid), and a dark spot (the eye), with the latter containing a light spot (the eyeball) which itself contains a dark spot (the iris) which finally contains a yet darker spot (the pupil). We call these light and dark spots, at whatever scale, <u>extremal regions</u>, since they each include a local intensity maximum or minimum.

<u>Hierarchical Descriptions from Multiresolution Processing</u>. The image description in terms of extremal regions can be produced by following the paths of extrema in a stack of images in which each higher image is a slightly blurred version of the previous one. Progressively blurring an image causes each extremum to move continuously and eventually to annihilate as it blurs into its background. An <u>extremum path</u> is formed by following the locations of an extremum across the stack of images.

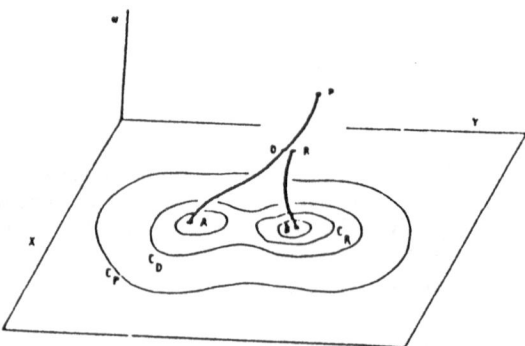

Figure 1: Extremum paths and associated isointensity contours.

Intensity change must be monotonic (increasing for dark spots and decreasing for light spots) as one moves along an extremum path from the original image towards images of increased blurring. As illustrated in Figure 1, while following each extremum path one can associate each path point with the isointensity contour that is at that point's intensity and that surrounds that extremum in the original image (Koenderink, 1984). The points (pixels) in the original image thus associated with each extremum path then form an extremal region (see Figure 2). Equivalently, each contour (non-extremum) point in the original image can be associated with its extremum path by linking the point to the closest point with its intensity level at the next level in the stack and continuing this linking through the levels until the extremum path is reached (see Figure 3). This process defines an <u>isointensity path</u>.

As indicated above, extrema annihilate when the blurring is sufficient to make the light or dark spot blur into an enclosing region. The amount of blurring necessary for an extremum to annihilate is a measure of the importance or scale of the extremal region, including the subregions that it contains. The intensity of the topmost point on an extremum path is the path's annihilation intensity. This is the intensity of the isointensity contour that forms the boundary of the associated extremal region. The annihilation intensity bounds from below (above) the intensities in the extremal region if the associated extremum is a maximum (minimum) and if there are no extremal sub-regions enclosed.

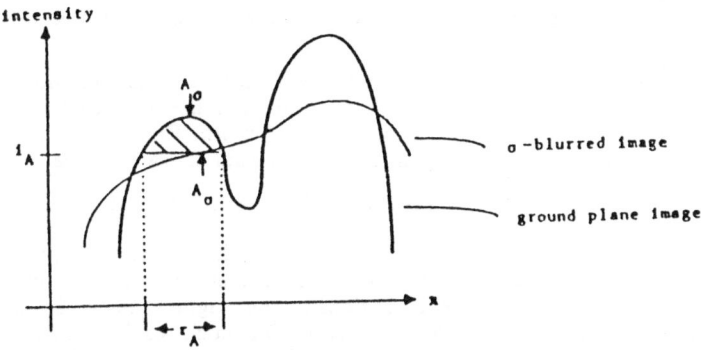

Figure 2: Extremum annihilation by blurring and the consequent extremal region. If the extremum at $A_o$ has moved to $A_\sigma$ at annihilation time, $r_A$ gives the extremal region and $i_A$ its minimum intensity.

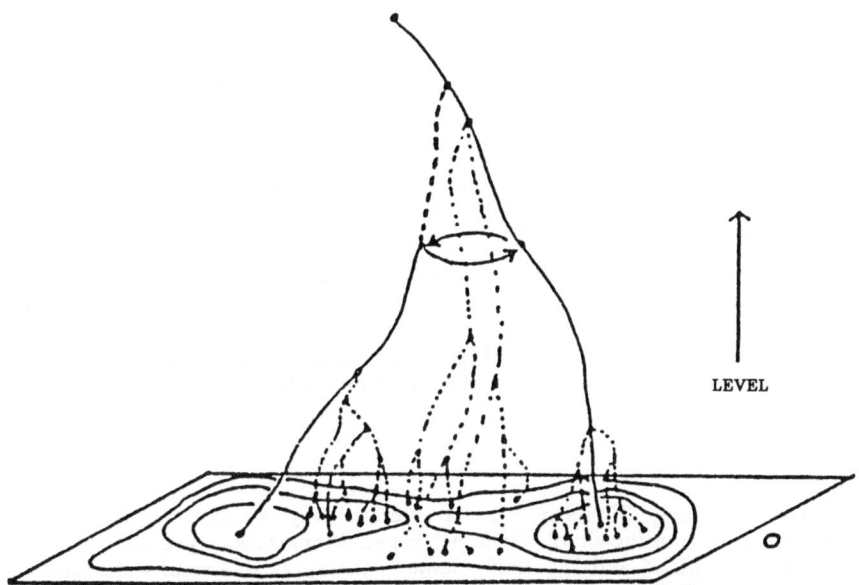

Figure 3: Extremum paths (solid lines) and isointensity paths (broken lines). Isointensity contours are indicated in the original image (level 0). The left extremal region is a subregion of the right extremal region.

A Tree of Extremal Regions for Image Description. As illustrated in Figure 1, when an extremum annihilates at some annihilation intensity, another region's isointensity contour at that intensity encloses the region associated with the annihilating extremum (Koenderink, 1984). Thus, a containment relation among extremal regions is induced by the process. This set of extremal regions together with their containment relations can be represented by an extremal region tree in which nodes represent extremal regions and a node is the child of another if the extremal region that it represents is immediately contained by the extremal region represented by the parent (see Figure 4). The root of the description tree represents the entire image.

Each node in the extremal region tree can be labeled with its scale, i.e. the total amount of blurring necessary for its extremum to annihilate. Furthermore, each node can be labeled with the annihilation intensity of the associated extremum. Finally, the node can be labeled with its size, shape, orientation, location, or other spatial characteristics.

## SECTION 2 - MATHEMATICAL PROPERTIES OF THE BASIC STACK

Our interest is in determining how maxima and minima behave when an image is blurred. Maxima and minima are of interest because these are the basic structures to which nonextremum points link and thereby define extremal regions in the original image. Several properties of extrema stem from basic results in Morse theory. One such result is that the number of minima, maxima, and saddle points cannot change (at least in the "typical" case) except through a bifurcation which causes both an extremum and a saddle point to appear (or annihilate). They both appear or annihilate at the same blurring level and same position (e.g.,

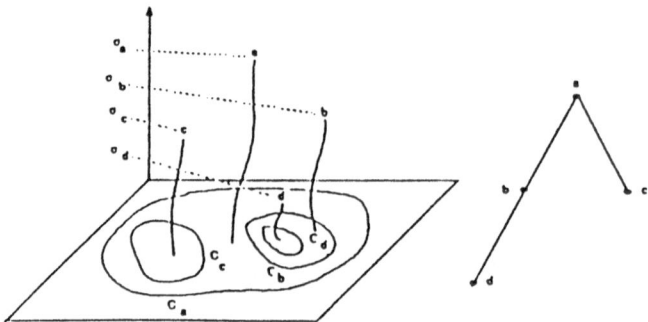

Figure 4: Left: Extremum paths, with their regions and scales. The vertical direction represents blurring. Right: The associated extremal region tree.

they must meet to annihilate). Similarly, the characteristic way in which the bifurcation occurs can be studied by examining simple "generic" cases. Morse theory precisely defines the meaning of the terms "typical" and "generic". Some of the applicable results of Morse theory are presented below. Differences between the results for the canonical cases presented and our particular case (which has the additional restriction of having to satisfy the heat equation) have some important theoretical implications which will be presented following the canonical exposition.

Morse Theory Basics for the Generic Case

Figure 5 shows the intensity of the extrema for $I(x,t) = x^3 + tx$. The way the maximum and minimum (when $t < 0$) in this particular function move towards each other (as $t$ increases) and annihilate (when $t = 0$) is "typical". $I(x,y,t) = x^3 + tx \pm y^2$ is the "typical" or generic description in two dimensions (with a maximum or a minimum annihilating with a saddle). Although Morse theory considers this function to be equivalent to all other generic extrema annihilations, the theory's notion of equivalence is too flexible for our purposes. It hides differences between functions that are of considerable importance to the extremal region definition. In the following section we describe the blurring scheme used to create the stack of lower resolution images from an initial image. It is then shown that the generic annihilation presented above does not evolve over time in a manner consistent with this blurring scheme.

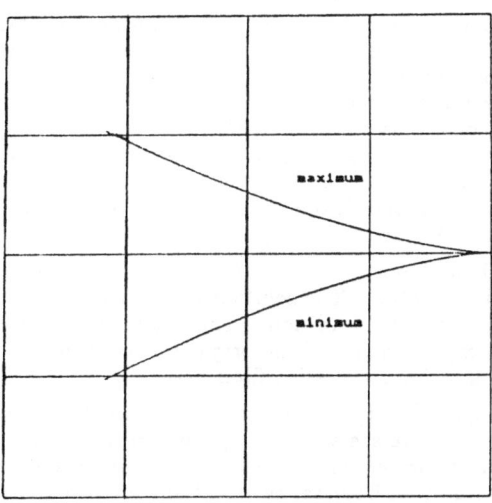

Figure 5: Extremum intensities (ordinate) for $x^3 + tx$ as a function of time (abscissa). The abscissa ranges from $-20$ to $0$, the ordinate from $-10$ to $10$. The two paths meet at time $t = 0$.

Modification of the generic annihilation to create a new function that does satisfy this constraint yields a function with important differences in the way extremal regions are allowed to form.

Embedding an Image in a Family Based Upon Gaussian Blurring

The most important property guiding the choice of a convolution kernel with which to create a stack of images is one of causality. We are concerned with extremal paths when creating the tree representation from a stack of images; ideally an extremum should not be allowed to be created (i.e., an extremal path to start) at any resolution level except the original one.

Another important property of the embedding is that it should be smooth. This means that intensity changes occur in a continuous manner as scale space is traversed. This implies that extremal paths and isointensity paths are smooth curves in position-scale space.

Koenderink (1984) examines the specific case of intensity creation. No intensity should exist at a low resolution level which cannot be traced (in a continuous manner) to an identical intensity at a higher resolution. Applying the constraints of causality, homogeneity, and isotropy, he derives the following necessary and sufficient relationship at the locations of the extrema: $I_{xx}(x,y,s) + I_{yy}(x,y,s) = \alpha^2 I_s(x,y,s)$, where $I(x,y,s)$ is intensity, $s$ is scale or resolution, $\alpha$ is a constant, and a subscript denotes a partial derivative. If this equation holds everywhere in an image the constraints are also maintained. This is the heat (or diffusion equation).

Despite the fact that no new intensity levels are created, extrema can be created in images of dimension greater than one. An easy example to help in the visualization of how this can occur in two dimensions is as follows. Imagine two broad, high mountains with a deep wide valley between them. One mountain is higher than the other. Connect these two mountains with a thin ramp bridge between their tops. The heights of the mountains, the valley, and the bridge represent intensity levels. The shorter mountain is not a local maximum because the ramp connects it with the higher mountain. But as diffusion occurs on the intensity distribution represented by this geography, the intensities of points represented by the bridge will decrease, since the deep valley is on both sides of it. It will quickly turn into a bridge with a deep dip in the middle. This will turn the smaller mountain into a local maximum.

111

The diffusion (heat) equation seems to be the best alternative available to guide blurring, since it does not create new intensity levels. The ability to create extrema is undesirable; features exist at low resolution levels which do not exist at higher ones. Nevertheless, this method of extrema creation is preferable to others which may also create new intensity levels. There are several additional reasons for desiring that the embedding satisfy the heat equation everywhere. First, if the image satisfies the heat equation, the solution of the equation will depend continuously on the data, i.e., the original image and boundary conditions (Zachmanoglou and Thoe, 1976). Second, if the image satisfies the heat equation, $I(x, y, t > 0)$ is infinitely differentiable (in $x$ and $y$) even if $I(x, y, 0)$ is not.

To blur an image, one should convolve it with the filter kernel that is the Green's function for the diffusion differential equation. The solution to a differential equation depends upon its initial conditions and boundary conditions. The initial condition is $I(x, y, 0) = H(x, y)$, where $H(x, y)$ is the original image. If the original image has no boundaries (i.e., takes up all of $R^2$), the solution yields a Gaussian filter kernel.

Unfortunately, if the image is not infinite in extent, the simple result of a Gaussian filter kernel is not necessarily correct. There are several ways the original image might be modified to eliminate its boundaries, and thereby maintain a Gaussian kernel solution to the diffusion equation. Mirroring of the image at its boundaries essentially creates an infinite image. An alternative approach to eliminating boundaries is to wrap-around an image at the boundary. This means that points outside a boundary are interpreted as being inside the boundary on the opposite side of the image. Both of these approaches create undesirable artifacts (Lifshitz, 1987) and are therefore not used.

A third method of handling the boundary conditions is to solve the diffusion differential equation explicitly for the finite plane with the given initial conditions (the initial image). The general solution to the finite domain heat equation is (John, 1982)

$$
\begin{aligned}
I(\varsigma, T) = & \int_\Omega K(\mathbf{x}, \varsigma, T) I(\mathbf{x}, 0)\, d\mathbf{x} \\
& + \int_0^T dt \int_{\mathbf{x} \in \partial\Omega} \left( K(\mathbf{x}, \varsigma, T - t) \frac{dI(\mathbf{x}, t)}{dn} - I(\mathbf{x}, t) \frac{dK(\mathbf{x}, \varsigma, T - t)}{dn} \right) dS_x .
\end{aligned}
\tag{1}
$$

Here $I(\varsigma, T)$ is the image at time $T$. $K(\mathbf{x}, \varsigma, T)$ is a Gaussian of width $T$. $\Omega$ is the region the image is defined on, and $\partial\Omega$ is its boundary. $dS_x$ is just the length element along the boundary, and $\frac{d}{dn}$ is the derivative in the direction normal to the boundary. This solution reduces to a convolution of the image with a Gaussian kernel if only the first term is nonzero. The conditions under which this is so will now be discussed.

The second term in the second integral will be equal to zero if the intensity of the image is zero along the boundary. An image which obeys the diffusion equation and has boundary values of zero can be created from the initial image (assuming the boundary conditions of the initial image are time independent). This is done by subtracting off an image which is invariant under blurring and has the identical boundary conditions.

The first term in the second integral will be nonzero unless an additional constraint is added, that the image be insulated, i.e., have $\frac{dI(x, t)}{dn} = 0$ at the boundary. This is not an unreasonable constraint to impose. The image is already discretely sampled in space. We can therefore always assume that the unknown intensity distribution between a boundary pixel and its neighbor in the interior is such that the constraint is satisfied without contradicting any known data or forcing the interpixel intensity distribution to be unnatural.

We can conclude that convolution of a bounded image with a Gaussian kernel (whose contribution is set equal to zero if outside the image boundary) can indeed be considered to be an appropriate solution to the diffusion equation for an insulated bounded image with zero intensity along its boundary. Since this approach is valid, it is the method used in this research. Toet (1986) also uses this technique but did not show that it was in fact valid.

## Containment for Extremal Region Paths in the Generic Case

Deciding on an embedding (blurring) scheme for the original image in a family of lower resolution images is not enough. Points in the image at one resolution level must also be associated with points in the image at another resolution level. This will define a path through resolution space for each point in the original image. The way that these paths (links) join up with each other will induce a decomposition of the original image into nested regions. All those paths which link to the same extremal path define the extremal region associated with that extremal path. Criteria for linking both nonextremum points and extremum points at one level to the appropriate pixels at the next level are needed to guide the creation of this path structure.

There are two criteria a path of a nonextremum point should satisfy. First, the intensity should stay constant along the path; the path of a nonextremum is therefore also called an isointensity path. Second, the point should move along the isointensity surface (in $x, y, s$ space) in a path of steepest ascent (where $s$, the resolution dimension, is up). Let the direction in which a path should move be defined as $\vec{v} = (v_1, v_2, v_3)$, where the three components are in the $x$, $y$ and $s$ directions respectively. These constraints then imply (Koenderink, 1984) $\vec{v} = \left(-I_s I_x, -I_s I_y, (I_x)^2 + (I_y)^2\right)$ . This is the direction the path of a nonextremum point should take. At an extremum $I_x$ and $I_y$ are both equal to zero, so $\vec{v}$ is a null vector. In other words, once a nonextremum path meets an extremum, $\vec{v}$ no longer specifies the direction in which to proceed. Criteria for the path direction of an extremum hold from then on. The extremal region associated with an extremum path is just all those points whose paths eventually join with the extremal path.

The path criterion for extrema is very simple. Each extremum is isolated in the typical case. That is, there are no other extrema in some neighborhood around each extremum. In addition, their positions move continuously through scale space. It is therefore always immediately evident what path each extremum should take. Contrary to isointensity path criteria, intensity along an extremal path changes. Intensity along the path of a maximum will decrease with decreasing resolution, while intensity of a minimum will increase. When an extremum annihilates, its path continues on as an isointensity path (see Figure 3). The path criteria for nonextremum and extremum points determine which regions in the original image become associated with each extremal path.

Let us now examine the generic case of extremum annihilation in an attempt to understand the rules guiding extremal region formation. The generic description of a saddle and a minimum annihilating was shown at the beginning of this section to be $I(x, y, t) = x^3 + tx + y^2$. The simplest way to visualize this (see Figure 6) is to imagine a second minimum (which will not annihilate) existing on the other side of the saddle point. The saddle exists between the two minima so that the isointensity curve through the saddle point surrounds the two minima. Annihilation of the saddle with one minimum takes place at $x = 0$, $y = 0$, $t = 0$. The annihilation intensity is zero. At some initial time $t_o < 0$ the zero intensity contours surrounding the minima lie inside the isointensity contour of the saddle. As time progresses, the minimum which will annihilate and the saddle point move towards each other. The lobe of the saddle isointensity contour which surrounds this minimum gets smaller, as does the zero intensity contour which surrounds the minimum. The zero intensity contour remains inside the saddle intensity contour the entire time. The zero intensity contour surrounding the annihilating minimum and the lobe of the saddle contour surrounding the annihilating minimum become identical for the brief instant as annihilation occurs. To determine the nature of the extremal region such a scenario will produce, one must examine which nonextremum paths link to the annihilating extremum. Nonextremum paths are isointensity paths. Those starting out inside the zero intensity contour surrounding the extremum have intensities less than zero. They can not cross the zero intensity surface represented by the zero contour in scale space. Yet the zero intensity contour eventually collapses into the extremum point, enclosing no area at annihilation time. The only place for the nonextremum paths to go is to link up with the extremum path. This means that all isointensity paths through resolution space that start off inside the zero intensity contour must eventually link up to the annihilating minimum. This region represents the extremal region associated with the annihilating extremum.

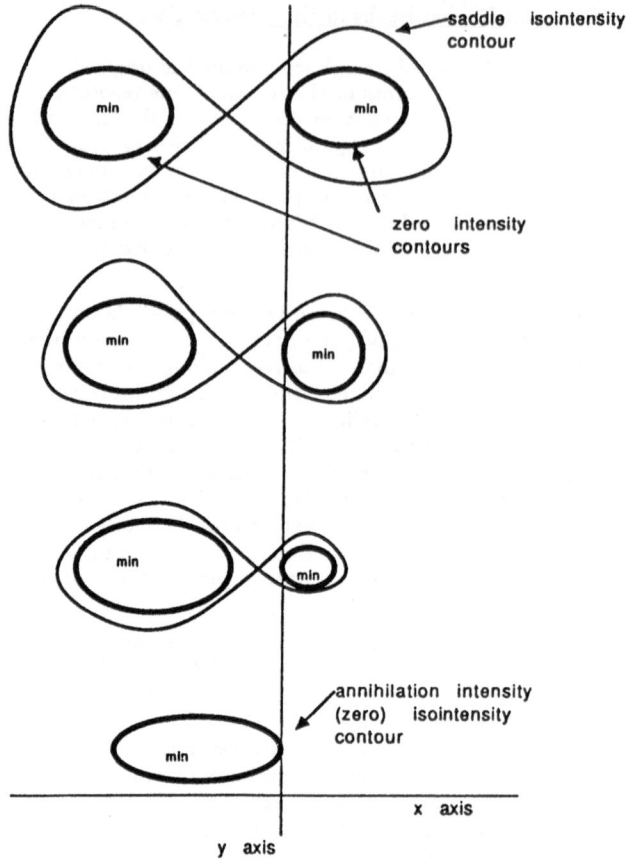

saddle isointensity contour

zero intensity contours

annihilation intensity (zero) isointensity contour

x axis

y axis

Time increases (more blurring) as we move downwards from one plot to the next.

Figure 6: Saddle and zero intensity contours at various times until annihilation. Nondiffusion case.

## Noncontainment for Extremal Region Paths in the Gaussian Case

Imposing the constraint of satisfying the heat equation (i.e., convolution with a Gaussian) modifies the conclusions reached above about the manner in which extrema annihilate. Once we restrict the embeddings to a particular class of smooth embeddings, namely those satisfying the heat equation, it becomes very difficult to know which descriptions are typical in this restricted subclass. Nevertheless, specific cases can and will be examined which must fit into the diffusion framework.

Blurring $x^3/6 + tx$ with a Gaussian produces the prototypical diffusion annihilation. In the one-dimensional case nothing changes significantly from the canonical (nondiffusion) description given above. The time parameter in the formalism gets replaced by $\sigma^2/2$, where $\sigma$ is the total standard deviation of the Gaussian blurring done so far. The $x^3$ term gets a factor of $1/6$ in front of it so that the prototype equation satisfies the one-dimensional heat equation.

The two-dimensional annihilation via a diffusion process changes from the generic annihilation in a subtle but very important way. The annihilation equation representing the diffusion case is $I(x, y, t) = x^3/6 + tx + t + y^2/2$. We have been forced to add a term solely in $t$ to preserve the diffusion characteristic! This has many important consequences. We will now examine this equation, which is for a saddle and a minimum annihilating, in detail; identical conclusions can be drawn from looking at the $-y^2/2$ case which is for a saddle and a maximum.

The intensities of these critical points differ from the nondiffusion case (compare Figure 5 with Figure 7). $I(\hat{x}, 0, t) = \pm\frac{(-2t)^{3/2}}{6} \pm t(-2t)^{1/2} + t$, where $\hat{x}$ is the position of a critical point, + is used for $\hat{x} > 0$ $\;(I(\hat{x}) < 0)$, whereas for $\hat{x} < 0$ $\;(I(\hat{x}) > 0)$ − is used; the square root is interpreted as being the positive root. This equation is valid for $t \leq 0$. Now examine $I(\hat{x},0,\hat{t}) = 0$, i.e., those times when the critical point intensity equals zero. We find that, as before, both the saddle and the minimum intensities equal zero at $t = 0$, the annihilation intensity and time. But we also now have zero intensity at $\hat{t} = -9/8$ for the saddle intensity! The saddle intensity, which starts out greater than zero (for time $< -9/8$), gradually decreases becoming less than the annihilation intensity when $t > -9/8$ . This is confirmed by setting $\frac{\partial I(\hat{x},0,t)}{\partial t} = 0$ and noting that the saddle (but not the minimum) has a turning point in intensity at $t = -1/2$. From $t = -1/2$ to $t = 0$ the saddle intensity is increasing, as is the minimum intensity.

There are significant consequences of the saddle intensity dipping below the annihilation intensity and then rising back up to it. In the canonical case analyzed previously, when a saddle existed between two minima, the isointensity curve through the saddle point surrounded the two minima (see Figure 6). The saddle intensity contour remained outside the zero intensity contour until annihilation time. This is not true for the diffusion case (see Figure 8). The

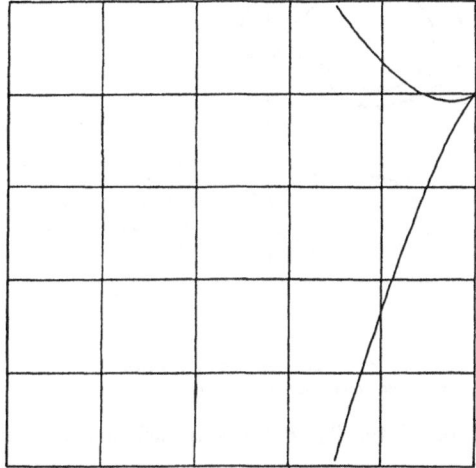

Figure 7: Saddle (upper curve) and minimum (lower curve) intensities (ordinate) with respect to time (abscissa). The time axis ranges from $-10$ to $0$, and the intensity axis ranges from $-8$ to $2$. Diffusion case.

zero intensity contour, which starts out inside the saddle intensity contour, ends up outside the saddle intensity contour! The saddle intensity contour and the zero intensity contour become identical at the instant the zero intensity contour surrounding the annihilating minimum joins the zero intensity contour surrounding the other minimum. After this time the zero intensity contour surrounds the saddle intensity contour and both of the minima. The "lobe" of the zero intensity contour that surrounds the minimum that will annihilate gradually contracts and "pinches off" at $x = 0$, $t = 0$ (see Figure 8).

The fixed point of $I(x,0,t)$, which does not change intensity with time, is now at $x = -1$ (see Figure 9). Intensities for all $x < -1$ continuously decrease, while those for points $x > -1$ continuously increase. Hence, if an isointensity path is at a particular $x > -1$ at some $\tilde{t}$, then at time $\tilde{t} + \delta t$ it will have to move towards the minimum, to compensate for the fact that all the intensities around it are rising. There are points with $x < -1$ that have negative intensities. These points will move away from the minimum even though their intensities are less than the annihilation (zero) intensity! The annihilation isointensity surface in $(x,y,t)$ space is still a concave cap, but now it has a hole in its side where it joins up with the other zero intensity surface; isointensity paths can escape from under the cap by sneaking out through this hole, so they are not forced to join the annihilating minimum's path!

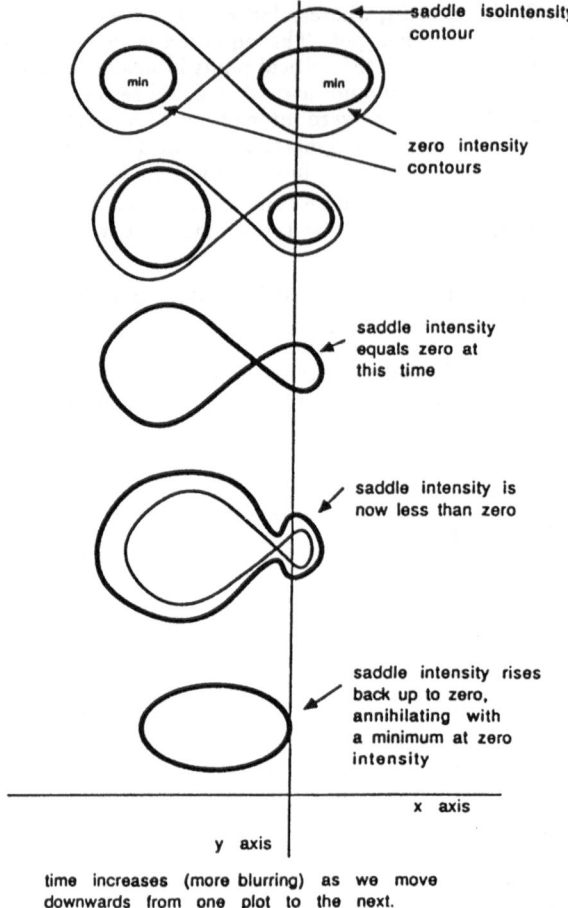

saddle isointensity
contour

zero intensity
contours

saddle intensity
equals zero at
this time

saddle intensity is
now less than zero

saddle intensity rises
back up to zero,
annihilating with
a minimum at zero
intensity

x axis

y axis

time increases (more blurring) as we move
downwards from one plot to the next.

Figure 8: Saddle and zero intensity contours at various times until annihilation. Diffusion case.

It is difficult to describe mathematically the nonextremum paths which escape through this hole. The isointensity paths are integral curves of the vector field $\vec{v} = (-I_x I_t, -I_y I_t, I_x^2 + I_y^2)$. What needs to be done is to substitute into this the formula for $I(x, y, t)$ and solve analytically for the isointensity paths. Unfortunately, an analytical solution of these differential equations is intractable. Nevertheless, qualitative examination of the vector field <u>directions</u> can yield a simple proof that some nonextremum paths do escape. The proof is as follows. For the prototypical diffusion case we have $\vec{v} = (-(\frac{x^2}{2} + t)(x + 1), -y(x + 1), (\frac{x^2}{2} + t)^2 + y^2)$. This means that any point with $x < -1$ and positive $y$ coordinate will have a positive $y$ component in $\vec{v}$, and such points will move away from the $x$ axis, which is where the saddle and minimum are. Furthermore, if such a point should happen to try to move towards an $x$ coordinate greater than $-1$, it will not get there. This is because at $-1$ both the $x$ and $y$ components of $\vec{v}$ are zero and the point will stay fixed at $x = -1$ for all future time. By showing that all points with $x$ coordinates less than $-1$ move away from the $x$ axis (if not on it to begin with) and that these points can never move to an $x$ value greater than minus one, we have shown that these points (paths) can never meet either the saddle or the minimum path. Yet many of these points have intensity between that of the minimum and the annihilation intensity (zero). Therefore, some points inside the annihilation intensity contour do not link to the minimum path.

By simulating the blurring and linking process, We have been able to display isointensity paths which start out inside an annihilation intensity contour, and yet do not link up to the extremum path of the annihilating minimum. In order to make the simulation as accurate as possible, an analytic model of the blurring process was used.

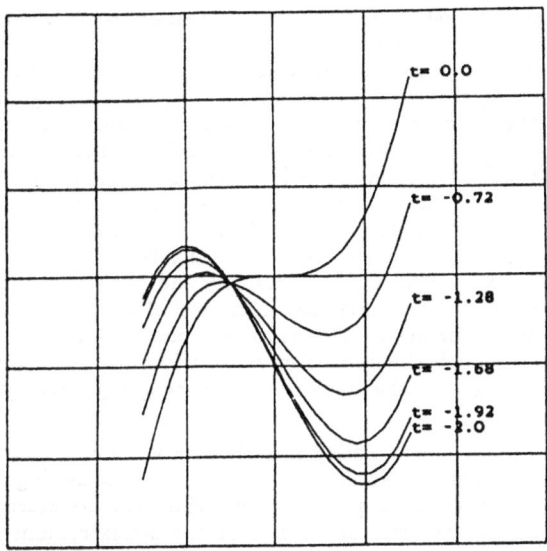

Figure 9: The prototypical annihilation satisfying the diffusion equation. $I = x^3/6 + tx + t$ is graphed for various values of $t$. The abscissa ($x$ axis) and the ordinate (intensity axis) both range from $-6$ to $6$.

Despite the surprising theoretical result that nonextremum paths can escape from the extremal region they originate in, we have yet to observe any clear examples of escaping paths when working with actual images. This is most likely due to the fact that extremal regions are not sufficiently isolated from other regions to display the type of behavior shown in the "prototypical diffusion" annihilation case. The behavior of that case stemmed primarily from the fact that all points with $x$ coordinate less than $-1$ continually decreased in intensity. In an actual image this would not occur since there would be another minimum at some $x$ less than $-1$ and this would tend to cause intensities in the region to increase under blurring. In addition, our sampling resolution may be coarse enough to miss some small regions.

## SECTION 3 - THEORETICAL ISSUES DUE TO DISCRETENESS

The entire theory upon which the stack algorithm is based applies to continuous Morse images embedded continuously in resolution space. Unfortunately images of this form cannot be handled by a digital computer. The continuous image must be approximated by one which is spatially discrete (i.e., made up of pixels). The smooth embedding of the image in resolution space is approximated by a stack of images each derived from the previous one by convolution with a blurring kernel of non-infinitesimal width and finite extent. Nonextremum and extremum paths, which theoretically are continuous paths, become represented by a chain of links from a pixel in one image to a pixel in the next image to a pixel in the next image and so on. The best manner in which to create these approximations and the complications such approximations create are the subjects of this section.

### Linking Criteria

As mentioned in the previous section, the nonextremum paths are theoretically integral curves of the vector field $\left(-I_t I_x, -I_t I_y, I_x^2 + I_y^2\right)$. This is equivalent to the requirement that a nonextremum path stay on an isointensity surface and move along it in the steepest path possible. This theoretical goal can only be approximated by a computer algorithm due to the discrete nature of the image representation and the non-infinitesimal amount of blurring occurring at each stage. The linking criteria employed should enable the discretely linked path to closely approximate the continuous path.

While in the theoretical case all paths are continuous and a point can always link to an arbitrarily nearby location with intensity identical to its own in an arbitrarily nearby image

117

plane, it is not uncommon for pixels to fail to satisfy this property in the discrete case. There are three main causes for this phenomenon.

1. Areas of an image with high contrast tend to change intensity more rapidly for a fixed amount of blurring than regions of low contrast. Hence the change in the intensities of all the pixels in the region may be too large for any good match in intensities to be found in a small local region around the current position of the linking path.

2. The image manipulated by the computer is a sampled version of the the continuous image dealt with in theory. The samples chosen may not be identical in intensity to that of an isointensity path being followed, even though the continuous image does, in fact, include that exact intensity between the sampled pixels.

3. Nonextremum regions very close in both intensity and position to an extremum will have no intensity to link up to (in the next level of the stack), due to the non-infinitesimal amount of blurring which has to take place. This is because the extremum intensity has passed through the desired intensity without ever having explicitly represented that intensity in one of the stack levels. These near-extremum points should be linked to the extremum.

Spatial discreteness caused by sampling is dealt with via a combination of two methods: use of an "original intensity" field and interpolation. Instead of searching for a parent pixel of intensity identical to the intensity of the pixel through which the nonextremum path currently passes, one is sought which has the original intensity of the nonextremum path as an inter-polant of its local neighborhood. By not associating the intensity of the pixel through which a path passes at any particular level with the path itself, the intensity value along the path is kept from changing and gradually drifting away from the desired original intensity. If a check for interpolation is not performed, the linking process becomes captive to the vagaries of the sampling process, and strange artifacts can occur. Particularly damaging would be the escape of a nonextremum path from the extremal region it should remain in by passing through an isointensity surface due to quantization artifacts. This would result in a nonextremum pixel becoming associated with the wrong extremal region.

If the intensity of the nonextremum path is above (below) the intensity of the current local neighborhood, the steepest path up (down) hill is traversed. Hill walking is terminated when a region is reached in which the nonextremum path intensity is an interpolant, or when a local extremum is reached.

A subtle problem which must be addressed in the implementation of the linking strategy occurs when multiple nonextremum path pixels link up to the same pixel on a lower resolution image. It would introduce significant error into the nesting structure to consider all paths which link to one pixel to be the same path from there on. Each of these nonextremum paths possess their own "original intensity". These values may be quite different from each other. The pixels are all linking to the same pixel because, due to spatial quantization, their preferred interpolated positions are nearest it. Therefore, the ability is provided to allow several distinct paths to pass through one pixel, without the paths becoming merged. The paths may eventually separate, and possibly even end up in different extremal regions.

Blurring

The blurring process itself is complicated by the discreteness of the implementation. Instead of a continuous Gaussian kernel of infinite extent a discrete approximation of finite extent must be used. Since blurring is not performed with an exact Gaussian, the theory which Koenderink derived no longer precisely applies. Conclusions that new intensity levels cannot be created do not necessarily apply when convolution is not with a Gaussian.

Spatial Sampling

The sampling in space should, by normal sampling practice, decrease as you move up the stack, that is, as the amount of blurring increases. More precisely, the inter-pixel sampling distance should be proportional to the standard deviation of the total amount of blurring due to both imaging and the convolution with Gaussians done to create the lower resolution image. Pizer (1983) uses an argument based on the aliasing error at the Nyquist frequency to suggest a specific proportionality constant. However, changing the spatial sampling at lower resolution levels in the stack complicates the extremum and isointensity path following processes. As a result the spatial sampling in all resolution levels has been left the same as in the original image. Part of the efficiency of resampling is still achieved since only extremum paths and isointensity paths that have not yet joined an extremum path are followed to the next resolution level.

## Extrema Creation

Several mechanisms can create extrema during blurring. One mechanism was mentioned earlier. If the neighborhood around a nonextremum point decreases (increases) in intensity faster than the point itself does, the nonextremum point becomes a maximum (minimum). This cannot happen in the one-dimensional case under Gaussian blurring. In higher dimensions it can occur.

Another possible cause of extrema creation is the non-Morse nature of an original image. Plateaus in intensity oftentimes exist in the initial image. These plateaus are non-Morse and hence unstable. Any slight perturbation of the image (e.g., blurring) will cause these plateaus to break up. In the process many extrema will get created. The most common time this occurs is during the initial blurring of the image. This phenomenon is minimized by blurring the initial image slightly before analyzing it. This new image (which would be Morse if the blurring kernel was of infinite extent, and has fewer plateaus in the finite kernel case) is the one which the stack algorithm is applied to. The intensity values of the original image are still used for display purposes.

A third way extrema can be "created" is due to the spatial sampling. If an extremum is of very small spatial extent, the extremum may be missed completely at one resolution level and sampled into at another.

Two precautions are taken in order to mitigate the consequences of extremum creation. First, nonextremum paths are allowed to turn into (as opposed to link to) an extremum path. Second, extremum paths which appear but are not on any path which started in the original image plane are still tracked. Since the extremum exists, nonextremum paths may very well eventually need to link into this extremum.

## Disconnected Extremal Regions due to the Discrete Implementation

A single isolated pixel can link to a distant object in instances in which it would not be isolated in the spatially continuous case. This occurs because the region that would also link to the object, and keep this isolated pixel from becoming isolated, is not represented in any pixel. An example will make this clearer. Suppose we have a group of pixels with initial intensities as follows:

| 100 | 100 | 100 |
| --- | --- | --- |
| 100 | 75 | 100 |
| 50 | 50 | 50 |

Now suppose there is a nearby maximum with an initial intensity of 90 and an annihilation intensity of 60. Then the only pixel in this group which is between 60 and 90 and thus may link to this maximum is the center one. It might do this because as lower resolution images are created an isointensity path to the maximum might appear. If this is the case, it will be the only pixel in this three by three neighborhood to link to this maximum. Since original intensities are kept for each nonextremum path and regions are always examined to determine if the original intensity is an interpolant, the path linking algorithm would have no problem correctly linking the isolated pixel (the one with intensity 75) to the correct extremum path. If the image was not discretely sampled, this pixel would not be an isolated region linking up to the maximum. Between the pixel at 100 on the center-right and the pixel at 50 on the bottom-right there would be a thin region at an intensity such that it would link to the same maximum as the center pixel.

## SECTION 4 - EXTENSIONS TO THE STACK - EMBEDDING SCHEMES

The basic stack algorithm does not always segment an image in the most preferred manner. It can take pixels that, visually, all belong to one region and link them to different extremum paths (and hence different regions). It may also join pixels together in one region that visually are very similar but semantically should not be joined (i.e., they are in different organs which happen to abut each other). The algorithm works well, but not always well enough. It therefore seems reasonable to try to adjust it in a way which would improve its performance. The aforementioned problem is one of accuracy in segmentation. An accurate tree description implies the existence of subtree structures whose leaves represent completely an area of the image which we subjectively determine to be meaningful, and only that region (e.g., it would include all pixels in the liver, and none not in the liver).

The question is how the stack algorithm should be modified to produce a more accurate image segmentation. There are two modifications to the algorithm which come immediately to mind. One is to alter the way the original image is embedded in the multiresolution stack. A different embedding should cause different extremal regions to form. The second approach is to alter the linking criteria. Modification of the linking criteria has not been investigated but would be an area for promising research in the future. Of course, both of these modifications could be applied concurrently.

Intuitively one would expect that modifying the shape of the blurring kernel to reflect the shapes of the regions of interest would yield better segmentation results than always performing stationary, isotropic Gaussian blurring. Any blurring scheme adopted should still be required not to create any new intensity levels as blurring proceeds. Koenderink's main criterion for this is that $I_{xx} + I_{yy} = \alpha^2(x,y,t)I_t$ at the extrema. Of course, the embedding should also remain smooth. This allows for considerable flexibility in choosing a blurring strategy. Let us first examine the effects of stationary, but anisotropic, blurring, and then those of nonstationary blurring.

### Anisotropic Stationary Blurring

It is fairly easy to show that for anisotropic Gaussians with $\sigma_{xy} = 0$, convolution of that Gaussian with a polynomial is equivalent to a rescaling of the coordinate axes, isotropic blurring, and then rescaling the coordinates back. This means that the properties of isotropic Gaussian blurring of images discussed in section 2 (no creation of new intensity levels, theoretical ability of paths to leave their original extremal region) should apply to the anisotropic case also. It does not mean that the extremal regions formed are identical in the isotropic and anisotropic cases.

A way to study the extremal regions formed is to investigate the analytical form of an anisotropic Gaussian convolved with the generic $\frac{x^3}{6} + tx + t + \frac{y^2}{2}$ polynomial. The result of convolving this polynomial with a two-dimensional Gaussian with variances in the $x$ and $y$ directions of $\sigma_x^2$ and $\sigma_y^2$, yields

$$x^3/6 + (t_{ox} + \sigma_x^2/2)x + (t_{oy} + \sigma_y^2/2) + y^2/2. \qquad (2)$$

This new formula changes which pixels are associated with an extremal region as compared with those associated in the isotropic case. Nonextremum pixels link to form nonextremum paths by following an isointensity path through resolution space. The vector field, $\vec{v}$, defining the direction of the isointensity paths changes because of differences between equation 1 and that for the isotropic case. Recall that the defining equation for $\vec{v}$ is $(-I_t I_x, -I_t I_y, I_x^2 + I_y^2)$.

Modification of the simulation program (see section 2) to perform anisotropic convolutions has permitted simulation of isointensity paths for anisotropic Gaussian blurring. Comparisons of Figure 10 (anisotropic paths) to Figure 11 (isotropic paths) clearly show that the isointensity paths are able to move more quickly in the $y$ direction when blurring is faster in the $y$ direction. In addition, paths which before headed away from the minimum (which has

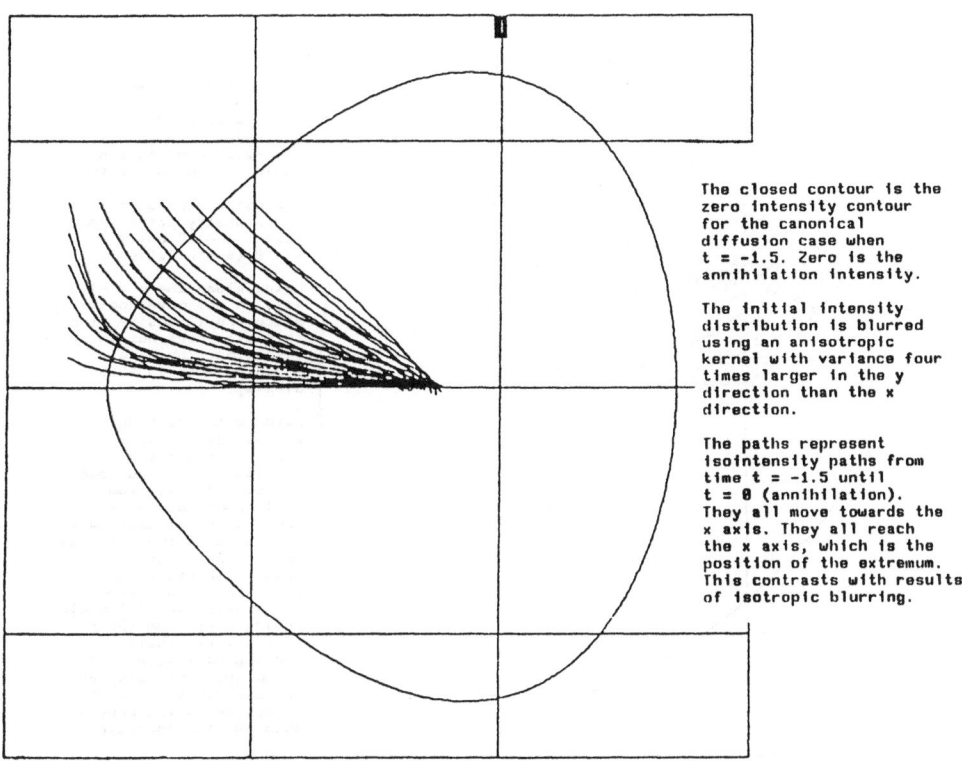

The closed contour is the zero intensity contour for the canonical diffusion case when t = -1.5. Zero is the annihilation intensity.

The initial intensity distribution is blurred using an anisotropic kernel with variance four times larger in the y direction than the x direction.

The paths represent isointensity paths from time t = -1.5 until t = 0 (annihilation). They all move towards the x axis. They all reach the x axis, which is the position of the extremum. This contrasts with results of isotropic blurring.

Figure 10: Isointensity paths under anisotropic blurring. Compare these paths with those in Figure 11. Note that many paths which do not reach the $x$ axis in the isotropic case do reach it (and join the extremum which is on the axis) in this case. The abscissa $(x)$ ranges from $-2$ to 4, the ordinate $(y)$ from $-3$ to 3.

$x > 0$ and $y = 0$ and moves towards $x = 0$ as time progresses) now head <u>towards</u> it. The extremal region associated with the minimum is clearly different in the anisotropic case from the isotropic blurring case.

Figure 12 shows the effect of isotropic and anisotropic blurring schemes on a synthetic image of ellipses. This demonstrates that segmentation results vary depending upon the orientation of the Gaussian kernel used to blur the image. Convolution of the image with an isotropic Gaussian finds each ellipse as an extremal region. When this image is convolved with a Gaussian which has four times the standard deviation in the $y$ direction (up-down axis on the page) as in the $x$ direction, each ellipse is not found as a single extremal region. As one would expect, the results are worse since the ellipses are oriented at a 90 degree angle to the Gaussian kernel. The algorithm is robust enough not to merge pixels from several neighboring ellipses into one region, but it also does not link all the pixels in one ellipse into one region. Each ellipse is represented by several regions, each of which independently links up to the last remaining extremum (instead of to each other). The second image in Figure 12 shows several of these regions. Despite this fragmentation of ellipses into multiple regions, the postprocessing discussed in section 5 ("displaying a union of subtrees") would allow us to view each ellipse in its entirety.

Nonstationary Blurring

Spatially variant blurring based upon local image content should improve the correspondence between the extremal regions and the semantically meaningful regions in the image. This statement is motivated by the human visual model of Cohen and Grossberg (1984), which indicates that object perception is performed via an intensity diffusion process (i.e.,

121

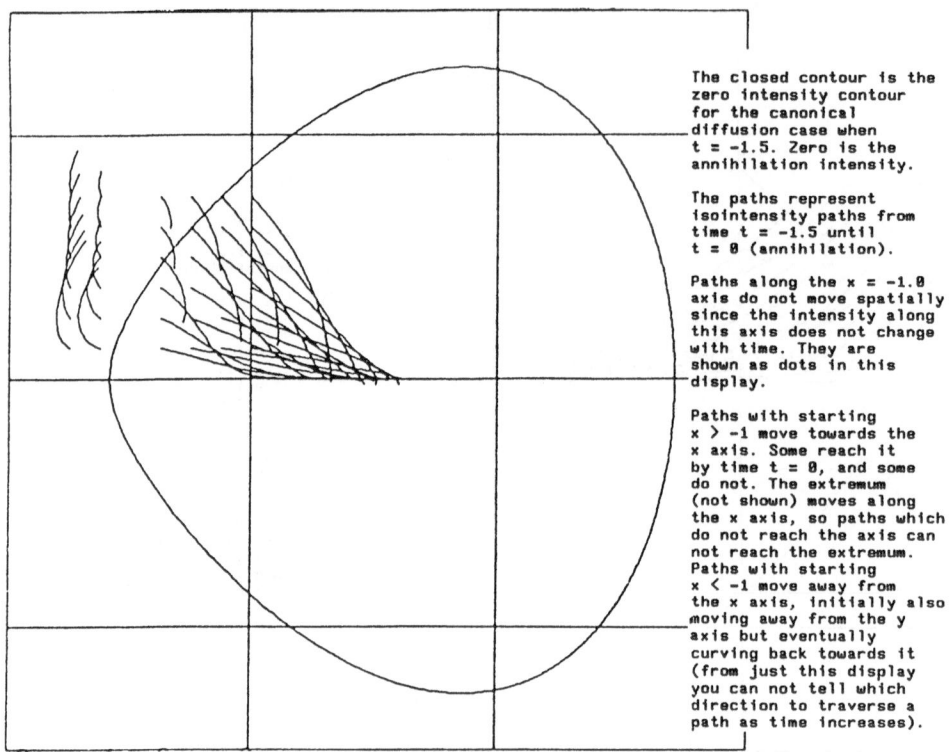

The closed contour is the zero intensity contour for the canonical diffusion case when t = -1.5. Zero is the annihilation intensity.

The paths represent isointensity paths from time t = -1.5 until t = 0 (annihilation).

Paths along the x = -1.0 axis do not move spatially since the intensity along this axis does not change with time. They are shown as dots in this display.

Paths with starting x > -1 move towards the x axis. Some reach it by time t = 0, and some do not. The extremum (not shown) moves along the x axis, so paths which do not reach the axis can not reach the extremum. Paths with starting x < -1 move away from the x axis, initially also moving away from the y axis but eventually curving back towards it (from just this display you can not tell which direction to traverse a path as time increases).

Figure 11: Isointensity paths under isotropic blurring. The abscissa ($x$) ranges from $-2$ to $4$, the ordinate ($y$) from $-3$ to $3$.

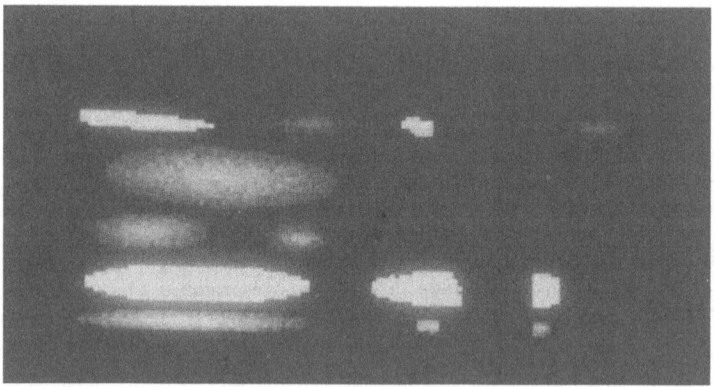

Figure 12: Original image (left) and anisotropic segmentation of ellipses (right). All pieces of each ellipse are found (but not joined together), only some are displayed here.

blurring) which is moderated by edge strength measures in the image (i.e., it is nonstationary). Many nonstationary blurring schemes can satisfy the causality and smooth embedding constraints. There is no simple coordinate transformation between embeddings produced by nonstationary blurring schemes and stationary blurring schemes. We have investigated several techniques, most of them based upon the premise that there should be minimal blurring across a region which is believed to contain an edge (Lifshitz, 1987). No completely satisfactory method has been found yet.

## SECTION 5 - USE OF THE STACK PROGRAM

Implementation Performance

The implementation of the stack and display algorithms has not been optimized for speed of execution or minimization of space requirements. Some indications of the speed and size of the implementation are nevertheless in order. The stack program has been applied to about 15 two-dimensional CT images of the upper abdomen. Approximately five one-dimensional and three-dimensional images have been analyzed also. To provide faster results for testing purposes, most of the CT images have been reduced from an initial size of 512 by 512 pixels to 64 by 64 pixels. Running on a moderately loaded VAX 780, it takes approximately 30 to 45 seconds to create each level in the stack, together with all of its associated data structures. The 64 by 64 images tend to need about 30 levels of blurring before only one extremum remains. Thus the program runs about 20 minutes. The image description tree created is approximately 250 kbytes.

All of the above numbers scale approximately linearly with image area. Of course, an image with a lot of noise or very many objects will tend to take longer and create a larger data structure. If it is known in advance that the structures of interest in an image are of small scale, the processing may be terminated before only one extremum remains, saving time.

The table below lists typical subroutine execution times when applied to a 128 by 128 pixel image.

### Typical Subroutine Execution Times

| % time* | total secs | # of calls | ms/call | name |
|---------|-----------|-----------|---------|------|
| 42.2 | 6,695.52 | 59 | 113,483.40 | blur image |
| 18.8 | 9,675.96 | 1 | 2,980.44 | calc. invariant image |
| 13.9 | 11,876.58 | 1,294,414 | varies | linking overhead |
| 8.1 | 13,169.04 | 59 | 21,906.16 | diagnostics |
| 6.4 | 14,182.78 | 592,108 | 1.71 | link nonextrema |
| 4.2 | 14,848.05 | 60 | 11,157.89 | find extrema |
| 1.7 | 15,117.32 | 65,248 | 4.12 | link extrema |
| 0.1 | 15,135.14 | 5,273 | 3.38 | annihilate extrema |

* Not all routines are shown, so times may not add to 100%

Note that the vast bulk of the time is spent performing the blurring. A large percentage of time is also spent calculating the image that is invariant under Gaussian blurring and has the same boundary values as the initial image. This algorithm was chosen for ease of implementation without regard to execution speed. We believe that the stack program execution time can be decreased by at least a third to a half without the use of any special hardware.

Typical relative frequencies of link types for a particular blurring level are shown below (not all link types are shown so numbers may not add exactly).

### Typical Relative Frequencies of Link Types and Link Distances

| Level 15 of 38 levels for a 64 by 64 image | | | |
|---|---|---|---|
| link type | # of links | avg dist | max dist |
| nonextremum to extremum | 147 = 4% | 3.22 | 11.00 |
| extremum continuing | 170 = 5% | 0.12 | 3.00 |
| extremum annihilating | 6 = 0% | 4.83 | 9.00 |
| nonextr. to appearing extr. | 24 = 0% | 1.25 | 2.00 |
| nonextremum continuing | 2,555 = 86% | 0.42 | 9.00 |
| total of all links | 2,946 = 100% | 0.56 | 11.00 |

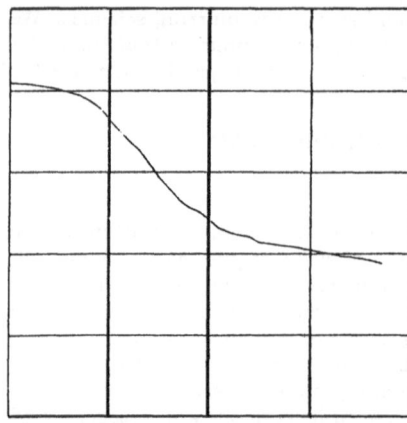

Figure 13: The number of paths remaining in each level. The abscissa is the stack resolution level and ranges from 0 to 40. The ordinate is the number of paths remaining and ranges from 0 to 5000 (this data is from a 64 by 64 pixel image).

The path link types maintain approximately the same relative frequencies through a wide resolution range.

Average link distances for nonextremum paths are kept less than one pixel (by keeping the blurring rate slow), this minimizes possible error in following isointensity paths. The number of paths remaining at each level in the stack decreases since isointensity paths link up to extremum paths (see Figure 13).

### Interactive Display Based on the Image Description Tree

We have investigated several different interaction methods with the data structure produced by the stack algorithm. The display techniques developed permit easy specification of the region of interest to be examined and also yield insight into why certain subregions nest the way they do. The display program initially reads in the image description tree from a file produced by the stack algorithm. A user can then interactively control which regions in the image (subtrees in the data structure) are displayed. Several methods for specifying these regions are provided. These methods are discussed at length below.

The image is displayed on an Adage 3000 raster graphics system. A vector representation of the tree of extremum paths (along with the nonextremum paths they turn into) can be displayed simultaneously with the raster image. The vector image is displayed in three dimensions $(x, y, t)$ on an Evans and Sutherland Picture System 300. This is a color vector graphics system. Paths of minima and maxima are displayed in different colors (see Figure 14). This tree can be interactively rotated using knobs to specify the rotation about each axis. This display gives the user a very good feel for the way the extrema in the image have moved and merged together during the blurring process. This tree can be interrogated by picking any branch using a light pen. The extremal region associated with this branch will then be displayed on the raster display device. This has turned out to be a very powerful tool for visualizing the relationship between the tree structure produced and the original image. Frequently a major organ can be displayed quickly by using a light pen to choose the major tree branch (i.e., a branch that exists until very low resolution levels) in the location of interest. A visual examination of the tree structure sometimes focuses attention on high interest areas. For instance, noting that the extremum path representing the stomach region has a smaller branch (subregion) associated with it can focus attention on that subregion, which may be a tumorous mass.

The tree data structure can be examined more globally via various A/D devices. Two sliders are used to specify a scale range of objects which should be displayed. The two sliders specify the low and high scale limits of the range of interest. The scale of a region is defined to be the blurring level at which its associated extremum path annihilates. All extremum paths which annihilate within the scale range specified by the sliders have their associated extremal regions displayed on the raster display. This method of choosing regions has been very

124

useful. Organs in the CT images can frequently all be chosen simultaneously simply by setting the sliders to display only regions of large scale. The length of time it takes to display the specified regions depends upon the number of regions specified. Typical display times range from about two to five seconds.

Similarly, two other sliders specify the intensity range of objects to be displayed. Even if the annihilation level of an extremum path lies within the specified scale range, it is only displayed if the average intensity of its associated region lies within the intensity window selected by the intensity sliders. Intensity windowing is useful when the regions of interest (or regions of disinterest) are most easily distinguished based upon their intensity. This would be used, for example, to select bright objects like the spinal column in the abdominal CT images or eliminate dark regions such as bowel gas. The display of extremal regions can also be constrained based upon the $(x, y)$ position of the annihilation point of the associated extremum

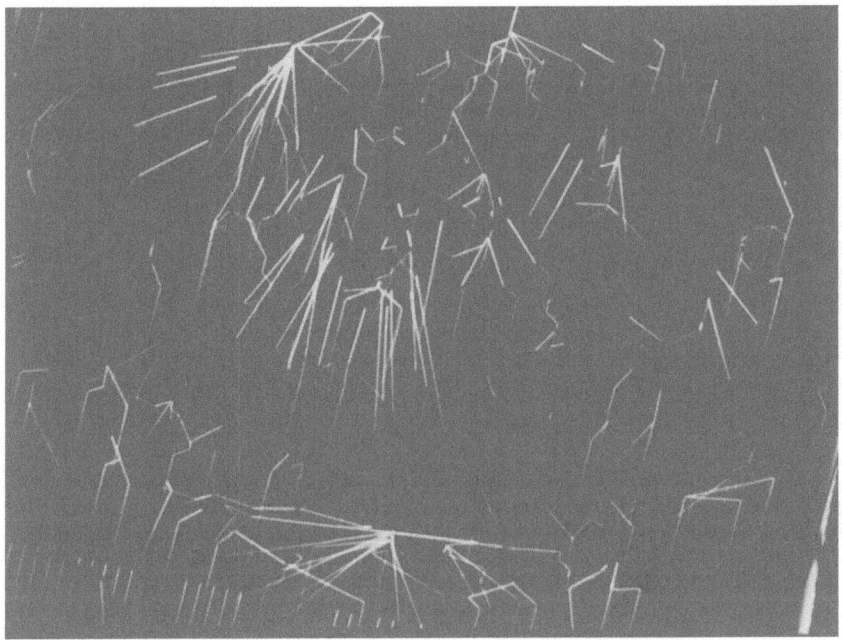

Figure 14: Paths of maxima and minima. Roughly half of these paths are minima and half maxima. The actual display is in color; this clearly differentiates between the two types.

path. Four knobs are used to specify the range of spatial locations (maximum and minimum $x$ and $y$ coordinates) within which extremum paths must annihilate in order to be candidates for display. The chosen extremum paths can also be highlighted on the Picture System 300 display for better visualization. Intensity and spatial windowing have not been used extensively. It is not yet clear how useful they will be in a production (e.g., clinical) setting.

There is a difficulty in displaying some of the lowest resolution (largest scale) structures in an image. This is easiest to explain by use of an example. The spinal column and its associated musculature are oftentimes the largest object in an abdominal CT scan. In this case an intensity maximum in the spinal column will become the extremum path in the image which lasts the longest under blurring. If this extremum path is picked with the light pen and its associated extremal region is displayed, the entire image appears. This is so because all pixels in the image eventually link up to the last remaining extremum path. There is no subtree which explicitly represents just the spinal column region. We have attempted to deal with this problem by providing more flexibility in the display mechanism. Entire regions associated with an extremum path do not have to be displayed. Subsections can be specified. Instead of following down all links from an extremum path, the user can specify that only links which join up before a certain blurring level be traversed. By picking this level low enough (high enough resolution), much of the image can be eliminated from the display. This often allows the isolation of the region of interest (e.g., the spinal column). The spinal region shown in Figure 15 was specified in this manner (Figure 18 is a schematic of organ positions in an abdominal CT scan). This method works since the true object of interest is usually spatially the closest to the extremum which forms the longest extremum path. As such, pixels in this region usually join the extremum path sooner than the other pixels in the image. Alternatively, if a resolution level is specified which is not as high as one used for the spinal region, the entire body in the CT image may be displayed without any of the surrounding image (e.g., the table the person is resting on).

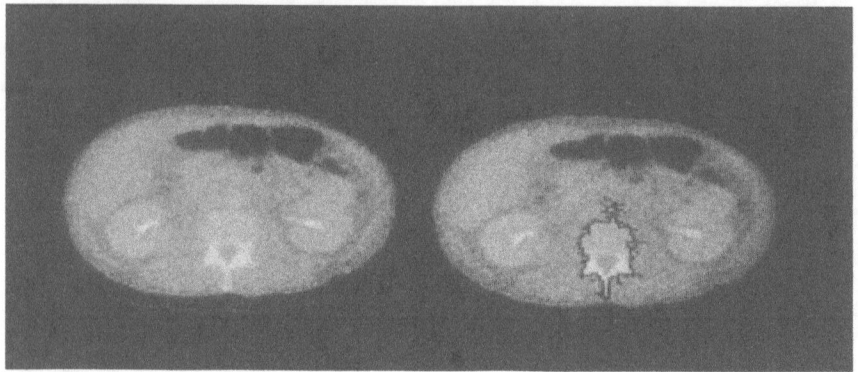

Figure 15. Left: Original image. Right: Spinal region. A 128 by 128 pixel noisy image created by adding Gaussian white noise with a mean of 0 and a standard deviation of 30 added to a CT image (which ranged in intensity from 0 to 1023).

Instead of displaying regions, the user has the option of displaying edges of regions superimposed over the original image. This is often useful since the interpretation of an isolated region displayed out of context can be difficult. Superimposing the edge of a region over the original image takes slightly more time than simply calculating the region itself. The time taken is highly variable depending upon the number of objects in the image, the number of objects specified to be displayed, and system load. The slower update rate does not significantly hamper interaction unless a large number of regions is specified.

Perhaps the most natural region specification method is via a cursor on the raster graphics console. By moving the puck on a data tablet, the user can position the cursor over a pixel in a region of interest (perhaps a pixel in the kidney). When a button on the puck is depressed, the smallest extremal region this pixel is in is displayed. Upon display, information about the region is shown on the user's terminal. This includes region size in pixels and average intensity of pixels in the region. The next larger extremal region is displayed when another button is pressed. Each successively larger region can be displayed until the root node of the entire tree is reached. This display method is the easiest to use, and will probably dovetail well with the future post-processing techniques.

Future Post-Processing Techniques

The difficulties with the algorithm as it stands now are:

1. A region of interest might not be precisely represented by an extremal region.

2. A region of interest does not always show up as one explicit subtree in the tree structure. It may be two subtrees with no common root except the last extremum.

An example of the first case might be an extremal region which includes the liver, but also includes part of the chest wall near the liver (see Figure 16). An example of the second type might be the kidney. Due to its shape, the two halves of the kidney may be represented as separate extremal regions. If the kidney is far enough from other organs, these two region

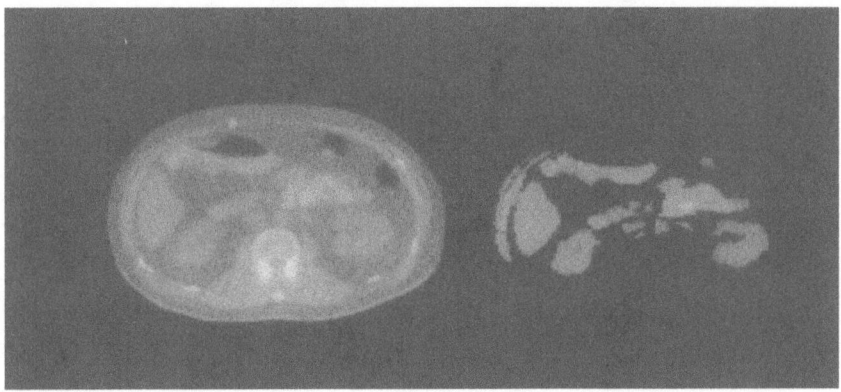

Figure 16. Left: Original image. Right: Segmented image. The liver and part of the chest wall are on the left side of the segmented image. The kidneys, intestine, pancreas, and a few blood vessels are also shown. A 128 by 128 pixel image.

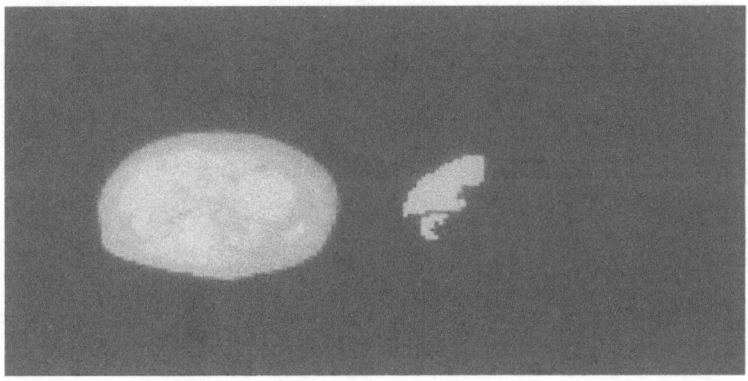

Figure 17: Left: Original image. Right: The liver and a piece of the kidney. The other piece of the kidney links to the liver at a higher level and is not shown. A 64 by 64 pixel image.

will join together (with one extremum path remaining) and be represented as one subtree. But proximity to the liver may cause each subtree to separately link to the liver extremum path instead of to each other (see Figure 17). If this is the case, there is no single subtree which will display just the kidney.

One way of dealing with these problems is to modify the basic stack algorithm. Various different blurring strategies based upon a priori and edge information seem promising (see section 4). An interactive post-processing step may be a simpler way to handle these difficulties.

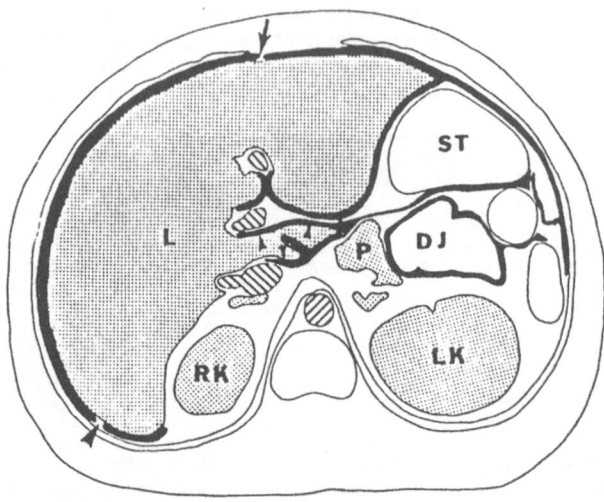

Figure 18: An anatomical model. RK-right kidney. LK-left kidney. L-liver. ST-stomach. P-pancreas. DJ-duodenojejunal flexure (part of the intestine). The white object in lower center is the spinal column. The cross-hatched region above it is the aorta. This figure is from Lee et al., (1983).

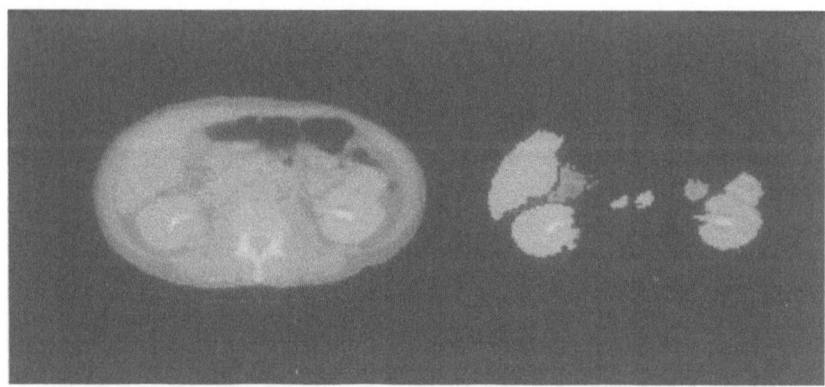

Figure 19: The kidneys, liver, and some blood vessels (the aorta and inferior vena cava, running perpendicular to the image plane near the center of the image). The dark region near the kidney and the liver is a part of the intestine, as is the region near the left kidney (right side of image). The region extending out from the top of the left kidney is a large tumor, as is the very small region extending out from the bottom right part of the right kidney. A 128 by 128 pixel image.

Various post-processing capabilities might be provided. A few of the most promising ones are discussed below.

Difficulties presented by the first case listed above could be mitigated by use of a simple pixel editor. This editor would allow use of the cursor to delete or add pixels to a region displayed on the console. If the region displayed is accurate except for a few pixels, it would be a simple matter to delete or add those pixels to the display. If desired, it would also be simple to actually change the corresponding links in the data structure so that the data structure remains in accord with the display.

Problems arising from the second case (multiple disconnected subtrees) could be minimized by building a simple graphical editor for the tree data structure which is displayed on the Picture System 300. Using the light pen as a dragging device, the branch representing

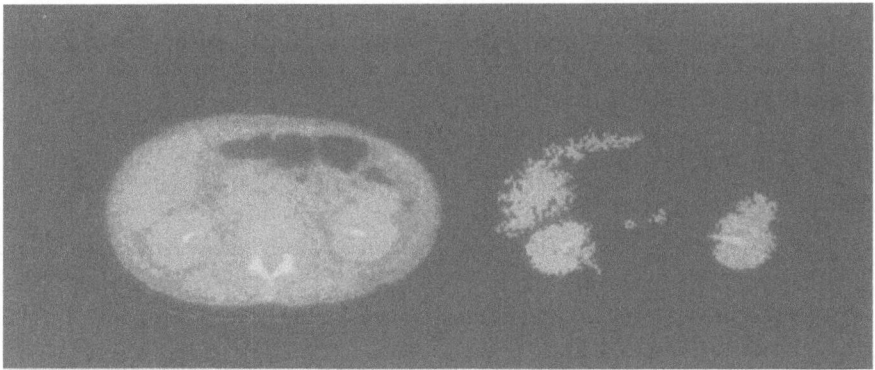

Figure 20: The kidneys, liver, aorta and inferior vena cava. This image is the image in Figure 19 with Gaussian white noise of mean 0 and standard deviation 30 added to it. The original image ranged in intensity from 0 to 1023.

one of the kidney subtrees could be picked and dragged over to the other subtree and graphically joined to it. This graphical operation could then be used to guide a similar change in the actual data structure. Alternatively, disconnected subtrees can be dealt with by finding connected regions in the displayed image (as opposed to in the data structure). Even if the kidney is represented as two subregions which do not link to each other in any way, the capability currently exists to display both subregions simultaneously. This is done by picking each subregion separately while specifying that the previously picked region remain on the display. Once the entire kidney is displayed, it would be a simple matter to automatically find all the pixels which are in the one connected region representing the kidney. As long as the pixels in the region of interest can be displayed on the console as a connected, isolated region, that region could be easily be defined to be one object and information about it calculated.

## Results

The results obtained so far have been encouraging. Many correct image segmentations have been produced. Figures 19 and 20 are two typical segmentation examples; the images on the left side of each photograph are the originals. CT scans are oriented so that the view presented is as if the viewer is standing at the foot of a table that the patient is lying on (face up), looking toward the patient's head. Thus the left side of the image is the right side of the person and the spinal column is towards the bottom of the image. High density objects (such as bone) show up as higher intensity (whiter) regions in the image. A schematic of the organ locations is shown in Figure 18. Which organs are actually present in a particular CT slice, and their size, depends upon the axial position of the slice and whether disease is present.

## Conclusions

Stack-based image segmentation correctly isolates anatomical structures in abdominal CT images. Both small vessels running perpendicular to the image plane and large organs are successfully identified in many instances. The inaccurate segmentations are frequently close enough to the desired result so that a simple interactive post-processing step might produce a correct segmentation. Post-processing is necessary because sometimes two nearby objects are represented as one extremal region, or a few pixels are missing from (or added to) a desired object. It remains to be seen whether a system with simple post-processing abilities will be accurate enough, often enough, to be employed on a routine basis.

The main problem remaining is the incorporation of additional, probably imprecise, knowledge about the image into the stack segmentation algorithm. The knowledge might be edge strengths from the image itself, or perhaps model-based information. The challenge is to use this information in a manner which produces a more accurate segmentation without forcing the result to mimic the input knowledge.

REFERENCES

Cohen, M. A. and Grossberg, S. (1984). Neural Dynamics of Brightness Perception: Features, Boundaries, Diffusion, and Resonance, Perception and Psychophysics, 36(5),428-456.

John, F. (1982). Partial Differential Equations, Springer-Verlag, New York.

Koenderink, J. J. (1984). The Structure of Images, Biological Cybernetics, 50,363-370.

Lee, J. K. T., Sagel, S. S., and Stanley, R. (1983). Computed Body Tomography, Raven Press, New York.

Lifshitz, L. M. (1987). Image Segmentation via Multiresolution Extrema Following, Dissertation, University of North Carolina at Chapel Hill.

Pizer, S. M. (1983). "Stack Sampling in the Resolution Direction", Personal notes, The University of North Carolina at Chapel Hill.

Pizer, S. M., Koenderink, J. J., Lifshitz, L. M., Helmink, L., and Kaasjager, A. D. J. (1986). An Image Description for Object Definition, based on Extremal Regions in the Stack, in: "Information Processing in Medical Imaging: Proceedings of the IXth International Conference on Image Processing in Medical Imaging, Washington, D.C., 1985,"S. L. Bacharach (ed.), Martinus Nijhoff , Boston.

Toet, L., Koenderink, J. J., deGraaf, C. N., and Zuidema, P. (1986). "The Treatment of Image Boundaries in the Case of Progressive Defocussing", Internal Report, The Department of Medical and Physiological Physics, The State University of Utrecht, Netherlands.

Zachmanoglou, E. C. and Thoe, D. W. (1976). Introduction to Partial Differential Equations with Applications, Williams and Wilkins Co., Baltimore.

# MULTIRESOLUTION SHAPE DESCRIPTIONS
# AND THEIR APPLICATIONS IN MEDICAL IMAGING

John M. Gauch*, William R. Oliver*†, Stephen M. Pizer*‡

Depts. of Computer Science*, Pathology†, and Radiology‡
University of North Carolina
Chapel Hill, NC, USA

## INTRODUCTION

The recognition of objects in medical images and the analysis of their properties in space and time requires a representation that reflects properties of shape. These representations are independent of position, orientation and size. They can be based on ad hoc features, object boundaries, object interiors (figures), or object deformations.

Our work is based on exploiting an inherent relationship between boundary and figure based shape descriptions. In both of these categories, noise and small image details often confound shape analysis. Therefore, it is essential to generate descriptions that are hierarchical by scale using multiresolution techniques. In the following we develop techniques of this kind which are applicable to shape description of both grey-scale images and binary objects. In the sequel we describe two applications which are based on these shape descriptions.

## GREY-SCALE IMAGE DESCRIPTION VIA LEVEL CURVES

Two dimensional grey-scale images can be viewed as a surface in three space defined by the graph $(x, y, I(x,y))$. One obvious way to describe the shape of such graphs is to use the tools of differential geometry to describe the surface. Another alternative is to describe the two regions of space separated by the surface.

Unfortunately, the intensity dimension is incommensurate with the spatial dimensions. There is no natural choice as to what intensity change is equivalent to what spatial distance. Shape descriptions which vary with a particular choice of equivalency must therefore be avoided. This can be accomplished by treating the intensity and spatial dimensions separately in our shape description. We do this by describing shape in terms of the level sets of the graph (see Figure 1).

The level sets for a two dimensional grey-scale image are the planar curves defined by $I(x,y) = C$, for all intensities in the image. These level sets act like boundaries. They partition each level into an inside and an outside. Specifically, the image surface is the union of its level sets at their respective intensity levels. The the volume below the surface is the union of all regions which have $I(x,y) \geq C$. Similarly, the volume above the image surface is the union of all regions where $I(x,y) \leq C$.

Thus, it is possible to represent the image surface and the regions on either side of the surface in terms of the level curves or regions defined by level curves. To describe

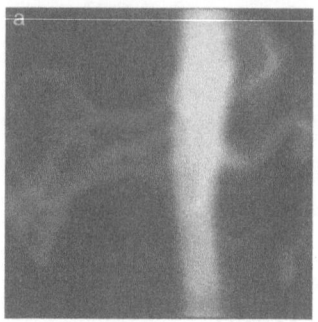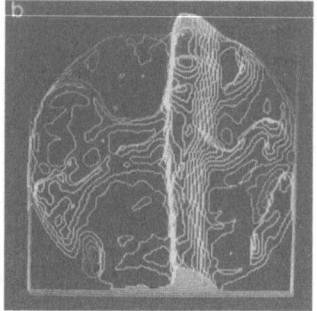

Figure 1. A digital subtraction angiogram and corresponding level sets.

the shape of these level curves we use existing figure based and boundary based shape descriptions for binary images.

## BASIC SHAPE DESCRIPTIONS

### Axes of Symmetry

We begin our analysis with figure based shape descriptions for two dimensional binary images. Object symmetry is a key to understanding shape. Circles are perfectly symmetrical, so the axes of symmetry defined by circles capture this property best. When the set of circles tangent to the object's boundary is considered, we derive axes of symmetry which describe the branching and bending of the object. Several methods use this approach.

Chords of tangent circles are used to define smoothed local symmetries (Brady and Asada, 1984). Arcs of tangent circles are used to define process inferred axes (Leyton, 1986). Centers of tangent circles are used to define the symmetric axis (Blum, 1974). The internal symmetric axis is defined by centers of tangent circles which are entirely within the object while the external symmetric axis is defined by centers of tangent circles which are outside the object. The global symmetric axis is defined by the centers of all tangent circles. When the radius of each of these circles is also considered, we have the symmetric axis transform (SAT) (Blum and Nagel, 1978).

The SAT has three attractive properties. First, the branching structure of the object is reflected by the branching of the axis. This yields a natural correspondence between components of the object and components of the shape description. Second, the bending and flaring of the object is reflected by changes in the curvature of the axis and the radius of the tangent circles. This gives us a way to compare and contrast similar shapes. Finally, this shape description is unique for an object and can be used to re-create the object.

One of the problems with the SAT is that it is very sensitive. Noise and small detail in the object can cause "unimportant" branches to appear in the axis. These confound shape analysis by introducing large numbers of axis segments and by breaking up main branches into numerous small sections. One solution is to use multiple resolution analysis to determine the scale of the individual components of the shape description. This approach yields the multiresolution symmetric axis described by (Pizer et al., 1986).

To compute this shape description requires that we measure the importance of each branch in the symmetric axis. As we lower the resolution the tendency is for an object to simplify, eventually becoming an ellipse. Because the symmetric axis varies smoothly with the figure it represents, the branching structure of the axis also simplifies as we lower the resolution. Thus, we can follow axis branches to annihilation through a multiple resolution sequence of binary images. The importance of each

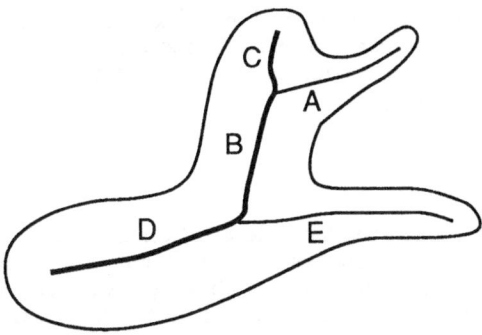

Figure 2. Branching hierarchy imposed on the symmetric axis by resolution reduction. When axis A annihilates it is labeled as a sub-branch of a new branch CB. Later, when axis E annihilates it is labeled as a sub-branch of the major axis CBD.

branch is then determined by its annihilation resolution. This process also imposes a hierarchy on axis branches (see Figure 2).

The order of annihilation of axis branches decomposes the SAT into limbs and twigs. When branch A annihilates two things happen. The adjacent branches C and B combine to form a single branch CB. Then branch A is labeled as a sub-object of this branch; much like a twig on a limb. When we do this for all axis branches, we obtain a description which reflects the shape of an object and also the hierarchy of sub-objects which make up the object. This multiresolution shape description can then be used to focus on image structure as a function of scale.

Now we return to the problem of obtaining a multiresolution sequence of binary images. The two alternatives we consider are boundary blurring and figure blurring. Both techniques yield acceptable results, but there can be problems. When boundary blurring is used, object topology is maintained but figural similarity is frequently not preserved. As a result, two shapes with different topologies may look similar at one scale yet look quite different at another scale (see Figure 3). This problem can be avoided by blurring the object figure.

When the characteristic function representing the object figure is blurred with a Gaussian, it gives us a grey-scale image. To obtain a binary image again requires an arbitrary selection of a level curve. To us, the most natural choice is to select the level curve which preserves the object's area, but all choices we know of can result in topological changes in the boundary. Thus, two objects may look similar at different resolutions yet have quite different topologies (see Figure 3). The problem of selecting a single level curve leads us to an important observation.

Binary images are a special case of grey-scale images; they are images which just have two values. As a consequence, binary images should be treated like grey-scale images. In particular, grey-scale shape descriptions should be applied to describe the

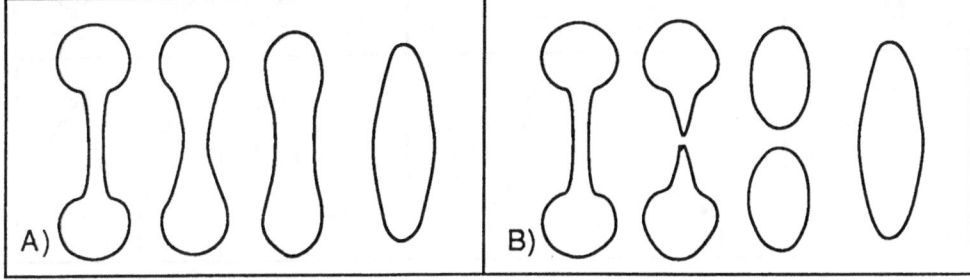

Figure 3. Three stages of a) boundary blurring and b) figure blurring. Notice the changes in topology in the object for figure blurring.

figure. To preserve causality under resolution reduction, Gaussian blurring of the intensities should be used to impose a resolution hierarchy (Koenderink, 1984). While this further motivates our investigation of grey-scale shape descriptions, we now return to level curve shape description.

## Boundary Curvature

The second major approach to shape description is based on boundary properties. Several researchers have focused on boundary curvature because it reflects the bending of the object, an essential aspect of shape (Brady and Asada, 1984). Extreme points of curvature (local maxima and minima) on the boundary can be used to characterize shapes.

If we decompose an object's boundary into sections bounded by two adjacent curvature minima, we obtain curve segments which (Richards and Hoffman, 1985) call codons. Each codon contains a single curvature maxima and can be classified into five types, depending on the signs of these curvature extrema (see Figure 4). By considering sections bounded by two adjacent curvature maxima, we obtain the codon duals described by (Leyton, 1986). These can be classified by simply changing the sign and type of each curvature extrema in our codon classification (see Figure 4).

Boundary curvature is also sensitive to image detail. As a result, two objects can appear quite similar yet have different codon decompositions. Conversely, objects can have the same codon decomposition yet appear quite different. To resolve this problem, we label each codon with a measure of its importance. At the same time, we impose a hierarchy on the codons which can be used to distinguish object shapes.

Under resolution reduction, the boundary will tend to simplify. This will cause two adjacent curvature extremum (a local maximum and a local minimum) to move together and annihilate into an inflection point. When this happens, the number of curvature extremum is decreased by two. Thus two adjacent codons become a single codon. The problem is to determine which codon annihilated into which.

Recall that a codon is a boundary segment bounded by two curvature minima with a curvature maxima somewhere between these points. When we have two adjacent codons, we have a sequence of five curvature extrema of the form: (1min, 2max, 3min, 4max, 5min), where codon A consists of (1min, 2max, 3min) and codon B consists of (3min, 4max, 5min). We say that codon A annihilates into codon B if 2max and 3min are blurred into an inflection point. Here, two of the three curvature extrema which comprise codon A have disappeared (see Figure 5). Similarly, we say that codon B annihilates into codon A when 3min and 4max are blurred together.

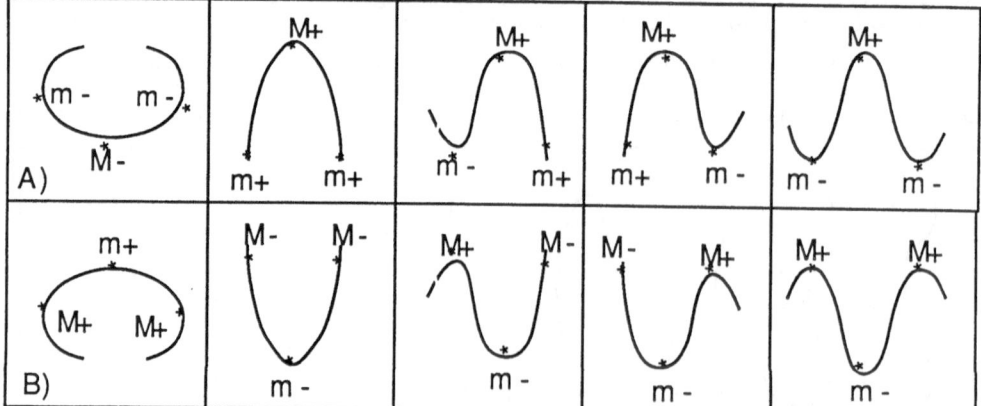

Figure 4. Boundary segments representing a) five types of codons and b) the five corresponding codon duals. The curvature extrema are labeled: M+ positive maxima, M- negative maxima, m+ positive minima, m- negative minima.

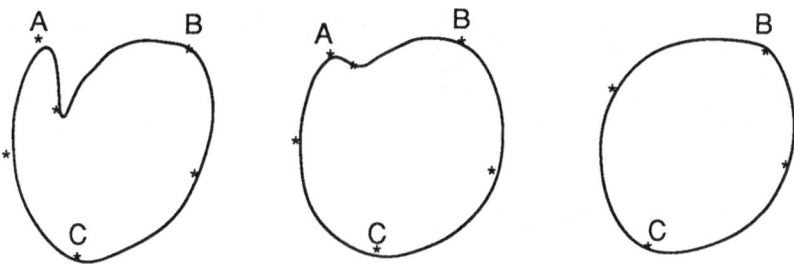

Figure 5. Codon annihilation under resolution reduction. Here codon A is determined to be a sub-object of codon B.

We record the level of resolution required to annihilate a codon as its scale. By also recording which codon blurred into which, we establish a codon hierarchy. This multiresolution shape description can then be used to focus on object curvature as a function of scale to compare and contrast objects.

Relationship Between Symmetric Axis and Boundary Curvature

Leyton has described an important relationship between these shape description methods. He has shown that each codon has associated with it a unique axis of symmetry and that this line terminates at or near the point of maximal curvature for the codon. Similarly, each codon dual has an symmetry line which terminates at a local curvature minima.

The type of symmetric axis associated with these boundary segments depends on the type and sign of the curvature extrema. Internal symmetric axes terminate at positive maxima, external symmetric axes terminate at negative minima, and global symmetric axes are associated with negative maxima and positive minima (see Figure 6).

This gives us a tool for studying the symmetric axis. Once we have decomposed the object boundary into codons (or at least located the curvature extrema), we know how many branch endpoints there are and also their locations. This information could be helpful for computing the SAT, but it is more important when we consider multiple resolution techniques.

We have seen that blurring imposes a scale based hierarchy on symmetric axis branches and on codons. If we recall the relationship between points of maximal curvature and axis endpoints, it is clear that these hierarchies are also related. The scale which causes the annihilation of an axis branch is equal to to the annihilation scale for the associated codon and vice versa.

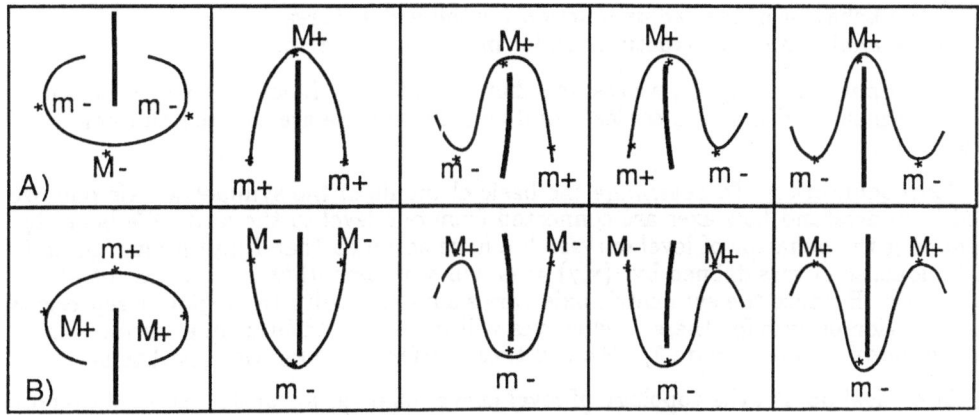

Figure 6. Relationship between the symmetric axis and a) five types of codons and b) the five types of codon duals. The axis is marked in bold.

We can use this fact to our advantage when computing these shape descriptions. Our work to date indicates that codons are easier to compute and follow through scale space than the symmetric axis. Thus, to compute the axis hierarchy we follow codons through multiple resolutions and use the correspondence between branches and codons to determine the scale of the components of the symmetric axis.

## GREY-SCALE SHAPE DESCRIPTION

Now we return to our main task, to describe the shape of grey-scale images. In the second section, we saw the need to treat the intensity and spatial dimensions separately when describing grey-scale images. This led us to an investigation of shape description methods for level curves in the third section. In the following section we bring these ideas together. This results in two methods to describe grey-scale shape in terms of the shape of individual level curves.

### Pile of Axes

First, we consider the behavior of axes of symmetry for the collection of level curves which represent a grey-scale image. To visualize this description, we embed this collection of axes in three dimensions at their respective intensity levels. This yields a figure based shape description we call the symmetric axis pile. When scale information is also recorded, we obtain the multiresolution symmetric axis pile.

What does this pile of axes describe? Because the level curves of the graph (x, y, I(x,y)) partition each level into an inside and an outside, we can describe two things. The volume below the image surface can be described by the internal symmetric axis for each level. Similarly, the volume above the image surface can be described by the external symmetric axis for each level. What do these volumes represent? Since image intensity corresponds to the height of the image surface, the volume below the image surface can be used to describe the shape of light structures in the image. The volume above the image surface can be used to describe the shape of dark of regions in the image.

One of the strengths of the symmetric axis is its ability to describe the shape of individual components of an object, and combine this information to describe the whole object. Naturally, we are interested in how our new shape description behaves in this respect. This requires us to focus on four aspects of our representation:
1) the basic elements of the symmetric axis pile,
2) the bending and branching behavior of these structures,
3) the behavior of the radius function for these structures,
4) the annihilation of structures under multiple resolutions.

To simplify our analysis, we assume that the intensity function I(x,y) is smooth and continuous and that the critical points on this surface are isolated and non-degenerate.

Axis Connection. To determine the basic elements of the symmetric axis pile, we need to understand how axes are connected from one level to the next. We begin by examining the behavior of level curves. We have assumed that I(x,y) is smooth and continuous, so curves defined by I(x,y) = C will vary smoothly with C, except at critical points. Because the symmetric axis varies smoothly with the region it represents, the collection of axes for these level curves will form smooth branching surfaces in three dimensions (see Figure 7). We call these surfaces symmetric axis sheets.

At critical points, the topology of level curves changes abruptly. At local extrema, level curves reduce to a point and then disappear (depending on the direction from which the extremum is approached). At saddle points, level curves come together, cross and then come apart again. The symmetric axis pile near these regions also

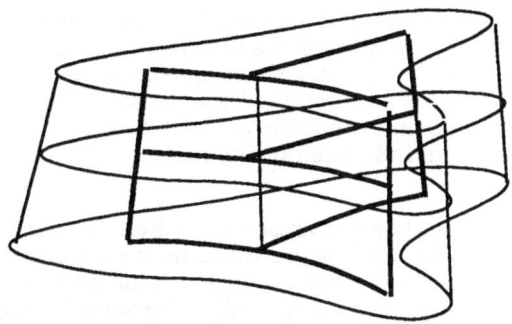

Figure 7. The level curves and corresponding symmetric axis pile for part of a synthetic grey-scale image. The shaded branching surfaces are called symmetric axis sheets.

changes abruptly. The remainder of this section investigates sheet behavior near critical points and the early indications of shape this behavior provides.

At a local maximum, the symmetric axis sheet for the region under the image surface shrinks with the level curve until it disappears at the critical point. The axis sheet above the surface near a local minimum behaves similarly. These points are called <u>sheet terminations</u> (see Figure 8). They are an indication of locally lightest or darkest spots in the image. The behavior of sheets on the opposite side of the image surface near these extremum is more complicated. Consider what happens to the symmetric axis for an object with a hole, as the hole gradually shrinks and then disappears. Initially, the axis for the object loops around the hole. This loop shrinks slightly as the hole shrinks, but suddenly disappears when the hole disappears. At the same time, a new piece of axis down the center of the object appears. This is exactly the situation we observe near local extremum in an image.

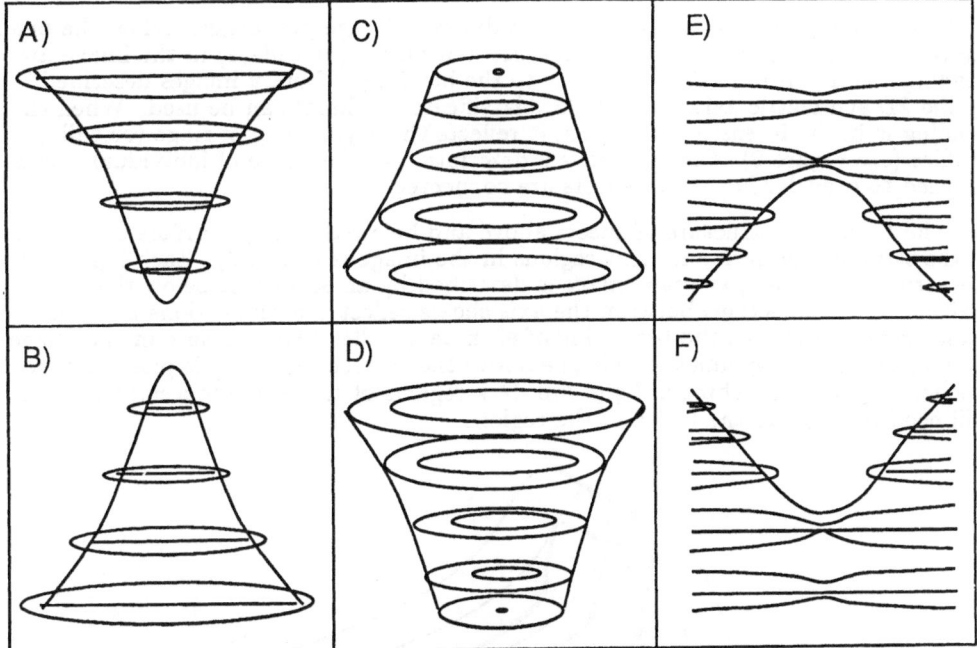

Figure 8. Symmetric axis behavior near critical points. Sheet terminations a) above and b) below the image surface. Loop terminations c) above and d) below the image surface. Axis tears e) above and f) below the image surface.

If we look at the symmetric axis just above a local minimum, we find that the symmetric axis sheet forms a loop around the indentation near the minimum, and that this loop disappears and another axis sheet appears as we move below the extremum. Similar axis behavior is also observed for the axis above the surface near a local maximum. These changes in symmetric axis sheets are called loop terminations (see Figure 8). They give us an indication of the nesting of dark regions within light regions and vice versa.

The level curves near a saddle point cross each other. If we calculate the symmetric axis pile for the region under the image surface near such crossing points, we find that the axis sheet separates into two pieces at the saddle point as we move up in intensity. These are called axis tears (see Figure 8). The same behavior is observed for the axis pile above the image surface except that the sheets tear apart as we go down in intensity. Thus, we call saddle points tear points of the symmetric axis. These points are special for two other reasons.

First, level curves through saddle points describe the nesting of hills and valleys in the image (Blicher, 1985). Thus, the axis sheets can be partitioned at these levels to obtain descriptions of local light and dark regions of the image. Second, saddle points are the only points in common to both axis piles, so they act as connection points between the axis pile below the surface and the axis pile above the surface. This adds coherence to our shape description which can be exploited to describe the relationship between local light and dark regions in the image.

Axis Bending and Branching. While critical point behavior yields a basic understanding of the relationships between light and dark regions in the image, additional information about the shape of these regions is conveyed by the branching and bending of symmetric axis sheets. How individual sheets bend gives us an indication of the shape of individual light and dark regions of the image. How these sheets combine to form branching surfaces captures the global branching structure of the image being described. By combining these shape properties, we can describe the general shape of the grey-scale image.

The bending of axis sheets reflect two different image properties. When the bending is in the spatial dimensions, it captures how ridges (or valleys) in the image are bending (see Figure 7). This is similar to the bending of binary images described by the 2D symmetric axis, so a similar classification scheme can be used. When the bending is in the intensity dimension, it reflects the asymmetry of ridge (or valley) profiles (see Figure 9). Once we have a description of the shape of individual sheets, we need to consider how these sheets are connected.

The branching structure of sheets above and below the image surface corresponds to the structure of dark and light regions in the image respectively. Each light ridge-like structure in the grey-scale image is described by an axis sheet below the image surface. The connections between the axis sheets reflect the connections between these ridges. Similarly, the branching of each dark valley-like structure in the image is described by the symmetric axis pile above the surface. While axis piles capture the bending and branching of light and dark regions of the image in a natural way, we still need to consider the width of the regions.

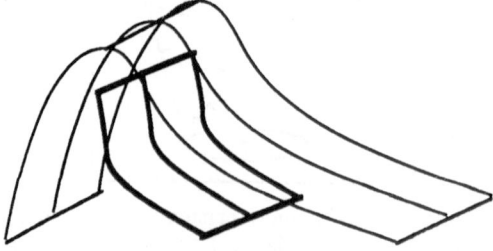

Figure 9. Asymmetry of ridge profiles reflected by axis bending.

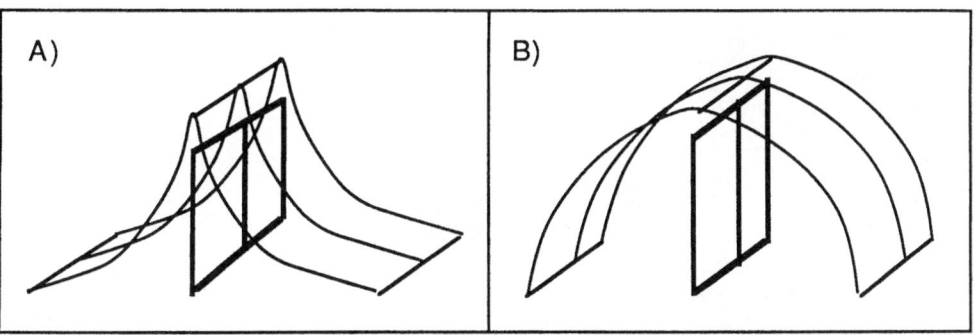

Figure 10. Roundness properties determined by second derivative behavior in the intensity direction. Second derivative is a) positive and b) negative for the ridge shown.

Axis Radius Function. Recall that each point on the 2D symmetric axis has associated with it the radius of the maximal circle at that point. This function is used to describe the widening and narrowing of individual axis branches. When this notion is extended to our symmetric axis pile, we have a radius function defined for each point on our axis pile which describes the width of the image at that point. Changes in the radius function along axis sheets gives us two indications of the shape of the grey-scale image.

Width changes in the spatial dimensions reflect the widening and narrowing of ridges and valleys. This happens when the first derivative of the radius function is positive and negative respectively. The second derivative behavior describes the flaring and cupping of ridges and valleys. The seven combinations of these derivative properties correspond to those described by Blum and Nagel for the radius function of the 2D symmetric axis.

The sharpness and roundness of ridges or valleys corresponds to width changes in the intensity dimension (see Figure 10). Consider the radius function as we go down the sheet for a ridge. Because the image surface is described by a function, the radius increases monotonically as we go down. Hence, the first derivative is always positive. When the second derivative is positive, the ridge appears sharp at the top, because it is flaring as we do down. Conversely, ridges which appear round have a negative second derivative; they are cupping as we go down. This analysis extends to valleys by considering the radius function as we go up the sheet corresponding to the valley.

When the shape properties provided by the radius function are combined with the other properties we have described, we obtain an overall description of the shape of a two dimensional grey-scale image at a single resolution. Next, we discuss the means of imposing a hierarchy on the symmetric axis sheets by multiresolution analysis.

Axis Hierarchy. The symmetric axis pile we have described captures many aspects of an image's shape. Unfortunately, as with the ordinary symmetric axis, it is too sensitive. Noise and small image details often produce "unimportant" axis sheets in our shape description. Our solution is to label each sheet with a measure of its importance and define a hierarchy on axis sheets. Then application programs can focus on image structure as a function of scale.

We determine the scale of axis sheets by continuously blurring the grey-scale image with a Gaussian and detecting the level of blurring required to cause each sheet to annihilate. After a small amount of blurring, the image structures corresponding to noise and small details will be annihilated. Because the symmetric axis pile varies smoothly with the region it represents, the axis sheets for these unimportant details will also disappear. Larger image structures persist and so do their corresponding axis sheets (see Figure 11). We continue this blurring until only one axis sheet remains (this occurs when the image becomes an elliptical blob). This process is also used to define a hierarchy on axis sheets.

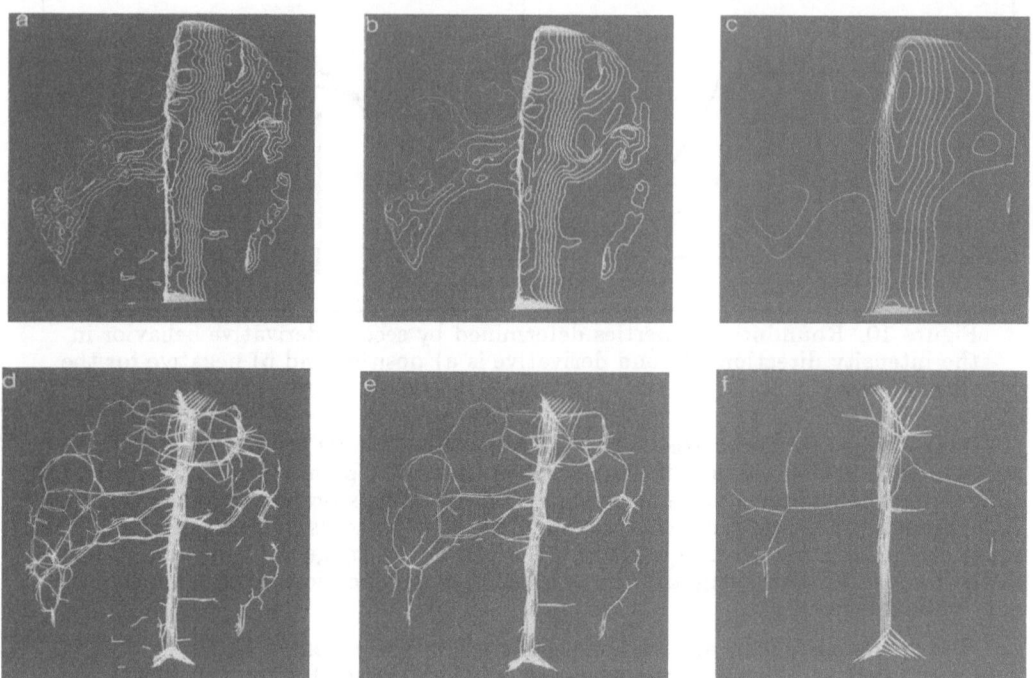

Figure 11. Level curves and corresponding symmetric axis piles for a digital subtraction angiogram reflecting three levels of blurring.

When one sheet blurs into another, the former sheet is defined to be a sub-object of the latter. When this is applied to every sheet in the pile, we obtain a hierarchical representation of the branching of axis sheets. While this hierarchical shape description yields a useful tool for studying an object's shape as a function of scale, it is difficult to compute because of the high dimensionality of the symmetric axis pile followed through scale space. To simplify this computational problem, we can exploit the relationship between axes of symmetry and boundary curvature.

<u>Vertex Curves</u>

We need to extend our analysis of boundary curvature to handle grey-scale images. To study curvature properties of the image surface, we extend our analysis of boundary curvature to all the level curves which represent the image. Again, we use the extreme points of boundary curvature (vertices) to characterize the image surface. By following the movement of vertices from one level curve to the next, we obtain curves on the image surface we call <u>vertex curves</u>. Since curvature extrema are the endpoints of codons, these curves define the boundaries of an image decomposition we call <u>codon districts</u>. Multiresolution analysis then yields an image representation which describes the spatial curvature properties of the image as a function of scale.

To understand the structure of vertex curves and the shape information they convey, we must examine the following:
   1) the connection of curvature extrema from one intensity level to the next,
   2) the branching of vertex curves,
   3) the surface partition defined by vertex curves,
   4) the behavior of vertex curves under multiple resolutions.

Again, we simplify our analysis by assuming that the intensity function is smooth and that critical points are isolated and non-degenerate.

<u>Connection of Curvature Extrema</u>. First, we investigate the behavior of curvature extrema. When the surface $(x, y, I(x,y))$ is smooth and continuous, the level curves

140

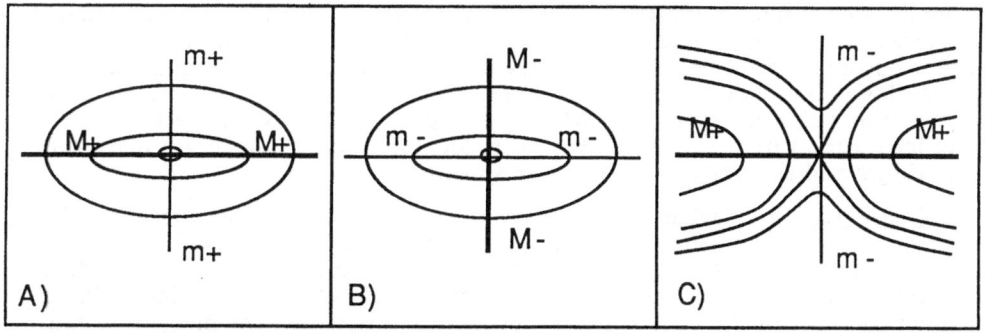

Figure 12. Vertex curve behavior near a) intensity maxima, b) intensity minima, and c) saddle points in an image.

defined by I(x,y) = C also vary smoothly, except at critical points. It follows that the curvature for these level curves will vary smoothly and that the points of local maximum and minimum curvature are connected and form curves on the image surface.

Since vertex curves are based on level curve behavior, they reflect the spatial curvature properties of the image. They tell us where the bending of level curves is most extreme. Vertex curves consisting of points which have positive maximal curvature correspond to tops of ridges in the image. Similarly, the bottoms of valleys in the image are marked by vertex curves consisting of negative curvature minima. The relationships among ridges and valleys are reflected in the branching structure of the vertex curves.

Branching of Vertex Curves. We begin our analysis of branching by considering vertex curve behavior near critical points (see Figure 12). At local intensity extrema, the topology of level curves changes. Slightly below a local intensity maxima, the level curve is generally elliptical. Thus, it contains four curvature extrema, two maxima and two minima. As we move up in intensity, the level curves shrink and these four vertices approach each other. At the local maximum, the level curve becomes a point and the four vertex curves defined by these points meet. Similarly, four vertex curves meet at each intensity minima in the image.

At saddle points, the topology of level curves also changes abruptly. The level curves at the saddle point cross while the level curves slightly above and below each saddle point are generally hyperbolic. Thus, we have two points of locally maximal curvature on the level curves above the critical point and two points of locally minimal curvature on the level curves below. As a result, four vertex curves meet at each saddle point in the image. Two curves of local curvature maxima go uphill and two curves of local curvature minima go downhill.

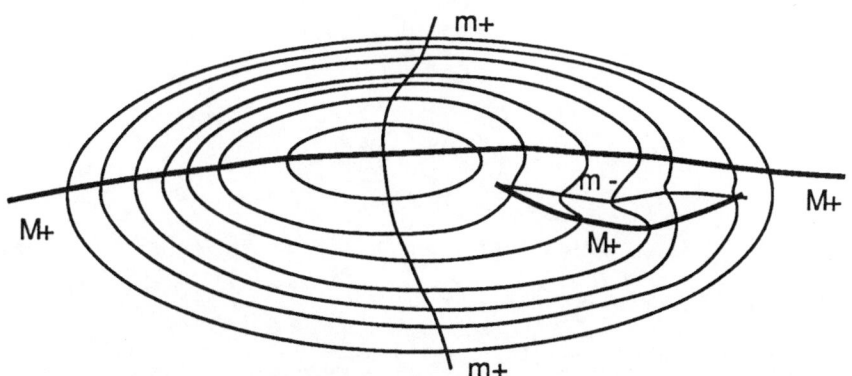

Figure 13. Vertex curve behavior near curvature inflection points. Here we have a small valley on the side of a hill whose extent is marked by two vertex curves.

141

Finally, we consider curvature inflection points on level curves. If we consider the level curves slightly above and below a level curve which has an inflection point, we find that one curve has two curvature extrema (one maxima and one minima) near the inflection point while the other has none. Thus, two vertex curves originate at each inflection point on the image surface (see Figure 13). Since one vertex curve consists of local curvature maxima and the other local minima, these curves mark the tops of ridges and the bottoms of valleys respectively.

Surface Partition. Marking ridge tops and valley bottoms vertex curves partition the image into regions which are similar to the slope districts described by (Nackman, 1984). Maxima vertex curves mark ridge tops much like the ridge lines which define watersheds. Similarly, minima vertex curves behave like course lines. Thus, vertex curves through the critical points in the image partition the image into hills and valleys. Vertex curves through inflection points reflect a different type of nesting of ridges and valleys.

Consider a small valley on a ridge side. In this case, a new maxima vertex curve marks the sub-ridge while the sub-valley is marked by a new minima vertex curve. The vertex curves defining this sub-region emerge at one curvature inflection point and disappear at another on the image surface (see Figure 13). Because these vertex curves do not pass through intensity extrema, this type of image structure would not be captured by slope districts. This is one of the advantages of our shape description.

More natural subdivision in terms of ridge areas and valley areas rather than sides of them is given in terms of the codon structure centered on vertex curves. These codon districts are each bounded by two vertex curves of the same type (either maxima or minima) and contain one vertex curve of the opposite type. This decomposition captures the extent of ridges and valleys in the image. Fundamental changes in the codon structure for level curves occur as we pass through saddle points. In particular, four minima vertex curves above the saddle point terminate at the level curve through the saddle point. Two new minima vertex curves start at the saddle point (see Figure 12). Hence, the topology change in the level curves at this point is reflected by the reduction of the number of level curve codons by two.

Multiresolution Analysis of Vertex Curves. The complexity of this new shape description and its sensitivity to small structures or noise can again be avoided by imposing a scale based hierarchy on the vertex curves and codon districts. Applications can then focus on the curvature properties of an image as a function of scale.

When we use Gaussian blurring to obtain a multiresolution sequence of grey-scale images, two things happen to simplify the image structure. First, the critical points of the image move together and annihilate in pairs (one saddle and one extremum).

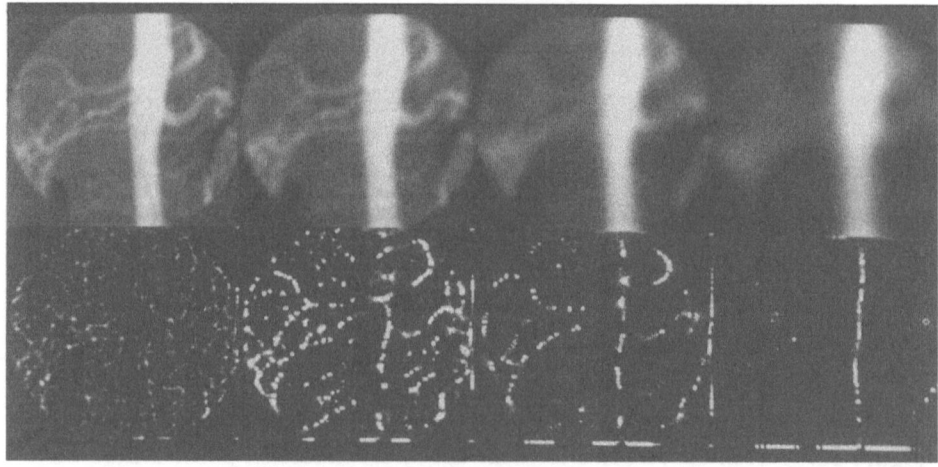

Figure 14. Images and corresponding vertex curves under blurring.

Second, the curvature of the surface is smoothed. Hence, the branching structure of vertex curves simplifies with blurring (see Figure 14).

While much work remains to categorize vertex curve behavior under blurring, it appears that the annihilation of vertex curves corresponds to the annihilation of branching structures in the image. This observation is explained by the relationship between our two grey-scale shape descriptions.

## Relationship Between Axis Piles and Vertex Curves

Both the symmetric axis pile and codon districts reflect the shape of grey-scale images on a level by level basis. For this reason, these methods retain the fundamental relationships between codons and axes of symmetry. In particular, each codon district has associated with it an axis sheet which terminates at or near the interior vertex curve. Thus, positive maxima vertex curves mark the ends of the branches of the symmetric axis pile under the image surface. Similarly, negative minima vertex curves mark the ends of branches above the image surface. The other vertex curves mark the extent of image surface associated with each axis branch.

As a result, this correspondence gives us a way to impose a scale based hierarchy on one description given the other. We have found that following the symmetric axis pile through scale space is a difficult task compared to computing surface curvature properties. It is our hope to calculate the annihilation scale of each axis branch by following the annihilation of the corresponding vertex curves. Then, the one to one correspondence between the original vertex curve segments and axis sheets can be used to derive the scale of axis sheets. Thus, we can compute the axis hierarchy.

Finally, this correspondence gives us two ways to look at the shape of an object. We can focus on the symmetric axis to get an understanding of the branching and bending of image components, or we can focus on the codon districts to partition the image surface into nested ridges and valleys. Both methods allow us to study the branching structure of ridge tops and valley bottoms.

# APPLICATIONS OF SHAPE DESCRIPTION METHODS

The two shape descriptions described in the previous section capture many aspects of grey-scale shape which can be exploited by computer vision applications. In this section we describe how these shape descriptions can be used to segment images and study the deformation of binary objects.

## Segmentation

Segmentation is the process of partitioning an image into "natural" regions. Lifshitz (Lifshitz, 1987) and others have shown that multiresolution analysis can be applied to obtain more successful segmentations than conventional techniques based on local pixel properties or measures of edge strength (Ballard and Brown, 1982).

Following Crowley (Crowley and Parker, 1984), we suggest that yet better segmentations can be obtained by taking image shape into account. Therefore, we propose to use our multiresolution shape descriptions as a tool for segmenting two dimensional images. These segmentation techniques hinge on our association of pixels to components of the shape description for these images. We begin with techniques to segment binary images and then extend these techniques to grey-scale images.

Binary Image Segmentation. To segment a binary image, we use the multiresolution symmetric axis. The association between pixels and segments is of prime importance. Consider a point on the symmetric axis. If we draw the maximal circle centered at that point, we define the region of the figure associated with that point of the axis. Extending this notion to a branch of the two dimensional symmetric axis, we find that the union of all maximal circles centered on the axis defines the region of the object associated with that axis segment.

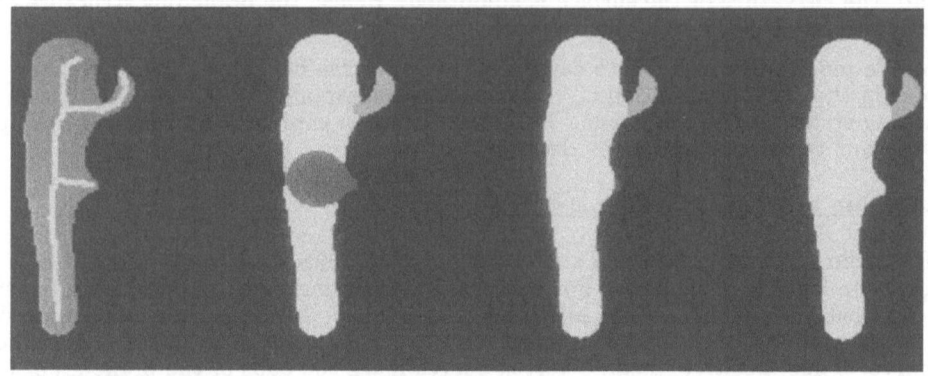

Figure 15. Symmetric axis for a binary object and three segmentations based on pixel associations to axis segments: a) pixels displayed as part of smallest scale axis, b) pixels displayed as largest scale axis, and c) small scale regions displayed as part of larger scale regions.

A problem with this technique is that axis regions can overlap. Pixels near branch points in the axis can be covered by several maximal circles. One solution is to use the scale of each symmetric axis component to determine which axis the point is associated with. There are several options here. We can associate pixels with the largest scale axis or the smallest scale axis of which it is a part. These result in quite different image segmentations (see Figure 15). When pixels are included as part of the largest scale axis to which they belong, the object is naturally decomposed into branches and sub-branches. When the pixels are associated with the smallest scale axis, we obtain a less natural decomposition because sub-branches subsume part of larger scale branches.

The axis hierarchy our shape description imposes can be used to segment the image into regions according to scale. Once a scale is specified, objects with smaller scales can be ignored or associated with the segment they belong to. We use the axis hierarchy to determine this relationship. In this way, pixels which reflect small image detail can be omitted or displayed as part of larger scale segments in a natural way (see Figure 15). This technique can be generalized to handle grey-scale images.

Grey-Scale Image Segmentation. The figure of a grey-scale object (the region above or below the image surface) can be segmented using the multiresolution symmetric axis pile. The key to this process is associating voxels in these regions with sheets of the symmetric axis pile. Extending the ideas from binary images, we define the region associated with an axis sheet to be the union of all maximal circles for all points on the sheet. To associate this volume with the original grey-scale image requires that we project this region in the intensity dimension onto the x-y plane and integrate its volume. This technique will give us a grey-scale image $R(x,y)$ which represents the region.

Just as the regions associated with branches in the two dimensional symmetric axis can overlap, we find that the volumes associated with axis sheets can also overlap. Again, we solve this problem by using the scale of axis sheets to associate voxels in the figure with only one axis sheet. Now, the sum of all volumes in our segmentation defines the figure of the grey-scale object. As a consequence, the sum of all region images $R(x,y)$ equals our original image $I(x,y)$. This is an important result. It gives us two novel ways to segment grey-scale images.

When voxels are associated with the largest scale axis sheet to which they belong, we obtain image segments which factor out small image details. When voxels are associated with the smallest scale axis sheet, the image decomposition looks less natural because small scale objects subsume larger scale objects. When the hierarchy on symmetric axis sheets is exploited, we can derive two segmentations based on scale. Objects below a specified scale can either be ignored or displayed as part of their parent objects. This approach is compelling because noise and small detail can be filtered ot or displayed as part of the larger scale objects.

## Deformation Analysis of Binary Images

A singularly interesting avenue of investigation in medical imaging is the question of shape deformation. While the diagnostic applicability of the extraction of shape data as vectors for structural or statistical pattern recognition and shape comparison are obvious, in many instances it would be illuminating to have tools to describe how one shape is transformed into another — the change from carcinoma in situ of the skin to invasive cancer, for instance, or the examination of developmental processes and abnormalities.

Examination of shape change as deformation was proposed in the biologic literature as early as the beginning of this century by Sir D'Arcy Thompson. Bookstein has described this deformation in terms of tensors, the "biorthogonal grid" (Bookstein, 1984, 1985, 1986). The applications of the statistical evaluation of shape change described in this manner have been elegantly demonstrated in such diverse systems as craniofacial growth and post-ischemic cardiac kinetics. Such applications are limited, however, in that the objects being evaluated must have recognizable landmarks, either inherent in the object itself (such as the anatomic landmarks of the skull) or imposed (as by surgical implantation of radiodense pellets onto the surface of the heart).

This is a severe limitation in areas of medical diagnosis which examine morphologic changes in soft tissues, such as anatomic pathology, because true or at least recognizable landmarks do not exist — there are no fins on a neoplastic gland. The application of the multiresolution symmetric axis transform may provide a method of allowing the investigator to use tools such as biorthogonal grid deformation analysis, however, by allowing the imposition of pseudo-landmarks based on the SAT.

As described previously, progressive blurring of any image allows the establishment of a hierarchy of SA limbs and twigs and in turn a hierarchy of vertex curves. In binary images, each vertex curve collapses into a point, the vertex, in the original unblurred image. Similarly each pile of SA branch points collapses into a single branch point. As a result, the hierarchy imposed can be taken to apply to the vertices and branch points. These landmarks may then provide shape-based, if not truly biologic landmarks that can serve as the requisite data for biorthogonal grid evaluation.

Inherent in the concept of a hierarchical object description is that the higher level descriptions contain both more important and more global information about the shape than the lower limbs and twigs of the hierarchy. Similarly, changes in the higher level landmarks provide relatively more information for deformation analysis. Of course, using only the highest levels of the SA provides an incomplete description of the shape deformation.

Transforming one symmetric axis into the other does not provide the true deformation, because the SA of the figure after deformation is not equal to the deformed SA. An iterative method of approximating the true shape deformation was recently suggested to us by Bookstein. This approach has the following steps:

1) Establish pseudo-landmarks in the original and deformed shapes by utilization of the hierarchical SAT.

2) Utilize the Bookstein method of geometric construction for the establishment of shape deformation tensors.

3) Perform the inverse of that deformation on the deformed shape to achieve a first approximation of the original shape. A deformation measure for boundary points which are not SAT derived landmarks is interpolated from the existing landmarks.

4) Calculate another SAT for the approximation of the original shape calculated in step 3. The difference between this SAT and the original SAT is used to measure object similarity.

5) Take as a new deformed shape the result of applying the approximate inverse deformation to the previous deformed shape. Repeat steps 1 – 4, and continue the process until the approximation converges.

The overall deformation is obtained by concatenating the series of SA-based deformations from the successive repetitions. An example of the application of this method is given in Figure 16.

Our continued work in this area will involve the following considerations:

1) Utilization of the first one or two levels of the hierarchy ignores the contribution of the lesser limbs of the SA to the deformation. While the lowest level twigs of the hierarchy may indeed be only noise, a way must be developed to integrate secondary information into the deformation analysis.

2) The current method of interpolation of deformation ignores that part of shape information carried by the width properties of the SA. For instance, shapes 1 and 2 in Figure 16 contain the same landmark data. A way must be found to integrate SA width properties into the iterative deformation algorithm.

3) Another possible complication with the hierarchical shape description method of imposing landmarks in a time series is a discontinuous change of hierarchy induced by a large shape change, e.g. when a previously dominant axis segment which would survive as part of a surviving limb decreased in importance, while a previously less important limb becomes dominant. Two answers immediately present themselves. The first is that in dealing with some processes, such as time series, the changes which occur between frames may be small enough to make the point moot. The second possibility is that in a given biologic system such as cell shape change, the change in the shape hierarchy may in fact reflect a concomitant change in the biologic importance of that portion of the cell, and that the change in hierarchical dominance is biologically appropriate.

We have currently investigated the iterative reverse deformation on only a few selected shapes, and need to pursue further experience to investigate whether the progressive approximation of shape features does, in fact, converge for an arbitrary figure.

In addition to providing a method of evaluating shape change, the SA also provides a convenient coordinate system for shape space. In a manner similar to that described for SA hierarchy-based segmentation, one may describe a location within the shape in terms of distance along the most dominant limb and distance along that radius of the tangent circle associated with the limb position which intersects the boundary. By use of the iterative inverse transformations, it is possible to describe the location of a subobject within a deformed shape in terms of the SA of the original shape. The description of subobject location in terms of the original SA provides a description of subobject movement which is invariant over shape change.

An application of this deformation analysis to a biologic process is the tracking of subobjects that move within the primary object while the primary object itself is undergoing a deformation. For instance, consider the subclass of white blood cells, the polymorphonuclear leukocyte, or neutrophil. The neutrophil is that cell which is concerned with finding and destroying various types of contaminants (bacteria, foreign bodies, senescent and dead somatic cells) within the body. As such, it is one of a small number of classes of cells which is capable of independent amoeboid movement within the body, and the ability of this cell to move in an appropriate manner is essential to its function in fighting disease. An organelle called the centriole is the origin of much of the cytoskeleton of the cell, and is thought to interact intimately, if not control, the dynamics of both cell movement and movement of organelles within the cell. As the cell moves or is otherwise activated, the centrioles themselves move within the cell. An understanding of the movement of the centrioles within the cells while the cell in turn is undergoing shape deformation may increase our understanding of cell motility. We plan to attempt to use the methods described above to examine the movement of the centrioles within the cell.

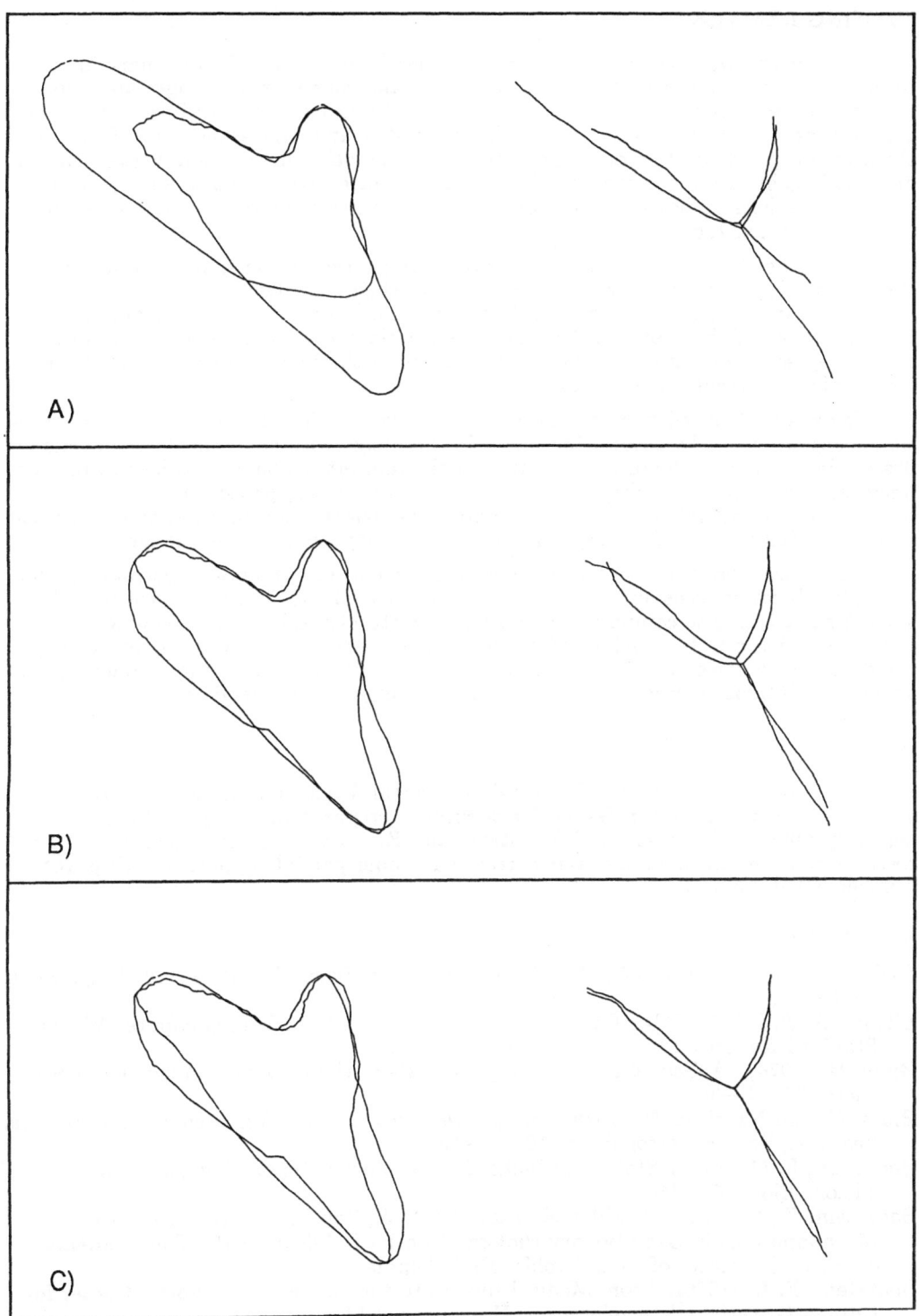

Figure 16. Deformation analysis based on pseudo-landmarks, a) original and deformed objects with corresponding symmetric axes, b) result after one iteration, c) result after convergence.

## CLOSING REMARKS

In summary, we have extended two shape description methods for binary images to describe grey-scale images hierarchically by scale. Since binary images are a special case of grey-scale images, these descriptions also describe binary images hierarchically by scale. One shape description, the symmetric axis pile, allows us to focus on the branching and bending of image structures. The other description, vertex curves, gives us insight into the curvature of the image surface. We have also demonstrated that the relationship between these methods can be exploited to obtain a powerful shape description tool.

We still need to analyze the behavior of vertex curves under multiple resolutions. We also need to complete our implementation of the symmetric axis pile, incorporating the hierarchy information provided by multiresolution vertex curves. Following the completion of this work for 2D images, we could extend these shape descriptions to 3D grey-scale images by studying the behavior of the higher dimension level surfaces which represent the 3D image.

We have prototyped two applications of the symmetric axis pile. Image segmentation is accomplished by associating pixels in the image with components of the shape description. Then the hierarchical nature of the representation is exploited to produce image segments based on shape and scale. We have also suggested how landmarks based on axis endpoints can be used to determine deformation maps. These can then be used to define a coordinate system for studying aspects of shape change.

Our future work will also address new applications of our shape descriptions. For example, object analysis applications could make use of the descriptive features of the symmetric axis pile to compare and contrast the structures of grey-scale objects. Object recognition could be facilitated by defining a metric on shape space (to measure the difference between two shapes) and using the scale based hierarchy defined by our shape descriptions to implement top down matching of object models.

## ACKNOWLEDGEMENTS

We are indebted to Fred L. Bookstein for useful discussions on deformation analysis. Many thanks to Susan Gauch for document preparation — a job which is deceptively difficult. We also thank Bo Strain and Karen Curran for photography. This research reported in this paper was carried out under partial support of NIH grant number R01-CA39060.

## REFERENCES

Ballard, D. H. and Brown, C. M. (1982). Computer Vision, Prentice Hall, Englewood Cliffs, NJ.

Blicher, A. P. (1985). Edge Detection and Geometric Methods in Computer Vision, Stanford Report STAN–CS–85–1041, 189–205.

Blum, H. (1974). A Geometry for Biology, Annals of the New York Academy of Sciences, 231, 19–30.

Blum, H. and Nagel, R. N. (1978). Shape Description using Weighted Symmetric Axis Features, Pattern Recognition, 10, 167–180.

Bookstein, F. (1984). A Statistical Method for Biological Shape Comparisons, J. Theor. Biol. 107,475-520.

Bookstein, F., Chernoff, B. Elder, R. Humphries, J., Smith, G., Stauss, R. (1985). Morphometrics in Evolutionary Biology. Special Publication 15. The Academy of Natural Sciences of Philadelphia, Philadelphia, PA.

Bookstein, F. L. (1986). From Medical Images to the Biometrics of Form, Center for Human Growth and Development, University of Michigan.

Brady, M. and Asada, H. (1984). Smoothed Local Symmetries and their Implementation, MIT AI memo 757.

Crowley, J. L. and Parker, A. C. (1984). A Representation for Shape Based on Peaks and Ridges in the Difference of Low-Pass Transform, IEEE PAMI, 6, No. 2, 156–170.

Koenderink, J. J. (1984). The Structure of Images, Biological Cybernetics, 50, 363–370.

Leyton, M. (1986). Smooth Processes on Shape, Draft Report, Harvard University.

Lifshitz, L. M. (1987). A Multiresolution Hierarchical Approach to Image Segmentation based on Intensity Extrema, Proceedings of the Xth IPMI International Conference, Plenum Publishing, New York.

Nackman, L. R. (1984). Two-Dimensional Critical Point Configuration Graphs, IEEE PAMI, 6, No. 4, 442–450.

Pizer, S. M., Oliver, W. R., Gauch, J. M., and Bloomberg, S. H. (1986). Hierarchical Figure-Based Shape Description For Medical Imaging, Chapel Hill Technical Report 86-026.

Richards, W. and Hoffman, D. D. (1985). Codon Constraints on Closed 2D Shapes, Computer Vision, Graphics, and Image Processing, 31, 265–281.

# APPLICATIONS OF STATISTICAL DECISION THEORY IN NUCLEAR MEDICINE

H.H. Barrett[1,2,3], J. N. Aarsvold[3], H. B. Barber[2], E. B. Cargill[1],
R. D. Fiete[1], T. S. Hickernell[1], T. D. Milster[4], K. J. Myers[5],
D. D. Patton[1,2], R. K. Rowe[1], R. H. Seacat, III[1], W. E. Smith[6], and
J. M. Woolfenden[2]

[1] Optical Sciences Center, University of Arizona, Tucson, AZ
[2] Dept. of Radiology University of Arizona, Tucson, AZ
[3] Program in Applied Mathematics, University of Arizona, Tucson, AZ
[4] IBM Corp., General Products Div., Tucson, AZ
[5] Corning Research Lab., Corning NY
[6] University of Erlangen-Nuremberg, Erlangen, W. Germany

## ABSTRACT

Over the last several years, Bayesian decision and estimation theory has become a central theme in the nuclear medicine research program at the University of Arizona. We have used concepts from this theory for image reconstruction, evaluation and optimization of imaging systems, position arithmetic in scintillation cameras, and in decision making in the operating room. In this paper, a brief review of Bayesian theory is given, followed by a survey of all of these applications, with emphasis on points of commonality among them.

## INTRODUCTION

Any experimental measurement yields random data since a repetition of the test will invariably give at least slightly different results. Medical diagnostic tests are certainly no exception. In a radiographic image, for example, the gray value at some pixel will fluctuate from image to image because of Poisson noise even if the patient and all other conditions are kept constant. Anatomic variations among patients with similar diseases often constitute a still greater source of variability. Thus a clinician is forced to make a diagnosis on the basis of uncertain data. Statistical decision theory is a formal and optimal approach to such decisions.

Included in statistical decision theory are the more specialized topics of signal detection theory, statistical pattern recognition and estimation theory. Signal detection theory arose from research on optimal radar receivers. In this problem, a known signal waveform is transmitted, reflected from a target, and received by a noisy receiver. The problem is thus basically to detect the presence of a known signal, but with unknown amplitude and arrival time, in the presence of noise. This problem has had a considerable influence on the field of medical imaging, where it is taken as at least a rough prototype for the detection of nodules in chest radiographs or metastatic lesions in liver scans. Much of the current research in the assessment of image quality in radiographic imaging is based on signal detection theory.

Pattern recognition is closely related to signal detection, though there is little recognition of the relationship in the literature. In both cases we are given a random data set and must *classify it into two or more categories*. In signal detection theory, the categories are signal-absent and signal-present, while in pattern recognition they may be more complicated, but as we shall see below this is not an essential difference. The more pertinent difference that seems to divide the two literatures is that the signal is well specified but buried in noise in the usual treatments of signal detection theory, while the "signal" itself, the pattern to be recognized, is quite variable in pattern recognition theory. Frequently no consideration is given to additional noise in the data. This dichotomy is unfortunate for two reasons. First, the problems are basically the same and should be treated in a common mathematical framework. Second, in radiology we are not justified in going to either extreme position. Our signals are not as precisely specified as a radar waveform, but we also cannot neglect Poisson fluctuations and other noise sources.

Estimation theory is the branch of statistical decision theory aimed at determining optimum values for numerical parameters. Examples from nuclear medicine include estimation of organ volumes, cardiac ejection fraction and uptake of iodine in the thyroid. SPECT image reconstruction is also an estimation problem where one wants to determine the activity in small volume elements or voxels. Less obvious examples of interest to our group include estimation of covariance matrices and image texture.

Though statistical decision theory is quite powerful, it is seldom used rigorously in the clinic. A major goal of our group at the University of Arizona is to bridge this gap and to make statistical decision theory a practical working tool in clinical nuclear medicine. This paper is both a brief review of the theory and a survey of those efforts.


REVIEW OF DECISION THEORY

General considerations

We begin with the assumption that scientific decisions are based on numbers. Of course, in our everyday lives we continually make decisions on information that we cannot or do not express as numbers, but medical and scientific decisions should have a more quantitative foundation. Even subjective observations ("The patient is jaundiced") can be expressed numerically ("How jaundiced, on a scale of 1 to 10?"). Thus we assume that our decision is based on a set of N numbers, which we can express as an N-dimensional "data vector" $\mathbf{g}$. (Boldface type denotes vectors throughout this paper.)

We further assume that the decision can be reduced to selecting one alternative or hypothesis from a specified set of M possibilities. In medical terms, we can diagnose the patient as either being normal or having one of M-1 possible diseases. If M=2, there are just two possible hypotheses (e.g., normal and abnormal), and we say the decision is binary. In the general case, we refer to an M-ary decision.

With these broad assumptions, the decision problem may be expressed as follows: Divide the N-dimensional data space into M regions such that when a data vector in the $m^{th}$ region is observed, hypothesis $H_m$ (m = 0,1,2,...,M-1) is chosen. An important special case is binary decisions with two simply connected regions. In this case a single scalar function $t(\mathbf{g})$ can be defined such that $t(\mathbf{g})=t_c$, where $t_c$ is a constant, is the equation of the boundary between the two regions. The decision task then reduces to calculating this scalar "test statistic" and comparing it to $t_c$ . If smaller values of $t(\mathbf{g})$ correspond to hypothesis $H_0$ and larger values to $H_1$, the decision rule is

$$\text{Choose } H_0 \text{ if } t(\mathbf{g}) < t_c ,$$
$$\text{Choose } H_1 \text{ if } t(\mathbf{g}) > t_c . \tag{1}$$

The test statistic $t(\mathbf{g})$ is thus a sufficient statistic for making the binary decision. The general M-ary decision task may be decomposed into a sequence of binary tasks, and at most M-1 test statistics are needed to partition the space into M simply connected regions. In the literature on pattern recognition, these test statistics are known as features, and the set of them is called a feature vector.

## Decision rules

The formulation above is very incomplete because it does not include any prescription for partitioning the data space into regions. All we have said so far is that, for the binary problem, we must calculate a scalar test statistic and compare it to a threshold; we have not specified how to define the test statistic or determine the threshold. There are three generic approaches to this problem: classical statistics, the likelihood principle, and Bayesian decision theory. For an excellent comparison of these approaches, see Berger (1985).

Classical statistics encompasses the familiar significance tests, such as $\chi^2$ or Student's t. More generally, it is the collection of statistical methods that do not involve formal consideration of prior information about the problem or the consequences of incorrect decisions. Classical methods are usually designed to test a null hypothesis $H_0$. All alternatives to $H_0$ are lumped into a hypothesis $H_1$, which is simply that $H_0$ is false. The decision problem is therefore binary, and it is based solely on the data g and knowledge of the statistics of g if $H_0$ is true. In other words, the data space is partitioned into two regions purely on the basis of the conditional probability density function $p(g|H_0)$, which is then the test statistic for this problem.

Methods based on the likelihood principle go one step further and consider the statistics of the data under alternative hypotheses. The decision is thus based on the set of probability density functions $p(g|H_m)$, $m = 0,1,...,M-1$. The quantity $p(g|H_m)$ is called the likelihood of the data under $H_m$, and the ratio of $p(g|H_m)/p(g|H_n)$ is the likelihood ratio for deciding between $H_m$ and $H_n$. In a pure likelihood test one simply selects the hypothesis with the greatest likelihood. For a binary problem (M=2), there is just one ratio to be considered, the likelihood ratio L defined by

$$L = \frac{p(g|H_1)}{p(g|H_0)} .$$

(2)

The binary likelihood test thus fits the paradigm of eq. (1), with the test statistic being L and the threshold being unity.

For M>2, there are M-1 likelihood ratios, which serve as the features for making the decision. Thus we have a direct way of extending the problem to M>2, but in any case we can make a more informed decision because we are considering the statistical behavior of the data under all possible hypotheses.

Still missing from our decision rule is any consideration of the probabilities of occurrence of the various hypotheses, for example the proportion of patients in our population who have a particular disease. These probabilities are referred to as prior probabilities or simply "priors" because they reflect what we know before acquiring the data g. Also missing is a consideration of the penalties for incorrect decisions. Bayesian methods bring in these missing ingredients.

## Bayesian decision-making

Consider the binary problem of deciding between $H_0$ and $H_1$, for example whether a disease is present ($H_1$) or absent ($H_0$). Since either $H_0$ or $H_1$ is true, the decision may be correct in two ways, namely if we select $H_1$ when the disease is in fact present or if we select $H_0$ when the disease is in fact absent. We refer to these outcomes as true positive (TP) and true negative (TN) decisions, respectively. Similarly, there are two possible incorrect decisions, choosing $H_1$ when disease is absent and choosing $H_0$ when disease is present. These are the false positive (FP) and false negative (FN) decisions, respectively.

We may assign a "cost" to each of these outcomes, perhaps on the basis of their influence on patient care, with negative costs for correct decisions and positive costs for incorrect ones. Let $C_{mn}$ be the cost of selecting hypothesis $H_m$ when $H_n$ is true. In the binary case the costs form a 2x2 matrix, and in general they form an MxM matrix. The Bayesian strategy is to minimize the "risk" or average cost, averaged over all possible decisions and all possible hypotheses.

For all forms of the cost matrix, the appropriate test statistic for a binary Bayesian decision is the likelihood ratio L defined above. Since L is independent of the costs and the prior probabilities of $H_0$ and $H_1$, the test statistic in all Bayesian tests is the same as in a likelihood test. The priors and the costs do, however, influence the choice of the threshold against which L must be compared to make a decision.

## Signal detection

Signal detection is a special case of a binary decision where the data vector $g$ is just random noise $n$ under $H_0$, while under $H_1$ there is also a specified (nonrandom) signal vector $s$ present:

$$H_0: g = n \qquad H_1: g = s + n . \tag{3}$$

We presume that the probability density functions for the data under the two hypotheses, $p(g|H_0)$ and $p(g|H_1)$, are known, so that we can form the likelihood ratio L. Often it is convenient to work with the logarithm of the likelihood ratio,

$$\lambda = \ln L , \tag{4}$$

where $\lambda$ is called the log-likelihood ratio. The optimal Bayesian decision rule is then:

Choose $H_1$ if $\lambda \geq \lambda_c$

Choose $H_0$ if $\lambda < \lambda_c$ , $\qquad\qquad\qquad$ (5)

where $\lambda_c = \ln L_c$ is the threshold value of $\lambda$.

If the noise is multivariate Gaussian, the probability density function $p(g|H_0)$ is completely specified by the covariance matrix K. If the data set consists of N measurements (pixels in the case of an image), then K is an NxN matrix. Furthermore, if the noise is independent of the signal, $p(g|H_1)$ is just a shifted version of $p(g|H_0)$ since the signal vector $s$ is not random. In this case, K is also the covariance matrix for $p(g|H_1)$ and the log-likelihood ratio is given by

$$\lambda = s^t K^{-1} g , \tag{6}$$

where the superscript t denotes the transpose of a vector. This form of the log-likelihood function is known as a "prewhitening matched filter". If the noise is stationary and spatially uncorrelated ("white"), then $K = \sigma^2 I$, where I is the identity matrix and $\sigma^2$ is the noise variance, and

$$\lambda = \frac{1}{\sigma^2} s^t g , \tag{7}$$

which is the usual matched filter. The expression $s^t g$ represents the scalar product of the two vectors, so the matched filter of eq. (7) may be implemented by multiplying the data point-by-point with the expected signal and summing. Equation (6), on the other hand, requires the additional step of matrix multiplication with $K^{-1}$ before forming the scalar product.

## Linear test statistics

Equations (6) and (7) show that the optimum test statistic, the log-likelihood function $\lambda$, is a linear function of the data in the problem of signal detection in Gaussian noise, but it must be emphasized that this linearity is the result of the assumption that the signal is nonrandom. Any uncertainty in the signal leads to a log-likelihood ratio that is a nonlinear function of the data (Barrett et al., 1986). In fact, a linear test statistic is almost never optimal in a Bayesian sense in real-world problems. Nevertheless there is a very large literature on them.

One reason for considering linear, and hence suboptimal, test statistics is that they are easy to implement. For electronic signal detection as in radar, the output of a linear filter sampled at a particular time is the linear test statistic. In pattern recognition the test statistics must be determined from a limited set of prototypical patterns (the "training set"), and it is difficult to get enough patterns to define complicated surfaces through the data space. Thus, so-called linear classifiers receive considerable attention in the literature on pattern recognition.

A less obvious reason for consideration of linear test statistics is that perhaps human observers are restricted to linear operations on the data. In other words, the human may make classification decisions by some sequence of matched-filtering operations. This conclusion is by no means firmly established, but some support for it is given by our results on the Hotelling trace criterion discussed below.

## Performance measures

We have presented above a general framework for making decisions. In the binary case the prescription is always to calculate a scalar test statistic and compare it to a threshold. Of course, not all of the decisions are correct since the data are noisy, and the threshold controls the trade-off between the two types of errors, false positives and false negatives. This trade-off is usually presented as a receiver operating characteristic (ROC) curve, which is a plot of the true positive fraction versus the false positive fraction. Although the full ROC curve is in general needed to describe this trade-off, useful summary measures or figures of merit (FOMs) such as the area under the curve or a detectability index d′ are often reported. The area under the curve is particularly useful since it is equal to the probability of making a correct decision in a two-alternative, forced-choice experiment. Other common FOMs are the accuracy, sensitivity and specificity, but they have the drawback of depending on the choice of decision threshold (i.e. on the operating point on the ROC curve). For more detail on ROC curves, see Swets and Pickett or Metz.

For the problem of signal detection in Gaussian noise, d′ and area under the ROC curve (AUC) are given by:

$$d'^2 = s^t K^{-1} s ,\tag{8}$$

$$AUC = \frac{1}{2} + \frac{1}{2} \mathrm{erf}(d'/2)\tag{9}$$

where erf(...) is the error function. Either of these FOMs is sufficient to determine the ROC curve in this case.

## REVIEW OF ESTIMATION THEORY

## Likelihood revisited

Suppose we wish to estimate the value of some scalar parameter $\theta$ on the basis of a data set $g$, and that we wish to report the results to three significant figures. This is really an M-ary decision problem with M=1000, namely we must decide which of the 1000 possible combinations of the three significant figures to report. A likelihood test is then to determine the probability density or likelihood $p(g|\theta)$ for each of the 1000 possible values of $\theta$ and report the value that gives the largest likelihood as the estimate of $\theta$. There is, of course, nothing magic about the choice of three significant figures, and we could as well regard $p(g|\theta)$ as a continuous function of $\theta$. The maximum-likelihood estimate of $\theta$ is then the value that maximizes $p(g|\theta)$ for the given $g$.

It is straightforward to extend this concept to multivariate estimation problems. If we wish to estimate the values of K parameters, we can express them as a K-dimensional vector $\mathbf{f}$. (The mnemonic is that $\mathbf{g}$ is the given or data vector, while $\mathbf{f}$ is the unknown parameter vector to be found.) The estimate of $\mathbf{f}$, denoted by $\hat{\mathbf{f}}$, is then the point in the K-dimensional space where the likelihood $p(\mathbf{g}|\mathbf{f})$ is maximum.

## Estimation errors

Because of errors in the data, $\hat{\mathbf{f}}$ will not exactly equal $\mathbf{f}$. Instead $\hat{\mathbf{f}}$ will be a random variable that will vary from repetition to repetition of the experiment, even if $\mathbf{f}$ is exactly the same each time. The average difference between $\mathbf{f}$ and $\hat{\mathbf{f}}$ is called the bias B:

$$B = <\mathbf{f}-\hat{\mathbf{f}}> , \tag{10}$$

where <...> denotes an average over the data $\mathbf{g}$. An estimate is called unbiased if B=0.

The variance of the estimate, $< |\mathbf{f}-\hat{\mathbf{f}}|^2 >$, is another important measure of the accuracy of the estimate. For any estimation rule, the variance can be no less than a fundamental limit known as the Cramer-Rao bound, expressions for which may be found in many standard texts (for example, Melsa and Cohn (1978), van Trees (1968), or Sakrison (1970)). An estimate that attains the Cramer-Rao bound is called efficient, though there is no guarantee that such an estimate exists. If an efficient estimate does exist, then it must be the maximum-likelihood estimate, which is one reason for the importance of this estimation rule.

## Bayesian estimation

The discussion above assumed that the data vector $\mathbf{g}$ was a random variable, but the parameter vector $\mathbf{f}$ was not. As in Bayesian decision theory, we can improve our estimates by recognizing that $\mathbf{f}$ itself may also vary and taking account of its prior probability density $p(\mathbf{f})$. To get an estimation rule in this case, we again define a cost $C(\mathbf{f},\hat{\mathbf{f}})$, which this time is a continuous function of both $\mathbf{f}$ and $\hat{\mathbf{f}}$. The Bayesian strategy is to minimize the risk R defined by

$$R = < C(\mathbf{f},\hat{\mathbf{f}}) > , \tag{11}$$

where now the average is with respect to two random vectors, $\mathbf{f}$ and $\mathbf{g}$. (Of course, $\hat{\mathbf{f}}$ is also random, but it depends only on $\mathbf{g}$, so a separate average is not required.)

Different forms of the cost functional lead to different Bayesian decision rules, two of which deserve attention here. The maximum a posteriori or MAP rule results from a cost functional that does not penalize very small errors, but assigns an equal cost to all errors exceeding some small value. Minimizing the risk in this case shows that the optimal estimator is the value of $\mathbf{f}$ that maximizes the posterior probability $p(\mathbf{f}|\mathbf{g})$, which is the probability density for the unknown $\mathbf{f}$ after we have collected the data $\mathbf{g}$. Application of Bayes' rule shows that MAP estimation is equivalent to maximizing $p(\mathbf{g}|\mathbf{f})p(\mathbf{f})$; it is therefore a weighted maximum-likelihood procedure that does not rely solely on the data as expressed in the likelihood, but rather weights it with the prior knowledge of $\mathbf{f}$. If the data are very noisy, the likelihood function $p(\mathbf{g}|\mathbf{f})$ is very broad and the maximum of the product $p(\mathbf{g}|\mathbf{f})p(\mathbf{f})$ will be determined mainly by the prior density $p(\mathbf{f})$. On the other hand, if the data are very precise, $p(\mathbf{g}|\mathbf{f})$ is a very sharply peaked function of $\mathbf{f}$ and the prior will be unimportant. We are then back to a maximum-likelihood procedure. Similarly, if the prior $p(\mathbf{f})$ is very broad, meaning that we do not have much prior information about $\mathbf{f}$, we again get a maximum-likelihood rule.

Another common cost functional for Bayesian estimation is the mean-square error, defined by

$$MSE = < |\mathbf{f}-\hat{\mathbf{f}}|^2 > , \tag{12}$$

where here again the average is over both $\mathbf{f}$ and $\mathbf{g}$. The estimation rule is clearly to select the $\mathbf{f}$ that minimizes this MSE, so the estimator is called an MMSE (minimum-MSE) estimator.

In general, Bayesian estimators are nonlinear functions of **g**, but there is one important exception to this statement. If both **f** and **g** are described by multivariate Gaussian densities, then the MMSE estimator turns out to be linear. That is, one can find a matrix, called the generalized Wiener filter, that relates the data vector **g** to **f̂**.

## Performance measures

Since the goal of Bayesian estimation is to minimize the risk, the only logical FOM for how well we have succeeded is the risk itself. For example, an MMSE estimator should be judged only by the MSE it attains. This metric is, however, often criticized on the grounds that it does not give proper weight to the important features of **f**. In medical image processing, for example, the MSE measures the agreement between the original object **f** and its image **f̂** averaged (in a mean-square sense) over all points in the image, all realizations of the noise, and all possible objects. An imaging system with a very small MSE could therefore completely miss small lesions because they do not occur in many objects and do not contribute much to the squared error when they do occur. The Bayesian would argue that this is simply because you have not chosen the correct cost functional, that you should have properly weighted the features you wanted to see. This does not really solve the problem, however, computational difficulties aside. The basic problem is that medical image processing is neither pure estimation nor pure decision. Ultimately what is desired is a diagnosis, perhaps only a single bit specifying whether the patient is sick or well. For the foreseeable future, however, this diagnosis will be made by a physician, not by a machine. The image processing or reconstruction problem is therefore aimed at providing the images that will be most useful for the physician. It is very much an open question whether a suitable cost function can be found to fit this problem into the mold of Bayesian estimation.

## APPLICATIONS OF DECISION THEORY

### Image quality and the ideal observer

Since considerable effort is expended to make better medical images, it is essential that we be able to define "better", but this is far from a trivial problem. Ultimately the best image is the one that leads to the best diagnosis or even the best care for the patient, but we do not yet know enough about the diagnostic process to predict these outcomes. Instead, many workers have suggested that we pose simple, prototypical tasks, such as detection of a disk signal in a uniform noise background, and ask how the ideal Bayesian observer would perform on this task. The Bayesian performance, as measured by d' or area under an ROC curve, is then taken as a measure of image quality. The idea is that a human will not perform as well as the ideal Bayesian observer, but perhaps at least the rank ordering of different imaging systems will be the same for the Bayesian and the human.

This approach is subject to several criticisms (Barrett et al., 1986). For one thing, the human falls short of the Bayesian ideal in several respects. It is now well established that human observers do not perform well in correlated noise. Myers et al. (1985), for example, have shown a dramatic reduction in human performance relative to the ideal observer when the noise is passed through certain high-pass filters, which introduce correlation. As noted above, the optimal test statistic for detection of a known signal in correlated Gaussian noise is the prewhitening matched filter of eq. (6), but it seems that the human cannot perform prewhitening, apparently using a test statistic like eq. (7) even when it is not optimal.

Even in uncorrelated or white noise, human observers do not attain the ideal level. These limitations are sometimes described as "observer efficiency" or "internal noise", but they have been investigated for only a few tasks, and their relevance to the assessment of the quality of clinical images is not clear.

Another serious objection to the ideal-observer approach is that the tasks considered are very stylized, and their relevance to the real clinical world is not obvious. Examining a chest radiograph for a nodule is definitely not the same task as trying to find a disk in a stationary noise field. One simple way to make this point is to note that the ideal observer would have perfect performance on the disk-detection task in the limit of an infinite number of photons, while no radiologist would claim to be able to detect every nodule in a chest radiograph if only the dose were large enough. Instead, the diagnostic task in this case is to separate the nodule from a confusing tangle of normal anatomical structures. In radar parlance, the limitation is the signal-to-clutter ratio, not the signal-to-noise ratio. The problem is more pattern recognition than signal detection.

Of course, there are some radiological tasks where noise is more important than clutter; detection of a cold nodule in a liver scan is perhaps an example. Then signal detection theory becomes a more relevant discipline. In most diagnostic tasks, however, it is not clear at the outset whether the main limitation is noise or clutter. What is needed is a synthesis of pattern recognition and signal detection. Our efforts in that direction are described in the next section.

## The Hotelling trace

Many treatments of pattern recognition are based on the so-called scatter matrices (see, for example, Fukunaga, 1972). Suppose we want to separate a set of objects into M classes on the basis of N measured features for each object. We can observe a training set of objects with known classification (supervised learning) and determine the mean feature vector and its covariance matrix for each of the classes. From these data we form two NxN matrices $S_1$ and $S_2$. The interclass scatter matrix $S_1$ is a measure of how widely separated the class means are, while the intraclass scatter matrix $S_2$ is just a weighted covariance matrix that gives the average spread of feature values in each class about the mean vector for that class. A useful scalar figure of merit, the Hotelling trace, can then be defined as

$$J = \text{Tr} \left( S_2^{-1} S_1 \right) , \tag{13}$$

where Tr denotes the trace (sum of the diagonal elements) of the matrix. The Hotelling trace has the desirable intuitive property that it gets larger as the class means become more widely separated (larger $S_1$) or when the individual classes cluster more tightly about their means (smaller $S_2$).

The Hotelling trace can be calculated for any features, including the original data vector **g** itself and linear or nonlinear functions of **g**. If, however, we restrict attention to linear transformations of **g**, then it can be shown that the optimum feature vector (the one that gives the largest J) is given by

$$h = B^t g , \tag{14}$$

where the matrix B is obtained by solving an eigenvalue problem:

$$S_2^{-1} S_1 B = B\Lambda , \tag{15}$$

with $\Lambda$ being a diagonal matrix of eigenvalues. The rank of B is M-1, where M is the number of classes. Thus for a binary decision problem, h is simply a scalar, which is a test statistic analogous to the log-likelihood ratio $\lambda$; it is, however, inferior to $\lambda$ in general since it is a linear function of the data while, as we have noted, $\lambda$ is usually nonlinear.

Though J is frequently used in the pattern-recognition literature as a figure of merit for features (see, for example, the excellent work of Insana et al. elsewhere in this volume), we are more interested in its use as a figure of merit for imaging systems. We assume the image can be described by a linear matrix equation of the form

$$g = Hf + n , \tag{16}$$

where the matrix H describes the system, **f** is the object being imaged, and the vector **n** is the noise in the image **g**. As in Bayesian estimation, the object is considered to be a random vector, and we may define scatter matrices and a Hotelling trace for both **f** and **g**.

Our basic suggestion is then to use the "Hotelling observer" in place of the ideal observer in assessing image quality. The best system is taken to be the one that yields the best classification when the Hotelling test statistic h is used. Classification performance for the Hotelling observer can be measured either by J itself or by d' or some similar metric derived from an ROC curve. This approach takes account of object variability or clutter through its use of the scatter matrices for **f**, yet it also includes noise since the scatter matrices for **g** depend on the covariance matrix of the noise **n**. It is not trivial to calculate J or h for realistic imagery, but we have developed an iterative procedure for doing so (Fiete et al., 1987).

Note that we are not proposing to actually use the Hotelling feature for automatic diagnosis, but rather to use it as a predictor of how well the human can perform. Thus it is crucial to establish that there is in fact a correlation between the performances of the human and Hotelling observers, and we have performed two rather extensive psychophysical studies with this goal.

We have previously reported the first study (Fiete et al., 1987) in which we generated 64 test objects crudely resembling a liver; 32 of the objects had a small, dark region simulating a cold nodule and 32 did not. Each of these objects was degraded by blurring it and adding noise, with nine combinations of blur width and noise level, so there were 576 images in all. These images were submitted to nine observers for psychophysical evaluation using the rating-scale method, and an ROC curve was derived for each level of noise and blur. The same images were used in a Hotelling analysis in which the test statistic h was compared to a sliding threshold to generate an ROC curve for the Hotelling observer. The human and Hotelling observers were compared on the basis of an ROC parameter $d_a$, which is similar to d'. Astonishingly good correlation was found (r=0.99), as shown in Fig. 1.

Encouraged by these earlier results, we have now performed a more realistic study based on the mathematical liver model described below. Again the task was to detect the presence of a cold nodule, but this time the images corresponded to different collimators that might be used for liver imaging. The simulations took account of normal variations in size and shape of the liver, variations in size, shape and location of the lesion, attenuation of the gamma rays, the intrinsic resolution of the detector and, of course, the resolution of the collimator. In sum, it was a very realistic simulation, and it was difficult to tell the resulting images from real, clinical liver scans.

The experimental protocol was the same as in the earlier study. Again a total of 576 images, 32 normals and 32 abnormals imaged through 9 different collimators, were presented to 9 human observers and also to the Hotelling observer. The results are shown in Fig. 1. Although not quite as high as in the earlier study, the correlation between human and Hotelling performance is still quite good (r=0.83).

Though the Hotelling feature h, being a linear function of the data, is inferior to the log-likelihood in classification performance, it does substantially better in predicting human performance (Fiete et al., 1987). We may speculate on this basis that the human observer is not able to use nonlinear test statistics, but further investigation would be required to establish this point.

### Bayesian decision-making in the operating room

We are developing a novel, hand-held radiation detector for use in intraoperative tumor localization. This probe, which we have designated the "dual probe," is actually two separate concentric detectors. The inner detector is most sensitive to the volume directly in front of it, while the outer detector is relatively insensitive to this central volume. Thus, if the dual probe is placed directly over a small tumor, the inner detector will receive counts from both the tumor and the background activity, while the outer detector will receive counts only from the background. A normalized difference between the two counts is then an ad hoc indicator of the presence of a tumor, but in the spirit of this paper we would like to find a Bayesian test statistic for this problem.

The data vector in this problem is two-dimensional, with the components being the counts in the inner and outer detectors, $C_i$ and $C_o$ , respectively. The likelihood ratio is thus

$$L = \frac{P(C_i, C_o | H_1)}{P(C_i, C_o | H_0)} ,$$

(17)

where $H_0$ denotes the null hypothesis that no tumor is present and $H_1$ denotes the alternative that a tumor of some size and activity is present. Note that we are using capital $P(..)$ here to

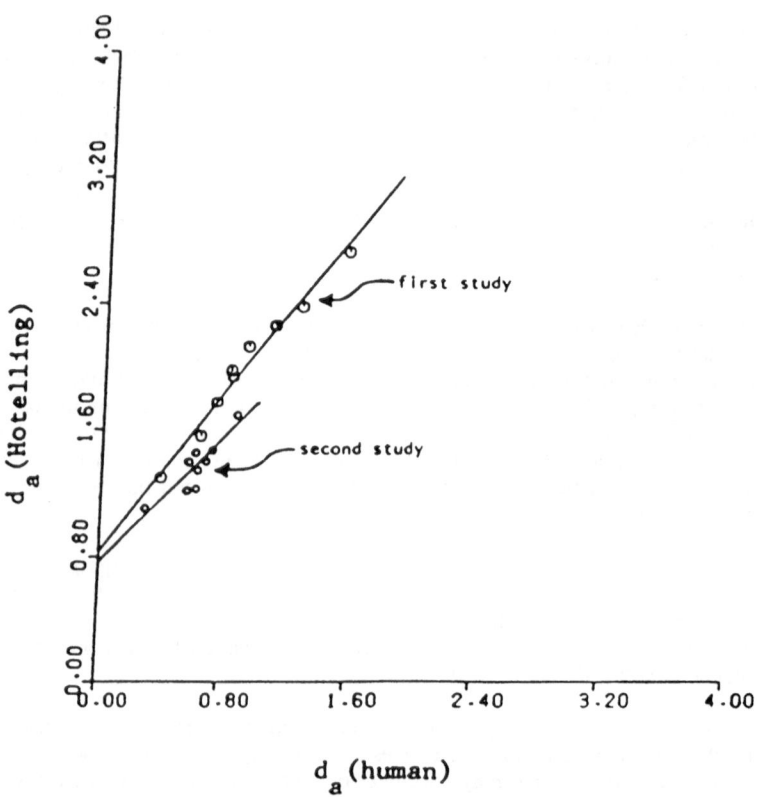

Fig. 1. Plot of $d_a$(Hotelling) versus $d_a$(human) with a linear fit to the data points. The correlation is 0.989 for the first study and 0.829 for the second study.

denote a probability, as opposed to $p(..)$ which signifies a probability density, since $C_i$ and $C_o$ are discrete random variables. The difficulty is in finding accurate expressions for these probabilities.

There are three primary sources of randomness in the data: Poisson counting statistics, normal anatomical variations in the configuration and activity of organs, and variations in size and activity of the tumor if one is present. For simplicity, let us assume that the tumors of interest are so small that they are "seen" only by the inner detector, in which case they are

160

fully specified by their activity A, a random variable with density p(A). There are many ways to specify the random character of the normal anatomical variations, but here we are concerned only with their effect on the measured counts $C_i$ and $C_0$, so we define two <u>mean</u> count rates $R_i$ and $R_0$. It is important to understand the sense in which the rates are means. If we make repeated measurements, each for an exposure time T, <u>over the same point on the body of the same patient</u>, then the mean value of $C_i$ will be $R_iT$, and similarly for $C_0$. If, however, we move about from point to point within the patient or from patient to patient, then these rates will vary. Even though they are means for purposes of describing the Poisson statistics at one point in one patient, they are nevertheless random variables. More formally, we may write

$$P(C_i,C_0|H_j) = \int_0^\infty dR_0 \int_0^\infty dR_i \int_0^\infty dA \; P(C_i,C_0|H_j,A,R_i,R_0) \; p(A) \; p(R_i,R_0) \; . \quad (18)$$

To reiterate the meaning of each factor is this equation, the conditional probability of $C_i$ and $C_0$, conditional on everything else, is the usual Poisson probability law, p(A) is the probability density on the tumor activity, and $p(R_i,R_0)$ describes the point-to-point and patient-to-patient variability in mean count rate, exclusive of Poisson statistics. To be able to apply a Bayesian decision rule, we must find reasonable expressions for these last two factors.

Since the density $p(R_i,R_0)$ would be very difficult to determine from first principles, our approach is to use mathematical modelling. We begin with a torso model derived from an atlas of cross-sectional anatomy, which represents a prototype organ configuration for one particular normal patient. The mean uptake for each organ of interest and the organ-to-organ covariance matrix is calculated from animal data, and this information is then used in a computer to simulate a large number of "normal patients" with the specified uptake statistics. These models are then used, along with measured spatial response characteristics of the probe, to generate an approximation to $p(R_i,R_0)$.

There are several possible approaches to finding p(A). One interesting one is to assume that tumors grow as the cube of their age $\tau$. This assumption is supported by a considerable body of experimental evidence for tumors without necrotic centers. If we assume that the tumor age is a random variable uniformly distributed from zero to some maximum value, then it is straightforward to show that

$$p(A) = \text{const} \; x \; A^{-2/3} \quad (19)$$

We now have all of the ingredients for determining the likelihood ratio and making optimal Bayesian decisions about the presence or absence of tumors. To summarize, the density for tumor activity follows from an assumed growth law, the normal anatomical variations are determined from a combination of mathematical modelling and animal data, and of course the Poisson law for counting statistics is well known. Some early results obtained in this way are shown in Fig. 2.

## APPLICATIONS OF ESTIMATION THEORY

### Modular scintillation cameras

We are developing a small, modular scintillation camera consisting of a 10x10 cm NaI crystal, a light guide, four 5cm square photomultipliers, 5-bit analog-to-digital converters for each photomultiplier, and digital electronics. Since each module is mechanically and electronically independent and easily replicated, this approach allows us to implement a variety of novel SPECT imaging geometries. For purposes of this paper, however, it affords a good opportunity to implement various aspects of estimation theory.

The data vector **g** has four components in this case, namely the digitized photomultiplier outputs, which we denote by A, B, C, and D. The quantity to be estimated is the position of each scintillation flash, given by its Cartesian coordinates x and y. The analog photomultiplier outputs are proportional to the number of photoelectrons generated by each light flash. To a good approximation, this number follows a Poisson law, which means that the digitized outputs are independent random variables. Thus the likelihood function factors as

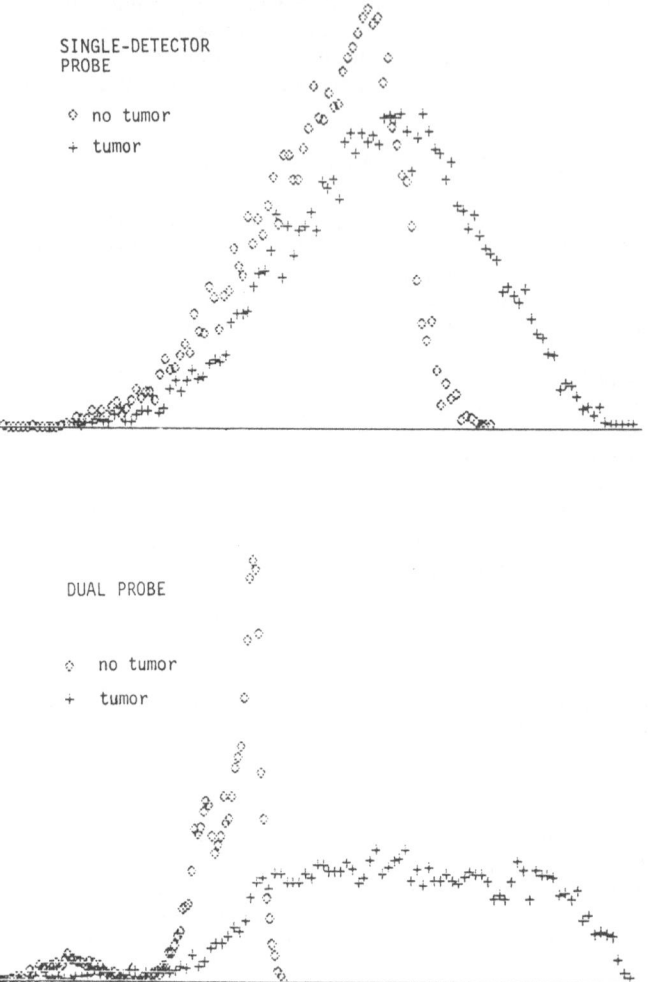

Fig. 2. Probability density functions for surgical probes. 2000 simulated patients were generated on the computer using our torso phantom and an organ-uptake covariance matrix derived from rabbit studies of cobalt-57 bleomycin. Half of the "patients" had simulated tumors and half were normal. We then used measured spatial response characteristics of the probes to determine the values of a certain test statistic for each probe at 14 sites in each patient. For the single probe this statistic was simply the actual counts in the probe minus the counts in the same time at a nearby point. For the dual probe the test statistic was a normalized difference between the counts in the inner and outer detectors. The upper graph shows histograms of the values of the test statistic for the single probe for patients with and without tumor. Note that there is substantial overlap between these two histograms, so the single probe is rather ineffective in determining the presence of tumor. The lower graph shows the corresponding histograms for the dual probe. Here there is considerably less overlap, demonstrating that the dual probe is far more effective than the single one.

$$P(A,B,C,D|x,y) = P(A|x,y)P(B|x,y)P(C|x,y)P(D|x,y) \ . \tag{20}$$

Each of the factors in this expression is fully determined (within the Poisson approximation) by knowledge of the mean number of photoelectrons generated in the tube by a flash at position x,y. We refer to this function as the mean detector response function (MDRF); for tube A it is denoted by $\bar{a}$, and similarly for tubes B, C, and D. Thus

$$P(A|x,y) = P(A|\bar{a}(x,y)) \ . \tag{21}$$

Note that this expression is not itself a Poisson law because of the coarse digitization (5 bits), but it may be readily calculated from the Poisson law.

It is now straightforward to compute the maximum-likelihood estimator of x and y for all possible combinations of A, B, C, and D; we simply find the values of x and y that maximize the product in eq. (20) by searching a 64x64 grid of xy points. The results are tabulated in a look-up table indexed by ABCD. Since each output is digitized to 5 bits, there are $2^{20}$ locations in this table. In operation, each flash generates an ABCD, and the corresponding xy is quickly fetched from the look-up table.

This approach works very well in practice. The estimator turns out, so far as we can tell, to be both unbiased and efficient (which means that the camera has good spatial linearity and resolution), though neither of these attributes could have been guaranteed in advance. There does not seem to be any advantage to other estimators for this problem. The MAP estimator is equivalent to maximum likelihood since we have no prior information about the locations of the flashes. The MMSE estimator is not mathematically equivalent, but it gives images almost indistinguishable from those obtained with maximum likelihood.

## Organ modelling

Our program involves the generation of a large number of carefully controlled images for system evaluation and psychophysical studies. This task is not practical, for several reasons, if the images have to be generated on actual imaging systems. For one thing, realistic imagery would require the existence of a large number of phantoms, since repeated images of the same object does not mimic the clinical situation well. It is difficult to build even one phantom that has any resemblance to clinical reality. For another thing, we want to simulate systems that have never been built, or even cannot be built, so that we can understand the fundamental limits of radionuclide imaging. Therefore we are using mathematical modelling or "mathematical phantoms" as an attractive alternative to plastic ones.

Two mathematical organ models are now being used routinely in our group, the torso model mentioned above and a liver model. The liver model was constructed by first tracing a prototype normal liver outline from a CT atlas and then fitting the outline to a series of spherical harmonics. A set of normal anatomical variants was generated by systematically varying the coefficients in this series, and the outlines were then filled in with activity, including tumors, fine structure and other pathology. Images generated from these models include the effects of attenuation, scatter, collimator or aperture blur, intrinsic camera resolution, and image processing. The most important application of the liver model to date was in the psychophysical validation of the Hotelling trace, but it is currently being used in a study to define the optimum collimator for rotating-camera SPECT.

## Image texture

In the course of developing the liver phantom, a question arose as to how to model the fine structure or "texture" of the liver. Since texture is often well characterized by the Fourier power spectrum of the image, we measured this quantity on 70 consecutive radiocolloid liver scans. In every case we found that the power spectra were excellent straight lines (r>0.99) when plotted on log-log paper (Fig. 3). This behavior is characteristic of fractal objects, and the slope on these plots is related to the fractal dimension. (For an exposition of fractals, see Mandelbrot, 1983 or Pietronero, 1986.) Furthermore, the fractal dimension is significantly different between normal and abnormal livers (32 well confirmed cases, t-test, p<0.001). When fractal dimension alone is used to separate normal and abnormal livers, the

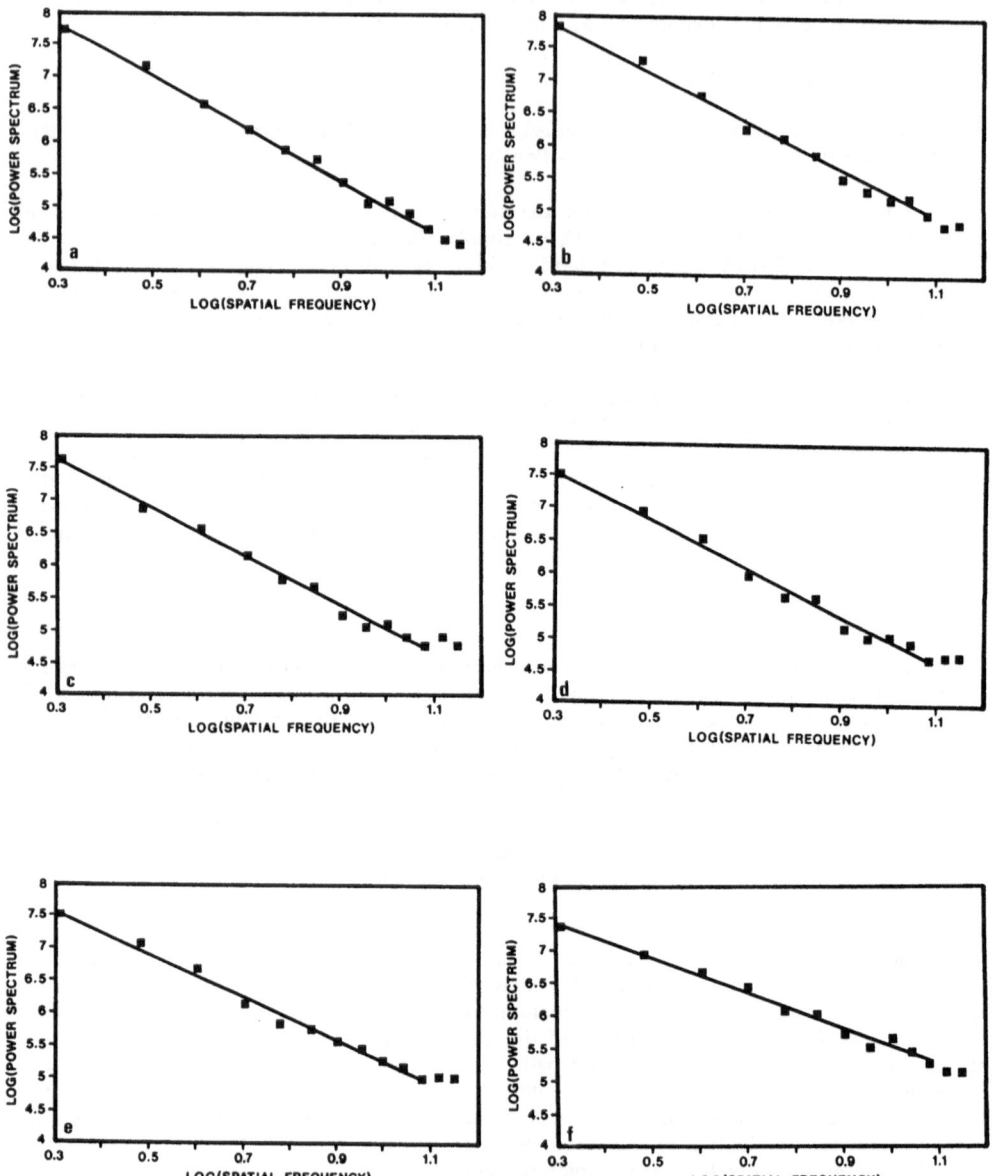

Fig. 3. Representative Fourier power spectra of radiocolloid liver scans, plotted on log-log paper. A straight line on this kind of plot, which we have found on all 70 liver scans we have plotted, is characteristic of fractal objects, and the slope is related to the fractal dimension. (a) normal liver, slope = -3.95; (b) normal liver, slope = -3.82; (c) diffuse disease, slope = -3.72; (d) diffuse disease, slope = -3.69; (e) metastatic disease, slope = -.3.34; (f) metastatic disease, slope = -2.90.

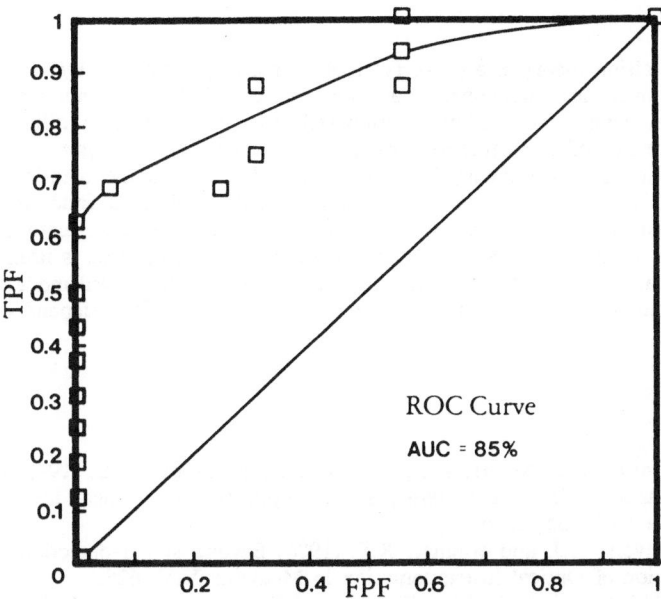

Fig. 4. Receiver operating characteristic (ROC) curve for liver diagnosis on the basis of fractal dimension alone. The slope of a log-log plot such as Fig. 3 was calculated for 32 well confirmed radiocolloid liver scans, 16 normal and 16 abnormal. Because of the limited number of abnormal cases, no attempt was made to distinguish different disease types, though we did notice that metastatic livers tended to have smaller slopes than those with diffuse disease. The slopes were conpared to various thresholds to generate the true positive fraction (TPF) and false positive fraction (FPF) for the different points on the ROC curve; no human observers were involved. The area under the ROC curve is a measure of how effective the test is. This area would be 1.0 for a perfect test and 0.5 for a worthless test. Here it is 0.85.

objects, and the slope on these plots is related to the fractal dimension. (For an exposition of fractals, see Mandelbrot, 1983 or Pietronero, 1986.) Furthermore, the fractal dimension is significantly different between normal and abnormal livers (32 well confirmed cases, t-test, $p<0.001$). When fractal dimension alone is used to separate normal and abnormal livers, the area under the resulting ROC curve is 0.85 (Fig. 4). To make matters even more interesting, we find that we can measure the fractal dimension with an accuracy of 1% with just 5000 counts, which is 1% of the usual number of counts in a liver scan. It remains to be seen whether fractal dimension can distinguish different abnormalities, such as cirrhosis vs. multifocal metastases, but at least it is a very good indicator of the presence of some disease.

Image reconstruction

Image reconstruction from projections is perhaps the most celebrated estimation problem in the radiological literature. For a detailed review of Bayesian approaches to this problem, see Hanson (1987).

## Conclusions

Bayesian decision theory is a powerful tool in many application. We have found it particularly useful in nuclear medicine, where we have used it for assessment of the quality of imaging systems, pattern recognition, position estimation in modular scintillation cameras, intraoperative detection of small tumors, image reconstruction, and analysis of image texture. In all of these applications, a unifying theme is likelihood. The likelihood ratio is the appropriate test statistic for all binary Bayesian decisions, and the likelihood function is the starting point for Bayesian estimation. A key difficulty in applying Bayesian methods is knowing accurately what the likelihood is in a particular problem. Indeed, this is itself an estimation problem, one that we approach through heavy reliance on mathematical modelling. Ultimately the success of our applications of Bayesian principles will, therefore, depend on the accuracy of our models.

## REFERENCES

Barrett, H.H., Smith, W.E., Myers, K.J., Milster, T.D., and Fiete, R.D. (1985) Quantifying the performance of imaging systems, SPIE, Application of Optical Instrumentation in Medicine XIII, 535, 65-69.

Barrett, H.H., Myers, K.J. and Wagner, R.F. (1986) Beyond signal-detection theory, SPIE, Application of Optical Instrumentation in Medicine XIV, 626.

Berger, J.O., 1985, Satistical Decision Theory and Bayesian Analysis, 2nd Ed., Springer-Verlag, New York.

Fiete, R.D., Barrett, H.H., Smith, W.E., and Myers, K.J. (1987) Hotelling trace criterion and its correlation with human-observer performance," J. Opt. Soc. Am. A, 4, 5.

Fukunaga, K. (1972) Introduction to Statistical Pattern Recognition, Academic Press, New York.

Hanson, K.M. (1987) "Bayesian and related methods in image reconstruction from incomplete data", in "Image Recovery: Theory and Applications", H. Stark, ed., Academic Press.

Melsa, J.L. and Cohn, D.L. (1978) in "Decision and Estimation Theory", McGraw-Hill, New York.

Metz, C.E. (1978) Basic principles of ROC analysis, Sem. Nucl. Med., 8, 283-298.

Myers, K.J., Barrett, H.H., Borgstrom, M.C., Patton, D.D., and Seeley, G.W. (1985) Effect of noise correlation on detectability of disk signals in medical imaging, J. Opt. Soc. Am. A., 2, 1752-1759.

Sakrison, D.J. (1970) Notes on Analog Communication, G.L. Turin, Ed., Van Nostrand Reinhold Company, New York.

Swets, J.A., and Pickett, R.M. (1982) Evaluation of Diagnostic Systems, Academic Press, New York.

Van Trees, H.L. (1968) Detection, Estimation, and Modulation Theory, Vols. I, II, and III, John Wiley, New York.

# Image Reconstruction and Restoration

# NEW TECHNIQUES FOR TRULY THREE-DIMENSIONAL IMAGE RECONSTRUCTION

M. Defrise

Division of Nuclear Medicine
Akademisch Ziekenhuis, VUB
Brussels, Belgium

R. Clack

Department of Mathematics
Dalhousie University
Halifax, Canada

D. Townsend

Division of Nuclear Medicine
University Hospital
Geneva, Switzerland

## INTRODUCTION

Three dimensional medical images are usually obtained by stacking several parallel slices, each slice being reconstructed separately, using any classical 2 dimensional reconstruction algorithm. This method allows an efficient implementation of the reconstruction, and can be used whenever the measured projection data can be factorized into independent sets, each relative to one single 2 dimensional slice. This is the case, in particular, with multi-ring positron cameras, or with SPECT systems with parallel holes collimators.

This approach, however, requires some form of shielding or collimation, in order to reject oblique rays, which would "mix" several slices and, therefore, would prevent the factorization of the 3 dimensional reconstruction problem. In emission tomography, collimation results in a rather inefficient utilization of the emitted radiation. A better geometrical efficiency is obtained in the absence of shielding, or, more generally, with any tomographical device accepting all available oblique rays. Note that the absence of shielding also influences other physical parameters, like the sensitivity to scattered radiation, or the uniformity and isotropy of the spatial resolution.

With such a system, the 3 dimensional image must be reconstructed as a whole, rather than as a stack of slices. This can be done using series expansion algorithms : from a conceptual point of view, these algorithms are not modified by the 3 dimensional character of the problem; indeed, they only require the translation of the physical reconstruction problem into some set of linear equations or inequalities, or, more generally, into a multi-parametric optimization problem which is then solved by means of adequate iterative techniques (Herman, 1980; Censor, 1983). The computational complexity, of course, is considerably increased in three dimensions; in fact, in some applications, the number of line integrals sampled by the detectors is so large that the iterative reconstruction techniques are unpractical.

This paper is devoted to the so-called "transform methods", which are based on the discretization of analytical inversion formulae for the X-ray transform, and allow more efficient numerical implementations. Contrary to the series expansion techniques, transform methods must be specifically developped to cope with the truly 3 dimensional character of the reconstruction problem. Such algorithms have been proposed by several authors in the last ten years; most of them rely on the shift invariance of the system point spread function, i.e., on the uniformity of the detectors geometrical efficiency all over the field of view. This condition, however, is satisfied only when the detectors subtend the full solid angle sector, which is never the case in the practice. Usually, shift invariance is recovered by rejecting a certain fraction of the measured projection data; this will be further discussed in section 3. The resulting loss of effective efficiency may be important when the object under study is large with respect to the detectors field of view.

The "Extended Truly 3 Dimensional Reconstruction" method proposed by Cho, Ra and Hilal (1983) allows a better utilization of the available data, but can only be applied when the measured projections are explicitely available. This is not the case, for instance, with positron cameras based on one or several pairs of multi-wire proportional chambers (Bateman et al., 1980; Jeavons et al., 1983; Perez-Mendez et al., 1983): the number of line integrals sampled by such cameras may be larger than $2^{33}$, i.e., much larger than the number of coincidences effectively recorded in a typical study (around $2^{21}$); the coincidence data must then be acquired in list-mode, and the projections are never explicitely available. In fact, in such a case, the first step of any practical reconstruction algorithm should be the backprojection of the list-mode data onto the image volume.

In sections 4 and 5, we present two 3 dimensional reconstruction algorithms which have been proposed recently (Clack et al., 1987; Defrise et al., 1987) to overcome the requirement of shift invariance, and which can be applied to list-mode data.

When the detectors subtend the full solid angle $4\pi$ , the projections of the unknown 3 dimensional density i,

$$p_u(\mathbf{s}) = \int du\; i(\mathbf{s} + u\mathbf{u}) \qquad \mathbf{u}.\mathbf{u} = 1,\; \mathbf{u}.\mathbf{s} = 0 \qquad\qquad (1)$$

can be measured for all directions $\mathbf{u}$. The reconstruction problem is then a straightforward generalization of the well-known 2 dimensional case. A specific feature of the 3 dimensional problem, however, is that 4 parameters (2 for the direction vector $\mathbf{u}$, 2 for the vector $\mathbf{s}$ in the projection plane perpendicular to $\mathbf{u}$) are necessary to identify a projection line, whereas the unknown image depends only on 3 spatial coordinates. This means that the 3 dimensional projection data present some redundancy, which is reflected by the existence of a large number of non-equivalent reconstruction algorithms. This is to be compared with the situation in 2 dimensions, where both the image and the data depend on 2 parameters.

Having the application to list-mode data in mind, we first backproject the data onto the image space :

$$b(\mathbf{x}) = \iint_{4\pi} d^2\mathbf{u}\; p_u(\,\mathbf{x} - (\mathbf{x}.\mathbf{u})\,\mathbf{u}\,) \qquad\qquad (2)$$

where $\mathbf{x} - (\mathbf{x}.\mathbf{u})\mathbf{u}$ is the projection of the point $\mathbf{x}$ onto the plane normal to $\mathbf{u}$.

Applying this expression to the data corresponding to a point source at $\mathbf{y}$ then leads to a point spread function

$$\mathrm{psf}_y(\mathbf{x}) = \frac{1}{|\mathbf{x}-\mathbf{y}|^2} \qquad\qquad (3)$$

which is shift invariant, at least if we consider ideal detectors. This function decreases more rapidly than its 2 dimensional equivalent, $1/|\mathbf{x}-\mathbf{y}|$. The advantage in terms of spatial resolution is only apparent, however, since the point spread function is integrated with a volume element proportional to $|\mathbf{x}-\mathbf{y}|^2$, instead of the surface element $|\mathbf{x}-\mathbf{y}|$. In fact, the fundamental similarity between the 2 and 3 dimensional reconstruction problems with complete angular acceptance, clearly appears by computing (in the framework of the theory of generalized functions) the 3 dimensional Fourier transform of the PSF, the modulation transfer function (MTF), which has the same frequency behaviour as in 2 dimensions :

$$mtf \ (\mathbf{v}) = \frac{1}{|\mathbf{v}|} \tag{4}$$

This function is everywhere non zero; it is therefore possible to reconstruct the image by means of Fourier space filtering techniques, using e.g. a 3 dimensional rho-filtered layergram algorithm, which reads just as its 2 dimensional equivalent :

$$backproject \ the \ data \Rightarrow b(\mathbf{x})$$
$$\Downarrow$$
$$Fourier \ transform \Rightarrow \tilde{b}(\mathbf{v})$$
$$\Downarrow$$
$$divide \ by \ the \ MTF \Rightarrow |\mathbf{v}| \ \tilde{b}(\mathbf{v})$$
$$\Downarrow$$
$$inverse \ Fourier \ transform \Rightarrow i(\mathbf{x})$$

Note that a whole family of reconstruction algorithms can be obtained by introducing a strictly positive integration weight $w(\mathbf{u})$ in the integral defining the backprojection (2); the modulation transfer function, of course, has to be modified accordingly.

The discussion of the numerical implementation of this algorithm ( side effects of the discrete Fourier transform, necessity of an apodizing filter, etc...) is beyond the scope of this paper.

3 DIMENSIONAL RECONSTRUCTION WITH RESTRICTED ANGULAR ACCEPTANCE

The limited angle problem is particularly important for 3 dimensional applications, the construction of a detector subtending the full solid angle being unpractical. Just as in 2 dimensions, incomplete angular coverage generally leads to the invalidation of the two conditions necessary to reconstruct the image by Fourier space filtering :

1. the point spread function is no longer shift invariant, since the solid angle subtended by the detectors now depends on the position in the camera's field of view. Thus, instead of a convolution problem, one faces a general Fredholm integral equation, which can no longer be solved by the efficient Fourier space filtering techniques.

2. the modulation transfer function may vanish in some sectors of frequency space; this means that the Fourier transform of the image within those sectors cannot be recovered from the available projection data. The reconstruction problem is severely ill-posed in such a case, and its solution requires the use of analytic continuation techniques, based usually on iterative algorithms (Tam and Perez-Mendez, 1981 a,b).

Let us now describe how these two difficulties have been solved by several authors (Chu and Tam, 1977; Colsher, 1980; Clack et al., 1984), who developed the 3 dimensional reconstruction algorithm which has been used until now with MWPC positron cameras.

Neglect first the shift invariance problem, and suppose that the projections $p_u(s)$ are measured for a set of directions $u \in \Omega$ ($\Omega$ is a subset of the unit sphere). The backprojection of a point source then has the same $1/r^2$ behaviour as in the case of complete acceptance, but with a support limited by $\Omega$ :

$$\text{psf}(r) = \frac{1}{|r|^2} \quad \text{if} \quad \frac{r}{|r|} \in \Omega$$

$$0 \qquad \text{otherwise} \tag{5}$$

The Fourier transform yields the modulation transfer function, which can be written as (Schorr et al. 1983) :

$$\text{mtf}(v) = \frac{1}{|v|} \iint_\Omega d^2u \ \delta(u.\frac{v}{|v|}) \tag{6}$$

where $\delta$ is the Dirac distribution.

This function will be everywhere non zero iff any equatorial circle on the unit sphere intersects the acceptance region (Orlov, 1975). This is the condition for a complete sampling of the image spectrum in frequency space. Let us discuss two examples :

1. A stationnary pair of planar detectors does not verify the previous condition; such a geometry therefore requires the use of analytic continuation techniques.

If the plane detectors are both normal to the axis $1_x$, for instance, one easily checks that the modulation transfer function vanishes for any frequency $v = |v| \ 1_x$

2. A truncated cylindrical detector, which can be simulated in the practice by a rotating pair of planar detectors, fulfils the condition :

Consider the central point on the rotation axis $1_z$, and denote by R the radius and 2H the length of the cylindrical detector. The acceptance region is then :

$$\Omega = \{ u \mid |u.1_z| < \sin \theta_0 = \frac{H}{\sqrt{H^2 + R^2}} \} \tag{7}$$

One then evaluates the integral in (6) :

$$\text{mtf}(v) = \frac{2\pi}{|v|} \qquad \text{when } \Psi < \theta_0$$

$$\frac{4}{|v|} \arcsin\{\frac{\sin \theta_0}{\sin \Psi}\} \qquad \text{when } \Psi > \theta_0 \tag{8}$$

where $v_z = |v| \cos \Psi$. This result was derived by Colsher (1980).

Thus, complete angular sampling is not necessary, in 3D, to ensure a complete sampling of the image in frequency space. This should be opposed to the situation in 2D, where the MTF does vanish as soon as some projections are not measured.

We now come back to the problem of shift invariance : different points $x$ in the field of view have different angular acceptance regions $\Omega_x$, which prevents the use of Fourier deconvolution. The usual solution consists of defining a Universal Acceptance Region (UAR) $\Omega$, as the intersection of the individual $\Omega_x$ for all points $x$ of the support D of the image, i.e., in emission tomography, of the region containing activity. This means that the line integrals $p_u(s)$ corresponding to a direction $u$ belonging to the UAR are measured for all values of $s$; the projections outside $\Omega$, on the other hand, are only partially sampled by the detectors. Shift invariance can be restored by backprojecting only the projections belonging to the UAR. The resulting backprojected image can be deblurred by Fourier space filtering (if the UAR satisfies the condition defined above) :

$$i = F_\Omega \, b_\Omega \tag{9}$$

where i is the reconstructed image estimate, $b_\Omega$ is the image obtained by backprojecting all coincidences measured within $\Omega$ :

$$b(x) = \iint_\Omega d^2u \, p_u(\, x - (x.u)u\,) \tag{10}$$

and $F_\Omega$ is the filtering operator corresponding to the UAR $\Omega$ :

$$\{ F_\Omega \, b_\Omega \}(x) = \iiint d^3v \, e^{2\pi i \, v.x} \, \frac{1}{mtf(v)} \iiint d^3y \, e^{-2\pi i \, v.y} \, b_\Omega(y) \tag{11}$$

This reconstruction algorithm can be implemented efficiently using the 3 dimensional Fast Fourier Transform; when the measured projections are explicitly available, an alternative approach consists of applying the same filter $1/mtf(v)$ to the projections, prior to the backprojection.

A NEW ALGORITHM FOR A BETTER UTILIZATION OF THE PROJECTION DATA

We have seen how the requirement of shift invariance leads to the rejection of a certain fraction of the data, which may become unacceptably large when the region D containing activity becomes large with respect to the camera's field of view. The statistical fluctuations in the reconstructed image i may be important in such a case.

Consider a more central region of interest D', contained within D. Line integrals passing through this internal region have been measured, which are not lying within $\Omega$, and, therefore, cannot be used in the standard reconstruction. We shall see how these supplementary data can be included in the algorithm so as to improve the reconstruction.

Denote by $\Omega'$ the UAR corresponding to the internal region D'. One easily checks, from the definition of the UAR, that the relationship $D \supset D'$ implies $\Omega' \supset \Omega$ : a smaller spatial region corresponds to a larger angular aperture. If the whole activity was contained within D', the image could be reconstructed as $F_{\Omega'} b_{\Omega'}$, where $F_{\Omega'}$ and $b_{\Omega'}$ are defined in the same way as $F_{\Omega}$ and $b_{\Omega}$. This is not the case, however : there is activity outside D', in the region where the point spread function corresponding to the larger aperture $\Omega'$ is not shift invariant. Therefore, the image $b_{\Omega'}$, backprojected using this larger aperture, cannot be deblurred by Fourier space filtering. Let us stress that even the restriction of $F_{\Omega'} b_{\Omega'}$ to the internal region D' is not correct. Indeed, the filter $F_{\Omega'}$ is a non-local operator; therefore, *even within D'*, the values of $F_{\Omega'} b_{\Omega'}$ depend on the incomplete values of $b_{\Omega'}$ outside D'.

This problem can be solved by reconstructing an estimate of $b^{comp}_{\Omega'}$, the complete backprojection with aperture $\Omega'$, which would be obtained if larger detectors were available. This backprojected image, corresponding to a shift invariant PSF (even outside D'), could then be filtered to yield an image estimate equal, up to the statistical fluctuations, to the first image estimate reconstructed with the usual algorithm (i.e., with the true UAR $\Omega$)

$$F_{\Omega'} \, b^{comp}_{\Omega'} = F_{\Omega} \, b_{\Omega} \qquad\qquad (12)$$

Thus, $b^{comp}_{\Omega'}$ can be obtained by applying the inverse filter operator $F^{-1}_{\Omega'}$ to $F_{\Omega} b_{\Omega}$. This low statistics estimate can be used to correct the *measured* backprojection $b_{\Omega'}$, which, as we have seen, is not valid outside the internal region D' :

$$b^{comp}_{\Omega'} = \begin{array}{l} b_{\Omega'} \quad \text{within D'} \\ F^{-1}_{\Omega'} \; \{F_{\Omega} \, b_{\Omega}\} \quad \text{outside D'} \end{array} \qquad\qquad (13)$$

The application of the filter $F_{\Omega'}$ to this composite backprojection then yields an improved reconstructed image, which incorporates a larger fraction of the measured data. The algorithm can be summarized as follows :

determine the universal acceptance region $\Omega$ corresponding
to the region D containing activity
⇓

backproject the data belonging to $\Omega \Rightarrow b_\Omega$

⇓

apply the filter corresponding to the aperture $\Omega \Rightarrow F_\Omega\, b_\Omega$

⇓

choose some internal region of interest D', and determine
the corresponding acceptance region $\Omega'$

⇓

backproject the data belonging to $\Omega' \Rightarrow b_{\Omega'}$

⇓

apply the inverse filter corresponding to the aperture $\Omega'$
to the first image estimate $F_\Omega\, b_\Omega$

⇓

construct the complete backprojection $b^{comp}_{\Omega'}$ by
combining $b_{\Omega'}$
(within D') and $F^{-1}_{\Omega'}\,\{F_\Omega\, b_\Omega\}$   (outside D')

⇓

apply the filter corresponding to the aperture $\Omega'$ to
obtain the improved reconstruction.


Thus, the algorithm allows one to cope with the shift variant
character of the point spread function, while still using the
numerically efficient Fast Fourier Transform. The numerical
implementation is discussed by Defrise et al. (1987), as well as
an application to simulated list-mode data, which demonstrates the
efficiency of the method for the reconstruction of large
radioisotope distributions. Note, however, that the algorithm does
not yet fully utilize the available data; indeed, if a very large
second aperture $\Omega'$ is chosen (so as to incorporate most data into
the backprojection $b_{\Omega'}$), the corresponding region D' in which $b_{\Omega'}$
is effectively used, becomes extremely small. This problem can be
solved, in the practice, by iterating the algorithm with a
sequence of growing apertures $\Omega', \Omega'', \Omega''', \ldots.$


AN ALTERNATIVE APPROACH TO THE 3 DIMENSIONAL RECONSTRUCTION

The previous sections are based on the study of the 3
dimensional point spread function, and of the deconvolution of the
backprojected image.

A different approach to the reconstruction problem has been
proposed by Cho, Ra and Hilal (1983) and also allows to overcome
the requirement of shift invariance. We shall discuss the main
features of the method, as well as its applicability to list-mode
data.

The key idea consists of describing the 3 dimensional reconstruction as the combination of the 2 dimensional reconstructions of all oblique slices for which all projections are available, i.e. for which the detector yields a complete $2\pi$ acceptance. These slices are called "valid" slices.

The image i is then reconstructed as :

$$i\,(\mathbf{x}) = \frac{\displaystyle\iint_{A_{\mathbf{x}}} d^2\mathbf{o}\; i\,(\,\mathbf{x}\,|\,\text{in slice}\,\mathbf{o}\,)}{\displaystyle\iint_{A_{\mathbf{x}}} d^2\mathbf{o}} \tag{14}$$

where $\mathbf{o}$ is a unit vector normal to the plane of one slice, $A_{\mathbf{x}}$ is the set of orientation vectors of all valid slices containing the point $\mathbf{x}$, and $i(\mathbf{x}\,|\,\text{in slice}\,\mathbf{o}\,)$ is obtained by applying the usual 2 dimensional filtered backprojection algorithm in the plane normal to $\mathbf{o}$, and containing $\mathbf{x}$.

Consider for instance the case of a shift invariant acceptance region $\Omega = \{\,\mathbf{u}\ |\ |\mathbf{u}.\mathbf{1_z}| < \sin\theta_0\}$ corresponding to a truncated cylindrical detector with axis along $\mathbf{1_z}$. An oblique slice, normal to a unit vector $\mathbf{o}$, is then a valid slice if all directions perpendicular to $\mathbf{o}$ belong to the acceptance region $\Omega$ : $A = \{\,\mathbf{o}\ |\ |\mathbf{o}.\mathbf{1_z}| > \cos\theta_0\}$. In general, of course, both $\Omega$ and A are shift variant.

In the practice, it would be unpractical to reconstruct each oblique slice individually. As a given line integral $p_{\mathbf{u}}(\mathbf{s})$ belongs to several valid slices, a more efficient procedure consists of applying the integral over the slice orientation $\mathbf{o}$ directly to the one dimensional ramp filter. This leads to a composite 2 dimensional filter :

$$F_{\mathbf{x}}\,(\,\mathbf{u}, \mathbf{v}\,) = \frac{\displaystyle\iint_{A_{\mathbf{x}}} d^2\mathbf{o}\; \delta\,(\mathbf{o}.\mathbf{u}\,)\ |\mathbf{v} - (\mathbf{v}.\mathbf{o})\mathbf{o}|}{\displaystyle\iint_{A_{\mathbf{x}}} d^2\mathbf{o}} \qquad \mathbf{v}.\mathbf{u} = 0 \tag{15}$$

This expression is derived by noting that a particular slice contributes to the filter, for a given projection $\mathbf{u}$, only if $\mathbf{u}$ belongs to the slice, i.e. to the plane normal to $\mathbf{o}$ (hence the Dirac $\delta(\mathbf{o}.\mathbf{u})$). For each orientation $\mathbf{o}$, the ramp filter $|\mathbf{v} - (\mathbf{v}.\mathbf{o})\mathbf{o}|$ is obtained by projecting the 2 dimensional frequency $\mathbf{v}$ onto the slice normal to $\mathbf{o}$. In the case of a truncated cylindrical detector, the general expression (15) reduces to the form given by Cho et al. (1983).

Alternatively, each projection $p_u$ can be convolved in the projection plane normal to $\mathbf{u}$, with the 2 dimensional inverse Fourier transform of (15) :

$$K_x(\mathbf{u},\mathbf{s}) = \frac{1}{\displaystyle\iint_{A_x} d^2\mathbf{o}} \; \frac{k(|\mathbf{s}|)}{|\mathbf{s}|} \qquad \text{if the unit vector normal to } \mathbf{u} \text{ and } \mathbf{s} \text{ belongs to } A_x$$

$$0 \qquad\qquad \text{otherwise} \qquad\qquad (16)$$

where $k(s)$ is the usual 1 dimensional reconstruction kernel, i.e., the 1 dimensional inverse Fourier transform of the ramp filter (with an appropriate apodizing window).

The image is reconstructed by backprojecting the filtered (or convolved) projections. The method is still unpractical, since the filter depends, via $A_x$, on the point $\mathbf{x}$ under study : a different filtering would be necessary to reconstruct each point in the field of view. Thus, one faces the same shift variance problem as in the previous sections. The solution also is similar, and consists in restricting the integrals in (14) and (15) to the slice orientations that are valid for all points in the region containing activity. Unsurprisingly, this solution also requires the rejection of a fraction of the measured projections.

In the "Extended Truly Three Dimensional " algorithm proposed by Cho, Ra and Hilal, the utilization of the available data is improved by dividing the field of view into several sub-regions; in each sub-region $D'$, the image is reconstructed using the filter (15) evaluated for a set of slice orientations $A_{D'}$, valid throughout this region : $A_{D'} = \cap A_x$ , $\mathbf{x} \in D'$.

Let us briefly discuss the applicability of the algorithm to list-mode data. Contrary to the reconstruction filters derived using eq. (6), the filter (15) depends on the projection vector $\mathbf{u}$; this means that the filtering and backprojection steps cannot be commuted, and, therefore, that the filter cannot be applied to the backprojected image. In principle, the algorithm could nevertheless be applied to list-mode data, by means of the method proposed by McIntyre (1981) for 2 dimensional reconstructions : the discrete representation of the convolution kernel (16) is centred at each list-mode event, and then backprojected. The method is unpractical in 3 dimensions, however, since the convolution kernel (16) is 2 dimensional : for each detected event, a very large number of rays (corresponding to the number of points necessary to discretize the kernel) should be backprojected.

A more practical algorithm can be derived, however, by using only the subset of valid slices parallel to some appropriate fixed direction in space. For instance, in the case of a truncated cylindrical detector having its axis along $\mathbf{1}_z$, one could select valid slices parallel to $\mathbf{1}_x$ and $\mathbf{1}_y$. Most line integrals then belong to only one selected slice; as a consequence, the 2 dimensional kernel is reduced to 1 dimension, which allows a practical implementation of McIntyre's method for list-mode data. A complete discussion of this algorithm, and of its numerical implementation, is given by Clack et al. (1987).

CONCLUSIONS

We have described two new truly three dimensional reconstruction algorithms, which can be applied to list-mode data, and which overcome the requirement of shift invariance, thereby allowing a better utilization of the available projections. This is important when the object under study is large with respect to the detectors field of view, i.e. when the Universal Acceptance Region contains only a fraction of the measured data.

The propagation of the statistical fluctuations by these algorithms should also be analyzed, in order to objectively compare their efficiency at incorporating the available projection data.

The existence of a large class of non-equivalent reconstruction algorithms, reflects the redundancy of the 3 dimensional projection data. Only a few examples have been given in this paper; in fact, as far as we know, the most general linear inversion formula for the 3 dimensional X-ray transform with restricted angular acceptance, has not been derived.

ACKNOWLEDGEMENTS

This work is partially funded by the Swiss National Science Fundation (grant nbr. 3.853-0.85). M.D. is Research Associate with the National Fund for Scientific Research (Belgium).

REFERENCES

Bateman J.E., Connolly J.F., Stephenson R. et al, 1980, The Rutherford Appleton Laboratory's Mark I multiwire proportional counter positron camera, Nucl. Instr. Meth., 225:209.
Censor Y., 1983, Finite series-expansion reconstruction method, Proc. IEEE, 71:409.
Cho Z.H., Ra J.B. and Hilal S.K., 1983, True three-dimensional reconstruction - application of algorithm towards full utilization of oblique rays, IEEE Trans. Med. Imag. MI-2:6.
Chu G. and Tam K.C., 1977, 3 dimensional imaging in the positron camera using Fourier techniques, Phys. Med. Biol., 22:245.
Clack R., Townsend D.W. and Jeavons A.P., 1984, Increased sensitivity and field of view for a rotating positron camera, Phys. Med. Biol., 29:1421.
Clack R., Townsend D.W. and Defrise M., 1987, Three-dimensional reconstruction using all available cross-plane rays, in preparation.
Colsher J.G., 1980, Fully three-dimensional PET, Phys. Med.Biol, 25:103.

Defrise M., Kuijk S. and Deconinck F., 1987, A new three-
    dimensional reconstruction method for positron cameras using
    plane detectors, to be published in Phys. Med. Biol.
Herman G.T., 1980: "Image reconstruction from projections",
    Academic Press, New-York.
Jeavons A.P., Hood K., Herlin G. et al, 1983, The High Density
    Avalanche Chamber for PET, IEEE Trans. Nucl. Sc., NS-30:640.
McIntyre J.A., 1981, Computer assisted tomography without a
    computer, IEEE Trans. Nucl. Sc., NS-28:171.
Orlov S.S., 1975, Theory of three dimensional reconstruction,
    Conditions for a complete set of projections, Sov. Phys.
    Crystallogr., 20:312.
Perez-Mendez V., Schwartz G., Nelson W.R. et al, 1983, Further
    improvements in the design of a positron camera with dense
    drift space MWPC's, Nucl. Instr. Meth., 217:89.
Schorr B., Townsend D.W. and Clack R., 1983, A general method of
    three-dimensional filter computation, Phys. Med. Biol.,
    28:305.
Tam K.C. and Perez-Mendez V., 1981 a, Tomographical imaging with
    limited angle input, J. Opt. Soc. Am., 71:582.
Tam K.C. and Perez-Mendez V., 1981 b, Limits to image
    reconstruction with restricted angular input, IEEE Trans.
    Nucl. Sc., NS-28:179.

# MAXIMUM ENTROPY RECONSTRUCTION WITH CONSTRAINTS: ITERATIVE ALGORITHMS FOR SOLVING THE PRIMAL AND DUAL PROGRAMS

Grant T. Gullberg and Benjamin M. W. Tsui

University of Utah, Division of Medical Physics
Department of Radiology, Salt Lake City, UT 84132
University of North Carolina, Department of Radiology
and Curriculum in Biomedical Engineering, Chapel Hill
NC 27514

## ABSTRACT

Using constraints to better define regions of known intensity can improve the signal-to-noise ration in computed tomography (CT). This is accomplished in positron emission tomography (PET) by reducing the region of unknown activity with time-coincidence circuitry. Mathematically, constraints can be implemented into reconstruction algorithms using a priori information, such as the use of an x-ray CT image to define regions of radionuclide uptake in single photon emission computed tomography (SPECT) or PET imaging. In addition to regional constraints, intensity constraints can also be included into the model equations. This may be especially useful where the data has a high degree of contrast as in DSA limited-angle tomography.

The maximum entropy reconstruction problem with equality constraints can be formulated either as a primal optimization program whose optimum is determined from a solution to a system of nonlinear equations or reduced to a dual optimization program using duality principles. The dual program is an unconstrained optimization problem with an objective function that is nonlinear and nonquadratic, but is an essentially smooth function as feasible solutions approach boundary points. Therefore, a solution can be determined using gradient type of algorithms. Simulations using a Gauss-Seidel-Newton iteration to solve the primal program are compared with a conjugate gradient algorithm that solves the dual optimization program. Simulations show that the two approaches produce reconstructions with very different texture.

## INTRODUCTION

The maximum entropy technique has been proposed as a method to reconstruct images from projections. Gordon et al. (1970), Budinger (1971), and Zwick and Zeitler (1973), first proposed the use of a maximum entropy criterion to select the reconstructed image from a set of feasible solutions satisfying projection constraints. The entropy technique was first applied to image reconstruction by D'Addario (1975), Gullberg (1975), Wernecke (1975, 1977), Wernecke and D'Addario (1977). A maximum entropy algorithm was later incorporated as part of the RECLBL Library (Huesman, et al., 1977). Since then, others have pursued the application of maximum entropy to the reconstruction problem. It was conjectured by Gordan et al. (1970) that the MART algorithm gave a maximum entropy solution. It was later proved by Lent (1977), that with some modification of the multiplication factors, the MART algorithm does converge to a maximum entropy solution. Minerbo (1979) later showed that the MENT algorithm gave a maximum entropy solution without the calculation of the exponential multiplicative factors required in the MART algorithm. The MENT algorithm used a nonlinear Gauss-Seidel method to solve a system of nonlinear equations that were derived from projection equations that included one specific weighting scheme. Here we extend the work presented by Minerbo to include projections with arbitrary geometrical weighting factors.

The principle of maximizing information entropy embodies the assurance of minimizing bias or prejudice in choosing an estimate (Jaynes, 1957). The entropy concept is utilized in fields such as thermodynamics, statistical mechanics, and information theory as a measure of the uncertainty in the system. For example, in thermodynamics the entropy of a system increases as molecules become more randomly orientated. In computed tomography, uncertainty in the reconstructed image as well as nonuniqueness exist due to statistical noise and inadequate sampling. The maximum entropy criterion will, therefore, give an estimate for the image which avoids any bias while satisfying the imposed constraints.

The motivation behind our previous work (Gullberg and Ghosh Roy, 1986) was to develop a method that would improve the signal-to-noise ratio of the reconstruction by adding constraints and incorporating an appropriate noise model, so that a solution could be selected with a desired smoothness. Here, we continue to investigate the maximum entropy reconstruction problem with a study that compares one approach which solves the primal program using a Gauss-Seidel algorithm with another approach which solves the dual program using a conjugate gradient algorithm. Simulations of maximum entropy reconstructions are presented for both algorithms.

THEORY

The reconstruction problem is stated formally as the following convex program (P):

(P)   Find the minimum of

$$
h(A,N) = \begin{cases} \sum_i \dfrac{a_i}{T_D} \ln\left(\dfrac{a_i}{T_D}\right) + \sum_j \dfrac{n_j}{T_N} \ln\left(\dfrac{n_j}{T_N}\right) \\ \\ \text{if } a_i \geq 0,\ n_j \geq 0 \quad \sum_{i=1}^{N_u} a_i = T_D,\ \sum_{j=1}^{M_s} n_j = T_N \\ \\ +\infty \qquad\qquad \text{otherwise} , \end{cases}
\tag{1}
$$

subject to     $FA + N - N_M = P$                                               (2)

$GA = Q$                                                                       (3)

The solution to (P) gives unbias estimates $A_O$ for the reconstructed image and $N_O$ for the noise in the projections. The intensities $a_i$ are elements of the column matrix A representing the feasible reconstructed images which have a total intensity $T_D$, $n_j$ are elements of the column matrix N representing the noise vector which has a total intensity $T_N$, and P is the projection column matrix related to A by the matrix F and the noise term $N - N_M$. The vector $N_M$ is a bias term so that the noise terms $n_j$ are greater than zero. The equality constraints in Eq. (3) are additional model constraints to those given by the projections in Eq. (2). Without the constraints in Eqs. (2) and (3), the maximum entropy will occur when all values of $a_i$ and $n_j$ are the same. However, the constraints modify the set of feasible solutions for the program (P) and, likewise, reduce the entropy of the image by introducing structure.

The program (P) allows for noise perturbations in the projections, Eq. (2), so that the noise vector N is also a variable in the optimization problem. The vector $N_M$ has components equal to $n_M$. The constant $n_M$ is of sufficient size that it cancels the most negative going values of $P - FA$, so that for all j, $n_j \geq 0$. A reasonable choice is to select $n_M$ equal to the maximum of $2\,\sigma(p_j)$ for all j. This noise model was proposed by Frieden (1972, 1975, 1977, 1980) who suggested scaling the noise entropy function in order to adjust the solution for the desired smoothness. The larger the constant is made, the more emphasis is placed upon maximizing the noise entropy function, and hence upon making the reconstructed image less smooth. For simplicity, we have assumed that the scale factor is equal to one.

The Lagrangian is used to characterize the optimal solution for (P) in terms of a "saddle-point" extrema. The Lagrangian function for the convex program (P) is

$$
L(\lambda,\mu,A,N) = 
\begin{cases}
h_A(A) + h_N(N) + <\lambda,(P - N + N_M - FA)>/T_D \\
\quad + <\mu, Q - GA>/T_D \\
-\infty \qquad \text{if } A \in \text{dom}_A h \text{ , } N \in \text{dom}_N h \\
+\infty \qquad \text{if } A \in \text{dom } h_A \text{ or } N \in \text{dom } h_N
\end{cases}
\qquad (4)
$$

where $h_A(A)$ denotes the negative of the entropy function for the pixel activity with dom $h_A = \{A | h_A(A) < \infty\}$, $h_N(N)$ denotes the negative of the entropy function for the noise in the measured projections with dom $h_N = \{N | h_N(N) < \infty\}$ and $\lambda,\mu$ are the Lagrange multipliers for the constraints in Eqs. (2) and (3). The Lagrangian function L is a concave function in $(\lambda,\mu)$ and convex in (A,N). A saddle-point for (P) represents an optimal solution $(A_o,N_o)$ for (P) and a Kuhn-Tucker vector $(\lambda_o,\mu_o)$ for (P), such that the saddle-value $L(\lambda_o,\mu_o,A_o,N_o)$ is the optimal value in (P). The vector $(\lambda_o,\mu_o)$ is a Kuhn-Tucker vector for (P) if the function

$$
g(\lambda,\mu) = \inf_{(A,N)} L(\lambda,\mu,A,N) \qquad , \qquad (5)
$$

where $\inf_{(A,N)}$ is read infimum over A and N, attains its supremum at $(\lambda_o,\mu_o)$. The function g is the objective function for a dual concave program $(P^*)$.

Duality theory (Rockafellar, 1970) gives a correspondence between generalized convex programs with perturbations and associated dual programs which are particular concave programs with perturbations. The Lagrangian function for (P) can be expressed in terms of a generalized bifunction $B\lambda^*\mu^*(A,N)$ where L is equal to the infimum over all $(\lambda^*,\mu^*)$ of the function $<\lambda^*,\lambda> + <\mu^*,\mu> + B\lambda^*\mu^*(A,N)$. The dual concave program $(P^*)$ is formed from the adjoint bifunction

$$(B^*A^*N^*)(\lambda,\mu) = \inf_{(A,N)} \left\{ L(\lambda,\mu,A,N) - \langle A,A^* \rangle - \langle N,N^* \rangle \right\} \quad , \tag{6}$$

which is the conjugate of the bifunction $B\lambda^*\mu^*(A,N)$. The objective function for $(P^*)$ is equal to $(B^*O)(\lambda,\mu)$. We see from Eq. (6) and the definition of the Lagrangian in Eq. (4), that the adjoint bifunction is a functional which maps supporting hyperplanes of our original optimization problem into the real numbers. In this way, we form a dual problem which maximizes a functional of supporting hyperplanes. If the function $B^*$ is differentiable for all $A^*$, $N^*$, then from Theorem 4.5 (Rockafellar, 1970) the optimal solution to (P) is

$$a_i^o = - \left. \frac{\partial(B^*A^*N^*)(\lambda_0,\mu_0)}{\partial a_i^*} \right|_{(A^*,N^*) = 0} \quad , \tag{7}$$

$$n_j^o = - \left. \frac{\partial(B^*A^*N^*)(\lambda_0,\mu_0)}{\partial n_j^*} \right|_{(A^*,N^*) = 0} \quad . \tag{8}$$

This simplifies the problem by first determining a Kuhn-Tucker vector $(\lambda_0,\mu_0)$ which is an optimal solution to the program $(P^*)$. The optimal solution to the program (P) is then evaluated directly using Eqs. (7) and (8).

Formulas for the objective function g for $(P^*)$ in Eq. (5) and formulas for the solution to (P) in Eqs. (7) and (8) are obtained using the adjoint bifunction defined in Eq. (6). Substituting the Lagrangian function, Eq. (4), into Eq. (6), we have the following series of expressions:

$$(B^*A^*N^*)(\lambda,\mu) = \inf_{(A,N)} \left\{ h_A(A) + h_N(N) + \langle \lambda, (P - N + N_M - FA) \rangle / T_D \right.$$

$$\left. + \langle \mu, Q - GA \rangle / T_D - \langle A,A^* \rangle - \langle N,N^* \rangle \right\} \quad . \tag{9}$$

Rewriting, we have

$$(B^*A^*N^*)(\lambda,\mu) = - \sup_A \left\{ \langle F^T\lambda + G^T\mu + A^*T_D, A/T_D \rangle - h_A(A) \right\}$$

$$- \sup_N \left\{ \langle N^*T_N + \lambda T_N / T_D, N/T_N \rangle - h_N(N) \right\} \tag{10}$$

$$+ \langle \lambda, P \rangle / T_D + \langle \lambda, N_M \rangle / T_D + \langle \mu, Q \rangle / T_D \quad .$$

Taking the supremum, we can write

$$(B^*A^*N^*)(\lambda,\mu) = - \ln \left[ \sum_i \exp(z_i + w_i + T_D a_i^*) \right]$$

$$- \ln \left[ \sum_j \exp(n_j^* T_N + \lambda_j T_N / T_D) \right] \tag{11}$$

$$+ \langle \lambda, P \rangle / T_D + \langle \lambda, N_M \rangle / T_D + \langle \mu, Q \rangle / T_D \quad .$$

where $Z = F^T\lambda$ and $W = G^T\mu$.

The objective function $g(\lambda,\mu)$ for the dual program $(P^*)$ is obtained by setting $(A^*, N^*) = (0,0)$ in Eq. (11). This gives the dual program

$(P^*)$   Find the maximum of

$$g(\lambda, \mu) = - \ln \left[ \sum_i \exp(z_i + w_i) \right] - \ln \left[ \sum_j \exp(\lambda_j T_N / T_D) \right]$$

$$+ <\lambda, P>/T_D + <\lambda, N_M>/T_D + <\mu, Q>/T_D$$

(12)

Since the function $B^*$ is differentiable for all $A^*$, then from Eq. (7), the optimal solution $A_o$ to (P) is

$$a_i^o = \frac{T_D \exp(z_i^o + w_i^o)}{\sum_i \exp(z_i^o + w_i^o)} \quad , \tag{13}$$

where $Z^o = F^T \lambda_o$ and $W^o = G^T \mu_o$, and $(\lambda_o, \mu_o)$ is an optimal solution to Eq. (12).

### Example

The model equations in Eq. (3) represent any physical constraints that can be described by a system of linear equations. As an example, suppose that the concentration is restricted to a bounded region of the plane whose extent is known _a priori_. Then Eq. (3) can be formulated using the following expressions for G and Q:

$$G = \begin{pmatrix} g_{11} & & 0 \\ & g_{22} & \\ 0 & & g_{N_u N_u} \end{pmatrix} \quad , \tag{14}$$

where

$$g_{ii} = \begin{cases} 0 & \text{if } a_i \geq 0 \\ 1 & \text{if } a_i = 0 \end{cases} \quad , \tag{15}$$

and

$$Q = \begin{pmatrix} 0 \end{pmatrix} \quad . \tag{16}$$

### ITERATIVE ALGORITHMS

Duality offers alternative approaches for solving optimization problems. Two approaches are developed here for determining the maximum entropy reconstruction from projections. The first approach is to solve the primal program (P) by solving a system of nonlinear equations of Lagrange multipliers. An iterative Gauss-Seidel algorithm is used to determine the solution to the system of nonlinear equations. We extend the work presented by Minerbo (1979) to a more general formulation of the reconstruction problem that incorporates arbitrary geometrical weighting into the system of nonlinear equations. The second approach is to solve the dual program $(P^*)$ by maximizing the unconstrained nonlinear function of Lagrange multipliers in Eq. (12). The maximum is determined using a conjugate gradient algorithm. The following discusses these two approaches and gives examples for specific noise and model constraints.

## Gauss-Seidel Algorithms for Solving the Primal Program

The basic nonlinear Gauss-Seidel algorithm (Ortega and Rheinboldt, (1970) is to solve the ith equation

$$f_i(x_1^{k+1}, \ldots x_{i-1}^{k+1}, x_i^k, x_{i+1}^k, \ldots, x_n^k) = 0 \tag{17}$$

for $x_i$ and set $x_i^{k+1} = x_i$. The Gauss-Seidel-Newton iteration is used to solve Eq. (17). The explicit form of the iteration is

$$x_i^{k+1} = x_i^k - f_i(x^{k,i})/\partial_i f_i(x^{k,i}) \tag{18}$$

$$i = 1, \ldots, n \qquad k = 0, 1, \ldots.$$

where $\partial_i f_i$ is the partial derivative of $f_i$ with respect to $x_i$ and

$$x^{k,i} = (x_1^{k+1}, \ldots, x_{i-1}^{k+1}, x_i^k, x_{i+1}^k, \ldots, x_n^k) \quad . \tag{19}$$

The solution to the program (P) is formulated as a solution to a system of nonlinear equations in the form of Eq. (17) with the Lagrange multipliers as the unknown variables. The system of nonlinear equations are developed for different noise and model constraints. The iteration step in Eq. (18) is derived for each case.

**1. Without noise and without model constraints.** The first example is to determine densities $a_i$ that maximize the entropy of all feasible images A satisfying only the projection constraints. This is stated formally in the following program

$(P_A)$    Find the minimum of $h_A(A)$

$$\text{subject to} \quad FA = P \quad . \tag{20}$$

The Lagrangian function for $(P_A)$ is

$$L(\lambda, A) = \sum_i \frac{a_i}{T_D} \ln\left(\frac{a_i}{T_D}\right) + \langle\lambda, (P - FA)\rangle/T_D \quad . \tag{21}$$

An optimum solution for $(P_A)$ must be a "saddle-point" of the Lagrangian function. This means that a necessary condition for A to be an optimum solution is that the partial derivative of L with respect to $a_i$ must be zero. Taking the partial derivative and setting to zero

$$\frac{\partial L(\lambda, A)}{\partial a_i} = \frac{1}{T_D} \ln\left(\frac{a_i}{T_D}\right) + \frac{1}{T_D} - (F^T\lambda)_i/T_D = 0 \quad , \tag{22}$$

gives the following solution for $a_i$ in terms of the Lagrange multipliers $\lambda_j$

186

$$a_i = T_D e^{-1} \exp[(F^T\lambda)_i] \qquad , \qquad (23)$$

or

$$a_i = T_D e^{-1} \prod_j \exp(f_{ij}\lambda_j) \qquad . \qquad (24)$$

The notation $(F^T\lambda)_i$ in Eqs. (22) and (23) denotes the ith component of the vector $F^T\lambda$. The variable $\omega_j$ (Minerbo, 1979)

$$\omega_j = \exp(\lambda_j) \qquad , \qquad (25)$$

is substituted into Eq. (24) to obtain the following expression for $a_i$

$$a_i = T_D e^{-1} \prod_j^{M_S} \omega_j^{f_{ij}} \qquad . \qquad (26)$$

The product in Eq. (26) is a backmultiply operation analogous to the back-projection operation $F^T$. Substituting $a_i$ in Eq. (26) back into Eq. (20) gives the following system of nonlinear equations in terms of the variables $\omega_m$

$$T_D e^{-1} \sum_i f_{ij} \prod_m \omega_m^{f_{im}} = P_j \qquad . \qquad (27)$$

A solution to Eq. (27) is obtained using the nonlinear Gauss-Seidel-Newton iteration outlined in Eqs. (17) - (19). The iteration step is

$$\omega_j^{k+1} = \omega_j^k \left[1 - U_j(\omega^{k,j})/V_j(\omega^{k,j})\right] \qquad , \qquad (28)$$

where

$$U_j(\omega^{k,j}) = \sum_i \left( f_{ij} \prod_{m=1}^{j-1} (\omega_m^{k+1})^{f_{im}} \prod_{m=j}^{M_S} (\omega_m^k)^{f_{im}} \right) - P_j\, e/T_D \qquad (29)$$

$$V_j = \sum_i \left( f_{ij}^2 \prod_{m=1}^{j-1} (\omega_m^{k+1})^{f_{im}} \prod_{m=j}^{M_S} (\omega_m^k)^{f_{im}} \right) \qquad . \qquad (30)$$

$M_S$ is the total number of projection samples. After a sufficient number of iterations, the reconstructed image A is determined from Eq. (26).

2. **With noise and without model constraints**. The second example is to determine densities $a_i$ and $n_j$ that maximize the sum of the image and noise entropy functions. The densities $a_i$ and $n_j$ are chosen subject to projection constraints. This is stated formally in the following program

$(P_{AN})$. Find the minimum of $h(A,N)$           (1)

         subject to    $FA + N - N_M = P$          (2)

The Lagrangian function for $(P_{AN})$ is

$$L(\lambda, A, N) = \sum_i \frac{a_i}{T_D} \ln\left(\frac{a_i}{T_D}\right) + \sum_j \frac{n_j}{T_N} \ln\left(\frac{n_j}{T_N}\right)$$

$$+ <\lambda, (P - N + N_M - FA)>/T_D \qquad (31)$$

Taking the partial derivatives of the Lagrangian with respect to $a_i$ and $n_j$ and setting to zero, gives the following expressions for $a_i$ and $n_j$ in terms of the Lagrange multipliers $\lambda_j$

$$a_i = T_D e^{-1} \prod_j \exp(f_{ij}\lambda_j) \qquad , \qquad (32)$$

$$n_j = T_N e^{-1} \exp(T_N\lambda_j) \qquad , \qquad (33)$$

or in terms of $\omega_j$ in Eq. (25)

$$a_i = T_D e^{-1} \prod_j \omega_j^{f_{ij}} \qquad , \qquad (34)$$

$$n_j = T_N e^{-1} \omega_j^{T_N/T_D} \qquad . \qquad (35)$$

Substituting $a_i$ and $n_j$ into Eq. (2) gives the following system of nonlinear equations in terms of the variables $\omega_m$

$$T_D e^{-1} \sum_i \left( f_{ij} \prod_m \omega_m^{f_{im}} \right) + T_N e^{-1} \omega_j^{T_N/T_D} - n_M = p_j \qquad . \qquad (36)$$

Using the nonlinear Gauss-Seidel-Newton iteration step in Eqs. (17) (19), gives the following iterative algorithm

$$\omega_j^{k+1} = \omega_j^k [1 - X_j(\omega^{k,j})/Y_j(\omega^{k,j})] \qquad , \qquad (37)$$

where

$$X_j(\omega^{k,j}) = \sum_i \left( f_{ij} \prod_{m=1}^{j-1} (\omega_m^{k+1})^{f_{im}} \prod_{m=j}^{M_S} (\omega_m^k)^{f_{im}} \right)$$

$$+ (T_N/T_D)(\omega_j^k)^{T_N/T_D} - (p_j + n_m) e/T_D \qquad , \qquad (38)$$

$$Y_j(\omega^{k,j}) = \sum_i \left( f_{ij}^2 \prod_{m=1}^{j-1} (\omega_m^{k+1})^{f_{im}} \prod_{m=j}^{M_S} (\omega_m^k)^{f_{im}} \right)$$

$$+ (T_N/T_D)^2 (\omega_j^k)^{T_N/T_D} \qquad . \qquad (39)$$

**3. Without noise and with model constraints**. The third example is to determine densities $a_i$ that maximize the entropy of all feasible images A satisfying projection constraints and satisfying additional *a priori* information formulated as linear constraints. This is stated formally in the following program

$(P_{AC})$  Find the minimum of $h_A(A)$

$$\text{subject to} \quad FA = P \quad , \tag{20}$$

$$GA = Q \quad . \tag{3}$$

The Lagrangian function for $(P_{AC})$ is

$$L(\lambda,\mu,A) = \sum_i \frac{a_i}{T_D} \ln \left( \frac{a_i}{T_D} \right) + <\lambda,(P - FA)>/T_D$$

$$+ <\mu,(Q - GA)>/T_D \quad . \tag{40}$$

Taking the partial derivatives of the Lagrangian with respect to $a_i$ and setting to zero, gives the following expression for $a_i$ in terms of the variables $\omega_j$ (Eq. (25)) and $\Delta_\ell$

$$a_i = T_D \ e^{-1} \ \prod_j \omega_j^{f_{ij}} \ \prod_\ell \Delta_\ell^{g_{i\ell}} \quad , \tag{41}$$

where $\Delta_\ell = \exp(\mu_\ell)$. Substituting $a_i$ into Eqs. (3) and (20), gives the following system of nonlinear equations in terms of the variables $\omega_j$, $\Delta_n$

$$T_D \ e^{-1} \ \sum_i \left( f_{ij} \ \prod_m \omega_m^{f_{im}} \ \prod_n \Delta_n^{g_{in}} \right) = P_j \quad , \tag{42}$$

$$T_D \ e^{-1} \ \sum_i \left( g_{i\ell} \ \prod_m \omega_m^{f_{im}} \ \prod_n \Delta_n^{g_{in}} \right) = q_\ell \quad . \tag{43}$$

A solution to Eqs(42) and (43) is obtained using the nonlinear Gauss-Seidel-Newton iteration. The iteration step for Eq. (42) is

$$\omega_j^{k+1} = \omega_j^k \ [1 - S_j(\omega^{k,j},\Delta^k)/T_j(\omega^{k,j},\Delta^k)] \quad , \tag{44}$$

where

$$S_j(\omega^{k,j},\Delta^k) = \sum_i \left( f_{ij} \ \prod_{m=1}^{j-1} (\omega_m^{k+1})^{f_{im}} \ \prod_{m=j}^{M_s} (\omega_m^k)^{f_{im}} \ \prod_n (\Delta_n^k)^{g_{in}} \right)$$

$$- P_j \ e/T_D \quad , \tag{45}$$

$$T_j(\omega^{k,j},\Delta^k) = \sum_i \left( f_{ij}^2 \ \prod_{m=1}^{j-1} (\omega_m^{k+1})^{f_{im}} \ \prod_{m=j}^{M_s} (\omega_m^k)^{f_{im}} \ \prod_n (\Delta_n^k)^{g_{in}} \right) \tag{46}$$

The iteration step for Eq. (43) is

$$\Delta_\ell^{k+1} = \Delta_\ell^k \ [1 - \bar{S}_\ell(\omega^{k+1},\Delta^{k,\ell})/ \ \bar{T}_\ell(\omega^{k+1},\Delta^{k,\ell})] \tag{47}$$

where

$$\bar{S}_\ell(\omega^{k+1}, \Delta^{k,\ell}) = \sum_i \left( g_{i\ell} \prod_m (\omega_m^{k+1})^{f_{im}} \prod_{n=1}^{\ell-1} (\Delta_n^{k+1})^{g_{in}} \prod_{n=\ell}^{M_c} (\Delta_n^k)^{g_{in}} \right)$$
$$- q_\ell \, e/T_D \qquad , \tag{48}$$

$$\bar{T}_\ell(\omega^{k+1}, \Delta^{k,\ell}) = \sum_i \left( g_{i\ell}^2 \prod_m (\omega_m^{k+1})^{f_{im}} \prod_{n=1}^{\ell-1} (\Delta_n^{k+1})^{g_{in}} \prod_{n=\ell}^{M_c} (\Delta_n^k)^{g_{in}} \right). \tag{49}$$

$M_c$ is the number of constraint equations.

## Conjugate Gradient Algorithm for Solving the Dual Program

The explicit form of the conjugate gradient iteration is

$$\lambda^{k+1} = \lambda^k + \beta_k \, \alpha^k \qquad , \tag{50}$$

where

$$\alpha^\circ = -\nabla^\circ \qquad , \tag{51}$$

$$\alpha^{k+1} = -\nabla^{k+1} + \beta_k \, \alpha^k \qquad , \tag{52}$$

$$\beta_k = \frac{\langle \nabla^{k+1}, \nabla^{k+1} \rangle}{\langle \nabla^k, \nabla^k \rangle} \qquad , \tag{53}$$

and $\langle \nabla^{k+1}, \alpha^k \rangle = 0$. The symbol $\nabla$ denotes the gradient of the function to be maximized.

The conjugate gradient algorithm is used to approximate the maximum of the nonlinear function of Lagrange multipliers in Eq. (12). Thus, it is used to maximize a nonlinear concave function, whereas, the Gauss-Seidel algorithm was shown in the previous section to solve a system of nonlinear equations to obtain the maximum entropy solution. We repeat the examples presented in the previous section and give expressions for the gradient required by the conjugate gradient algorithm to define the iteration step in Eq. (50).

1. **Without noise and without model constraints**. The first example is to determine the densities $a_i$ that maximize the entropy of all feasible images A satisfying only the projection constraints. This is stated formally in the following program

$(P_A)$  Find the minimum of $h_A(A)$ ,

subject to    $FA = P$    . \hfill (20)

The dual program is

$(P_A^*)$  Find the maximum of

$$g(\lambda) = -\ln\left[ \sum_i \exp(z_i) \right] + \langle \lambda, P \rangle / T_D \qquad , \tag{54}$$

where $Z = F^T\lambda$ is the backprojection of the Lagrange multipliers $\lambda_j$. The dual program is an unconstrained optimization problem with a concave objective function g. Maximum solutions to g can be determined using a conjugate gradient algorithm or some other gradient algorithm.

The gradient of g in Eq. (54) is given by

$$\nabla g(\lambda) = -FE/\sum \exp(z_i) + P/T_D \quad , \tag{55}$$

where $E = [\exp(z_1), \exp(z_2),\ldots\ldots, \exp(z_{N_u})]$. An optimum solution $\lambda_o$ is determined after a sufficient number of iteration steps. The reconstructed image is given by

$$a_i^o = \frac{T_D \exp(z_i^o)}{\displaystyle\sum_i \exp(z_i^o)} \quad , \tag{56}$$

where $Z^o = F^T\lambda_o$, and $\lambda_o$ is an optimal solution to Eq. (54). The derivation of Eq. (56) is similar to that of Eq. (13) except without the noise and additional model constraints.

**2. With noise and without model constraints.** The second example is to determine densities $a_i$ and $n_j$ that maximize the sum of the image and noise entropy functions. The densities $a_i$ and $n_j$ are chosen subject to projection constraints. This is stated formally in the following program

$$(P_{AN}). \quad \text{Find the minimum of } h(A,N) , \tag{1}$$

$$\text{subject to} \quad FA + N - N_M = P \quad . \tag{2}$$

The dual program is

$$(P_{AN}^*) \quad \text{Find the maximum of}$$

$$g(\lambda) = - \ln \left[ \sum_i \exp(z_i) \right] - \ln \left[ \sum_j \exp(\lambda_j T_N/T_D) \right]$$

$$+ <\lambda, P>/T_D + <\lambda, N_M>/T_D \quad , \tag{57}$$

where $Z = F^T\lambda$ is the backprojection of the Lagrange multipliers $\lambda_j$.

The gradient of g in Eq. (57) is given by

$$\nabla g(\lambda) = -FE/\sum \exp(z_i) - E'T_N/T_D/\sum \exp(\lambda_j T_N/T_D)$$

$$+ P/T_D + N_M/T_D \quad , \tag{58}$$

where $E = [\exp(z_1), \exp(z_2),\ldots\ldots, \exp(z_{N_u})]$ and $E' = [\exp(\lambda_1 T_N/T_D),$ $\exp(\lambda_2 T_N/T_D),\ldots\ldots,\exp(\lambda_{M_s} T_N/T_D)]$. Once an optimum solution to g is determined, the reconstruction is calculated from Eq. (56).

191

**3. Without noise and with model constraints.** The third example is to determine densities $a_i$ that maximize the entropy of all feasible images A satisfying projection constraints and additional *a priori* information formulated as linear constraints. This is stated formally in the following program

$(P_{AC})$   Find the minimum of $h_A(A)$

subject to   $FA = P$                                    (20)

$GA = Q$                                    (3)

The dual program is

$(P^*_{AC})$   Find the maximum of

$$g(\lambda,\mu) = - \ln \left[ \sum_i \exp(z_i + w_i) \right] + <\lambda,P>/T_D + <\mu,Q>/T_D \qquad (59)$$

where $Z = F^T\lambda$ and $W = G^T\mu$.

The gradient of g, $\nabla g = (\nabla_\lambda g, \nabla_\mu g)$, is given by

$$\nabla_\lambda g(\lambda,\mu) = -FE/\sum \exp(z_i + w_i) + P/T_D \quad , \qquad (60)$$

$$\nabla_\mu g(\lambda,\mu) = -GE/\sum \exp(z_i + w_i) + Q/T_D \quad , \qquad (61)$$

where $E = [\exp(z_1 + w_1), \exp(z_2 + w_2),\ldots, \exp(z_{N_u} + w_{N_u})]$. Once an optimum solution for g is determined, the reconstruction is calculated from Eq. (13).

## RESULTS

Computer simulations were performed to evaluate the Gauss-Seidel and conjugate gradient algorithms for solving the maximum entropy reconstruction problem. The simulations assumed only projection constraints and did not incorporate other model constraints as in Eq. (3) nor a noise model given in Eq. (2). The Gauss-Seidel-Newton iteration in Eq. (28) was used to determine a solution of Lagrange multipliers to the system of nonlinear equations in Eq. (27). The reconstructed image was then determined from Eq. (26). These results were compared with those obtained using the conjugate gradient algorithm to maximize the function in Eq. (54).

The simulations used a 128x128 computer generated heart-lung phantom (Lewis, et al, 1982) shown in Fig. 1. Reconstruction of 128x128 images were obtained from 64 and 128 projections over 180° both with and without noise. The projections were formed by evaluating line integrals of the phantom shown in Fig. 1. For the simulations that incorporated noise, statistical noise of 1% and 5% were added to the projections $\bar{p}_j$. This gave statistically varying projections

$$p_j = \bar{p}_j + n_j \quad , \qquad (62)$$

where the noise random variable $n_j$ was generated with zero mean and with $\sigma(n_j) = .01\bar{p}_j$ for 1% noise. This gave a constant percent root-mean-square (RMS) error per projection of 1%.

## Gauss-Seidel Algorithm

The results for the Gauss-Seidel algorithm are shown in Figs. 2, 3, and 4. The results in Fig. 2 are reconstructions from 64 projections without noise after 2, 4, 6, and 12 iterations. The results in Fig. 3 are reconstructions from 128 projections without noise after 2, 3, 4, and 5 iterations. More than 5 iterations were not possible with 128 projections because of numerical overflow when calculating the division operation in Eq. (28). The solution appears to have nearly converged after 5 iterations. The results for 64 projections give a "salt and pepper" texture that becomes less noticeable for 128 projections. The results in Fig. 4 are reconstructions, after 10 iterations, from 64 projections with 1, 5, and 7% noise.

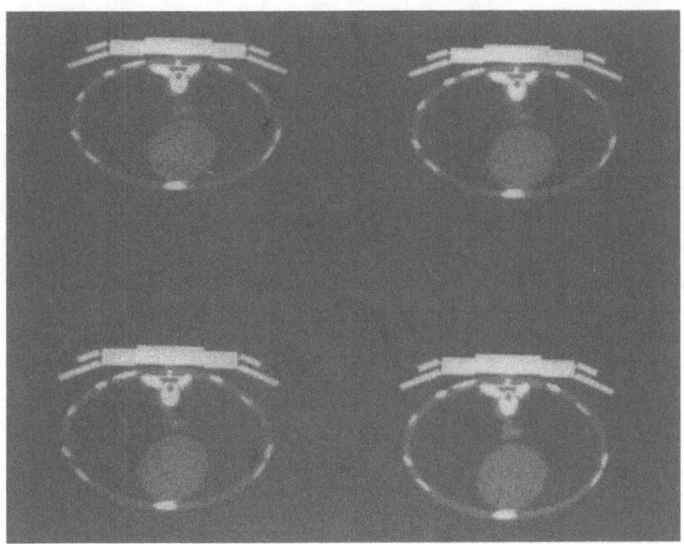

Fig. 1. A 128x128 computer generated transmission phantom representing a slice through the heart and lung.

The backmultiply operations in Eqs. (29) and (30) are similar to a backprojection operation, as far as the indexing is concern; except, the projection samples that backproject through a particular pixel are raised to powers equal to the geometrical weighting factors and then multiplied together. The geometrical weighting factors $f_{im}$ are determined by the specific model chosen for the projection operation. The summation operations in Eqs. (29) and (30) reproject the result of the backmultiply operation. Therefore, each iteration requires one projection and one backmultiply operation. The solution for $a_i$ in Eq. (26) is obtained by scaling the last backmultiply operation at the final iteration step. The simulations used geometrical weighting factors equal to the line length of the projection ray intersecting each pixel. The multiplication and exponentiation operations are computationally more time consuming than a multiply and an addition in the backprojection operation. Therefore, the Gauss-Seidel algorithm requires more time per backmultiply-projection operation than does the backprojection-projection operation used in the conjugate gradient algorithm.

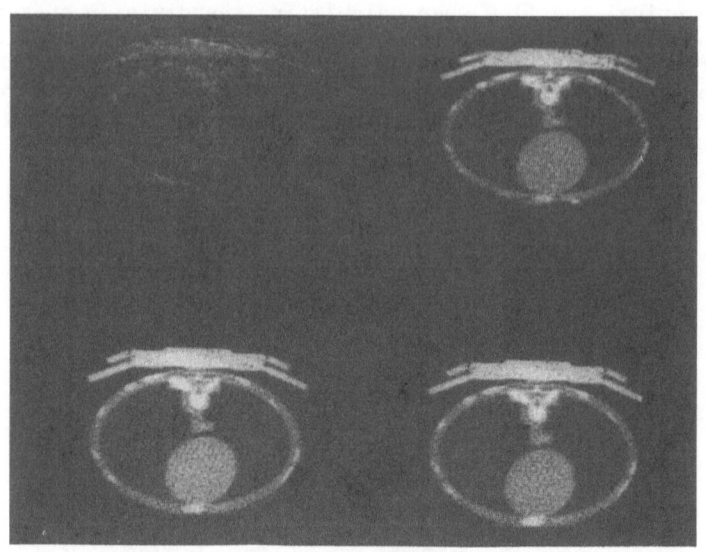

Fig. 2. The maximum entropy solution after 2, 4, 6,and 12
iterations for 64 projections using the Gauss-
Seidel-Newton algorithm.

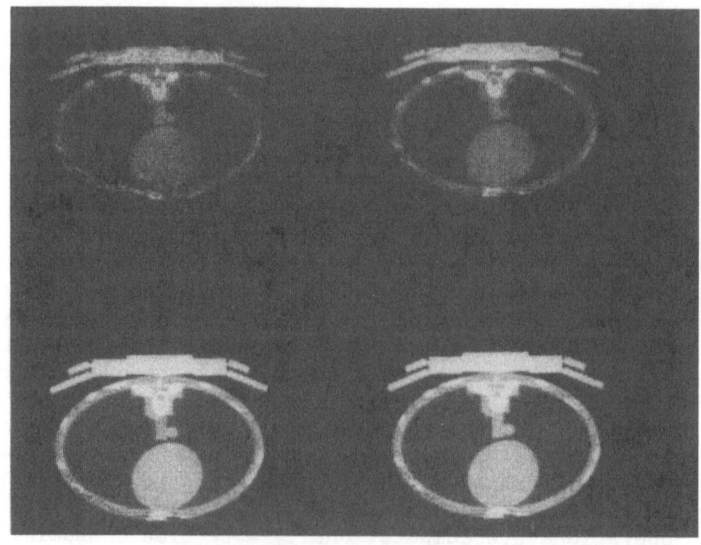

Fig. 3. The maximum entropy solution after 2, 3, 4, and 5
iterations for 128 projections using the Gauss-
Seidel-Newton algorithm.

## Conjugate Gradient Algorithm

The results for the conjugate gradient algorithm are shown in Figs. 5, 6, and 7. The results in Fig. 5 are reconstructions from 64 projections without noise after 2, 4, 6, and 12 iterations. The results in Fig. 6 are reconstructions from 128 projections without noise after 2, 3, 4, and 5 iterations. The reconstructions from both 64 and 128 projections do not give the same "salt and pepper" texture that is observed with the Gauss-Seidel algorithm. The results in Fig. 8 are reconstructions, after 10 iterations, from 64 projections with 1, 5, and 7% noise.

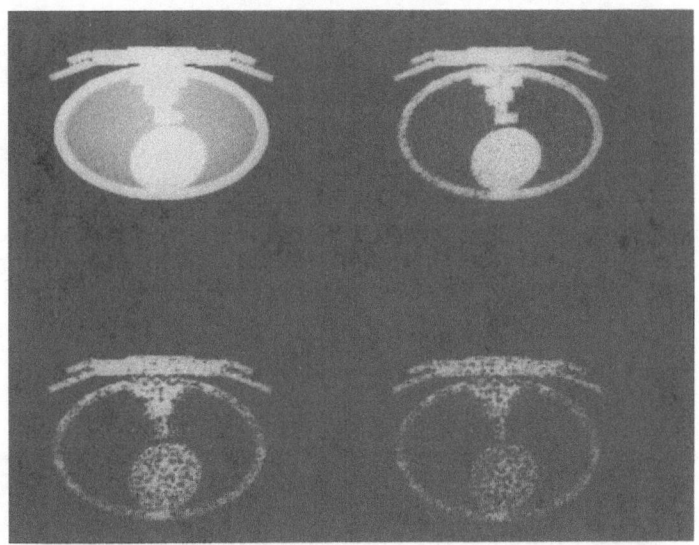

Fig. 4. Comparison of original image with the maximum entropy solution after 10 iterations of the Gauss-Seidel-Newton algorithm for projections with 1%, 5%, 7% noise.

The maximum entropy reconstruction program in the RECLBL library (Huesman, et al., 1977) was used to obtain the results for the conjugate gradient algorithm. The algorithm requires an expression for the gradient of g at each iteration to evaluate a new step direction. Note, that the evaluation of $\nabla g$ in Eq. (55) requires a projection operation FE and a backprojection operation $F^T\lambda$. Therefore, each iteration requires at least one projection and one backprojection operation to evaluate the gradient. Each iteration requires additional backprojection operations to determine the minimum of g in Eq. (54) along the conjugate gradient direction. For the simulations presented here, the projection and backprojection operations were accomplished using the PLL and BLL subroutines in the RECLBL Library (Huesman, et al, 1977). These routines weighted each pixel by the length of the ray passing through the pixel.

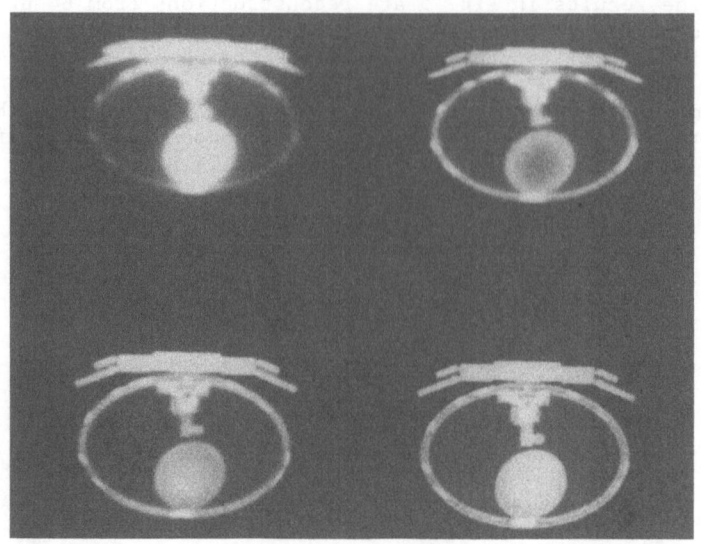

Fig. 5. The maximum entropy solution after 2, 4, 6,and 12 iterations for 64 projections using the conjugate gradient algorithm.

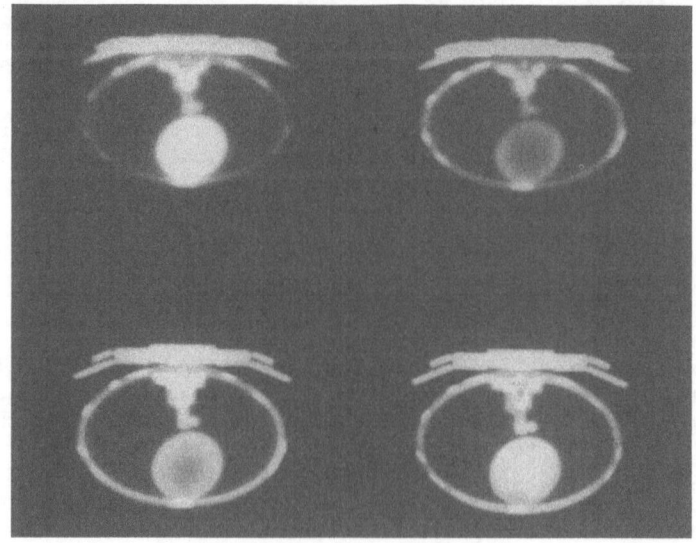

Fig. 6. The maximum entropy solution after 2, 3, 4,and 5 iterations for 128 projections using the conjugate gradient algorithm.

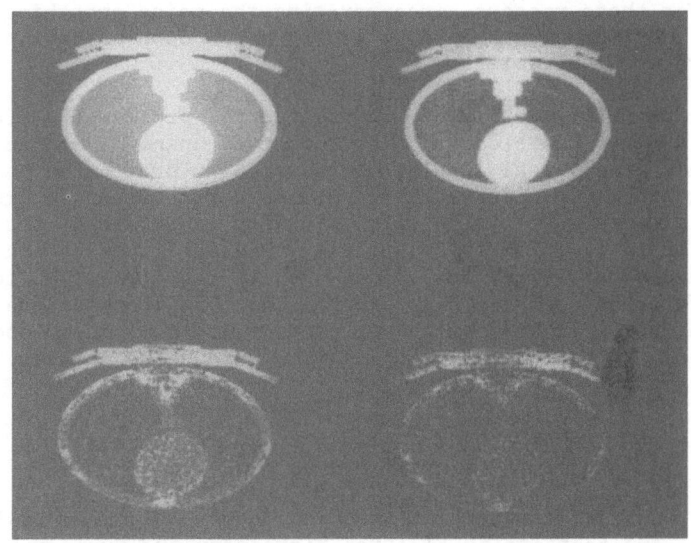

Fig. 7. Comparison of original image with the maximum entropy
solution after 10 iterations for projections with 1%,
5%, and 7% noise.

DISCUSSION

The results presented here demonstrate that a maximum entropy solution
is a feasible approach to reconstructing images from projections.  Compared
with other simulations (Gullberg and Malko, 1984) these results were similar in image quality yet seemed to converge in fewer iterations than the
maximum likelihood techniques (Shepp and Vardi, 1982, Lange and Carson,
1984).  The results give less artifacts than conjugate gradient (Budinger,
et al., 1979) and iterative convolution (Walters, et al., 1981) techniques.
It has previously been reported (Minerbo, 1979), in the case of a small
number of views, that the maximum entropy method does not result in
"streaking" artifacts common to backprojection of filtered projection and
other iterative algorithms.

A maximum entropy solution using a Gauss-Seidel algorithm gives
reconstructions with a "salt and pepper" texture which becomes less objec-
tionable with noisy data.  In fact, the results seem to show less correlated
structure than the conjugate gradient algorithm.  This isn't too surprising
seeing that the Gauss-Seidel algorithm makes corrections on a ray by ray
basis; whereas, the iteration updates for the conjugate gradient algorithm
are determined from all projection rays.  The Gauss-Seidel algorithm that
we have developed is able to reconstruct images from projections using
different weighting schemes for any desired geometrical configuration.

Work is progressing to evaluate solutions obtained using the noise
model in Eq. (1).  In the application of iterative algorithms to computed
tomography, as in nuclear medicine, the smoothing is accomplished after
stopping at an iteration which gives a reasonably perceived reconstruction.
This is a somewhat ad hoc technique for suppressing noise.  The algorithm
is not based upon any mathematics requiring a noise model to estimate the

solution. For these reasons, incorporating the noise smoothing or suppression within the iterative procedure itself based upon an appropriate noise model appears more suitable.

Duality principles are useful to reduce the problem to a form that is most easily handled numerically. The number of unknowns in the dual problem is less than in the primal problem if the angular projection samples are less than the number of pixels being reconstructed, which occurs with limited-angle tomography. Also, with equality constraints, the dual program is an unconstrained optimization program. Duality is not useful for constrained least squares problems, since duality principles applied to the sum of squares function yields a dual program that has an objective function in terms of the matrix inverse of the product of the projection operator and its transpose. The dimension of the matrix product is usually too large to invert numerically.

# REFERENCES

Budinger, T. F. (1971). "Transfer Function Theory and Image Evaluation in Biology: Applications in Electron Microscopy and Nuclear Medicine," Ph.D. dissertation, University of California, Berkeley.

Budinger, T. F., Gullberg, G. T. and Huesman, R. H. (1979). Emission computed tomography, in: "Image Reconstruction From Projections: Implementation and Applications," G. T. Herman, ed., Springer-Verlag, New York, 147-246.

D'Addario, L. R. (1975). Maximum a posteriori probability and maximum entropy reconstruction, in: "Image Processing for 2-D and 3-D Reconstruction from Projections," Technical Digest of Papers Presented at Topical Meeting on Image Processing for 2-D and 3-D Reconstruction from projections, Stanford Univ., Stanford, WAS-1-WAS-4.

Frieden, B. R. (1972). Restoring with maximum likelihood and maximum entropy, J Opt Soc Amer., 62, 511-518.

Frieden, B. R. (1975). Image enhancement and restoration, in: "Topics in Applied Physics-Picture Processing and Digital Filtering," T. S. Huang, ed., Springer-Verlag, New York, 177-248.

Frieden, B. R. (1977). Estimation--A new role for maximum entropy, in: "1976 SPSE Conference Proceedings," R. Shaw, ed., Society of Photographic Scientists and Engineers, Washington D.C., 261-265.

Frieden, B. R. (1980). Statistical models for the image restoration problem, Comput Graph and Image Process, 12, 40-59.

Gordon, R., Bender, R. and Herman, G. T. (1970). Algebraic reconstruction techniques (ART) for three-dimensional electron microscopy and x-ray photography, J Theor Biol., 29, 471-481.

Gullberg, G. T. (1975). Entropy and transverse section reconstruction, in: "Information Processing in Scintigraphy," C. Raynaud and A. Todd-Pokropek, eds., "Proceedings of the IVth International Conference," Orsay, France, 249-257.

Gullberg, G.T. and Malko, J.A. (1984). Attenuation correction for quantitative tomography-different methods, Europ J Nucl Med, 9, A24.

Gullberg, G.T. and Ghosh Roy, D.N. (1986). Maximum entropy reconstruction with constraints: Reducing the problem using duality principles, in: "Proceedings of the International Workshop on Physics and Engineering of Computerized Multidimensional Imaging and Process," SPIE 671, 25-33.

Huesman, R. H., Gullberg, G.T., Greenberg, W.L. and Budinger, T.F. (1977). "Users Manual Donner Algorithms for Reconstruction Tomography,"

Jaynes, E. T. (1957). Information theory and statistical mechanics, Phys Rev, 106, 620.

Lange, K. and Carson, R. (1984). EM reconstruction algorithms for emission and transmission tomography, J Comput Assist Tomogr., 8, 306-316.

Lent, A. (1977). A convergent algorithm for maximum entropy image restoration, with a medical x-ray application, in: "1976 SPSE Conference Proceedings," R. Shaw, ed., Society of Photographic Scientists and Engineers, Washington, D.C., 249-257.

Lewis, M. H., Willerson, J. T., Lewis, S. E., Bonte, F. J., Parker, R. W. and Stokely, E. M. (1982). Attenuation compensation in single-photon emission tomography: A comparative evaluation, J Nucl Med, 23, 1121-1127.

Minerbo, G. (1979). MENT: A maximum entropy algorithm for reconstructing a source from projection data," Comput Graph and Image Process, 10, 48-68.

Ortega, J. M., and Rheinboldt, W.C. (1970). "Iterative Solutions of Nonlinear Equations in Several Variables," Academic Press, New York.

Rockafellar, R. T. (1970). "Convex Analysis," Princeton University Press, Princeton.

Shepp, L. A. and Vardi, V. (1982). Maximum likelihood reconstruction for emission tomography, IEEE Trans Med Imaging, MI-1, 113-122.

Walters, T. E., Simon, W., Chesler, D. A. and Correia, J. A. (1981). Attenuation correction in gamma emission computed Tomography, J Comput Assist Tomogr, 5, 89-94.

Wernecke, S. J. (1975). Maximum entropy image reconstruction, in: "Image Processing for 2-D and 3-D Reconstruction from Projections," Technical Digest of Papers Presented at Topical Meeting on Image Processing for 2-D and 3-D Reconstruction from Projections, Stanford Univ., Stanford, WAG-1-WAG-4.

Wernecke, S. J. (1977). Maximum entropy techniques for digital image reconstruction, in: "1976 SPSE Conference Proceedings," R. Shaw, ed., Society of Photographic Scientists and Engineers, Washington, D.C., 238-243.

Wernecke, S. J. and D'Addario, L. R. (1977). Maximum entropy image reconstruction,IEEE Transactions on Computers, C-26, 351-364.

Zwick, M. and Zeitler, E. (1973). Image reconstruction from projections, Optik, 38, 550-565.

# THE MAXIMUM LIKELIHOOD ESTIMATOR METHOD OF IMAGE RECONSTRUCTION:

# ITS FUNDAMENTAL CHARACTERISTICS AND THEIR ORIGIN

Jorge Llacer and Eugene Veklerov

Lawrence Berkeley Laboratory
University of California
Berkeley, CA 94720 U.S.A.

## ABSTRACT

In this paper we review our recent work in characterizing the image reconstruction properties of the MLE algorithm. We have studied its convergence properties and confirmed the onset of image deterioration, which is a function of the number of counts in the source. By modulating the weight given to projection tubes with high numbers of counts with respect to those with low numbers of counts in the reconstruction process, we have confirmed that image deterioration is due to an attempt by the algorithm to match projection data tubes with high numbers of counts too closely to the iterative image projections. We have also developed a stopping rule for the algorithm that tests the hypothesis that a reconstructed image could have given the initial projection data in a manner consistent with the underlying assumption of Poisson distributed variables. The rule has been applied to two mathematically generated phantoms with success and to a third phantom with "exact" (no statistical fluctuations) projection data with results which confirm our understanding of the fundamental process of iterative image reconstruction. We conclude that the behavior of the target functions whose extrema are sought in iterative schemes is more important in the early stages of the reconstruction than in the later stages, when the extrema are being approached but the results are in contradiction with the Poisson nature of the measurement.

## INTRODUCTION

The non-linear iterative Maximum Likelihood Estimator (MLE) method of image reconstruction for tomography has received increasing attention in the last several years because it promises reconstructions with very low noise and sharp edges, even from incomplete sets of projections. In the last two years, instabilities or image deterioration with increasing number of iterations have been reported in the reconstruction of smooth activity fields. This could make the method rather useless for medical applications. Snyder and Miller (1985) have proposed stabilizing the solution by filtering with sieves along with the iterative process. Levitan and Herman (1986) have used a maximum a posteriori probability expectation maximization algorithm to constrain the MLE algorithm to solutions that do not deviate more than a certain measure from a pre-determined expected image. Although these approaches work at stabilizing the solution, they appear to visibly degrade the images from what may be called the "best" MLE solutions and they introduce some arbitrary parameters in the reconstruction process. For those reasons we chose to follow a different path and attempted to analyze the MLE process in sufficient detail to give us an understanding of the reason for the image deterioration. We hope that we can thereby develop an image-independent rule for stopping the iterative process at some optimum point and, perhaps, open the way for the development of better algorithms.

In this paper we shall review the work that we have carried out during the last year, including the development of an effective stopping rule, describe recent experiences in its use and discuss the implications that our work appears to have with respect to the choice of target functions for iterative algorithms.

CONVERGENCE PROPERTIES OF THE MLE ALGORITHM

We extract here the essential points reported in Llacer et al (1987) on the convergence characteristics of the unmodified original MLE algorithm proposed for PET by Shepp and Vardi (1982) and of a weighted algorithm proposed for analytical purposes in Llacer and Veklerov (1987).

The likelihood function that one seeks to maximize in the MLE method is defined as:

$$L(\lambda) = P(n^*|\lambda) = \prod_{d=1}^{D} e^{-\lambda^*(d)}\lambda^*(d)^{n^*(d)}/n^*(d)! \tag{1}$$

where $n^*(d)$ is the number of counts detected in projection tube d, and $\lambda^*(d)$ is the projection into tube d of the reconstructed image.

Since our purpose was to evaluate the behavior of the MLE algorithm exclusively, without being sensitive to effects due to the possible inaccuracies of the matrix p(b,d) in representing a particular detector instrument, we have generated and reconstructed images by computer in a self-consistent manner; the images were obtained first by random assignment of events to pixels according to a specific image pattern. We call these the "source images". The corresponding projections were then obtained by assigning each event in each pixel to a tube d by a random process using a previously computed set of probabilities p(b,d) that may correspond to a model of some specific instrument. The same set of probabilities was used subsequently in the reconstructions.

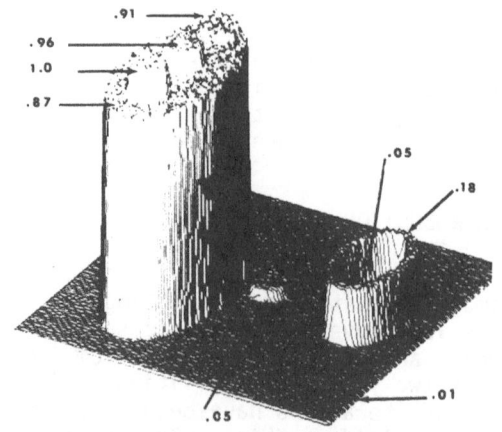

Figure 1 shows the source image used for the experiments for the particular case of 32 million counts in the image. The relative activities per

Fig. 1: Source image with 32 million counts obtained by a random process with probabilities corresponding to the relative activities indicated. Image discretized in 128x128 pixels.

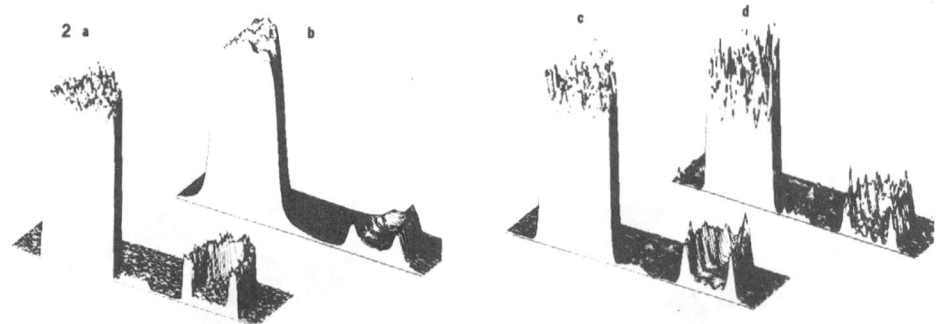

Fig. 2:  a) Cut through a line in the source image of 2 million counts.
b) ditto for a corresponding MLE reconstruction after 9 iterations.
c) ditto after 45 iterations.  d) ditto after 200 iterations.


unit area are shown in the figure.  The interior of the elliptical shell
has a relative activity of 0.05.  Random background was simulated by a
relative activity of 0.01 over the entire surface of the image.  The image plane has been discretized into 128 by 128 pixels.  The matrix of
$p(b,d)$ values used for projection generation and image reconstruction
was obtained following the algorithm described by Shepp and Vardi (1982)
and adapted to one ring of the UCLA ECAT-III, 512 detector tomograph, in
Hoffman et al (1983).

For a source image with 2 million counts (2M), Fig. 2a shows a cut
through a line in the source image and Figs. 2b - d show the MLE reconstructions with 9, 45 and 200 iterations, respectively.  The same experiment was repeated with the source image containing 8 million (8M) and 32
million (32M) counts.  The results are shown in Figs. 3 and 4.


An examination of the reconstructed images shows that:

a)  reconstructions improve towards a reasonable representation of
    the source images up to 30 - 50 iterations;
b)  the image quality remains virtually the same for a number itera-
    tions; and
c)  after that point, images begin to deteriorate.


It was also observed that images from sources with a higher number
of counts require more iterations to reach their best appearance and
they remain in that condition for more iterations.

We also carried out an analysis of the probability that the source
images could have generated their own projection data and compared the
results with the corresponding probabilities that the MLE reconstructed
images would have generated such data.  This was done by a straightforward application of the Poisson function to the projection of the images
as means and the projection data as instances of the distributions.  Figure 5 shows the results of the calculations.  We see that, as expected,
the probability that the MLE images would have generated the projection
data increases with iteration number.  After all, that is what the MLE
algorithm is supposed to do.  We see, however, that the source image
which actually generated the projection data is substantially removed
from having that maximum probability.  As the number of counts in the
source increases, the distance to that maximum decreases.

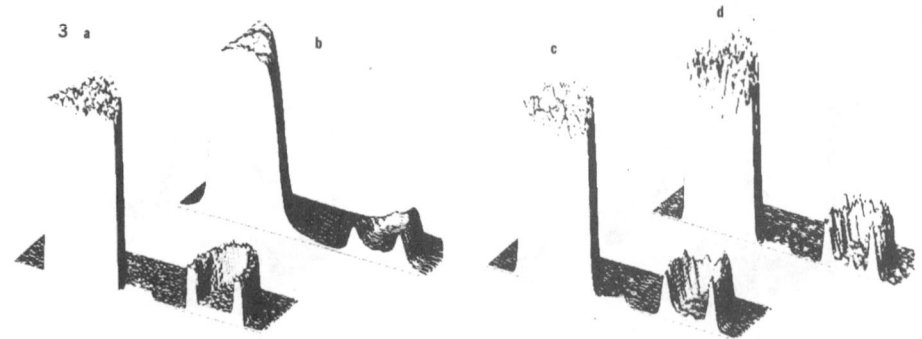

Fig. 3: a) Cut through a line in the source image of 8 million counts.
b) ditto for a corresponding MLE reconstruction after 9 iterations.
c) ditto after 45 iterations.  d) ditto after 200 iterations.

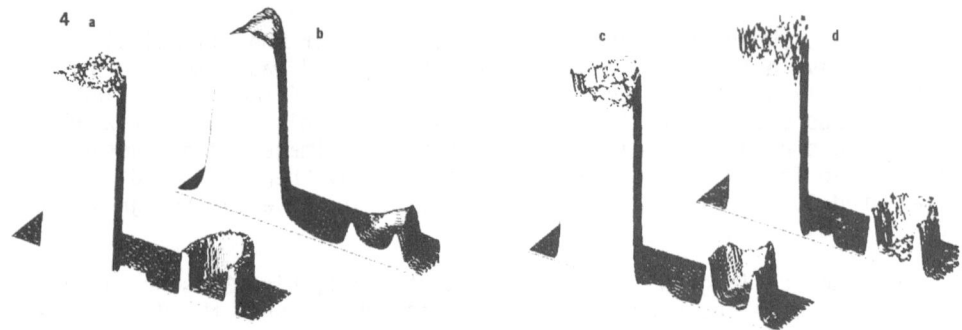

Fig. 4: a) Cut through a line in the source image of 32 million counts.
b) ditto for a corresponding MLE reconstruction after 9 iterations.
c) ditto after 45 iterations.  d) ditto after 200 iterations.

This last set of observations gave us the first indications of the origin of the image deterioration observed in the MLE solutions:  because of statistical uncertainty in the process of going from disintegrations in the pixels to detection in projection tubes, the projections present an inconsistent set of data to the matrix of p(b,d) values.  As the iterative process continues beyond a certain point, the algorithm tries to find an image that reconciles those inconsistencies as well as possible in the manner precribed by the target function chosen (the likelihood function L of Eq. 1).  In fact, it goes beyond the value of L corresponding to the source image.

We have obtained further confirmation of our hypothesis by developing a modified target function, which we call the Weighted Likelihood Estimator (WLE).  The function that we seek to maximize is:

$$WL(\lambda) = WP(n\star|\lambda) = \prod_{d=1}^{D} \left[ e^{-\lambda\star(d)} \lambda\star(d)^{n\star(d)} / n\star(d)! \right]^{s \cdot n\star(d)+t} \tag{2}$$

With s = 0 and t = 1, the function WL is identical to the likelihood function L of Eq. 1.  Keeping t = 1, s > 0 will give higher weight during the process of maximization to those tubes that have higher number of counts, while making s < 0 will decrease their weight.  The iterative formula for the maximization of Eq. 4 is:

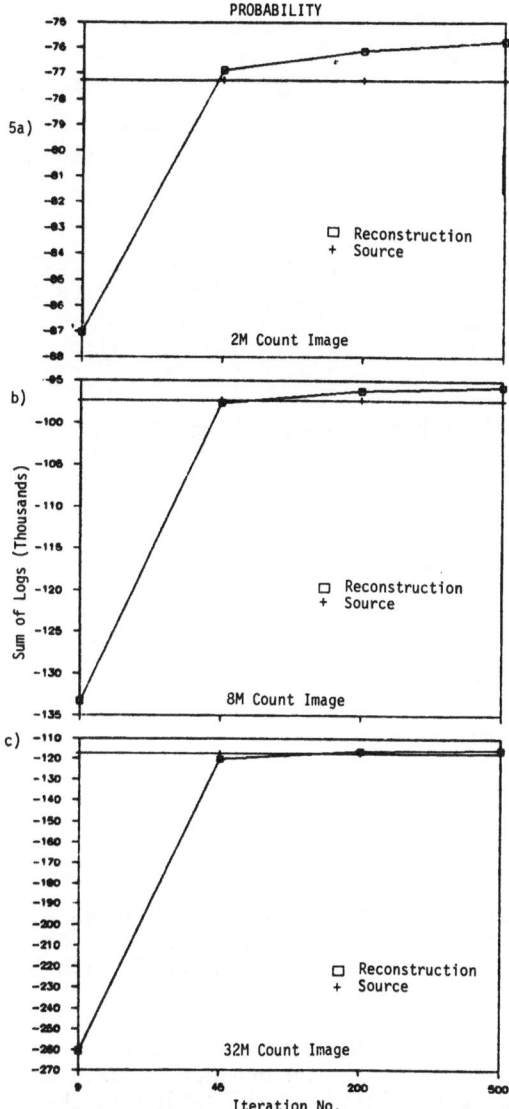

Fig. 5: Probability that the image obtained at a certain number of iterations has yielded the particular set of projection data used as input for the reconstruction; horizontal line indicates the probability for the source image that truly generated the input data. a) case with 2 million counts in the source image. b) case with 8 million counts. c) case with 32 million counts.

$$\lambda^{new}(b) = \lambda^{old}(b) \left[ 1 + \sum_{d=1}^{D} [s \cdot n^*(d) + t] \, p(b,d) \, \frac{n^*(d) - 1}{\sum_{b'=1}^{B} \lambda^{old}(b') p(b',d)} \right] \quad (3)$$

We have carried out reconstructions with the WLE target function with the source image of Fig. 1 with 2M counts, with values s = 0.0025, 0 and −0.0015. It is observed that the onset of image deterioration in regions of high activity comes early in the first case and is delayed in the last case, with respect to the s = 0 case. No substantial differences are

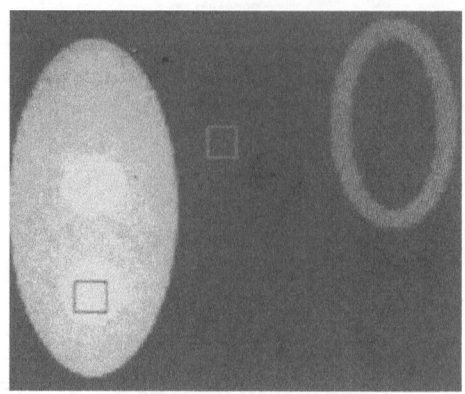

Fig. 6:  Source distribution showing Reg. 1 and 2 for noise evaluation.

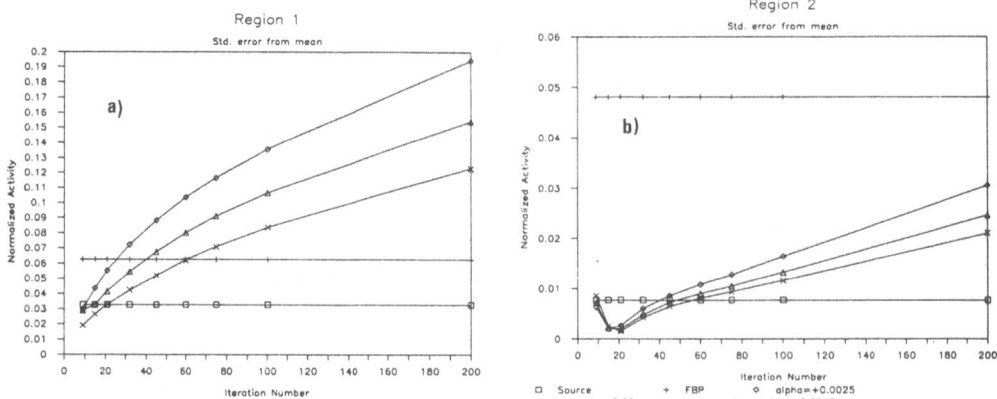

Fig. 7:  Plots of standard error σ from the mean as a function of iteration number for different values of parameter s in Eqs. 2 and 3.  a) Reg.
1, with high counts (1.0 relative).  b) Reg. 2, with low counts (0.05).

observed in regions of low activity, which have its corresponding tubes
with low counts reconciled with the projection data very early in the iterative process and suffer little modification in the later stages, seen
in Llacer et al (1986).  Figure 6 shows two regions (small squares) in
the source image chosen for investigation, one in the region of 100%
counts, the other in the region of 5% counts.  Figure 7 shows plots of
standard error from the mean σ, in each of two zones as a function of iteration number for the WLE reconstructions.  Also shown are the standard
errors for a filtered backprojection (FBP) reconstruction with the Shepp-
Logan filter and for the source image.  For the region with high counts,
Region 1, we observe that σ is a factor of 2 higher than the source image
error.  For the WLE reconstructions, we see a substantial influence of
the parameter s on the iteration number at which σ is equal to that of
the FBP method.  In the region of low counts, Region 2, the error of the
FBP is 0.05, of the same magnitude as the signal, while the WLE results
remain under 0.01 (near the source noise) up to iterations 40 to 60.

The observation that modulating the weight of tubes with high counts
on the likelihood function changes substantially the onset of image deterioration supports the above argument that image deterioration occurs
by an attempt by the MLE algorithm to match the projection tubes with
high numbers of counts to the statistically deficient projection data too

well.  The question then arises naturally:  is there a way to determine
an optimum stopping point that is image and number of count independent?
In the following a concise statement of the stopping rule which we have
devised in Veklerov and Llacer (1987) is presented.

## STOPPING RULE FOR ITERATIVE ALGORITHMS

We shall first show that the maximization of Eq. 1 and the underlying
assumption that the data are Poisson-distributed become contradictory to
each other beyond a certain number of iterations.  We propose a quantitative criterion that allows the user to catch the moment when they are
least contradictory.

It was noticed by Snyder, Lewis and Ter-Pogossian (1981) that $n^*(d)$
are independent and Poisson random variables and $\lambda^*(d)$ are their means.
Therefore, the image maximizing Eq. 1 must be such that $\lambda^*(d)$ are as
close to $n^*(d)$ as possible.  (This is also seen from Eq. 1 directly.)

This fact leads to a paradoxical situation.  The closer $\lambda^*(d)$ become
to $n^*(d)$, the higher the probability that the image generates the projection data as measured by the likelihood function L.  However, for Poisson
distributed data, if the two get too close for all or almost all tubes d,
it becomes statistically unlikely that the image could have generated the
data.  This paradox can be illustrated with the aid of the following simplified example.  Let us assume that each tube in the initial projection
data has exactly 100 counts and the algorithm is able to assign values
to the image pixels so that each image projection tube has a value between 99 and 101.  These values are means of Poisson distributed variables of which the 100 numbers are realizations.  The condition just described would be a very good match as measured by the L criterion or by
other criteria, such as the minimum least squares, for example.  We as-
sert, however, that the means are too close to the data to be consistent
with the underlying assumption that the data are Poisson distributed.
Indeed, now we have a situation with a large number of independent measurements each of which differs from the mean by less than 1.  However,
since the underlying distribution is Poisson, the standard deviation
should be approximately 10.  This contradiction demonstrates our point.

In order to avoid arriving at this contradictory condition during
image reconstruction, we propose to test, at the end of each iteration,
the hypothesis that the values of $n^*(d)$ for each d=1,...,D are jointly
statistically valid realizations of Poisson-distributed random variables
corresponding to their means $\lambda^*(d)$.  In other words, we test the hypothesis that $n^*(1)$ is a realization of a Poisson variable with the mean $\lambda^*(1)$
and $n^*(2)$ is a realization of another such distribution with mean $\lambda^*(2)$
and so on.  It is reasonable to require that only images passing the
test (for which the hypothesis is not rejected) be declared acceptable.
The development of the testing procedure is described in Veklerov and
Llacer (1987), to which we refer the reader for details.  The test is
based on an application of Pearson's chi-square test as shown in Canavos
(1984) adapted to our case.  It results in:

a)  A histogram of projection tubes with a number N of bins of equal
    probability which is flat if the projection data $n^*(d)$ are valid
    realizations of Poisson distributed variables with means $\lambda^*(d)$.
    If the histogram is relatively empty at the center, the itera-
    tive process has not yet gone far enough and maximization of the
    likelihood function (or another suitable target function) can
    continue.  If bunching occurs in the central bins, the iterative
    process has gone too far; the projection data are too close to
    the projection of the image whose validity is being tested.

b) A hypothesis testing function H which is obtained from the above tube histograms by Pearson's test applied to the results of successive iterations. This function should go through a minimum with values below 36.2 and 27.2, for an example with N = 20 bins, corresponding to significance levels of 0.1 and 0.01, respectively. The significance levels are the probabilities of rejecting the hypothesis, given that it is true.

EXAMPLES OF THE APPLICATION OF THE STOPPING RULE

The above stopping rule has been applied first to the MLE reconstructions of the activity distribution of Fig. 1, as reported in Veklerov and Llacer (1987). The results of the hypothesis testing function H for 2M, 8M and 32M counts in the source image are shown in Fig. 8, curves a), b) and c), respectively. They indicate that the images at iterations near 30, 50 and 90 are "best" in terms of consistency of the images with the Poisson nature of the PET process. This result agrees with our observations about image deterioration as a function of iteration number and counts in the source image, as discussed above. Figure 9 shows a comparison of the source image, an FBP image (Shepp–Logan filter) and MLE recontruction images at 9, 32 and 200 iterations for the 2M count case. At the three count levels tested, the "best" image represents compromises between some deterioration at the regions of high counts (Region 1 of Fig. 6, for example) and the attaining of reasonable sharpness and detail in the regions of low counts (Region 2).

A second test with a source distribution containing substantial detail, mimicking a brain phantom in some fashion, has also been carried out with 2M counts. The source image and projection data have been generated by the same computational method used for the phantom of Fig. 1. Figure 10, left to right, top to bottom, shows the source image, an FBP (Shepp–Logan filter), and MLE reconstructions from 21, 32, 45 and 100 iterations, presented with 16 levels of gray. The "best" image is near iteration 45, determined by the value of the hypothesis testing function H, of Fig. 11. Figure 12 shows the tube histograms for the same set of iterations; the contents of the histogram bins is flattest at 45 iterations.

We have also carried out another experiment to further confirm the correctness of our interpretation of the tube histograms and their relationship to the consistency of the Poisson distribution. Starting with an image of the Hoffman brain phantom in Hoffman et al (1983), supplied to us by the UCLA group, we have generated an exact set of projection data by multiplying the image pixels by the elements of a p(b,d) transition matrix which describes the ECAT-III tomograph in the Shepp–Vardi approximation (1982). The projection data are exact in the sense that no statistical fluctuations have been introduced in going from the pixel counts to the projections. The multiplications have been made in double precision and all fractional counts have been kept. The reconstructions were carried out in double precision using the same transition matrix.

In reconstructing the Hoffman brain phantom from such a set of data, we would expect the MLE process to be able to proceed without image deterioration for a very large number of iterations, since there are no statistical fluctuations in the projections; i.e., the projection data are fully consistent with the transition matrix (matrix of p(b,d)'s). In fact, the projection data contain the statistical accuracy of a nearly infinite number of counts in the source image, although in reality, most of the significant tubes have counts in the order of 100. We would also expect that the tube histogram obtained during the iterative process to

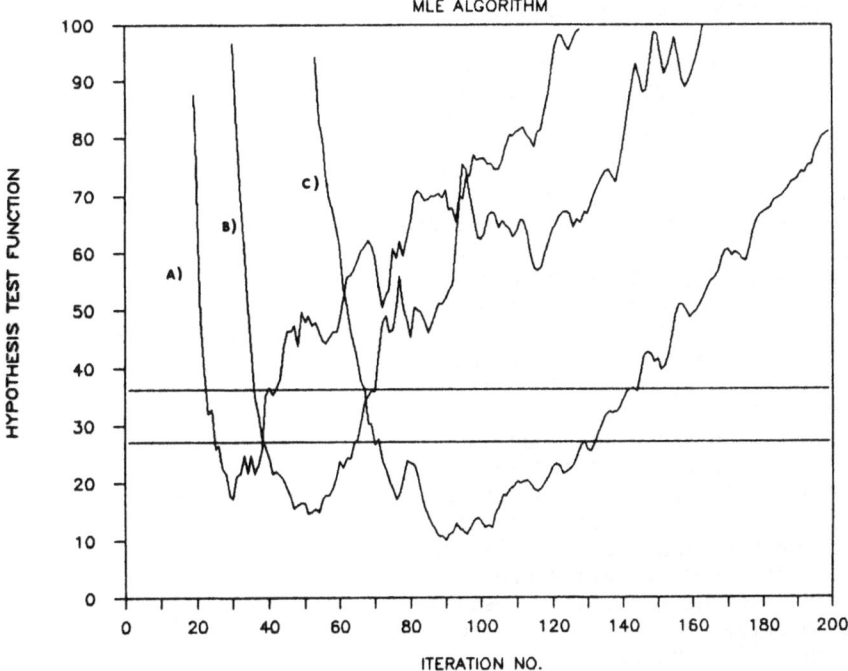

Fig. 8: Value of the hypothesis test function vs. iteration number for MLE reconstructions of the source distribution of Fig. 1. Curve a) is for 2 million counts in the source image, b) for 8 million and c) for 32 million counts. The line at a value of 36.2 is the limit below which the probability of accepting an image when it should be rejected is 0.1. The line at 27.2 is the corresponding limit for a a probability of 0.01.

be badly behaved. For tubes with approximately 100 counts, consistency with a Poisson distribution would require, like in our previous simplified example, that the projection data are all realizations of Poisson distributions with standard deviations of approximately 10. Instead, the reconstruction has an infinitesimally small standard deviation and the tube histogram can be expected to be bunched up in the middle. The results of our reconstructions confirm the above expectations: Fig. 13 shows the source image and the results of reconstruction at iteration 150, showing no deterioration. Figure 14 shows the tube histograms at several iterations. The hypothesis testing function never reaches a value low enough to be considered acceptable.

We intend to start applying our stopping rule to reconstructions from real data obtained from tomographs in the near future. We expect some difficulties due to:

a) the existence of background counts from random coincidences which are inconsistent with the transition matrix,
b) detector pair non-uniformities that will probably require applying corrections to the transition matrices directly so as not to modify the statistics of the raw data by a normalization,
c) absorption corrections that we also expect will have to be applied to the transition matrices, and
d) the transition matrix must represent the tomographic instrument with an as yet undetermined level of accuracy.

## DISCUSSION AND CONCLUSIONS

We feel that the most important result that we have obtained in the research reviewed in this paper is the realization that an iterative algorithm that seeks an extremum of some target function may lead to a contradiction with the underlying assumption that the generation of projection data follows Poisson statistics. This contradiction will clearly occur when the target function is one that has an extremum when the projections of the obtained images approach the projection data as the number of iterations increases, as is the case with the likelihood function L of Eq. 1, or a minimum least squares error function. In order not to violate the Poisson nature of the process, we have shown that it is necessary to stop the iterative process at some point and the hypothesis testing method described appears to be a suitable method of doing so.

Stopping the iterative process before reaching an extremum of a target function places the choice of such a function in a different light from the customary one, since we would seldom expect to attain the goal for which it was designed. What is most important is the behavior of the target function in the earlier stages of the iterative process, while it follows a path towards its extremum. In that respect, we have obtained a substantial amount of information about the MLE algorithm. In its useful range of iterations its behavior is determined principally by the fact that the magnitude of the derivative of the Poisson function with respect to its mean in the vicinity of the mean is higher for low means that for high means. During the iterative process, the likelihood function L of Eq. 1 gains more by matching $\lambda^*(d)$ to $n^*(d)$ for tubes with low numbers of counts than for tubes with high counts. It appears that this explains most of the observed behavior of the algorithm:

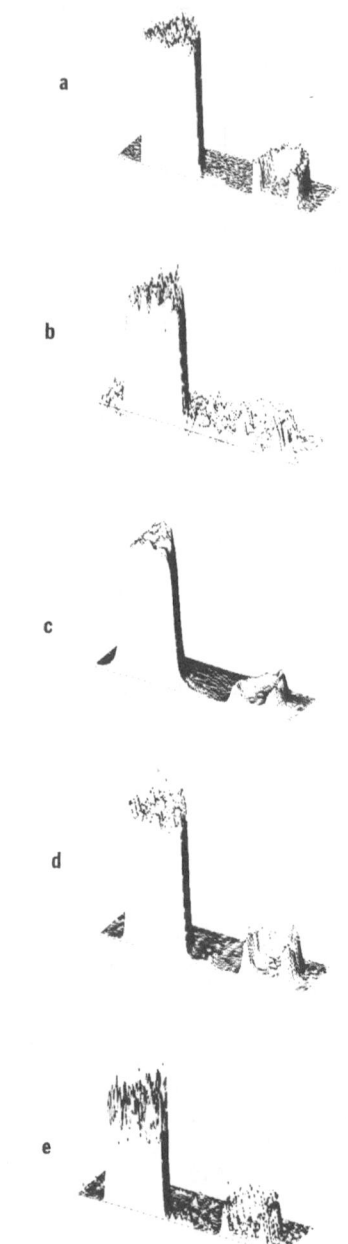

Fig. 9: Cuts through source and reconstructed images. a) source image with 2 million counts. b) reconstruction by filtered back-projection (Shepp-Logan filter). c) MLE reconstruction, 9 iterations. d) ditto, 32 it. ("best" image). e) 200 iterations.

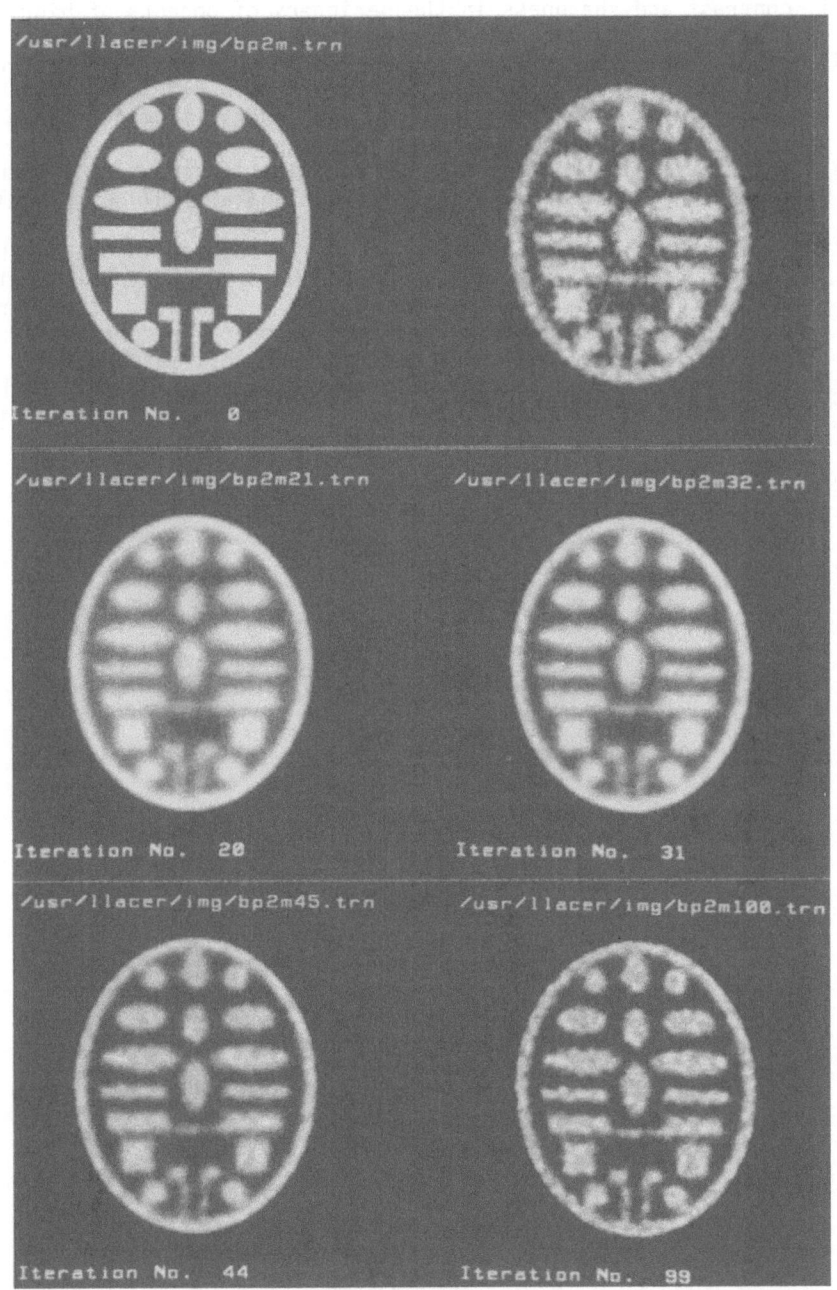

Fig. 10: Left to right, top to bottom: source image, FBP (Shepp–Logan filter) and MLE reconstructions for 21, 32, 45 and 100 iterations, presented with 16 levels of gray. The "best" image is near iteration 45, determined by the value of the hypothesis testing function H, of Fig. 11.

a) backgrounds in MLE reconstructions are very clean, with very little noise magnification.
b) the meaningful matching of tubes with high counts starts to occur after the low count tubes are already rather well matched.
c) contrast and sharpness in the periphery of objects of high activity are very good in MLE reconstructions.
d) ringing at edges is usually observed in the "best" reconstructions and it is a consequence of the finite size of pixels being traversed by tubes with low and high counts (from different projection angles) in the vicinity of edges.
e) contrast inside regions of high activity is somewhat difficult to attain, as already pointed out by Tanaka (1987), since all the projections involved may have high counts.
f) accurate reconstruction of low activity regions in the neighborhood of high activity regions may be hard to obtain since it involves tubes with both high counts and low counts. It appears then that the low activity region is properly reconstructed when the high activity region is getting very well matched, with image deterioration. In the case of Region 2 of Fig. 6, the proper average activity of 0.05 was only attained past the "best" image point, but could be modulated by using the WLE target function with $s < 0$.

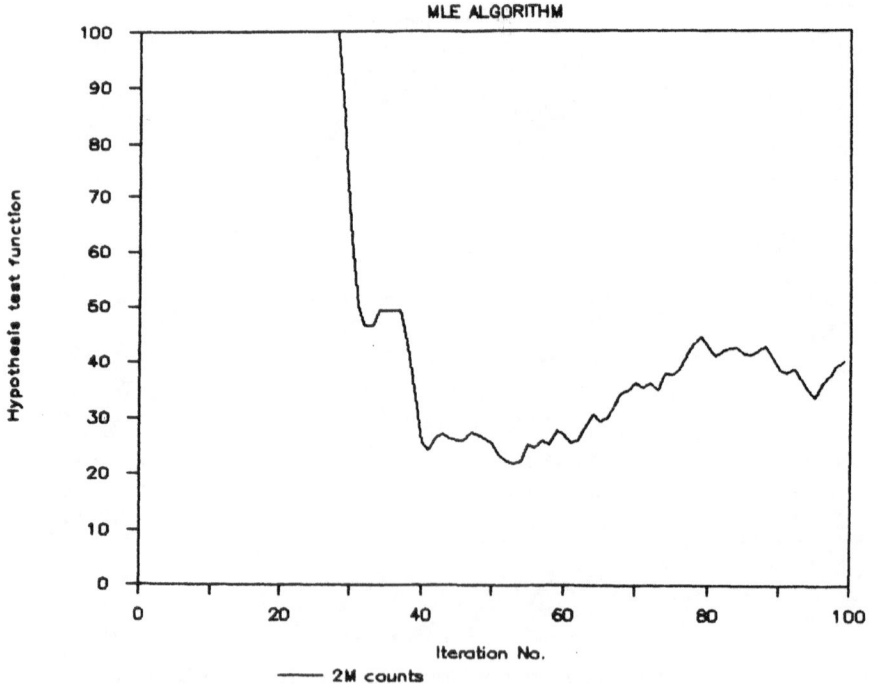

Fig. 11: Hypothesis testing function for the reconstructions of the phantom of Fig. 10, with 2 million counts in the source.

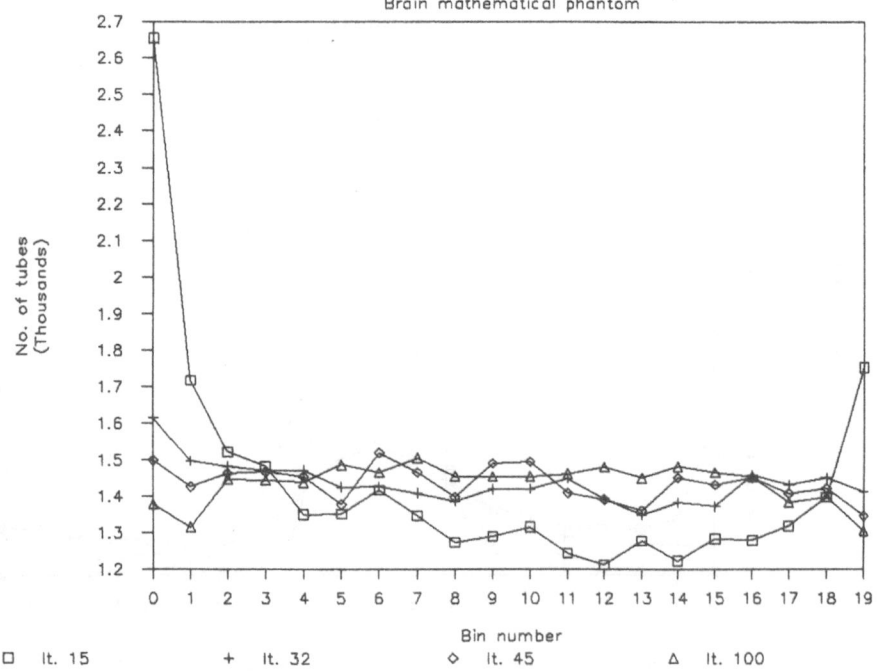

Fig. 12: Tube histograms for the MLE reconstructions with 15, 32 and 100 iterations. The flat distribution is attained near the "best" reconstruction.

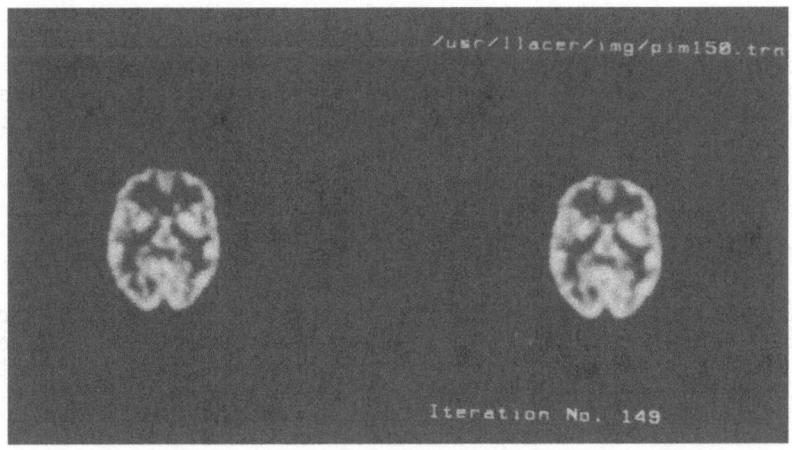

Fig. 13: Source image consisting of a reconstructed Hoffman brain phantom and MLE reconstruction at iteration 150. An exact generation of projection data (without statistical fluctuations) results in no image deterioration.

## Tube histograms for MLE reconstruction

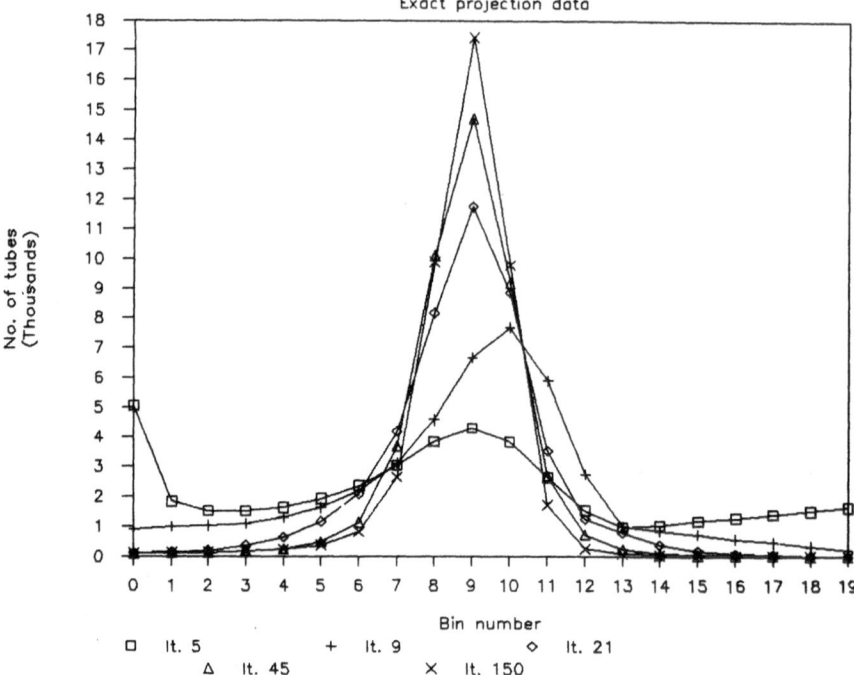

Fig. 14:  Tube histograms for the reconstruction of Fig. 14 at 5, 32 and 200 iterations.  A good flat histogram is never obtained for the "exact" (non-Poisson) projection data.


In conclusion, we see the likelihood target function of Eq. 1 as a very interesting one that may have usefulness in medical reconstructions, but it is not clear to these authors, at this time, that its virtues are important in clinical diagnosis.  Along with a continued study of a broader spectrum of target functions, we intend to test the usefulness of the MLE algorithm by a series of ROC studies in collaboration with the UCLA PET group.


## ACKNOWLEDGMENTS

The active collaboration of Edward J. Hoffman, UCLA Dept. of Radiological Sciences, in several aspects of our work is gratefully acknowledged.  This work was supported in part by the National Cancer Institute (CA-39501) and by the U.S. Department of Energy under Contract No. DE-AC03-76SF00098.

## REFERENCES

Canavos, G. (1984). Applied Probability and Statistical Methods, Little, Brown and Co., Boston, Toronto.

Hoffman, E. J., Ricci, A. R., Var der Stee, L. M. A. M. and Phelps, M. E. (1983). ECAT-III, basic design considerations, IEEE Trans. Nucl Sci., NS-30, No. 1, 729.

Levitan, E. and Herman, G. T. (1986). A maximum a posteriori probability expectation maximization algorithm for image reconstruction in emission tomography, Medical Image Proc. Group Tech. Report No. MIPG115, Department of Radiology, U. of Pennsylvania.

Llacer, J., Andreae, S. and Chatterjee, A. (1986). On the applicability of the maximum likelihood estimator algorithm for image recovery in accelerated positron emitter beam injection, SPIE, 671, 269.

Llacer, J., Veklerov, E. and Hoffman, E. J. (1987). On the convergence of the maximum likelihood estimator method of tomographic image reconstructions, Proc. Conf. on Medical Imaging, Newport Beach, CA SPIE, 767.

Llacer, J. and Veklerov, E. (1987). The high sensitivity of the maximum likelihood estimator method of tomographic image reconstruction, Proc. Int. Symposium on Computed Assisted Radiology (CAR '87), Berlin.

Shepp, L. A. and Vardi, Y. (1982). Maximum likelihood reconstruction for emission tomography, IEEE Trans. Med. Imaging, MI-1, No. 2, 113-121.

Snyder, D. L., Lewis, J. T. and Ter-Pogossian, M. M. (1981). A mathematical model for positron-emission tomography systems having time-of-flight measurements, IEEE Trans. Nucl. Sci., NS-28, 3575.

Snyder, D. L. and Miller, M. I. (1985). The use of sieves to stabilize images produced with the EM algorithm for emission tomography, IEEE Trans. Nucl. Sci., NS-32, No. 5, 3864.

Tanaka, E. (1987). A Fast Reconstruction Algorithm for Stationary Positron Emission Tomography Based on a Modified EM Algorithm, to be publ. in IEEE Trans. on Med. Imaging.

Veklerov, E. and Llacer, J. (1987). Stopping rule for the MLE algorithm based on statistical hypothesis testing, submitted to IEEE Trans. Medical Imaging for publication.

# A FILTERED ITERATIVE RECONSTRUCTION ALGORITHM

# FOR POSITRON EMISSION TOMOGRAPHY

Eiichi Tanaka

Division of Physics
National Institute of Radiological Sciences
Anagawa-4, Chiba-shi, Japan

## INTRODUCTION

Positron emission tomography (PET) has received increasing attention
for the use in physiological studies in medical diagnosis.  Most PET systems
have a circular array of bismuth germanate (BGO) detectors and the coincidence detection of two annihilation photons is employed to reconstruct
tomographic images.  The detector gantry usually undergoes some type of
scanning motion (wobbling, rotation, etc.) to achieve fine sampling of
projection data.  A recent trend of development in PET is to realize
stationary PET systems with a reasonable spatial resolution (Derenzo et
al.,1981; Burnham et al., 1984; Muehllehner and Karp, 1986).  A totally
stationary PET avoids the mechanical problems associated with accurate
movement of the heavy assembly and is particularly advantageous in gated
cardiac imaging or in fast dynamic studies.  Elimination of scan motion
along the detector plane allows one to scan the gantry quickly in the axial
direction so that continuous three dimensional imaging can be achieved with
a limited number of detector rings.

In the image reconstruction by means of an analytical method such as a
convolution backprojection (CBP) method, it is recognized that the linear
sampling interval should be smaller than or at least equal to half the
spatial resolution to be obtained (Brooks et al., 1979).  In a stationary
PET using discrete detectors, the effective linear sampling interval is
larger than the above required value by a factor of about 2 for the full use
of detector resolution.  Accordingly, narrower crystals have to be used in a
stationary mode than in a scanning mode to attain the same resolution.

The above sampling requirement arises from the use of an analytical
reconstruction method.  If we use an adequate iterative reconstruction
method, the sampling requirement may be relaxed and we may realize the full
use of detector resolution in the stationary mode.  Conceptually, the
essential requirement for the data collection is to sample the "object
plane" rather than to sample the "projections."  To improve the sampling of
the object plane, Tanaka et al.(1986) proposed a "bank array" of detectors.
The main objective of this paper is to propose a practical reconstruction
algorithm for the stationary PET.

There have been a number of studies on the iterative reconstruction
techniques (Herman and Lent, 1976).  These are algebraic reconstruction

technique (ART) (Gordon et al., 1970), simultaneous iterative reconstruction technique (SIRT) (Gilbert, 1972), iterative least-square technique (Budinger and Gullberg, 1974), conjugate gradient method (Kawata and Nalcioglu, 1985), maximum entropy method (Minerbo, 1979), etc. Although the fastest convergence is expected by the conjugate gradient method at present, it still needs more than several iterations to attain a reasonable spatial resolution.

Recently, maximum likelihood reconstruction based on an EM algorithm (Rockmore and Macovski, 1977; Shepp and Vardi, 1982; Lange and Carson, 1984) has received considerable attention for its use in the emission computed tomography. The algorithm incorporates the Poisson nature of data and has the following advantages: The reconstructed images are non-negative and the total image density is preserved at each iteration; the convergence is assured in theory and the image converges to the maximum likelihood estimate as iteration proceeds.

The algorithm, however, has several drawbacks, although these are more or less common properties of most iterative techniques. First the convergence is slow. The correction efficiency at each iteration step is not uniform over the image plane and it depends on the image pattern. The convergence speed is inversely proportional to the spatial frequency and accordingly the high frequency component of objects requires a larger number of iterations than the low frequency component. In addition, statistical noise tends to increase as iteration proceeds (Tanaka et al., 1985; Snyder and Miller, 1985; Llacer et al., 1986), and the iteration must be stopped at a certain criteria on the noise magnitude or another appropriate parameter. As a result, the spatial resolution depends strongly on the image pattern, on the number of iterations and on the point of interest in the image.

As an initial attempt to improve the convergence speed of the EM algorithm, a fast iterative reconstruction method has been developed (Tanaka, 1987a,1987b), in which the high frequency component of the ratio of measured to calculated projections is extracted and is taken into account to iterative correction of image density in such a way that the correction is performed efficiently over a wide range of spatial frequency. The algorithm is named "Filtered Iterative Reconstruction (FIR)" algorithm. This paper presents further improvement of the algorithm and the results of simulation studies on the performance for the application to PET studies.

FILTERED ITERATIVE RECONSTRUCTION ALGORITHM

Performance of the EM Algorithm

The development of the filtered iterative reconstruction (FIR) algorithm was initiated with an intention to improve the EM algorithm. We shall first describe an analysis of the properties of the EM algorithm. Assuming that data are binned first according to view angle $\theta$ and then according to projection bin for that angle (see Fig. 1), the iterative scheme of the EM algorithm is expressed by

$$s^{new}(b) = s(b) \sum_{\theta i} \sum \frac{n(i,\theta)}{m(i,\theta)} p(b;i,\theta) \qquad (1)$$

where

$$m(i,\theta) = \sum_{b'} s(b') p(b';i,\theta) \qquad (2)$$

where $s(b)$ and $s^{new}(b)$ are the old and the new image density of pixel b, respectively, $n(i,\theta)$ an observed projection, $m(i,\theta)$ the estimated projection, and $p(b;i,\theta)$ the probability that emission in b is detected in the i-th bin at angle $\theta$.

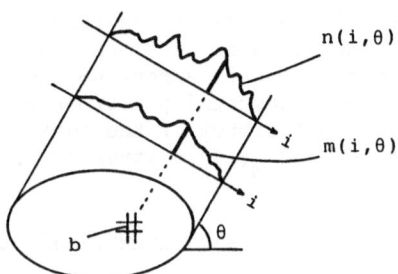

Fig. 1.  Illustration of a measured projection $n(i,\theta)$ and the estimated projection $m(i,\theta)$ at a view angle $\theta$.  "b" is an arbitrary pixel.


We use the following simplified notations hereafter:

$$n \equiv n(i,\theta), \quad m \equiv m(i,\theta) \tag{3}$$

$$\langle \cdot \rangle \equiv \sum_{\theta i}\sum(\cdot)p(b;i,\theta) \tag{4}$$

where $\langle \ \rangle$ implies backprojection operation.  Then Eq.(1) is rewritten as

$$s^{new}(b) = s(b)\langle n/m \rangle \tag{5}$$

$$= s(b) + s(b)[\langle n/m \rangle - 1] \tag{6}$$

The amount of correction on pixel b is given by

$$\Delta s(b) = s^{new}(b) - s(b)$$

$$= s(b)\langle e/m \rangle \tag{7}$$

where
$$e \equiv e(i,\theta) = n(i,\theta) - m(i,\theta) \tag{8}$$

is the difference between a measured and a calculated projection.  For a rough evaluation of the efficiency of the correction at each iterative step, we shall make the following assumption:

ASSUMPTION-A : Calculated projections, $m \equiv m(i,\theta)$, are nearly independent of angle for each pixel.

Then Eq.(7) reduces to

$$\Delta s(b) \simeq s(b)\langle 1/m \rangle \langle e \rangle. \tag{9}$$

This equation implies that the projection errors are backprojected into each pixel with a space dependent weight $s(b)\langle 1/m \rangle$.  The frequency response is given by

$$RSP_{EM}(f) = s(b)\langle 1/m \rangle/(\pi f) \tag{10}$$

where f is the spatial frequency (pixels$^{-1}$) in polar coordinates in the Fourier domain.  If we replace $m(i,\theta)$ in $\langle 1/m \rangle$ by its mean value, $\pi D s(b)/4$, for a uniform disc source having a diameter D, we have

$$RSP_{EM}(f) = 4/(\pi^2 D f). \tag{11}$$

Note that the value of Eq.(11) is 0.81 at the fundamental frequency, f=1/(2D), of the object. The value is less than unity and it is not inconsistent with the fact that the EM algorithm shows stable convergence. This equation represents the fundamental performance of the EM algorithm qualitatively. That is, the efficiency of the correction depends upon the position by $s(b)<1/m>$ and the $RSP_{EM}(f)$ is inversely proportional to the spatial frequency.

## Initial Approach to a Filtered Iterative Reconstruction Algorithm

To overcome the drawbacks of the EM algorithm, the FIR algorithm has been investigated. The algorithm is basically an accelerated EM algorithm combined with high frequency enhancement. The iterative scheme is expressed as

$$s^{new}(b) = s(b)C(b)^{\alpha} + [\beta/B(b)][U(b)-1] \tag{12}$$

where

$$C(b) = <n/m> \tag{13}$$

$$U(b) = <(nm')/(n'm)> \tag{14}$$

$$B(b) = <m'/(n'm)> \tag{15}$$

where $\alpha$ and $\beta$ are constants, and $n'$ and $m'$ are the smoothed projections filtered by a low pass filter $h(i)$:

$$n' = n(i,\theta) * h(i) \quad \text{and} \quad m' = m(i,\theta) * h(i) \tag{16}$$

where the asterisks denote convolution. The values of $h(i)$ are non-negative and are normalized by

$$\sum h(i) = 1. \tag{17}$$

The first term of Eq.(12) represents an accelerated EM algorithm which mainly deals with low frequency correction. $\alpha$ is the acceleration factor. The second term deals with the enhancement of high frequency correction, where $U(b)$ is the correction matrix. The factor $1/B(b)$ compensates the space-dependent correction efficiency as shown later.

A key point of the method is the way of extracting the high frequency component to be corrected. Any irregularity of detection probability $p(b;i,\theta)$ in projections does not appear directly in the matrix $U(b)$, because it is canceled between observed and estimated projections. Since $h(i)$ is non-negative, $U(b)$ is also non-negative.

We now consider the frequency response of the correction expressed by the second term of Eq.(12). Letting $e=n-m$ and $e'=n'-m'$, we can show that

$$U(b) = <\frac{1 + (m-m')/n'}{1 + (m-m')/m'} + \frac{m'}{n'm}(e - e')> \tag{18}$$

$$\simeq 1 + <[m'/(n'm)](e - e')>. \tag{19}$$

We now make the following assumption:

ASSUMPTION-B : $m'/(n'm)$ are nearly independent of angle for each pixel.

Equation (19) is then rewritten, using Eq.(15), as

$$U(b) \simeq 1 + B(b)<e - e'>. \tag{20}$$

220

The term $\langle e-e'\rangle$ implies the backprojection of the high frequency component of the projection errors. The second term of Eq.(12) becomes $\beta\langle e-e'\rangle$, and the frequency response of the correction is $\beta[1-H(f)]/(\pi f)$, where $H(f)$ is the Fourier transform of $h(i)$.

Since the first term of Eq.(12) is an accelerated EM algorithm, the frequency response of the correction is given by Eq.(11) multiplied by $\alpha$ under ASSUMPTION-A. The overall frequency response of the FIR algorithm is then given by

$$RSP(f) = 4\alpha/(\pi^2 Df) + \beta[1 - H(f)]/(\pi f). \tag{21}$$

The filter, $h(i)$, and the constants, $\alpha$ and $\beta$, are determined in such a way that $RSP(f) \simeq 1$ for $f>1/D$. In the FIR algorithm with $\alpha>1$, the total image density is not preserved at each iteration, and the convergence may become unstable at low spatial frequency. However, by normalizing the total image density after each iteration, a stable convergence is achieved with $\alpha \leq 2$. Then $\alpha=2$ was used throughout the present work.

In the practical implementation, to keep the non-negativity of images, a multiplicative correction is used when $U(b)<1$ as follows.

$$s^{new}(b) = \begin{cases} s(b)C(b)^\alpha + \dfrac{\beta}{B(b)}\dfrac{s(b)}{s(b)+\rho}[U(b) - 1] & \text{if } U(b)>1 \quad (22) \\[2ex] s(b)C(b)^\alpha U(b)^{\beta/[\{s(b)+\rho\}B(b)]} & \text{if } U(b)<1 \quad (23) \end{cases}$$

where $\rho$ is a small positive constant which is introduced to avoid too large correction for $s(b)\simeq 0$. The total image density is normalized after each iteration. The iteration is initiated from a flat image.

In the early stages of the simulation study on the FIR algorithm, the following drawback was found: If we use a $\beta$-value which optimizes the $RSP(f)$ given by Eq.(21), a large distortion of image due to overcorrection may occur at the second iteration. This overcorrection obviously arises from the strong ASSUMPTION-A and ASSUMPTION-B described above. For example, these assumptions do not hold at the edge of a high activity region, and the local correction efficiency may exceed unity intolerably.

However, if the first iteration is made with the optimal $\beta$-value and the following iterations are made with a $\beta$-value lowered by a factor of about 2, the algorithm shows a satisfactory performance, and a fairly good image is obtained by a few iterations. The results of the simulation study are described by Tanaka(1987b).

Another drawback of the algorithm is that each iteration involves three backprojection operations for calculating $C(b)$, $U(b)$ and $B(b)$. This is undesirable from a viewpoint of computational efficiency. To overcome these drawbacks, a new FIR algorithm has been developed, which will be described in the following.

## New Filtered Iterative Reconstruction Algorithm

In the new FIR algorithm, a correction matrix is generated after a constant value (pedestal) k is added to both the measured and calculated projections so as to improve the spatial non-uniformity of the correction efficiency. The number of backprojection operations per iteration is reduced to one by combining $C(b)$ and $U(b)$ and by using a constant, B, instead of $B(b)$.

The new algorithm is expressed, in an additive form, as

$$s^{new}(b) = s(b) + (\beta/B)[W(b) - 1] \tag{24}$$

where

$$W(b) = \langle \frac{n+k}{m+k}[\varepsilon + (1-\varepsilon)\frac{m'+k}{n'+k}] \rangle \tag{25}$$

$$\varepsilon = 4\alpha/(\beta\pi D) \qquad ( D = \text{object diameter} ) \tag{26}$$

$$k = \gamma \times (\text{mean value of projections}) \tag{27}$$

$$B = 1/[(1+\gamma) \times (\text{mean value of projections}) \times (\text{number of views})] \tag{28}$$

where $W(b)$ is a correction matrix, and $\gamma$ is a constant which determines the amount of pedestal to be added to projections. The amount of correction, $\Delta s(b)$, is given by

$$\Delta s(b) = \frac{\beta}{B}[\varepsilon\{ \langle \frac{n+k}{m+k} \rangle - 1\} + (1-\varepsilon)\{ \langle \frac{(n+k)(m'+k)}{(m+k)(n'+k)} \rangle - 1\}] \tag{29}$$

$$\simeq \frac{4\alpha}{\pi DB} \langle \frac{e}{m+k} \rangle + \frac{\beta(1-\varepsilon)}{B} \langle \frac{m'+k}{(n'+k)(m+k)}(e - e') \rangle. \tag{30}$$

If we choose k-value in such a way that $1/(m+k)$ and $(m'+k)/[(n'+k)(m+k)]$ are nearly independent of $\theta$ and $i$, we can assume that $\langle 1/(m+k) \rangle \simeq B$ and $\langle (m'+k)/[(m+k)(n'+k)] \rangle \simeq B$. Then Eq.(30) is rewritten as

$$\Delta s(b) = [4\alpha/(\pi D)]\langle e \rangle + (1 - \varepsilon)\beta\langle e - e' \rangle. \tag{31}$$

The frequency response of the correction is then expressed as

$$RSP(f) = 4\alpha/(\pi^2 Df) + (1 - \varepsilon)\beta[1 - H(f)]/(\pi f). \tag{32}$$

Equation (32) is similar to Eq.(21) expect the term $(1-\varepsilon)$, but it is important to note that no strong assumptions are made in this case, and accordingly, the spatial uniformity of the correction efficiency is greatly improved.

In the practical implementation of the algorithm, correction for pixel density is performed by either of additive or multiplicative correction scheme depending on the value of $W(b)$ as follows

$$s^{new}(b) = \begin{vmatrix} s(b)+(\beta/B)[s(b)/\{s(b)+\rho\}][W(b)-1] & \text{if } W(b)>1 & (33) \\ s(b)W(b)^{\beta/[B\{s(b)+\rho\}]} & \text{if } W(b)<1 & (34) \end{vmatrix}$$

where $\rho$ is a small positive constant which is introduced to avoid too large correction at $s(b) \simeq 0$. A typical $\rho$-value is 1% of the maximum image density.

Starting from a flat image as an initial guess, the recovery of a cold area at the first iteration is not sufficient, because the minimum density obtained by the multiplicative mode is about $1/e(=0.368)$ of the old image density even if the algorithm works properly. Then the first iteration is made by the additive correction scheme regardless of $W(b)$ value, and the obtained image $s(b)$ is then treated by the non-negative operation given by

$$s^{new}(b) = \begin{vmatrix} s(b) & \text{if } s(b)>s_t & (35) \\ s_t \exp[(s(b)/s_t)-1] & \text{if } s(b)<s_t & (36) \end{vmatrix}$$

where $s_t$ is a threshold value (typically 10% of the average image density). The correction matrix $W(b)$ may be smoothed by a 9-point 2-D filter (1:2:1 in X- and y-direction) before multiplying it to the old image to suppress progressive ringing.

## Implementation to Sparsely Sampled Data

In the previous discussion, we have implicitly assumed that a projection at each view angle is fully sampled. In some applications, however, the full sampling may not be achieved. An example is the application to a stationary PET using a circular array of discrete detectors. For the stationary PET, a "bank array" of detectors has been proposed, in which all the detectors are grouped into odd number banks, each bank consists of a closely packed detector array, and the gap between the banks is equal to a half the detector width. With this configuration, the object plane is more adequately sampled by coincidence lines than a uniform circular array (Tanaka et al., 1986). A part of the "t-θ map" of such a system consisting of 15 banks of 16 detectors is shown in Fig. 2, in which t represents sampling points (square dots) in the projection at view angle θ. The bin width is a quarter of the detector spacing, and the angular step is π/120. Note that about half of the projection bins are empty.

For implementation in the sparsely sampled data, the FIR method can be performed using only the measured data (Tanaka, 1987b), but in the present study, the following "interpolation method" has been used. First, the empty bins in the measured projections are filled by linear interpolation from the nearest neighbor data at the same view angle. In the iterations, forward projections are calculated only for the sampled bins and the empty bins are filled by interpolation in a similar way to that used for the measured data. Other procedures of the iteration are performed as if the data were fully sampled.

## Filter Function, h(i)

The filter function, h(i), is determined in such a way that the RSP(f) given by Eq.(32) is fairly flat and is nearly equal to unity in a frequency region f>1/D, where D is the largest diameter (in pixels) of objects. Using D=50 pixels and α=2, the following filter was obtained:

$$h_1(i) = \begin{cases} a_1/(i^2 - 0.5) & \text{for } |i| = 1 \sim 8 \\ 2.5\, a_1 & \text{for } i = 0 \end{cases} \tag{37}$$

where $a_1$ is a normalizing constant to satisfy Eq.(17). The value of h(0)

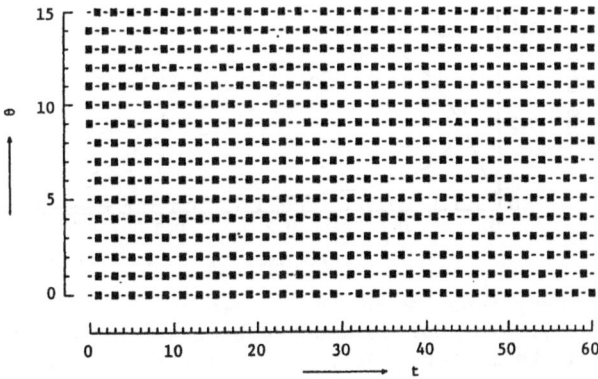

Fig. 2. A part of t-θ map of the stationary PET having 15 banks of 16 detectors. The projection bin width is a quarter of the detector spacing. The angular step is π/120.

affects the magnitude of high frequency correction but it does not affect the relative frequency response, and hence the h(0) value was determined so as to yield an appropriate correction efficiency with β=1. The frequency response is shown in Fig. 3(a).

Note that, h(i) for i≠0 has a similar form to the negative part of the Shepp–Logan filter (Shepp and Logan, 1974) except that h(i) has a limited spread. This seems to be reasonable because δ(i)−h(i) plays a similar role to the convolution kernel in the filtered backprojection method, where δ(i) is the delta function. The limited spread of h(i) causes the drop of the low frequency response which is compensated by the first term of Eq.(32).

When the correction matrix W(b) is smoothed by a 9-point 2-D filter, or when sparsely sampled projections are filled by interpolation, the loss of high frequency component can be partly compensated by modifying the filter, h(i). An example of such a deblurring filter is

$$h_2(i) = \begin{cases} a_2(i^2 - 0.5)^{-1.2} & \text{for} \quad |i| = 1 \sim 10 \\ 0.3a_2 & \text{for} \quad i = 0. \end{cases} \tag{38}$$

The frequency response of the FIR algorithm with $h_2(i)$ is shown in Fig. 3(b). The curve denoted by "RSP-S(f)" in the figure is the overall response including the smoothing effect which is assumed to be equivalent to 1:2:1 smoothing in projections.

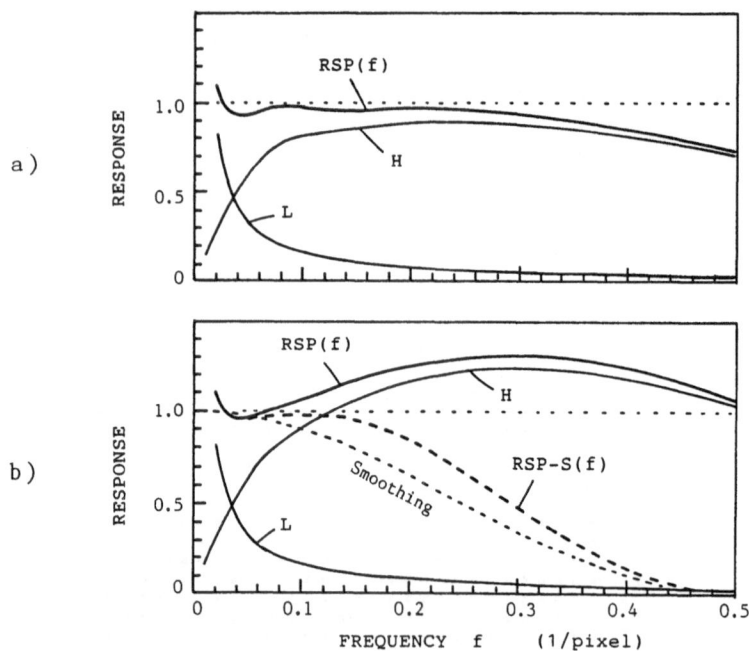

Fig. 3. Frequency response of the correction by the FIR algorithm. See Eq.(32). The curves denoted by L and H indicate the first and the second term of Eq.(32), respectively, with α=2 and β=1.
(a) : Normal filter defined by Eq.(37)
(b) : Deblurring filter defined by Eq.(38)
        The curve "RSP-S(f)" is the overall response including the smoothing effect of 1:2:1 filtering.

# SIMULATION STUDIES

## Phantoms and Projection Data

Simulation studies have been performed considering two PET systems: one is a scanning PET having a uniform array of 240 detectors and the other is the stationary PET having the bank array (16 detectors x 15 banks) described in the previous section. The crystal width is 5 mm, and the center-to-center spacing of the crystals is 6 mm. The imaging matrix is 62 x 62. The pixel size and the bin width of projections are 1.5 mm, a quarter of the crystal spacing.

The projection data were generated as follows: a mathematical phantom was digitized in a 62 x 62 matrix, and the projections were calculated from the phantoms by taking the detector response into account. The detector response was assumed to be a Gaussian function having a full-width at tenth-maximum of 5 mm (= crystal width) which corresponds to a full-width at half maximum of 2.74 mm(=1.83 pixels). The Gaussian function was defined in 1.5/4 mm pitch. Attenuation and scattering of photons were ignored. The mathematical phantoms used in this study and their images are shown in Fig. 4. The images were obtained by applying a 9-point 2-D filter (1:2:1 in X- and Y-direction) to the mathematical phantoms. The smoothed images are considered to be ideal images to be reconstructed taking into account the assumed detector resolution.

The detection efficiency, $p(b;i,\theta)$, was calculated as the overlapping area between the pixel and the rectangular strip having a width equal to projection bin width. Iteration was initiated with a flat image having a slightly larger diameter than the phantom. The total image density was normalized after each iteration. Throughout the work, $\alpha=2$ and $\beta=1$ were used.

## Effect of Projection Pedestal

Figure 5 shows the images of Phantom A obtained with different amounts of the projection pedestal. It is seen that excessive edge enhancement occurs at the second iteration when $\gamma$-value is small. The reason for this is that the assumption made in deducing Eq.(31) does not hold when $\gamma$ is small. Although the images with $\gamma=0.2$ are fairly good, all of the following studies were made with $\gamma=1$.

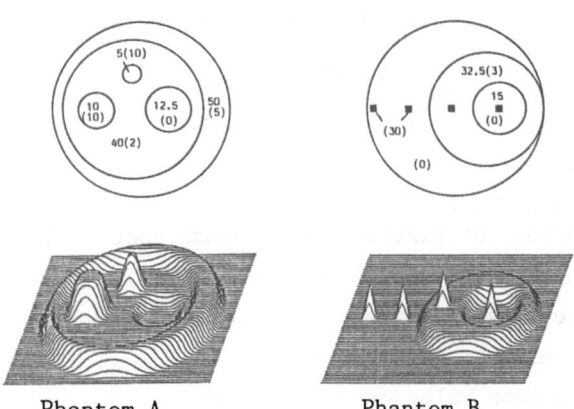

Phantom A                    Phantom B

Fig. 4. Mathematical phantoms and their smoothed images. The values are diameters (pixels) and the values in the parentheses are relative activity densities. Phantom B has four point sources for resolution test.

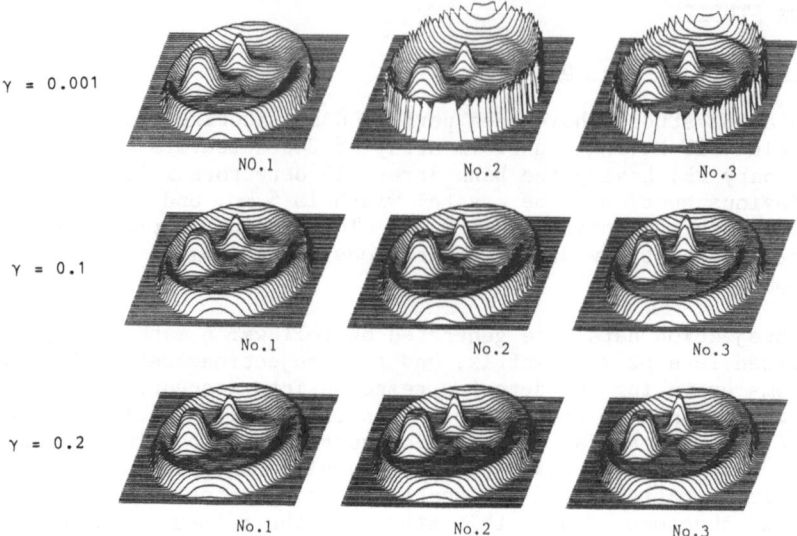

$\gamma = 0.001$    NO.1    No.2    No.3

$\gamma = 0.1$    No.1    No.2    No.3

$\gamma = 0.2$    No.1    No.2    No.3

Fig. 5. Effect of projection pedestal on the reconstructed images after 1, 2, and 3 iteration(s). The $\gamma$-value is the relative amount of the pedestal (See Eq.(27)). (The name code of the reconstruction defined in Table 1 is "sSII".)

## Convergence

To check the behavior of convergence, simulation studies were performed using Phantom A with various modes of reconstruction, and the following four quantities were monitored as a function of iteration number.

(a) Mean amount of correction at each iteration defined as

$$\text{MAC} = \frac{1}{N_b s_{max}} \sum_b |s^{new}(b) - s(b)| \qquad (39)$$

(b) Mean density error from the smoothed phantom defined as

$$\text{MDE} = \frac{1}{N_b s_{max}} \sum_b |s^{new}(b) - s_o(b)| \qquad (40)$$

(c) Root mean square error of projections defined as

$$\text{RMS-PROJ} = \frac{1}{n_{mean}}[\frac{1}{N_p} \sum_\theta \sum_i |n(i,\theta) - m(i,\theta)|^2]^{1/2} \qquad (41)$$

(d) Root mean square noise of image defined as

$$\text{RMS-NOISE} = \frac{1}{s_{max}}[\frac{1}{N_b} \sum_b |s_n(b) - s(b)|^2]^{1/2} \qquad (42)$$

where   $N_b$ is the number of pixels in the reconstruction area,

$N_p$ is the number of sampled projection bins,

$s_o(b)$ is the image density of the smoothed phantom,

$s_{max}$ is the maximum value of $s_o(b)$,

$n_{mean}$ is the mean value of $n(i,\theta)$, and

$s_n(b)$ is the image density with statistical noise.

The results are summarized in Fig. 6. The meaning of the name codes on the curves is defined in Table 1. In the evaluation of RMS-NOISE by Eq.(42), the difference of the image densities with and without noise at the same iteration number was used in order to avoid the error due to different resolution recovery. The total number of counts is 1,000,000. The values for CBP images are shown by arrows in Figs. 6(c) and (d).

From Fig. 6(a), it will be seen that the convergence is quite stable and satisfactory. The MDE curves for noise free data have a minimum value at 2 or 3 iterations where the detector resolution is almost recovered. Further iterations tend to deblur the image gradually. The RMS-PROJ value with noise decreases very rapidly to the value for the CBP image, and the following iterations decrease the value very slowly. It is interesting to note that a small decrease in RMS-PROJ is attained by a large increase in RMS-NOISE. The noise of the non-smoothed CBP image of the stationary PET is nearly equal to that of the smoothed CBP image of the scanning PET. Figure 7 shows the images obtained with the scanning mode at various iteration numbers. Figure 8 shows the FIR images after two iterations with various modes of reconstruction and the CBP images obtained with the standard Shepp-Logan filter. Figure 9 shows the images similar to those in Fig. 8 except that statistical noise is included assuming the total number of counts is 200,000.

## Spatial Resolution

The recovery of spatial resolution was investigated with Phantom B. Figure 10 shows the comparison of the FIR images and the EM images. The number of iterations are shown below each image. It will be recognized that the FIR algorithm yields fairly uniform resolution over the whole reconstruction area while the EM algorithm does not. Note that the resolution recovery of the EM images is particularly slow in a cold area surrounded by a hot area as expected from Eq.(9).

The spatial resolution of the FIR image was evaluated as the mean value of the following quantity, w, for the four point sources in the image.

$$w = [(\text{volume of PSF})/(\text{peak height of PSF})]^{1/2}/1.06 \qquad (43)$$

where PSF is the point source spread function and the factor, 1.06, is a normalizing factor by which the w-value presents FWHM in the unit of pixel width for a Gaussian point spread function. Figure 11 shows the resolution thus obtained as a function of iteration number for various modes. The stationary PET provides lower resolution than the scanning PET. This is due to the smoothing effect of interpolation applied to projections.

Table 1. Name code of simulation data

FIR data ( four letters )
  1-st letter -- "s": scanning PET;  "b": stationary PET (bank array)
  2-nd letter -- "S": W(b) smoothed;  "I": W(b) not smoothed
  3-rd letter -- "D": filter $h_2(i)$;  "I": filter $h_1(i)$
  4-th letter -- "N": with noise;  "I": without noise

CBP data
  "CBP"      : reconstructed with standard Shepp-Logan filter
  "CBP(S)"   : reconstructed with smoothed (1:2:1) Shepp-Logan filter
  "   -N"    : with statistical noise

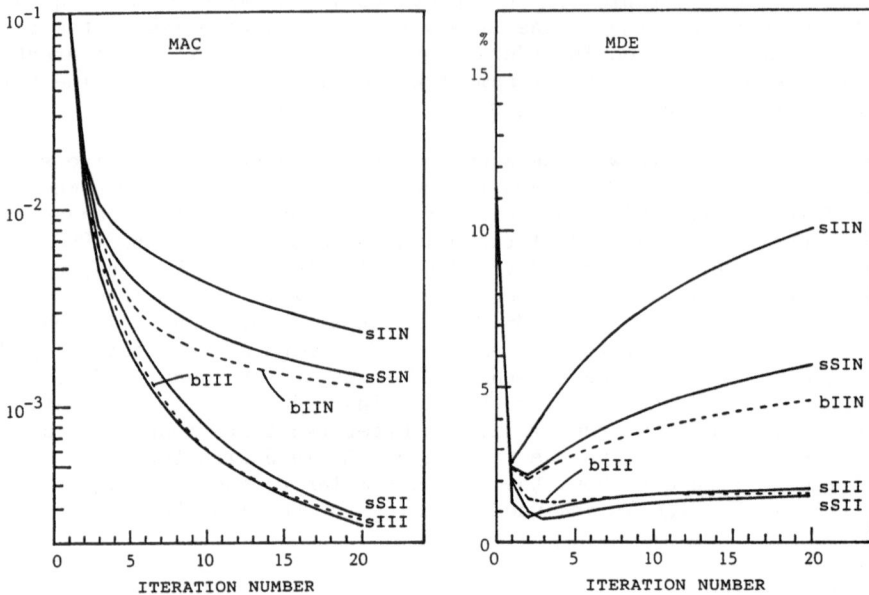

(a) Mean amount of correction
    at each iteration

(b) Mean density error from
    the smoothed phantom

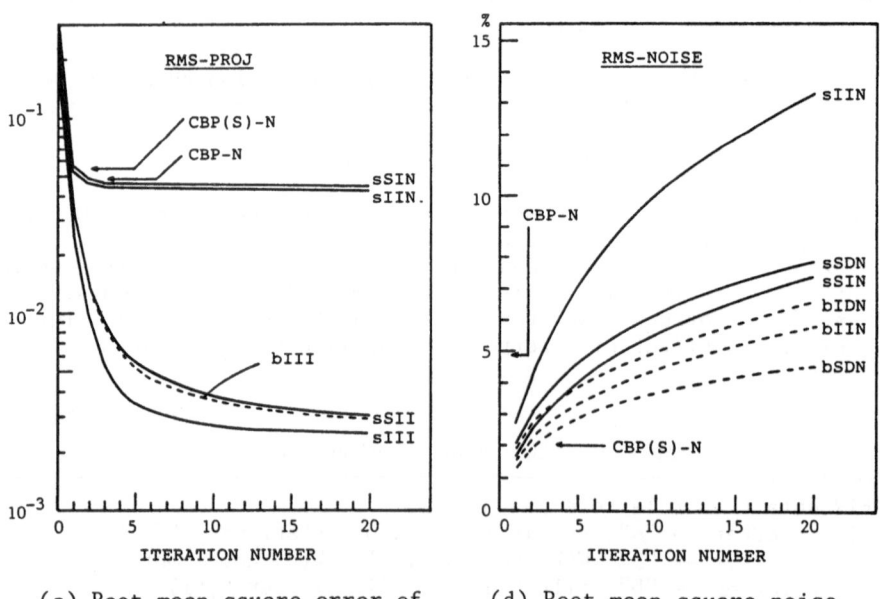

(c) Root mean square error of
    projections

(d) Root mean square noise
    of image

Fig. 6.  Behavior of convergence.  The name codes on the curves are
defined in Table 1.  The values for the CBP images are shown by
arrows.  Statistical noise was generated assuming the total
number of counts is 1,000,000.

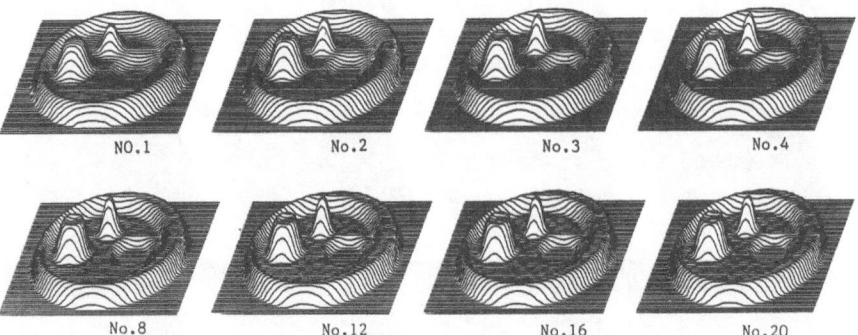

Fig. 7. Images of Phantom A after various iteration numbers. The name code is "sSII" in Table 1.

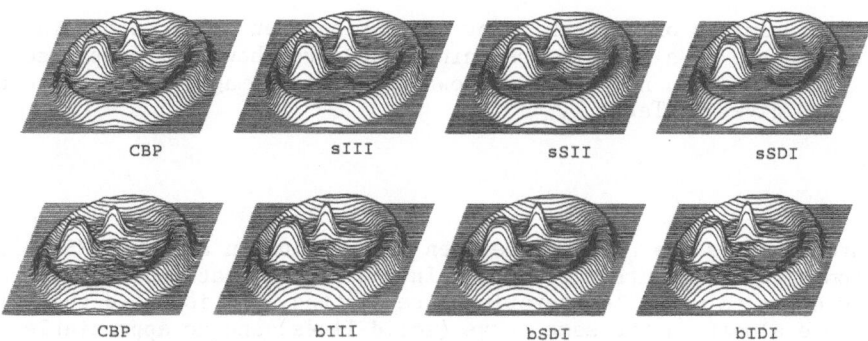

Fig. 8. Images after two iterations with various modes of reconstruction. The name codes are given in Table 1. Top row: scanning PET; Bottom row: stationary PET.

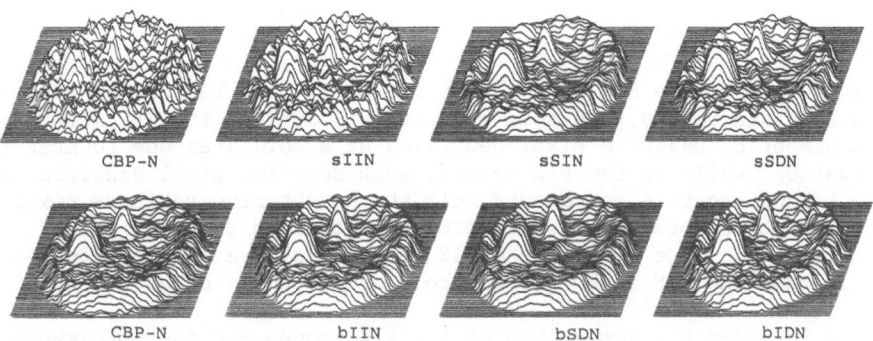

Fig. 9. Images similar to those in Fig. 8 except that statistical noise is included assuming that the total number of counts is 200,000.

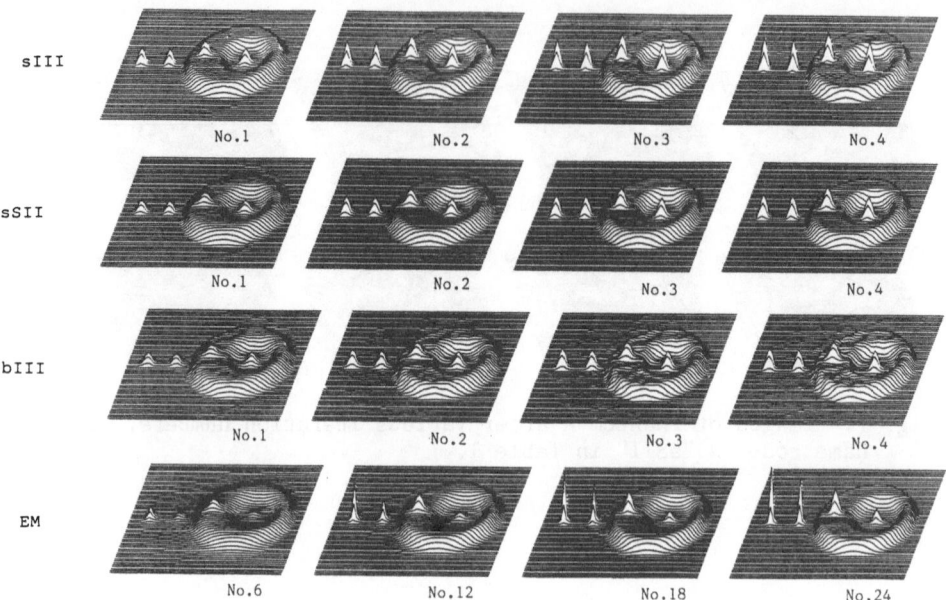

Fig. 10. Images of Phantom B for resolution test. Images obtained with the EM algorithm (scanning mode) are shown for comparison. The iteration numbers are shown under each image. The name codes are given in Table 1.

Figure 12 shows the relation between the resolution and the RMS–NOISE for Phantom A (total counts: 200,000). In the figure, data points for the FIR images obtained with 2∿4 iterations are plotted. It is noted that all the plots are almost on the same curve (solid lines) and no appreciable difference in the resolution-noise relationship is observed among the different modes. The dashed curve in Fig. 12(right) represents the fitting curve for the scanning PET. The small difference in the two fitting curves may be due to the non-uniformity in the sampling density over the reconstruction area in the stationary PET. The star marks in the figure show the data points for CBP images obtained with and without smoothing(1:2:1) on the Shepp-Logan filter. Note that the CBP data points are also on the same fitting curve in either case.

Non-Negativity

An advantage of the FIR method over the CBP method is the non-negativity of the obtained images. In poor counting statistics, the CBP method may produce a number of negative pixel densities at a cold area due to statistical fluctuation, while in the FIR method, such negative pixel densities are forced to be non-negative and accordingly the neighboring positive pixel values tend to be compressed toward zero so as to keep the mean local density unchanged. As a result, the FIR method yields a higher signal-to-noise ratio than the CBP method at the cold area (Tanaka et al., 1985).

Figure 13 shows the comparison of the FIR images and the CBP images of Phantom B obtained with various numbers of total counts. The FIR images were obtained by two iterations with W(b) smoothed. The CBP images were obtained from projections smoothed by a 1:2.5:1 filter so that the two methods provide the same spatial resolution. Note that the point sources are more clearly observable in the FIR images than in the CBP images.

230

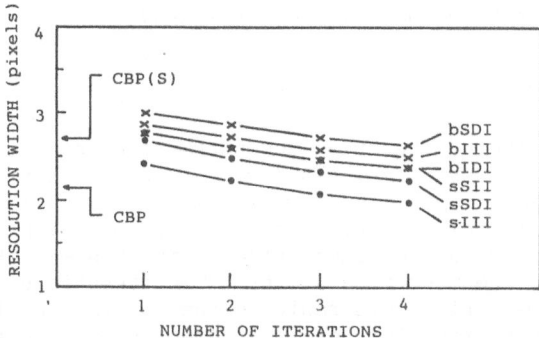

Fig. 11. Resolution width as a function of iteration number. The values for the CBP images are shown by arrows. The name codes are given in Table 1.

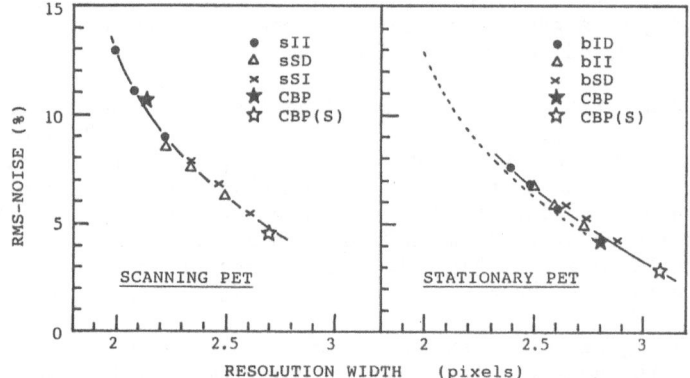

Fig. 12. Relationship between resolution width and statistical noise (RMS-NOISE) in scanning PET (left) and in stationary PET (right). The total number of counts is 200,000. The star marks are the data points for CBP images. The dashed curve is the fitting curve for the scanning PET.

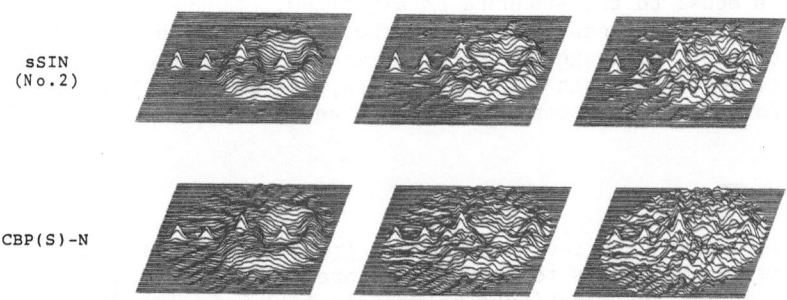

Fig. 13. Comparison of FIR images (sSIN, No.2) and CBP images of Phantom B in various counting statistics. The total counts are 100,000(left), 30,000(middle) and 10,000(right).

Calculations based on Eq.(42) showed that the RMS-NOISE of the CBP images are about 25% higher than that of the FIR images.

## DISCUSSION AND CONCLUSIONS

An improved filtered iterative reconstruction (FIR) algorithm and its performance have been described. The present studies have been made with an intention to realize a fast reconstruction method which is applicable to the routine use for scanning or stationary PET systems. With the optimized parameters, the reconstruction resolution is independent of image pattern and depends only on the iteration number. Two iterations are sufficient to obtain a spatial resolution comparable to that of the CBP images, and the successive iterations yield further improvement of resolution at a cost of noise increase.

The magnitude of statistical noise has been compared at various modes of reconstruction, but there is no essential difference in noise-resolution relationship among various modes of the FIR method or between the FIR method and the CBP method, although a slightly higher noise is observed with the stationary PET than with the scanning PET. In low activity regions, the FIR method yields higher signal-to-noise ratio than the CBP method due to the non-negativity involved in the FIR algorithm.

In the FIR algorithm, a lot of modifications are made to the original EM algorithm, and accordingly it is considered that the FIR algorithm does not seek the maximum likelihood estimate. With the EM algorithm, correction of image density is made by more accurate matching of projection data with low counts than by matching the data with high counts. This is the reason why the resolution recovery is much faster in a peripheral low activity region (see the EM images in Fig. 10) than in the other regions. The non-uniformity in resolution recovery will be unavoidable from the same reason.

In the FIR algorithm, on the other hand, the amount of correction is proportional to the average difference between measured data and calculated data as shown by Eq.(32), and accordingly the obtained images is expected to be similar to the CBP images as long as the projections are fully sampled. The main advantages of the FIR method over the CBP method are the applicability to incomplete projection data, non-negativity of the obtained images and the deblurring capability.

The present studies have been made with the optimized parameters, but the FIR algorithm is flexible, and the converging speed or other performance can be controlled by the suitable choice of the parameters, $\alpha$, $\beta$ and $\gamma$, and the filter function $h(i)$. If we use $\alpha=1$, $\beta=4/(\pi D)$ (hence $\varepsilon=1$) and $\gamma=0$ the algorithm is equal to the standard EM algorithm. In this sense, we feel that the FIR algorithm can bridge over the gap between the CBP method and the EM algorithm. Although the detailed studies on the performance with different parameters remain for future work, the new FIR algorithm appears promising for the image reconstruction in the emission computed tomography.

## ACKNOWLEDGMENTS

This work was supported in part by a grant from the Ministry of Education. The author wishes to thank N. Nohara, T. Tomitani, M. Yamamoto and H. Murayama of National Institute of Radiological Sciences, H. Toyama of Tsukuba University and T. Yamashita of Hamamatsu Photonics K.K. for their useful discussions.

# REFERENCES

Brooks, R.A., Sank, V.J, Talbert A.J. and DiChiro, G. (1979). Sampling requirements and detector motion for positron emission tomography, IEEE Trans. Nucl. Sci., NS-26, 2760-2763.

Budinger, T.F. and Gullberg, G.T. (1974). Three-dimensional reconstruction in nuclear medicine emission imaging, IEEE Trans. Nucl. Sci., NS-21, 2-20.

Burnham, C.A., Bradshaw, J., Kaufman, D., Chesler D. and Brownell G.L. (1984). A stationary positron emission ring tomograph using BGO detector and analog readout, IEEE Trans. Nucl. Sci., NS-31, 632-636.

Derenzo, S.E., Budinger, T.F. and Huesman, R.H. (1981). Imaging properties of a positron tomograph with 280 BGO crystals, IEEE Trans. Nucl. Sci., NS-28, 81-89.

Gilbert, P. (1972). Iterative methods for the three-dimensional reconstruction of an object from projections, J. Theor. Biol., 36, 105-117.

Gordon, R., Bender, R. and Herman, G.T. (1970). Algebraic reconstruction techniques(ART) for three-dimensional electron microscopy and x-ray photography, J. Theor. Biol., 29, 471-481.

Herman, G.T. and Lent, A. (1976). Iterative reconstruction algorithm, Comput. Biol. Med., 6, 273-294.

Kawata, S. and Nalcioglu, O. (1985). Constrained iterative reconstruction by the conjugate gradient method, IEEE Trans. Med. Imag., MI-4, 65-71.

Lange, K. and Carson, R. (1984). EM reconstruction algorithms for emission and transmission tomography, J. Comput. Assist. Tomogr., 8, 306-316.

Llacer, J., Veklerov, E. and Hoffman, E. J. (1987). On the convergence of the maximum likelihood estimator method of tomographic image reconstruction, in: Proc. of Conf. on Medical Imaging, Newport Beach, CA (1987), SPIE Vol.767.

Minerbo, G. (1979). Maximum entropy reconstruction from cone-beam projection data, Comput. Biol. Med., 9, 29-37.

Muehllehner, G. and Karp, J.S. (1986). A positron camera using position-sensitive detectors: PENN-PET, J. Nucl. Med., 27, 90-98.

Rockmore, A. and Macovski, A. (1977). A maximum likelihood approach to emission image reconstruction from projections, IEEE Trans. Nucl. Sci., NS-23, 1428-1432.

Shepp, L.A. and Logan, B.F. (1974). Fourier reconstruction of a head section, IEEE Trans. Nucl. Sci., NS-21, 21-43.

Shepp, L.A. and Vardi, Y. (1982). Maximum likelihood reconstruction for emission tomography, IEEE Trans. Med. Imag., MI-1, 113-122.

Snyder, D.L. and Miller, M.I. (1985). The use of sieves to stabilize images produced with the EM algorithm for emission tomography, IEEE Trans. Nucl. Sci., NS-32, 3864-3872.

Tanaka, E. (1987a). Recent progress on single photon and positron emission tomography - From detectors to algorithms, IEEE Trans. Nucl. Sci., NS-34, 313-320.

Tanaka, E. (1987b). A fast reconstruction algorithm for stationary positron emission tomography based on a modified EM algorithm, IEEE Trans. Med. Imag., MI-6, 98-105.

Tanaka, E., Nohara, N., Tomitani, T. and Yamamoto, M. (1985). Utilization of non-negativity constraints in reconstruction of emission tomograms, in: Proc. of the 9-th Conf. of Information Processing in Medical Imaging, Washington, D.C., June 10-14, 1985, S.L. Bacharach, ed., Martinus Nijhoff, pp.379-393.

Tanaka, E., Nohara, N., Tomitani, T., Yamamoto, M. and Murayama, H. (1986). Stationary positron emission tomography and its image reconstruction, IEEE Trans. Med. Imag., MI-5, 199-206.

ILL-POSEDNESS AND NON-LINEARITY IN ELECTRICAL IMPEDANCE TOMOGRAPHY

William Breckon and Michael Pidcock

Department of Computing and Mathematical Sciences
Oxford Polytechnic, U.K.

INTRODUCTION

Electrical Impedance Tomography (EIT) is a relatively new method of medical imaging which is being investigated by a number of research groups around the world. These studies have lead to the production of at least one prototype piece of apparatus which is currently under clinical evaluation. The development of the associated reconstruction algorithms is also being actively pursued by a number of groups including our own.

In EIT a number of current distributions are applied to the surface of a body and by making measurements of the resulting electrical potential on the surface one attempts to determine the conductivity within the body.

We will assume that the body $\Omega$ is an isotropic Ohmic conductor. Denoting the conductivity by $\sigma$, the electrical potential by $\Phi$ and the current density vector by $J$, Ohm's Law gives

$$J = -\sigma \nabla\Phi. \tag{1}$$

In the absence of current sources within the body we have

$$\nabla.J = -\nabla \cdot (\sigma\nabla\Phi) = 0. \tag{2}$$

This is a partial differential equation relating $\sigma$ and $\Phi$.

We hope to identify $\sigma$ from a knowledge of the voltage at certain points on the surface $\partial\Omega$ of $\Omega$ when various patterns of current density are applied to the surface. In practice the currents will be applied via some finite number of electrodes on $\partial\Omega$ and the voltage measurements made between other electrodes. It is possible that the same electrodes might be used for both purposes but this is not necessarily the best procedure.

Since in the potential $\Phi$ depends not only on the current densities applied to the boundary, but also on the conductivity $\sigma$, equation (2) is nonlinear in $\sigma$. If the current patterns we apply to $\sigma$ are $j_\alpha$ for $\alpha = 1\ldots n$ then let $\Phi_\alpha$ be a solution to the Neumann problem

$$\nabla \cdot (\sigma \nabla \Phi_\alpha) = 0 \tag{3}$$
$$-\mathbf{n} \cdot \nabla \Phi_\alpha = j_\alpha$$

where $\mathbf{n}$ is the outward unit normal to $\partial\Omega$. If we also specify the potential at some point on $\partial\Omega$ then this solution is unique. We also know that $\Phi_\alpha$ agrees with the voltage measurements $v_{\alpha\beta}$ which we make between the pair of measurement electrodes labelled by $\beta$. If we define $\chi_\beta$ to be the 'characteristic function' of the measurement electrode pair $\beta$, that is for x on the surface $\partial\Omega$

$$\chi_\beta(x) = \begin{cases} 1 & \text{if x is under the first electrode of pair } \beta \\ -1 & \text{if x is under the second electrode of pair } \beta \\ 0 & \text{otherwise} \end{cases}$$

then

$$v_{\alpha\beta} = \int_\Omega \chi_\beta(x) \Phi_\alpha \, dS. \tag{4}$$

If we define the 'measurement field' $\Psi_\beta$ to be a solution of
$$\nabla \cdot (\sigma \nabla \Psi_\beta) = 0 \tag{5}$$
$$-\mathbf{n} \cdot \nabla \Psi_\beta = \chi_\beta$$

then from the divergence theorem we have

$$v_{\alpha\beta} = \int_\Omega \sigma \nabla \Psi_\beta \cdot \nabla \Phi_\alpha \, dV. \tag{6}$$

This is a system of non-linear equations relating $\sigma$ to the voltage measurements $v_{\alpha\beta}$.

DISCRETE REPRESENTATIONS

If we are to solve these equations numerically we must first choose discrete spaces of allowable conductivities and potentials. One approach to this numerical representation is to use finite element spaces. To represent a function f on a region $\Omega$, we first divide the region into 'elements'. For a two dimensional region these might be triangles or quadrilaterals; for a three dimensional region tetrahedra, prisms, or bricks. These elements need not be regular and can be adapted to the geometry of the problem. On each element we represent the function f by linear combinations of polynomials $\eta_i$ (called shape functions) in such a way that the approximations to f (and possibly the derivatives up to a certain order) are continuous across the boundaries of the elements. If the finite element approximation to f is $\Sigma_i f_i \eta_i$ then we will denote the vector of coefficients $f_i$ by $\underline{f}$.

If $\Phi_\alpha$ and $\Psi_\beta$ are approximated on a finite element mesh then the Neumann problems (3) and (5) can easily and rapidly be solved by standard numerical techniques. Since (6) involves the gradients of $\Phi$ and $\Psi$ it is desirable to use a more accurate approximation for $\Phi$ and $\Psi$ than for $\sigma$ so that all the terms in (6) are approximated to the same accuracy. If $\underline{\sigma}$ represents the finite element approximation to $\sigma$ and $\underline{v}$ is the vector of voltage measurements $v_{\alpha\beta}$ then we can write (6) as

$$\underline{v} = F(\underline{\sigma}) \qquad (7)$$

where F is a nonlinear, vector valued function.

ALGORITHMS

The problem of determining $\underline{\sigma}$ from equation (7) is not only non-linear but it is also ill-posed in the sense that very small changes in the voltage measurements may be the result of large changes in the conductivity. This is essentially because (6) is a first kind integral equation. Since the voltage data will be subject to noise and the model we use will not exactly fit the physical situation it is unrealistic to expect to solve this equation exactly. Instead we seek the 'least squares' or best fitting solution, that is we seek a conductivity $\underline{\sigma}$ to minimize the mean-square error in the voltage measurements

$$\| F(\underline{\sigma}) - \underline{v} \|^2. \qquad (8)$$

Because of the ill-posedness mentioned above this process is numerically unstable and it is necessary to apply some kind of regularization procedure. There are essentially two possible approaches here. Either we can apply Newton's method to the original problem and regularize each of the linear steps or we can regularize the nonlinear problem and then solve the resulting well posed nonlinear problem by some variant of Newton's method. The former methods are generally referred to as Levenburg-Marquardt or Quasi-Newton methods (Marquardt, 1963) and the latter as penalized likelihood methods (Kristensen and Vogel, 1986).

The Quasi-Newton methods involve making the linear approximation

$$F(\sigma + \delta) = F(\sigma) + F'(\sigma)\delta + o(||\delta||^2) \qquad (9)$$

where $F'(\sigma)$ denotes the Fréchet derivative (or Jacobian matrix) of $F$ at $\sigma$. The algorithm can stated as follows:-

Given an initial guess for the conductivity $\sigma_0$
Repeat

1.  find a correction $\delta_n$ which satisfies
$$F'(\sigma_n)^* F'(\sigma_n)\delta_n = F'(\sigma_n)^*(y - F(\sigma_n)); \qquad (10)$$

2.  update the estimate of the conductivity
$$\sigma_{n+1} = \sigma_n + \delta_n;$$

until $||y - F(\sigma_{n+1})||^2$ is sufficiently small.

As we will allow fewer degrees of freedom in $\delta_n$ than the number of independent voltage measurements there may not be a solution to $F'(\sigma_n)\delta_n = (y - F(\sigma_n)$ so we have multiplied both sides of equation (10) by the transpose (denoted here by $*$) of the derivative matrix $F'(\sigma_n)$. This will give us the best fitting solution in the least squares sense. Step 1 is a linear ill-posed problem and a different Quasi-Newton method can be derived by using any regularization technique at this stage. The idea behind regularization techniques is to ask a well-posed question about an ill-posed problem. We will briefly discuss two possible regularization procedures: Tykhonov regularization and truncated singular value expansion. Both of these methods involve a parameterized sequence of well-posed problems whose limiting case is the original ill-posed problem. The value of the parameter actually used is determined by the level of noise present in the data and the inaccuracies involved in the numerical calculations.

Tykhonov regularization consists of minimizing the functional

$$T_\mu(\delta) = || F'(\sigma_n)\delta - y + F(\sigma_n)||^2 + \mu||\delta||^2 \qquad (11)$$

where $\mu>0$ is a regularization parameter. This is a well posed problem for $\mu$ sufficiently large. The minimizer $\delta_{min}$ can easily be shown to be

$$\delta_{min} = (F'(\sigma_n)^*F'(\sigma_n) + \mu I)^{-1} F'(\sigma_n)^*(y - F(\sigma_n)). \qquad (12)$$

The matrix $F'(\sigma_n)^*F'(\sigma_n) + \mu I$ is a positive definite symmetric matrix so $\delta_{min}$ can be calculated by a standard numerical method such as Cholesky factorization.

The singular function expansion is essentially a diagonalization of the symmetric matrix $F'(\sigma_n)^*F'(\sigma_n)$ in the form

238

$$F'(\underline{\sigma}_n)^* F'(\underline{\sigma}_n) = U \Lambda^2 U^* \tag{13}$$

where U is an orthogonal matrix. The columns $u_r$ of U are the right-hand singular vectors of $F'(\underline{\sigma}_n)$ and $\Lambda$ is a diagonal matrix of singular values $\lambda_i$ arranged in decreasing order

$$\lambda_1 \geq \lambda_2 \geq \ldots \geq \lambda_N > 0. \tag{14}$$

The vector

$$\underline{\delta} = \Sigma^N_{r=1} u_r < F'(\underline{\sigma}_n)^*(\underline{v} - F(\underline{\sigma}_n), u_r > /\lambda_r^2 \tag{15}$$

will then be a solution to (10).

Numerical studies show that the singular values decrease rapidly. This makes calculation of $\underline{\delta}$ from this formula unstable as we will be dividing by small numbers $\lambda_r$ which will amplify error in the voltage difference measurements $\underline{v}$. A suitable regularization procedure is to truncate the series at some value k and set

$$\underline{\delta}(k) = \Sigma^k_{r=1} u_r < F'(\underline{\sigma}_{n.})^*(\underline{v} - F(\underline{\sigma}_n)), u_r > /\lambda_r^2. \tag{16}$$

The truncation level k here plays the rôle of a regularization parameter.

In the penalized likelihood method a penalty function $\gamma p(\underline{\sigma})$ is added to (8) and one minimizes

$$L_\gamma(\underline{\sigma}) = \| F(\underline{\sigma}) - \underline{v} \|^2 + \gamma p(\underline{\sigma}) \tag{17}$$

The penalty function is usually chosen to be a quadratic function $p(\underline{\sigma}) = <\underline{\sigma}, W\underline{\sigma}>$ where W is a weighting function incorporating any a priori knowledge about $\underline{\sigma}$. The minimization is achieved by solving $\nabla L_\gamma(\underline{\sigma}) = 0$ using a Quasi-Newton method.

THE EFFECTS OF ERRORS

We will divide the errors which effect reconstruction algorithms for EIT into two categories. The first category consists of the errors in the voltage measurements caused by noise in the measurement apparatus. The second consists of the effect of errors in our mathematical model for the object being imaged. This second category includes inaccurate knowledge of the boundary shape and position of electrodes, errors due to the finite element approximation, and modelling errors caused by our simplifying assumptions about the electrical properties of the body. The first category will introduce errors into the vector $\underline{v}$ and the second will introduce errors into our predicted voltage measurements $F(\underline{\sigma}_n)$. Errors of the first category

239

can reasonably be modelled by assuming that the error in $y$ is a random variable $e$ with mean zero and components $e_{\alpha\beta}$ which are uncorrelated with variance $\varepsilon^2$. The covariance matrix is then $\mathrm{Cov}[e_{\alpha\beta},e_{\eta\zeta}] = \delta_{\alpha\eta}\delta_{\beta\zeta}\varepsilon^2$.

The Tykhonov parameter used should satisfy $\mu \geq 1/s^2$ where the signal to noise ratio $s$ is defined to be

$$s = \| y - F(\sigma_n) \| / \varepsilon. \tag{18}$$

For the truncated singular value expansion the truncation level $k$ should be such that $\lambda_k \geq \lambda_1/s$. The number $k$ may be thought of as the number of 'degrees of freedom' or number of parameters which can be reliably identified from data with the given amount of noise. Gisser et al (1987) have suggested a procedure for determining the optimal current patterns $j_\alpha$ which maximize $\| y - F(\sigma_n) \|$ for a given $\sigma_n$. If the technology can be developed to drive currents approximating these optimal patterns then it would be possible to use them to take a new set of readings $y$ at each iteration. This would give the maximum number of degrees of freedom in each iteration step $\delta_n$. However to our knowledge EIT apparatus currently in existence can only drive current in fixed patterns, typically only across a pair of electrodes.

Of the errors in the second category we discuss only the errors in $F(\sigma_n)$ caused by inaccurate knowledge of the boundary shape and electrode position since these are probably the most important. In a clinical environment it is extremely difficult to determine with any accuracy the electrode positions. Our knowledge of this data is likely to be much less accurate than our knowledge of the voltage measurements. In contrast to the errors in the first category these errors are correlated. If one electrode of the measurement pair $\beta$ is moved by a small amount $r$ then for all current patterns $\alpha$ the measurement $v_{\alpha\beta}$ will change in proportion to the average value over that electrode of $\nabla v_\alpha . r$ where $v_\alpha$ is the restriction of $\Phi_\alpha$ to the boundary $\partial\Omega$. If the positions of the electrodes are changed by a random amount with mean zero and variance $\kappa^2$ then the covariance matrix of the error $e$ in $y$ is is given by

$$\mathrm{Cov}[e_{\alpha\beta},e_{\eta\zeta}] = \delta_{\beta\zeta}\kappa^2 \int_{\partial\Omega} |\chi_\beta| \nabla v_\alpha . \nabla v_\eta \, ds. \tag{19}$$

From this formula we see that at points on the boundary where the voltage gradient is large, errors in electrode position will be amplified to produce large errors in voltage measurement. One approach to this difficulty would be to scale the voltage measurements so that this error is more 'evenly spread' over the data set. In the method used by Barber and Seagar (1987) a set of reference voltages $y'_{\alpha\beta}$ are used to scale the measurements, the quantities used in their calculation being essentially $(y_{\alpha\beta} - F(\sigma)_{\alpha\beta})/y'_{\alpha\beta}$. A more sophisticated approach might be to first take a set of 'calibration' measurements to determine the position of the electrodes and possibly some information about the boundary shape. This information would then be used to adjust the finite element model so that calculations of F would be in better agreement with the geometry of the system. To do this one would have to choose current drive patterns which were (in the terminology of Gisser et al) unable to distinguish between $\sigma$ and $\sigma_0$ given the accuracy of the measurements but which were sensitive to positional changes in a given electrode. If differences between the actual conductivity $\sigma$ and initial approximation $\sigma_0$ were largest far from the boundary (which is not unreasonable in clinical applications) then the current patterns least able to distinguish between them would have components of high spatial frequency and hence large gradients at some points. These would be most sensitive to positional changes in the electrodes. Since the impedances of various tissues vary with frequency it might also be possible to make these calibration measurements at a frequency for which $\sigma_0$ were closer to $\sigma$. To find the positional errors in the electrodes from the calibration measurements involves solving another system of non-linear equations. However for small positional errors it may be adequate simply to solve the linearized equations

$$v_{\alpha\beta} - F(\sigma) = \int_{\chi_\beta} \nabla v_\alpha \cdot r_\beta \tag{20}$$

for the positional changes $r_\beta$.

NUMERICAL RESULTS

We are able to present here some limited results of numerical simulations. Further results will be presented in a forthcoming paper. Our experiments have so far only used a two dimensional object. We expect that the algorithms will work as well in three dimensions although the computing time will be greater. The results we present here are for a square domain because although our finite element programs will work on arbitrary shaped domains, the results for the square are easier to present graphically. The finite element model we used consisted of eighty-one identical four node square elements. The same approximation space was used for the conductivity and potentials.

The current patterns used were two-electrode patterns as used by Barber and Seagar (1987), Tarassenko (1985). We chose to simulate current driven between opposite electrodes. As shown in Breckon and Pidcock (1987) the angle between the drive electrodes makes little difference to the ill-posedness of the problem. We used sixteen electrodes the width of each being the same as the inter-electrode distance. The current distribution over the electrodes was assumed to be uniform.

We used simulated data calculated using the same finite element model as the reconstruction algorithm. In addition to accurately calculated data

we generated data contaminated by errors. We simulated errors in the voltage
measurements by adding normally distributed pseudo-random numbers to the
accurate values. To simulate small random errors in electrode position we
added a pseudo-random number to the electrode position and interpolated the
voltage measurements which would result from this change. Error in boundary
shape where simulated by adding a random vector to the position of the nodes
on the boundary.

The algorithm we tested was a Quasi-Newton method using truncated
singular value decomposition. A graph of the logarithms of the singular
values obtained is given in Fig. 1. Note that the singular values decay
rapidly indicating the severe ill-posedness of this problem.
Fig. 2 (a) shows the original conductivity distribution $\sigma$ which we will reconstruct. At sixteen points on the edge of a square the conductivity is 50
units, elsewhere it is 100. We take the initial guess $\sigma_0$ to be uniform at
100 units. Fig. 2 (b) and 2 (c) give respectively $\sigma_1$ and $\sigma_5$.when the data is
not contaminated by any noise. As can be seen from Fig. 3 the convergence
rate is approximately quadratic, when using exact data. When errors of

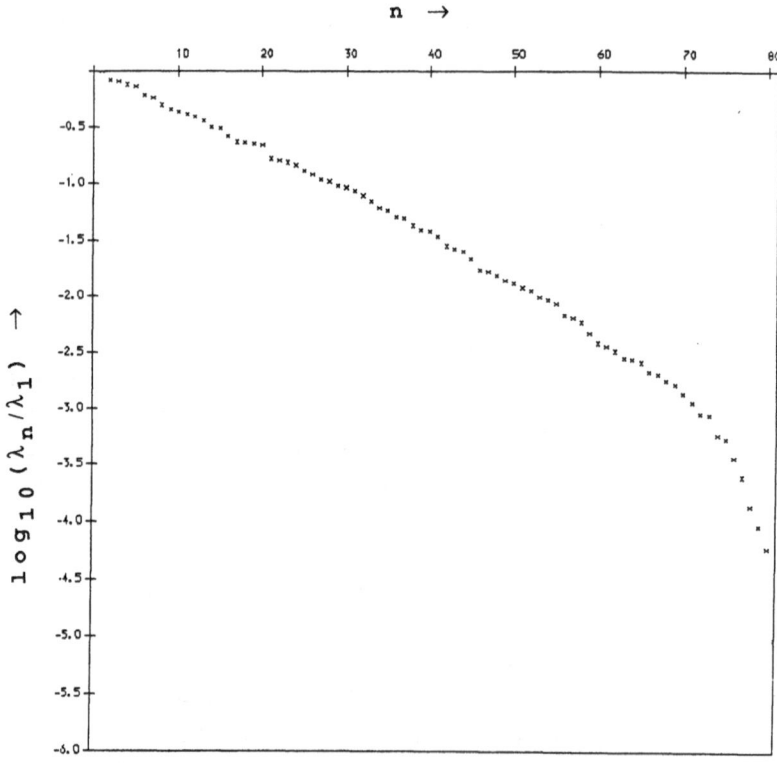

Fig. 1. Graph of the logarithm of the normalized singular
values $\log_{10}(\lambda_n/\lambda_1)$ of $F'(\sigma)$ for constant $\sigma$,
plotted against n. The graph shows that the number
of identifiable degrees of freedom decreases exponentially with the level of noise in the data.

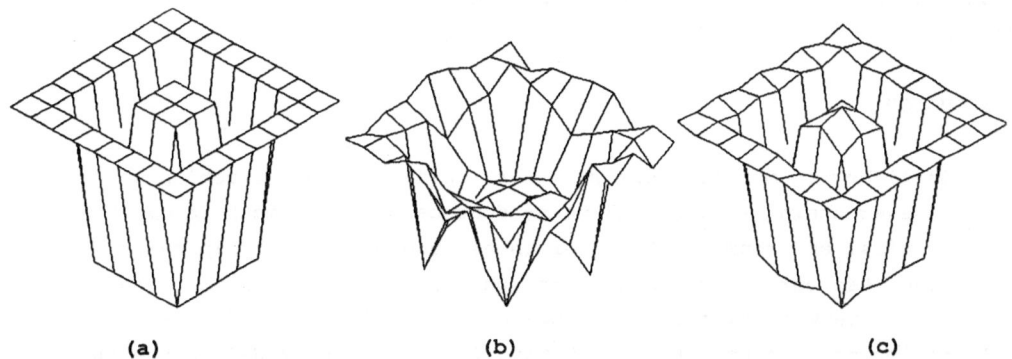

Fig 2.(a) The conductivity distribution we attempted to reconstruct. The lowest value is 50, the largest 100. (b) the
first iteration with exact data. (c) fifth iteration.

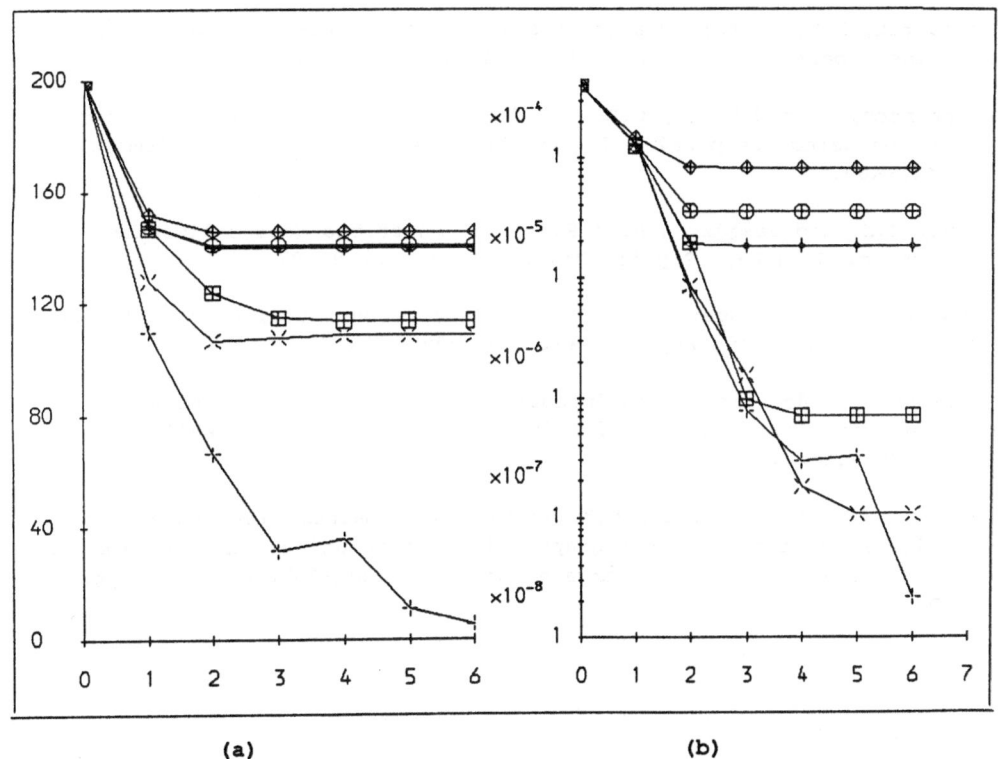

(a)                                        (b)

Fig 3. (a) The error in the conductivity $\|\sigma_n-\sigma\|$ for each iteration.
(b) The error in the voltage $\|F(\sigma)-v\|$ Exact data +. Error in
electrode position: 0.1% of inter-elecrode distance) ✕, 0.5%
+ . Error in boundary shape 0.1% inter-electrode distance +.
Noise added to voltage measurements 0.1% ⊕, 0.05% +

whatever type are introduced the quality of reconstruction is substantially degraded (see Fig. 3). This is to expected given the nature of the singular values.

CONCLUSION

Quasi-Newton methods work well for impedance reconstruction with exact data however there is much work to be done before such methods can be used in a clinical environment. We offer three suggestions for improving the technique. Use current drive patterns.which, at each iteration, can best distinguish between $\sigma_n$ and $\sigma$ (see Gisser et al, 1987). Find ways of making calibration measurements to adjust the finite element model to the physical system. Investigate ways of improving the tolerance of the algorithm to errors, for example try penalized likelihood methods which in similar problems have proved more tolerant to errors (see Kristensen and Vogel, 1987).

REFERENCES

Marquardt, D.W. (1963).An algorithm for least squares estimation of non-linear parameters, SIAM J. Appl. Math.,11,431-441.

Kristensen, G. and Vogel, C.R. (1986). Inverse problems for acoustic waves using the penalised likelihood method, Inverse Problems,2, 461-480.

Brown, B.H. and Seagar, A.D. (1987). The Sheffield data collection system, Clin Phys Physiol Meas.,8 Suppl. A, 91-97.

Barber, D.C. and Seagar, A.D. (1987). Fast reconstruction of resistance images, Clin Phys Physiol Meas., 8 Suppl. A, 47-54.

Tarassenko (1985) Electrical impedance techniques for the study of the cerebral circulation and cranial imaging in the newborn, DPhil. thesis, Oxford University.

Breckon, W.R. and Pidcock, M.K. (1987). Some mathematical aspects of electrical impedance tomography, in : Mathematics and Computing in Medical Imaging, M.A. Viergever and A.E. Todd-Pokropek, Springer, Berlin.

# A THEORETICALLY-CORRECT ALGORITHM TO COMPENSATE FOR A THREE-DIMENSIONAL SPATIALLY-VARIANT POINT SPREAD FUNCTION IN SPECT IMAGING

Barry R. Zeeberg[1,2], Alden N. Bice[2], Screcko Loncaric[2,3], and Henry N. Wagner, Jr.[2]

[1]Department of Radiology, George Washington University, Washington D.C., 20037, USA. [2]Divisions of Nuclear Medicine and Radiation Health Sciences, Johns Hopkins Medical Institutions, Baltimore, Md. 21205, USA. [3]Department of Nuclear Medicine, Clinical Hospital Center, Zagreb, Yugoslavia.

## INTRODUCTION

Three factors which degrade positional information and the quantitative potential of single photon emission computed tomography (SPECT) are finite detector size, Compton scatter, and the detector point spread function (PSF). We focus here on the PSF, which is modelled as a gaussian whose standard deviation depends on the perpendicular distance between the detector and the point being imaged. Thus the PSF is spatially-variant (SVPSF). The PSF is spatially-invariant, of course, within the plane of the detector for a fixed image point-detector distance.

The degrading effects of the SVPSF have been demonstrated in two-dimensional simulations (Eisner et al., 1984; Clausen et al., 1985; Loncaric et al., 1986) and a limited number of efforts have been made to compensate for this degradation (Hsieh and Wee, 1976; O Ying-Lie, 1983). We extend these approaches by first quantitating the effects of the SVPSF in three-dimensional simulations, with an emphasis on the frequency domain rather than the spatial domain. Second, an algorithm is presented which compensates for the SVPSF in a theoretically-exact way. This algorithm depends on a new transform, the Extended Radon Transform (ERT). Finally, we examine the implementation and limitations of the algorithm in a realistic imaging situation; this led to the derivation of a second new concept, a Truncated Central Section Theorem.

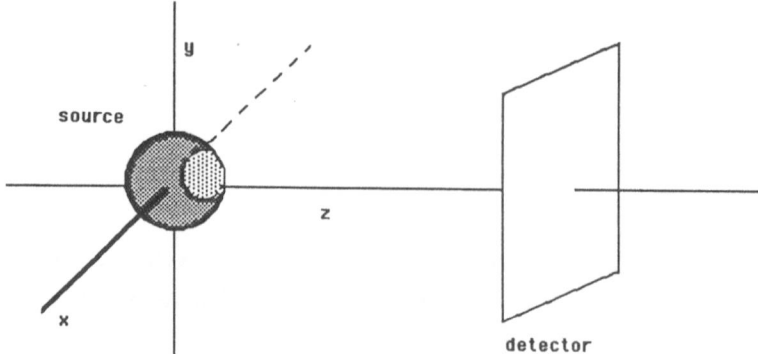

Fig. 1. Coordinate system illustrating the plane of the detector face and a sphere centered at the origin.

## THEORY

### Extended Radon Transform

Define the x-y plane as being parallel to the detector, the z axis as being perpendicular to the detector, and r as a vector in the x-y plane (Fig. 1). Then the detector response will be given by a three-dimensional convolution:

$$det(z,r) = \int_{-\infty}^{z} \int_{-\infty}^{\infty} im(z',r') \, g(z-z',r-r') \, dr' \, dz' \qquad (1)$$

where det is the detector response, im is the object being imaged, and g is the SVPSF. This is reduced to a one-dimensional convolution when the x-y plane is transformed to Fourier frequency space:

$$DET(z,R) = \int_{-\infty}^{z} IM(z',R) \, G(z-z',R) \, dz' \qquad (2)$$

Define the Extended Radon Transform ERT as a line integral of the line integrals:

$$ERT(R) = \int_{-\infty}^{\infty} DET(z,R) \, dz = \int_{-\infty}^{\infty} \int_{-\infty}^{z} IM(z',R) \, G(z-z',R) \, dz' \, dz \qquad (3)$$

By letting s = z-z', whenever $\int_{0}^{\infty} G(s,R) \, ds$ converges, we are able to separate the variables and transform the double integral equation into a simple equation involving ERT(R) which is experimentally measurable, F(R)

246

which can be precomputed numerically, and $\int_0^\infty IM(z,R)\, dz$, which is the Fourier transform of the undegraded line integral:

$$ERT(R) = \int_{-\infty}^{\infty} \int_0^{\infty} IM(z\text{-}s,R)\, G(s,R)\, ds\, dz = \int_0^{\infty} G(s,R)\, [\int_{-\infty}^{\infty} IM(z\text{-}s,R)\, dz]\, ds$$

$$= \int_0^{\infty} G(s,R)\, ds \int_{-\infty}^{\infty} IM(z,R)\, dz = F(R) \int_{-\infty}^{\infty} IM(z,R)\, dz \qquad (4)$$

where $F(R)$ is defined as $\int_0^{\infty} G(s,R)\, ds$. If G is a gaussian, then neither $F(0)$ nor $ERT(0)$ is defined. Finally, the desired Fourier transform of the undegraded line integral can be computed as:

$$\int_{-\infty}^{\infty} IM(z,R)\, dz = ERT(R)/F(R) \qquad (5)$$

## Truncated Central Section Theorem

In the absence of a PSF, and expressing $im(z',r)$ identically as the inverse Fourier transform of its Fourier transform with respect to $z'$, a truncated line integral from $\underline{a}$ to $z$ is given by:

$$det_a(z,r) = \int_a^z im(z',r)\, dz' = \int_a^z dz' \int_{-\infty}^{\infty} IM(Z,r)\, e^{2\pi i z'Z}\, dZ$$

$$= \int_{-\infty}^{\infty} dZ\, IM(Z,r) \int_a^z dz'\, e^{2\pi i z'Z} \qquad (6)$$

Taking the Fourier transform with respect to r and letting boldface $IM(Z,R)$ denote the Fourier transform with respect to both z and r:

$$DET_a(z,R) = \int_{-\infty}^{\infty} det_a(z,r)\, e^{-2\pi i rR}\, dr = \int_{-\infty}^{\infty} dZ\, IM(Z,R) \int_a^z e^{2\pi i z'Z}\, dz' \qquad (7)$$

Now when $\underline{a} = -\infty$ and $z = \infty$, the inner integral reduces to the generalized delta function with argument Z, so that Eq. 7 reduces to the Central Section Theorem (Bracewell, 1956):

$$DET(R) = IM(0,R) \qquad (8)$$

When $\underline{a}$ or $z$ is finite or zero, Eq. 7 reduces to the Truncated Central Section Theorem:

$$DET_a(z,R) = \int_{-\infty}^{\infty} dZ \; IM(Z,R) \; [e^{2\pi iZz} - e^{2\pi iZa}]/(2\pi iZ) \qquad (9)$$

Eq. 9 can be used to derive an expression for the missing portion of the ERT:

$$\int_0^x dz \; DET_a(z,R) = \int_0^x dz \int_{-\infty}^{\infty} dZ \; IM(Z,R) \; [e^{2\pi iZz} - e^{2\pi iZa}]/(2\pi iZ)$$

$$= \int_{-\infty}^{\infty} dZ \; IM(Z,R) \; [e^{2\pi iZx} - 1 - xe^{2\pi iZa}]/(2\pi iZ) \qquad (10)$$

where $x$ is minimum achievable radius of rotation for the detector.

Since $IM(Z,R)$ can be directly computed from Eq. 8 (and a simple radial to Cartesian transformation) applied to the full set of $DET(R)$ collected at all angles (about an axis of rotation which lies in the x-y plane), the transform of the truncated line integrals $DET_a(z,R)$ can be computed as an integral function of the physically-realizable $DET(R)$. That is, it is not necessary to explicitly perform the reconstruction of $IM(Z,R)$.

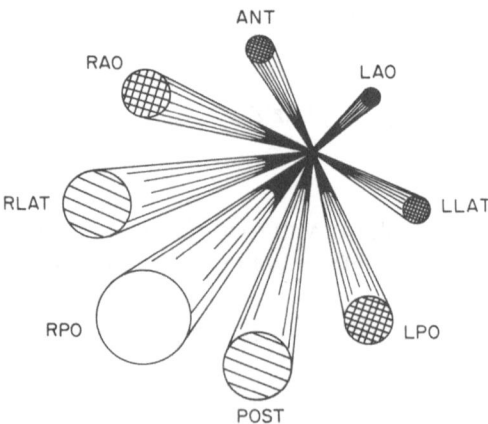

Fig. 2. Effect of the depth-dependent resolution on the projection images of a point source offset towards LAO (from Clausen et al., 1985).

METHODS

Although the algorithm is theoretically-correct for any arbitrary three-dimensional distribution of radioactivity, in the three-dimensional simulations we always used spheres centered at the origin since the resulting symmetry reduced the dimensionality of the problem. Thus, a (one-dimensional) Hankel transform (Bracewell, 1978) could be used instead of a two-dimensional Fourier transform; this made it possible to use a microcomputer with no floating-point hardware.

The SVPSF is represented as a gaussian whose standard deviation is given by $k_1 z + k_2$ where $k_1 = .05$ and $k_2 = .2$ cm, and z is the image point-detector distance in cm. Thus, at a 20 cm SPECT radius of rotation, the standard deviation of the gaussian would be 12 mm. The x-y plane was taken as parallel to the detector and the z axis as perpendicular to the detector. The Hankel transform was performed for the sphere and the gaussian in the x-y plane, and these two transforms were numerically convolved along the z axis throughout the spatial extent of the sphere (Eq. 2). The convolution was performed for each desired position of the detector along the z axis. The Hankel transform of the gaussian was $G(z,R) = \exp[-2\pi^2(k_1 z+k_2)^2 R^2]$, and the Hankel transform for the planes of the sphere were $rad \cdot J_1(2\pi\, rad\, R)/R$ for $R \neq 0$ and $\pi \cdot rad^2$ for R=0, where rad is the radius of the disk cross section of the sphere at a given position along the z axis, $J_1$ is the Bessel function of order one, and R is the radial frequency.

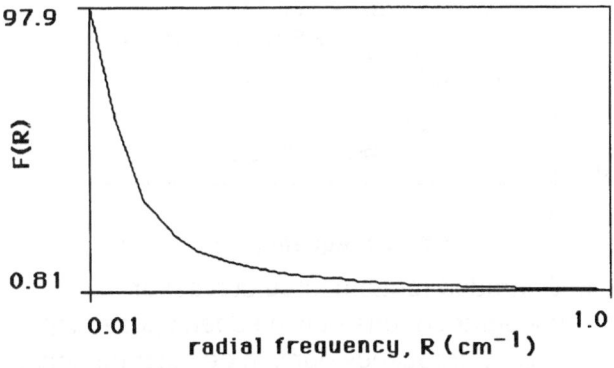

Fig. 3.  F(R) for a Gaussian SVPSF whose standard deviation is .05 z + .2 cm.

Direct numerical integration was used to compute the inverse Hankel transform of the simulated frequency domain projection data, and to compute the correction factor F(R) from the expression for G(z,R) (Eq. 4). The formula used to analytically computed the undegraded projection of the sphere in the spatial domain was $2(\text{rad}^2-r^2)^{1/2}$, $0 \le r \le \text{rad}$, where rad is the radius of the sphere and r is the radial distance from the z axis.

RESULTS AND DISCUSSION

As previously demonstrated (Clausen et al., 1985), the detector response PSF can lead to degradations in the tomographic projection data and consequently in the reconstruction of a radioactive source (Fig. 2). For an extended source the degradation in the projection image is the result of blurring with gaussians of many different PSF's, so that in theory Wiener filtering cannot be used for restoration.

Our approach was initially motivated by the idea that a weighted average of projections taken at two different detector radii of rotation might provide an improved reconstruction. The correct algorithm actually utilizes projection data from every nonnegative radius of rotation (Eqs. 1 - 5). Intuitively, the algorithm removes the spatial variation of the PSF since each point in the object is viewed at every possible detector distance; thus each point undergoes exactly the same distortion. The key

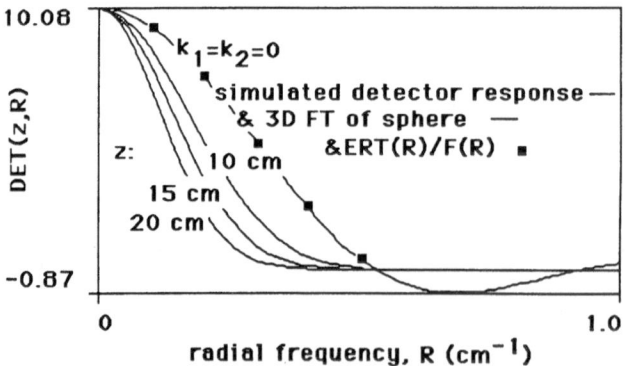

Fig. 4. Degraded (bottom three curves) or undegraded (one of two superimposed top curves) frequency domain detector response, and a radial line in the 3D Fourier transform (one of two superimposed top curves), for a 1.34 cm sphere (Bracewell, 1978). Squares indicate simulated values for ERT(R)/F(R).

step is in Eq. 4, where the infinite inner integral permits the separation of variables. Thus the transform of the undegraded line integrals can be obtained from the transform of the detector response divided by a numerically precomputed function of the radial frequency (Eq. 5 and Fig. 3).

We computed the frequency domain projection data at several detector positions along the z axis (Fig. 4) to show the degradations in the frequency domain resulting from the SVPSF. According to the Central Section Theorem, when $k_1$ and $k_2$ are equal to zero, the projection data should be identical with a radial line through the origin of the 3D Fourier transform of the source image. These were found to be in good agreement (Fig. 4). In accord with Eq. 5, the ratio ERT(R)/F(R) was in close agreement with the transform of the undegraded projection data (Fig. 4).

The corresponding projection data in the spatial domain (Fig. 5) illustrate the loss of positional and quantitative information. When $k_1$ and $k_2$ are equal to zero, the spatial projection computed this way is in good agreement with that computed analytically (Fig. 5).

The implementation of this algorithm requires the acquisition of data in some detector positions which are physically impossible (that is, the detector inside the object). This is not the first report of such a dilemma; Cormack (1980) reports in his Nobel Award Address: "The most interesting request for a reprint came from a Swiss Centre for Avalanche Research.

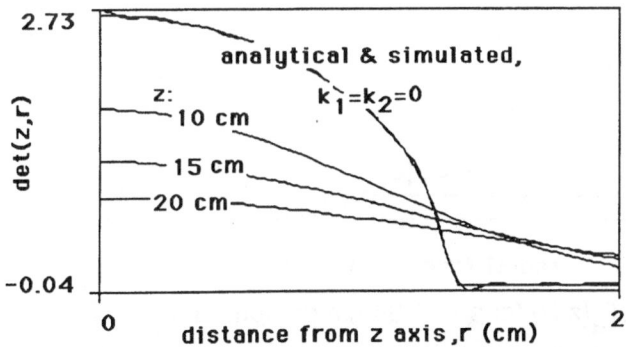

Fig. 5. Inverse Hankel transforms of simulated degraded (bottom three curves) or undegraded (one of two top curves) frequency domain detector response, and analytically-computed undegraded spatial domain detector response (one of two top curves), for a 1.34 cm sphere.

The method would work for deposits of snow on mountains if one could get either the detector or the source into the mountain under the snow!"

The study of techniques to extrapolate the obtainable data into the inaccessible region has led to the formulation of an appropriate counterpart of the Extended Radon Transform, namely the Truncated Central Section Theorem (Eqs. 6 - 9). An integrated version of this theorem (Eq. 10) permits undegraded projection data to be used to estimate the undegraded missing portion of the ERT (Fig. 6). Since the measured projection data are in fact degraded, the estimated portion of the ERT will also be degraded, and the theory is only approximately correct. Furthermore, the degradation in the estimate of the missing portion of the ERT will be based upon the SVPSF at the minimum achievable detector radius of rotation, not upon the proper SVPSF for each inaccessible detector position.

For example, in order to estimate ERT, we will add the measurable portion of the ERT from 10 cm to 50 cm (Fig. 7) to the missing portion estimated from the Truncated Central Section Theorem using the projection data acquired at a detector radius of rotation equal to 10 cm. When $k_1 = k_2 = 0$, this technique provides an accurate estimate of the missing portion of ERT (Fig. 7). For the values of $k_1$ and $k_2$ given in

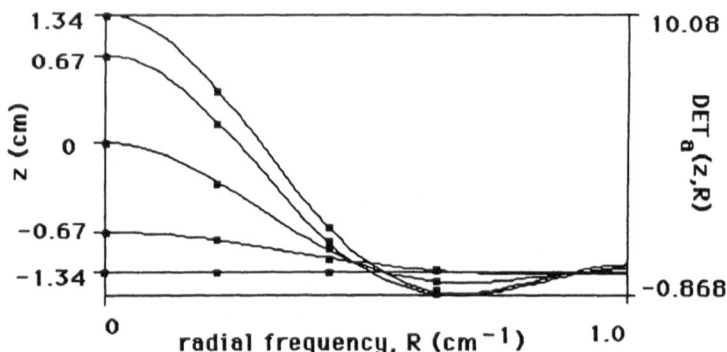

Fig. 6. $DET_a(z,R)$ for $a = -1.34$ cm computed by the Truncated Central Section Theorem (Eq. 9, squares) or by simulation (Eq. 2, solid lines). $IM(Z,R)$ in Eq. 9 was not computed explictly; rather Eq. 8 and DET(R) (the top curve of Fig. 4, extended to $R = 5$ cm$^{-1}$) were used to generate interpolated values of $IM(Z,R)$ as needed.

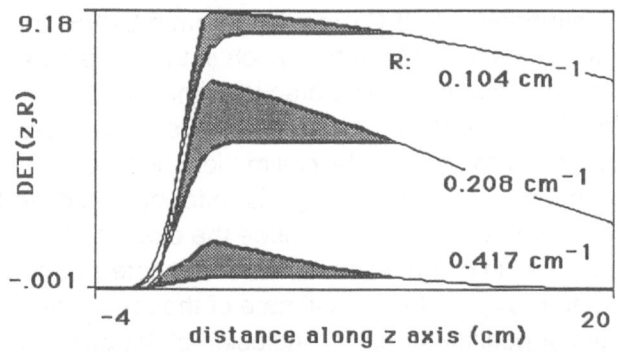

Fig. 7. Estimation of the detector response for inacessible detector positions by means of the Truncated Central Section Theorem. Shaded areas represent the difference between detector responses simulated using Eq. 2 (upper curve of each pair) and detector responses estimated by the Truncated Central Section Theorem (Eq. 9) from z = -4 to 10 cm with $a$ = -10 cm (lower curve of each pair).

Table 1

Estimation of a portion of the Extended Radon Transform
by the Truncated Central Section Theorem

| R (cm$^{-1}$) | ERT theoretical (Eq. 3) | ERT estimated (Eq. 9) | $\dfrac{\text{ERT(Eq. 9)}}{\text{ERT(Eq. 3)}}$ | $\dfrac{\text{DET(10,R), degraded}}{\text{DET(10,R),theoretical}}$ |
|---|---|---|---|---|
| 0.104167 | 319.53 | 314.54 | 0.9844 | 0.9002 |
| 0.208333 | 110.83 | 98.191 | 0.8860 | 0.6571 |
| 0.416667 | 11.772 | 5.2258 | 0.4439 | 0.1890 |

The ratios involving DET(10,R) are based on data from the top and the "10 cm" curves in Fig. 4.

Methods, the estimated missing portion of ERT is in error (Fig. 7). However, the error in the ERT estimated this way provides a considerable improvement over the error in the original projection data at 10 cm (Table 1).

Thus, the distortions in SPECT resulting from a SVPSF have been analyzed, we have derived an algorithm which in theory can exactly compensate for these distortions, and practical limitations have been examined and partially overcome. The algorithm is a 3D inversion of the degraded Radon transform for parallel collimation; Moore and Mueller (1986) have published a 3D inversion algorithm for point-focused collimation. Areas for future research include the examination of curve-fitting techniques in conjunction with the Truncated Central Section Theorem to provide a better estimate of the response at the inaccessible detector positions (Fig. 7), inclusion of the effects of attenuation and counting statistics, and simulations with more complex source distributions.

This work was supported by USPH grants CA09199 and NS22215.

REFERENCES

Bracewell, R. N. (1956). Strip integration in radio astronomy, Austr. J. Phys., 9, 198-217.

Bracewell, R. N. (1978), The Fourier Transform and its Applications, McGraw-Hill Book Company, New York.

Clausen, M., Bice, A.N., and Wagner, H.N., Jr. (1985). Resolution of Line Sources in SPECT with $180^o$ sampling (technical note), NUC Compact, 16, 449-454.

Cormack, A. M. (1980). Early two-dimensional reconstruction and recent topics stemming from it, Med. Phys., 7, 277-282.

Eisner, R. L., Gullberg, G.T., Malko, J.A., and Nowak, D.J. (1984). Effects of $180^o$ acquisition on tomographic image quality, J. Nuc. Med., 25, 30-35.

Hsieh, R. C., and Wee, W. G. (1976). On methods of three-dimensional reconstruction from a set of radioisotope scintigrams, IEEE Trans. Sys. Man. Cyb., SMC-6, 854-862.

Loncaric, S., Bice, A.N., Clausen, M., and Wagner, H.N., Jr. (1986). Recovery coefficients for quantitative imaging of small objects by $180^o$ and $360^o$ SPECT, J. Nuc. Med., 27, 1005-1006.

Moore, S. C., and Mueller, S. P. (1986). Inversion of the 3D Radon transform for a multidetector, point-focused SPECT brain scanner, Phys. Med. Biol., 31, 207-221.

Ying-Lie, O. (1983). An ECAT reconstruction method which corrects for attenuation and detector response, IEEE Trans. Nuc. Sci., NS-30, 632-635.

# STATISTICAL IMAGE RESTORATION AND REFINEMENT

Christopher Jennison and Michael Jubb

School of Mathematical Sciences

University of Bath, BATH BA2 7AY, U.K.

## SUMMARY

We consider the problem of reconstructing an image from a noisy record. We describe existing methods due to Geman and Geman (1984) and Besag (1986) which use a Markov random field model for the true scene but assume that each pixel consists of a single colour. In order to improve the quality of the restoration at the boundary of regions of different colours we extend these methods to allow pixels to contain two regions of colour separated by a single straight line. An algorithm for performing the reconstruction is presented and illustrated by an example.

## INTRODUCTION

We consider a rectangular region partitioned into pixels labelled $1,2,...,n$. Each pixel is coloured black or white and the colour of pixel $i$ is denoted by $x_i$ which takes the value 0 for white and 1 for black. The $x_i$ are unobserved. We work instead from the observed record $y_i$ which consists of $x_i$ plus added noise. We denote the whole scene by $x = \{x_i; i=1,...,n\}$ and the set of records by $y = \{y_i; i=1,...,n\}$. The noise distribution will be assumed to be known but if this were not the case, it could be established by studying training data.

Recent developments in statistical restoration methods use a Bayesian approach. The maximum a posteriori (MAP) estimate of the true scene is the value of $x$ which maximises $P(x|y)$, the conditional probability of $x$ given the record $y$. By Bayes' theorem

$$P(x|y) \propto l(y|x)\, p(x), \tag{1}$$

where $l(y|x)$ is the conditional likelihood of the observed record, $y$, given the true colouring, $x$, and $p(x)$ is the prior probability of $x$.

We assume the conditional density function $f(y_i|x_i)$ to be known and for the remainder of this paper we shall assume that the records, $y_i$, are independently distributed as Gaussian with mean $x_i$ and variance $\sigma^2$. Thus,

$$l(y|x) = \prod_{i=1}^{n} f(y_i|x_i) = (2\pi\sigma^2)^{-\frac{n}{2}} \exp\{ \frac{-1}{2\sigma^2} \sum_{i=1}^{n} (y_i - x_i)^2 \}.$$

To obtain a valid formula for $p(x)$, we assume that the true scene corresponds to a locally dependent Markov random field (MRF) with respect to a specified neighbourhood system, that is, the conditional distribution of pixel $i$ given the colourings of all other pixels depends only on the neighbours of pixel $i$. We shall use a second order neighbourhood system in which pixels are considered to be neighbours if they are horizontally, vertically or diagonally adjacent to each other. A detailed definition and further examples of Markov random fields may be found in Besag (1974).

The form of $p(x)$ is determined by the nature of the Markov random field. In our case, we have

$$p(x) \propto e^{-\beta Z(x)},$$

where $Z(x)$ is the number of discrepant pairs in the scene, $x$, i.e. the number of pairs of neighbours which are of opposite colour, and $\beta$ is a fixed positive constant (normally chosen to be between 0.5 and 1.5 ).

The maximisation of $P(x|y)$ now corresponds to the minimisation of

$$\frac{1}{2\sigma^2} \sum_{i=1}^{n} (y_i - x_i)^2 + \beta Z(x) \tag{2}$$

over values of $x = \{x_i; i=1,\dots,n\}$.

This expression may be regarded as a penalty, the first term penalising any difference between the record and the fitted value, the second term penalising excessive roughness in the reconstruction. Clearly, with $2^n$ possible values for $x$ this is a computationally large problem and necessitates the use of a sophisticated algorithm.

Geman and Geman (1984) use the method of simulated annealing which attempts to find the MAP estimate of $x$ given the record $y$. Their method is computationally extravagant and more recent developments by Greig, Porteous and Seheult (1986) show that the MAP estimate of any two colour scene may be found exactly using the Ford-Fulkerson labelling algorithm for maximising flow through a network.

Besag (1986) proposed the computationally simpler method of iterated conditional modes (ICM) which updates each pixel in turn, choosing for it the most likely colour based on its record and the current colouring of its neighbours. In updating pixel $i$ the new $x_i$ is chosen to minimise the sum of terms involving $x_i$ in the penalty (2), i.e.

$$\frac{1}{2\sigma^2}(y_i - x_i)^2 + \beta Z(x_i)$$

where $Z(x_i)$ is the number of neighbours of pixel $i$ in the current restoration which are of the opposite colour to $x_i$. The method proceeds by scanning the scene, successively updating each pixel until convergence is reached. This will normally occur at a local rather than global maximum of $P(x|y)$, but, given the possibility of undesirable long range dependencies in the MRF model, this is not a serious drawback and might even be an advantage.

## SPLIT PIXELS

So far we have considered scenes in which each pixel is coloured wholly one colour. We now allow pixels in the true scene to be coloured partly black and partly white. Each record $y_i$ is distributed as Gaussian with variance $\sigma^2$ and mean $p_i$, the proportion of pixel $i$ which is coloured black. The restoration methods that we have previously discussed can be used for this problem by proceeding as if the pixels were only of one colour but the quality of the restoration at the edges of objects or regions will obviously be poor. Instead, we can allow pixels in the restored image to be coloured partly black and partly white. The simplest form of this is to quarter each pixel and allow it to be filled with the most likely of the $2^4$ configurations. This method, proposed by Jennison (1986) uses a modified version of ICM, firstly iterating at full pixel size and subsequently restoring the quarters; in the second stage the same form of MRF model is used for the subpixels as is originally used for full pixels This method appears to work well and has prompted work into the further breakdown of pixels.

For further refinement we can either (i) consider an $m \times m$ breakdown of each pixel or (ii) use continuous lines within the pixel to represent the edge. The implementation of (i) requires the minimisation of

$$\frac{1}{2\sigma^2}\sum_{i=1}^{n}(y_i - \frac{1}{m^2}\sum_{j=1}^{m}\sum_{k=1}^{m}x_{ijk})^2 + \frac{1}{2}\beta\sum_{i=1}^{n}\sum_{j=1}^{m}\sum_{k=1}^{m}Z(x_{ijk}),$$

where the subscript $ijk$ refers to subpixel $j,k$ within pixel $i$; $x_{ijk}$ takes value 0 or 1 and $Z(x_{ijk})$ is the number of subpixel neighbours of subpixel $ijk$ in the current restoration which are of the opposite colour to $x_{ijk}$ (the factor $\frac{1}{2}$ is needed as each discordant pair is counted twice). Note that subpixels at the edge of a pixel will have some subpixel neighbours contained in an adjacent pixel. We can see that as $m$ increases this minimisation becomes computationally cumbersome. Also, it offers only an approximation to (ii) and it turns out to be easier to pass to the limit and work directly with continuous solutions.

The most basic form of (ii) allows a single straight line edge within each pixel and it is the implementation of this that we shall describe. It is no longer meaningful to talk of discrepant pixel or subpixel pairs and we replace the second term of (2) by a multiple of the total length of edge in the reconstruction $x$. Thus, the restored image is chosen to minimise

$$\frac{1}{2\sigma^2} \sum_{i=1}^{n} (y_i - p_i(x))^2 + \beta' L(x), \tag{3}$$

over images $x$ made up of pixels $x_i$, $i=1,\ldots,n$, either of a single colour or divided into two regions of different colours by a single straight line; $p_i(x)$ denotes the proportion of black in pixel $i$; $L(x)$ is the total edge length in scene $x$ and $\beta'$ is a fixed constant related to the $\beta$ used earlier.

An advantage of edge length as a measure is that the penalty is rotationally invariant, i.e. remains constant throughout all rotations of the scene within the region. This could not be obtained using discrepant pairs as a measure although it has been shown by our colleague Robin Sibson that this variability can be minimised using a down weighting of $1/\sqrt{2}$ for the diagonal adjacencies.

## THE RESTORATION ALGORITHM

The restoration is done in three stages, the first two of which have already been described :

Stage 1 : ICM to convergence on full size pixel grid.

Stage 2 : ICM to convergence on 2×2 pixel grid.

Stage 3 : Updating process on the line segments representing the edges.

Stage 3 requires that we now regard the reconstruction as a series of line segments separating the two colours. An initial representation is obtained in a straightforward way from the end product of Stage 2. The updating process treats pixels in pairs, selecting the best place for two edges to meet, given the current restoration of neighbouring pixels.

As an example, consider the configuration at pixels $i$ and $j$ shown in Figure 1. The distances $a$ and $b$ are determined by the current colouring of neighbouring pixels and treated as constant for the moment. The distance $W$ is chosen to minimise the contribution from pixels $i$ and $j$ to the total penalty (3), i.e.

$$g(W) = \frac{1}{2\sigma^2} \sum_{k=i,j} (y_k - p_{kW})^2 + \beta'(e_{iW} + e_{jW}), \tag{4}$$

where $e_{kW}$ is the length of edge in pixel $k$ when the join is at $W$ and $p_{kW}$ is the proportion of black in pixel $k$ when the join is at $W$.

For the case shown in Figure 1, this penalty is

$$g_1(W) = \frac{1}{2\sigma^2} \{(y_i - a - \tfrac{1}{2}(W-a))^2 + (y_j - b - \tfrac{1}{2}(W-b))^2\}$$
$$+ \beta'\{\sqrt{1+(W-a)^2} + \sqrt{1+(W-b)^2}\}.$$

This can not be minimised directly but the form of

$$\frac{dg_1(W)}{dW} = \frac{1}{4\sigma^2}(2W+a-2y_i+b-2y_j) + \beta'\left[\frac{(W-a)}{\sqrt{1+(W-a)^2}} + \frac{(W-b)}{\sqrt{1+(W-b)^2}}\right]$$

suggests an iterative approach. Given an approximate solution $W_{s-1}$ we solve

$$\frac{1}{4\sigma^2}(2W_s+a-2y_i+b-2y_j) + \beta'\left[\frac{(W_s-a)}{\sqrt{1+(W_{s-1}-a)^2}} + \frac{(W_s-b)}{\sqrt{1+(W_{s-1}-b)^2}}\right] = 0$$

to obtain

$$W_s = \frac{4\sigma^2\beta'\left[\dfrac{a}{\sqrt{1+(W_{s-1}-a)^2}} + \dfrac{b}{\sqrt{1+(W_{s-1}-b)^2}}\right] + (2y_i-a+2y_j-b)}{2+4\sigma^2\beta'\left[\dfrac{1}{\sqrt{1+(W_{s-1}-a)^2}} + \dfrac{1}{\sqrt{1+(W_{s-1}-b)^2}}\right]}.$$

Starting from any sensible initial value, $W_0$, accuracy to 3 decimal places was achieved after at most four iterations. In practice we take $W_0$ to be the value of $W$ prior to this update.

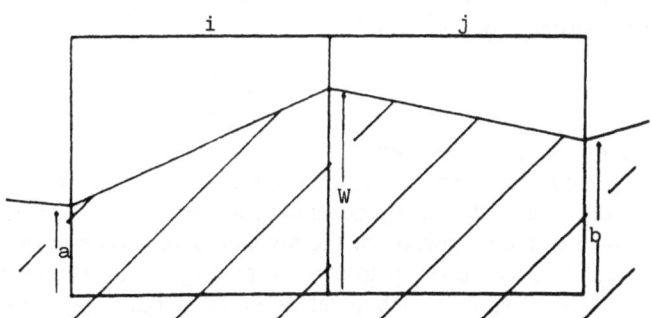

Fig. 1. Updating the position of edges in pixels $i$ and $j$.

Different forms of (4) are possible depending on which neighbours of pixels $i$ and $j$ contain both colours. There are only four distinct cases that may arise and these are shown in Figure 2.

We have shown the method of solution for case (i) and cases (ii) - (iv) are solved in a similar way. All other cases can be reduced to one of the above by means of exchanging and/or inverting the pixels and their colours.

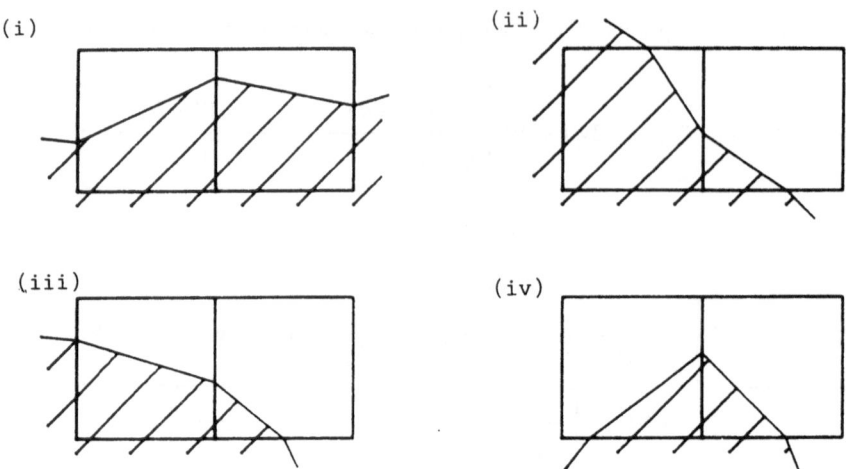

(i)

(ii)

(iii)

(iv)

Fig. 2. Possible configurations of edges in two neighbouring pixels.

The most natural order of updating the edge pixels would seem to be to follow an edge around, updating each join in turn, completing circuits of the edge until convergence. An alternative method is to update every $k^{th}$ join around the circuit, therefore completing $k$ laps before each pixel has been updated once. Initial results suggest that this provides additional stability in the updating process; we have found the value $k = 3$ to give particularly good results.

AN EXAMPLE

We illustrate the methods we have described with an artificial example. Figure 3a shows a true image and the superimposed pixel grid. The record from which a restored image was constructed was obtained by generating a Gaussian random variable for each pixel with mean equal to the proportion of the pixel coloured black in the true image and variance $0.01^2$. Figure 3b is the reconstruction after stage 1, in which the ICM method with $\beta=1$ has been used, treating each pixel as either completely black or completely white. Note that this is a rather poor approximation to the true image but it is the best that can be done without dividing pixels. Subdividing each pixel into four in stage 2 produces the reconstruction in Figure 3c: the amounts of black in each full pixel are now much closer to the corresponding records and the divisions of split pixels match up well with the true image. Proceeding to stage 3, we found that using $\beta'=50$ gave better results than those obtained using lower values of $\beta'$. The final reconstruction is shown in Figure 3d. Despite the coarseness of the original pixel grid and the addition of noise to the record, this reconstruction is barely distinguishable from the true image.

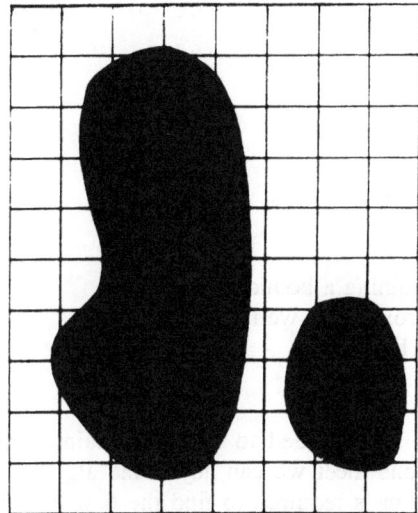

Fig 3a True image

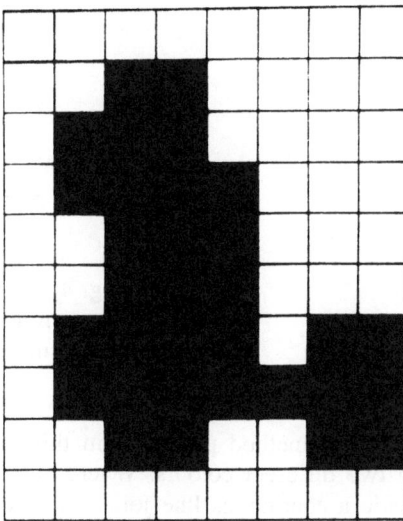

Fig 3b Reconstruction after stage 1

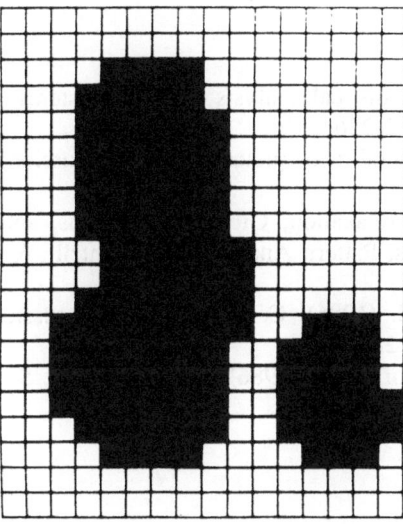

Fig 3c Reconstruction after stage 2

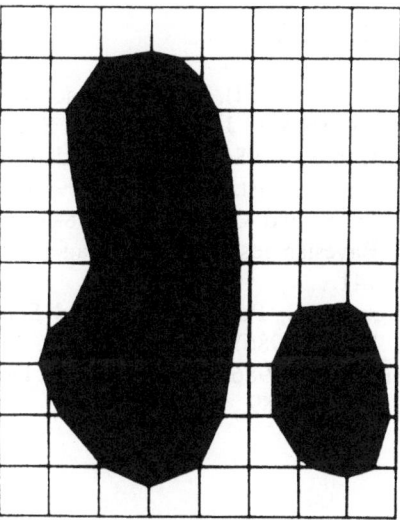

Fig 3d Final reconstruction

FURTHER EXTENSIONS

(a)      Consider a pixel which has true colouring as shown in Figure 4.  Clearly the straight line approximation to this edge will be poor and could have an adverse effect on the reconstruction of neighbouring pixels and pixels further along the edge. This may be overcome using a more intricate restoration method, e.g. allowing two straight lines meeting at some point within a pixel.

261

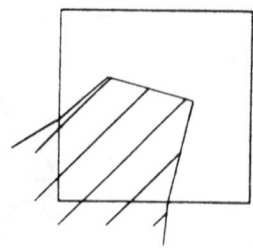

Fig. 4. A pixel containing a boundary
that can not be approximated well
by a single straight line.

(b)      The method presented in this paper can be extended to scenes containing more
than two different colours. Where any two regions meet we can adjust the algorithm to
provide a continuous line join. More computation is required to find the best colouring
for a pixel in which three or more regions meet.

REFERENCES

Besag, J. E. (1974). Spatial interaction and the statistical analysis of lattice systems (with
    discussion). J. Royal Statist. Soc. B, 36, 192-236.
Besag, J. E. (1986). On the statistical analysis of dirty pictures (with discussion). J.
    Royal Statist. Soc. B, 48, 259-302.
Geman, S. and Geman, D. (1984). Stochastic relaxation, Gibbs distributions, and the
    Bayesian restoration of images. IEEE Trans. Pattern Anal. Machine Intell., 6, 721-
    741.
Greig, D. M., Porteous, B.T. and Seheult, A.H. (1986). Contribution to Discussion of
    Besag (1986). J. Royal Statist. Soc. B, 48, 282-284.
Jennison, C. (1986). Contribution to Discussion of Besag (1986). J. Royal Statist. Soc. B,
    48, 288-289.

CONSTRAINED DECONVOLUTION TO REMOVE RESOLUTION DEGRADATION CAUSED BY

SCATTER IN SPECT

J C Yanch[+], S Webb[+], M A Flower[+], and A T Irvine[*]

[+]Joint Section of Physics, [*]Department of Nuclear Medicine
Institute of Cancer Research and Royal Marsden Hospital,
Downs Road, Sutton, Surrey.  SM2 5PT.   U.K.

## 1. INTRODUCTION

Although one of the ultimate aims of SPECT is to provide quantitative information concerning the radionuclide distribution in the object being scanned, it is essential to realize that much of the diagnostic information in Nuclear Medicine imaging is gained from visual examination of the image (Muehllehner, 1985).  An important goal in image enhancement or restoration is therefore to improve the accuracy and confidence of visual detection of small structures.

The ability to discern objects of a particular size depends on the contrast present in the image. Image contrast is a function of the original object contrast and of the modulation transfer function (MTF) of the entire imaging system.  The MTF can be used as a measure of the system spatial resolution (Beck et al., 1969; Metz et al., 1980) and in SPECT, is mainly determined by the physical dimensions of the collimator (Tsui et al., 1985; Muehllehner, 1985; Ehrhardt et al., 1974).   The unavoidable inclusion of scattered photons in the image will degrade the MTF (ie.  reduce resolution) (Beck et al., 1982; King et al., 1986; Todd-Pokropek, 1980) and since image contrast in small structures changes rapidly with only minor changes in spatial resolution (Muehllehner, 1985), it is expedient to eliminate the resolution loss introduced by scatter.

Several methods of eliminating or compensating for the effects of scattered photons have been proposed.  One approach has been to use an artificially low value of attenuation coefficient (eg. $0.12^{-1}$ cm rather than $0.15$ cm$^{-1}$ for $^{99}$Tc$^m$) with the assumption that a portion of unattenuated photons can be replaced by the same number of scattered photons (Jaszczak et al., 1984).   Most other procedures involve subtracting the scatter content from the acquired data but differ in their method of estimating the scatter contribution (eg. Lowry and Taylor, 1986; Jaszczak et al., 1984; Axelsson et al., 1984; Waggett and Wilson, 1977).

This paper describes the use of constrained deconvolution in removing the resolution degradation caused by scattered photons in projection data, or their effects in the reconstructed image. Acquisitions of both phantom and clinical data were carried out and the results of deconvolving these data are given. Presented for comparison are the results of simply using a reduced value of $\mu$ in the attenuation correction. This latter technique of scatter correction is currently used by many commercial SPECT system, primarily because it is quick and easy to implement. The assumption with this technique is that a portion of the attenuated primary photons can be replaced with the same number of scattered photons (Jaszczak et al., 1984).

The use of constrained deconvolution in correcting for scatter has also been compared with correction by scatter window subtraction (Jaszczak et al., 1984; Lowry and Taylor, 1986). This work is curently being prepared for publication and will not be discussed here.

## METHOD

### Background

To examine the effect of scattered photons on acquired data the image of a point source in air is often compared with that of a point in a scattering medium (Figure 1). This comparison can be misleading because the peak of the distribution of scattered photons is small compared with the height of the peak of the unattenuated photons (Beck et al., 1969) the FWHM changes only slightly. Greater difference is seen in the large FWTM (ie. scatter adds long tails to the point source response function) and it is therefore tempting to suggest that scatter removal could be effected simply by subtracting a constant background level from the data. While this subtraction would tend to remove the side tails from the PSRF, it would not affect the scatter peak that is a part of the full point source response. The ineffectiveness of background subtraction is demonstrated by noting that when only the scatter data are reconstructed, an image similar to the reconstruction of the primary photons is seen (Pang and Genna, 1979), and is not a uniform distribution spread across the image.

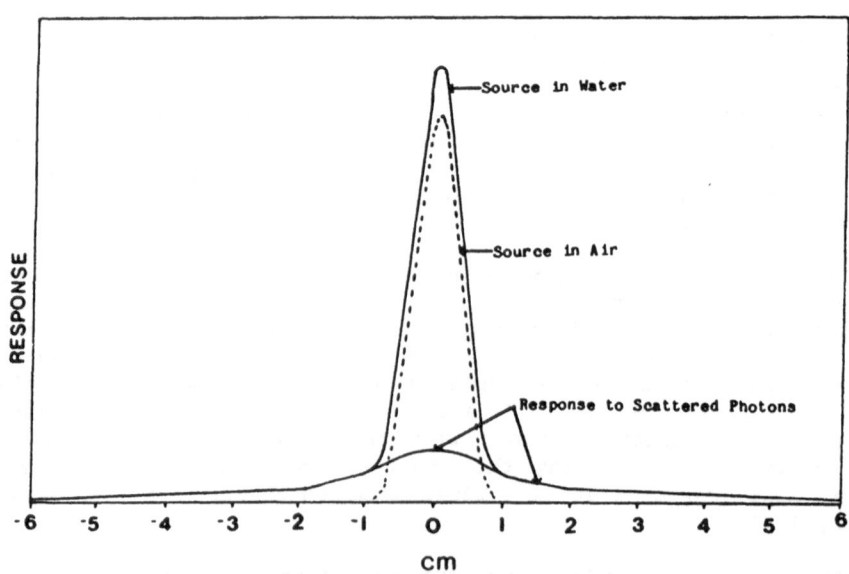

Figure 1: Schematic representatiohn of the response of the imaging system to a point source in air, and in water. [Redrawn from Beck et al., 1969]

264

The effect on resolution of scattered photons in the acquired data can be illustrated by examining the change in the modulation transfer function (MTF) that occurs when a scattering medium is present (Beck et al., 1969). The MTF is a measure of the efficiency of transferring the object modulation (or object contrast) of a distribution to an observed modulation in the image (or image contrast). It is a function of spatial frequency and can be expressed as the normalized Fourier Transform (FT) of a planar view of a point source. Figure 2 illustrates the MTF of a point imaged at a distance of 19.5 cm from the detector

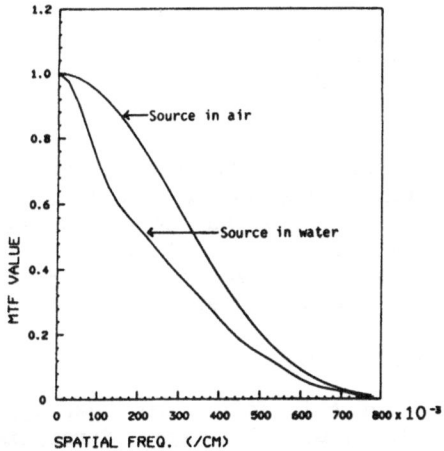

**Figure 2:** MTF of a point source at a fixed distance from the collimator in air (upper curve) and under 9.5cm of water (lower curve).

face, in air, and under 9.5 cm of water. The loss of efficiency of modulation transfer caused by scattered radiation reduces contrast and resolution in images of source distributions contained in a scattering medium (Beck et al., 1969; King et al., 1986). Note that subtraction of a constant background level from the data will not affect the MTF. The degradation of the MTF by scatter (and other causes) however, can be deconvolved from the projection data (King et al., 1986) or from the reconstructed image using an MTF acquired in a scattering medium.

## Deconvolution

Deconvolution is a direct inversion technique for solving a convolution integral. If the true object distribution is represented by $f(x,y)$ and the image data by $g(x,y)$ then in two dimensions:

$$g(x,y) = \int\int\limits_{-\infty}^{\infty} f(x',y') \, h(x-x',y-y') \, dx'dy' \qquad (1)$$

for a linear, space invariant system with point source response $h(x-x',y-y')$ (Andrews and Hunt, 1978).

The direct inverse of this equation would yield $f(x,y)$ by finding the inverse FT of G/H (where upper case letters represent the FT of the corresponding lower case quantity). Inversion however will lead to large fluctuations in the estimate of the object distribution due to the ill-conditioned nature of this equation. It is necessary to constrain the deconvolution to avoid this problem.

There are several ways to constrain deconvolution (eg Webb et al., 1985). It is desirable to do so in such a way that the inverse filter is followed as much as possible (ie. deconvolution), faithfully transferring as much of the data in frequency space as is practical before frequencies at which the noise begins to swamp the object occur. At this point noise suppression is effected by forcing the filter to rapidly decrease in value.

The procedure for constrained deconvolution discussed here uses the following equation to arrive at an estimate of F for the FT of equation 1:

$$F(u,v) = \frac{G(u,v) \ H*(u,v)}{\left|H(u,v)^2\right| + \gamma} \tag{2}$$

Here $\gamma$ is held constant. Equation 2 is a modification of the Wiener filter, in which $\gamma$ is a function of frequency and represents the ratio of power spectra of noise and signal. Because these spectra are difficult to determine in practice (King et al., 1986; Gonzalez and Wintz, 1977), modifying the filter by keeping $\gamma$ fixed becomes a useful approximation (Gonzalez and Wintz 1977).

Three deconvolution procedures

The general form of this filter has been applied to both phantom and clinical data in three separate ways. First, image deconvolution of a single transaxial frame was carried out. Alternatively each projection view was deconvolved prior to reconstruction. The third technique performed three dimensional deconvolution of the reconstructed image volume.

The first deconvolution technique, (called DecA), involved deconvolving a transaxial image with the reconstructed image of a point source in a scattering medium. Here the assumption of spatial invariance in the image of the point was made. It has been shown (Jaszczak et al., 1981) that spatial resolution, as a function of distance from the axis of rotation, is reasonably constant in the reconstructed section for parallel hole SPECT. This is due primarily to the addition of opposed views in the backprojection process (Ying-Lee 1983).

The shape of the DecA filter in frequency space changes with the value of $\gamma$ chosen. Examples are given in Figure 3. It is seen that an appropriate choice of $\gamma$ will control whether or not the filter acts as a low pass or high pass filter and to what extent. An optimum value of $\gamma$ ($5 \times 10^8$) was chosen as one producing a filter which gave a large numerical increase in image contrast, without creating a qualitatively undesirable image. The method of choosing the value of $\gamma$ is discussed in the following section.

In the second method of deconvolution, DecB, constrained deconvolution of each frame of projection data using the modified Wiener inversion produced 64 modified projection images of the object. This was followed by image reconstruction by filtered backprojection using a ramp filter. With DecB, the PSRF used in the calculation of equation 2 is the planar projection data of the point, and consequently the shape of the filter for different values of $\gamma$ will be different from that of the filter for DecA which used a transaxial slice reconstructed through the centre of the point. Figure 4 illustrates the DecB filter for

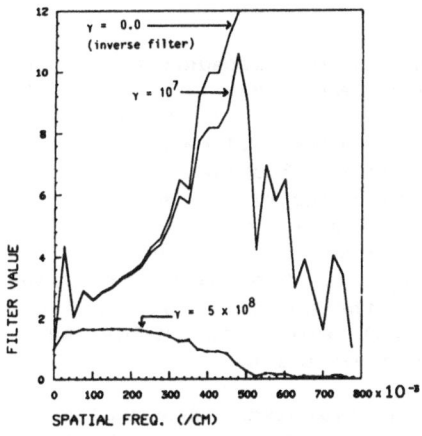

Figure 3:
Filters for DecA, produced (in order of increased smoothing) when $\gamma=0.0$ (inverse filter), $10^7$ and $5 \times 10^6$.

various values of $\gamma$. The procedure of choosing an optimum value of $\gamma$ was carried out as described below; a value of $5 \times 10^4$ was chosen.

For the third deconvolution method, DecC, equation 1 was extended to three dimensions:

$$g(x,y,z) = \int\!\!\!\int\limits_{-\infty}^{\infty}\!\!\!\int f(x',y',z')\, h(x-x',y-y',z-z')\, dx'dy'dz' \qquad (3)$$

Again spatial invariance throughout the object volume was assumed in order to validate the use of the transfer function. In equation 3, $g(x',y',z')$ is the 3D reconstructed image of the object and $h(x-x',y-y',z-z')$ is the 3D reconstruction of the point. Again, in order to obtain the three-dimensional object distribution, constrained deconvolution using the modified Wiener inversion was carried out. A value of $\gamma=5 \times 10^5$ was used.

The three methods of carrying out constrained deconvolution were applied to phantom and clinical data in an attempt to eliminate the degradation of the MTF caused by scatter. Also eliminated by the process of deconvolution will be other causes of resolution loss, the most important of which is the geometric response of the collimator.

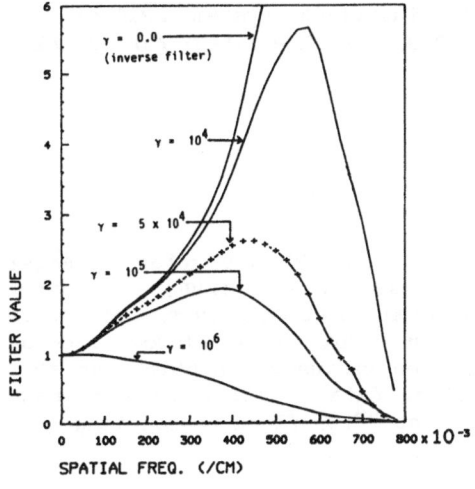

Figure 4:
Filters for DecB, produced (in order of increased smoothing) when $\gamma=0.0$ (inverse filter), $10^4$, $5 \times 10^4$, $10^5$ and $10^6$.

## Determination of γ and H

The optimum value of γ for each deconvolution procedure was chosen by measuring image contrast in reconstructed images of a phantom containing cold cylinders of various sizes (1.0 to 5.0 cm diameter). This phantom and the method of contrast assessment will be discussed in more detail in section 3. The data were processed several times, each time with a filter produced by a different value of γ. As expected, contrast measurements in images with high frequency components (eg. in the smallest cold spots) are improved when a smaller γ is used as this is a closer approximation of the inverse filter. The smaller the value of γ, however, the more mottled or grainy the hot areas of the image will appear. The image becomes more and more unacceptable as γ decreases and the method approaches pure deconvolution.

The larger cold spots showed more of an improvement when a slightly higher value of γ was used than that value giving highest contrast in the smaller cold areas. We chose this higher γ as the optimum value because, although improvement in contrast in smaller cold spots is more desirable than contrast improvement in large cold areas (which are already easily detected), the filter created by the larger γ produced qualitatively more acceptable images. This value was subsequently used for all implementations of the particular deconvolution method in question.

It was found that this optimum value of γ depended very little on the count density in the data to be processed. Repeating the procedure of γ assessment when the count density was more than an order of magnitude lower produced exactly the same estimate of optimum filter shape in each deconvolution procedure. Thus, if this filter were to be used for general image processing, a separate filter would not have to be calculated each time new data were acquired.

The effect of scatter on the system PSRF will change as a function of the scatter fraction included in the acquired data (Metz et al (1980)). The magnitude of the scatter fraction depends on the depth of the source in the scattering medium. Thus using the PSRF of a source placed at one point in the medium will be incorrect for a source placed elsewhere. It is necessary, however, to choose a single value for the PSRF in order to validate the use of the transfer function in the deconvolution. For the purpose of this study, a very small source was imaged in the centre of a water-filled cylindrical phantom (19.0 cm diameter x 12.0 cm height) in an attempt to estimate an average PSRF. Other researchers have found that using an average PSRF provides a reasonable approximation to a shift invariant system (Miller and Sampathkumaran, 1982; Miracle et al., 1979; Ying-Lee, 1983; King et al., 1983).

## IMPLEMENTATION AND TESTING

### Data Acquisition

Tomographic data were acquired on a GE 400 A/T rotating Anger camera fitted with a Low Energy High Resolution (LEHR) collimator (H2503BD). Sixty-four projections were obtained at equally spaced angles over 360 degrees. Data were collected in a 20% energy window (126-154 keV) centered on the $^{99}Tc^m$ photopeak. The radius of rotation was 19.5 cm (or as small as practical for patient data). All projection data were corrected with a single 30 x 10$^6$ count $^{99}Tc^m$ flood source image.

Reconstruction by filtered backprojection was carried out on the GE STAR computer; a Hanning window with cutoff value of 0.5 cycles/pixel applied to a ramp filter was used. The STAR implements an attenuation correction by fitting an ellipse to the object outline and correcting each view and ray prior to reconstruction. The attenuation coefficient used with this correction was 0.15 $cm^{-1}$ except in the case of reconstruction alone (no deconvolution) in which case it was 0.12 $cm^{-1}$. The threshold value, used to determine the patient outline, was 0.1 of the maximum pixel value in each projection.

Tomographic data were scatter corrected in three separate ways using the different applications of the deconvolution procedure already discussed. All Fourier Transforms were calculated using the multi-dimensional discrete FT routine supplied by the Numerical Algorithm Group (NAG) Library and run on a VAX 11/750 computer. The point source data necessary for the deconvolution procedure were obtained by imaging a very small (2mm x 1mm x 1mm) 600 MBq source of $^{99}Tc^m$ pertechnetate supported in the centre of a water-filled cylindrical phantom (19.0 cm diameter x 12.0 cm height). Sixty-four planar views containing approximately 7400 counts each were collected with the energy window set at 126–154 keV. The radius of rotation was again 19.5 cm.

## Phantom 1

The effect of constrained deconvolution on spatial resolution was assessed by imaging a pie-shaped 'cold spot' resolution insert placed in a large cylindrical phantom. The height of the insert was 6.0 cm and it was placed in the centre of a 21.0 cm (diameter) 20.0 cm phantom containing a solution of 650 MBq $^{99}Tc^m$ pertechnetate in water. Data were collected for 20 seconds/projecion resulting in a maximum pixel count of approximately 530 in each planar view. The diameters of the cold spots in the insert were 1.55, 1.25, 1.15, 0.95, 0.80, and 0.55 cm.

Resolution assessment of the final images of phantom 1 was by visual inspection and also by drawing profiles through the cold spots.

## Phantom 2

A phantom containing large cold spots of various sizes was imaged in order to numerically evaluate the effect of each deconvolution procedure on image contrast. Contrast in the image depends on the modulation transfer function which should be improved by the process of deconvolution. An improved MTF will therefore result in increased image contrast.

A 19.0 cm diameter x 12.0 cm thick cylindrical Perspex phantom filled with a solution of 500 MBq $^{99}Tc^m$ pertechnetate in water was imaged. The phantom was constructed such that fillable cylindrical inserts of various sizes could be placed at different radial and axial positions. In this experiment five water-filled cylinders were placed at similar radial positions (6.0 cm from the centre) and had outer heights and diameters of 5.0, 4.0, 3.0, 2.0, and 1.0 cm. Data were again acquired for 20 seconds/projection resulting in a maximum pixel count of approximately 1340 in each view. Because of the increased number of counts in these images (compared with phantom 1) a ramp filter with a very high cutoff value was used in all reconstructions.

Deconvolution procedures were carried out as described above. Evaluation of the effect of each procedure on image contrast involved the placement of inscribed square regions of interest (ROI) inside each of the circular cold spots. The location of the ROI for each cold spot was consistent from image to image and can be seen in Figure 7. ROI sizes are listed in Table 1. The background level was determined for a large irregular ROI by placing a rectangular box over the entire image and applying a threshold pixel value.

Image contrast for a particular cold spot was defined as the difference in average count density (counts/pixel) in the ROI within the cold spot and the average count density in the background, all divided by the background count denisty. Image mottle was determined by taking the ratio of the standard deviation of pixel values to the mean value in the background ROI. The concept of image mottle is included here so as to provide an estimate of the effect of constrained deconvolution on image quality. High values of mottle correspond to very grainy images; low values indicate images which are smooth in appearance.

## Clinical Data

The effect of constrained deconvolution on image quality was also evaluated using clinical data. Two cases are presented, both with Glioma affecting the brain.

Both patients were imaged with the GE STARCAM rotating $\gamma$ camera fitted with a LEHR collimator. Patients were injected with 750 MBq of $^{99}Tc^m$ – labelled hexamethyl propyleneamine oxime (HMPAO), a cerebral blood flow imaging agent. Data were accumulated for 20 seconds per view in each of 64 views. The energy window was again placed at 126–154 keV and projection data were uniformity corrected as mentioned above. Reconstructions of the transaxial images and constrained deconvolution were carried out exactly as for the phantom data except that a Hanning window with a cutoff value of 0.8 cycles/pixel was applied to a ramp filter in all reconstructions. All images were presented for qualitative analysis to a radiologist who was unaware of the procedures used to generate the images.

## RESULTS

## Phantom 1

Reconstructed images of the resolution pie phantom are seen in Figure 5. The 1.55 cm cold spots (largest size) can be seen in all of the images. Resolution of some of them is poor, however, when scatter compensation was by attenuation correction with $\mu$ = .12 $cm^{-1}$. Horizontal profiles drawn through the 1.55 cm cold spots (not shown) indicate that far greater image contrast is realized by the three-dimensional deconvolution technique.

## b) Phantom 2:

Values of image mottle and ROI contrast in phantom 2 were calculated for each of the deconvolution techniques and are listed in Table 1; they are compared with the values obtained when scatter correction is carried out simply by using an artificially low value of the attenuation coefficient. These results are also plotted in Figure 6. Figure 7 presents images produced by each of the methods on an equivalent slice through the phantom.

It is seen from Table 1 and Figure 6 that the three methods of deconvolution are successful in improving image constrast in cold areas larger than 2 cm. Only DecA (2-dimensional deconvolution of a single

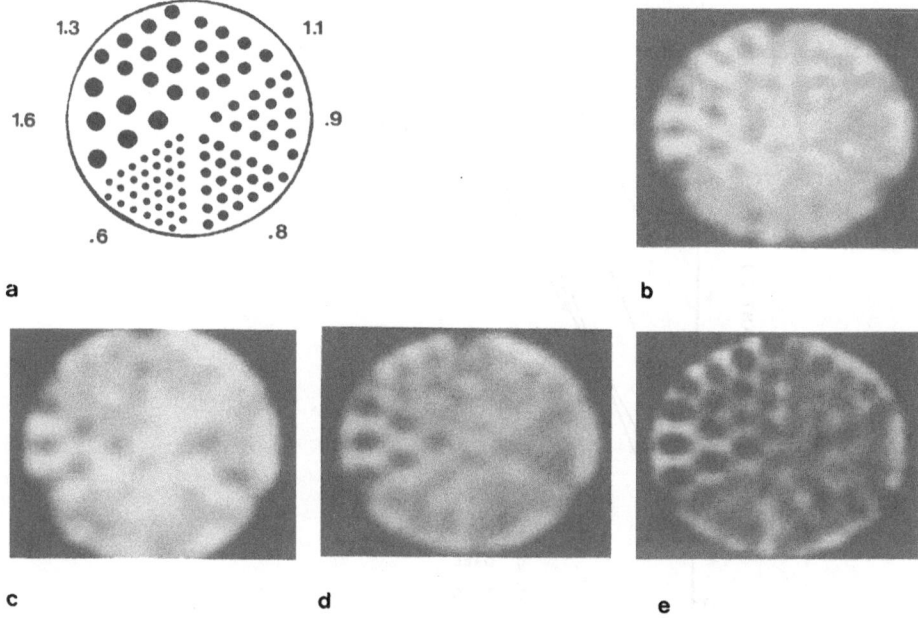

a                                                          b

c                                   d                          e

Figure 5: Results of scatter correction methods applied to data from
phantom 1. a) schematic representation of a transaxial slice,
including diameter of cold rods (cm), b) use of a reduced $\mu$
in attenuation correction, c) DecA, d) DecB, e) DecC.

transaxial frame) does not produce improvement in contrast in the 1 cm
cold spot. Choosing a value of $\gamma$ such that the filter used in DecA
acted more as a high pass filter (eg. a $\gamma$ of $5 \times 10^7$ rather than $5 \times 10^6$) resulted in improved contrast in the 1 cm cold spot over the $\mu$ =
.12 $cm^{-1}$ image for this procedure as well. This is done however, at
the expense of image mottle (increased from 8.4 to 10.7%) and at the
expense of contrast in the larger cold spots. For example the contrast
in the 4 cm cold spot fell from .95 ± .01 when $\gamma$ was $5 \times 10^6$, to .84 ±
.04 when $\gamma$ was $5 \times 10^7$.

## Clinical Data

Results of applying the different methods of deconvolution to
clinical data are given in Figures 8 and 9. An X-ray CT scan of patient
1 demonstrated a tumour of the corpus callosum with a cystic component.
Reconstruction using a $\mu$ of .12 $cm^{-1}$ in the attenuation correction
produced a transaxial image of limited value (Figure 8), the tumour
being poorly delineated. Deconvolving the projection data prior to
reconstruction (DecB) produced an image which was preferred by the
interpreting radiologist as that most clearly demonstrating the tumour
as well as enhancing the normal physiological and anatomical features.

A 4 cm mass with a necrotic centre was seen in the right
temporal-parietal region on an X-ray CT scan of patient 2. The
reconstructed SPECT image (Figure 9) shows an area of abnormal activity
in the parietal region peripherally with a region of low activity within
it. Again DecB was chosen as the method which best clarified the ring
of abnormal activity and the contained photon deficient area.

271

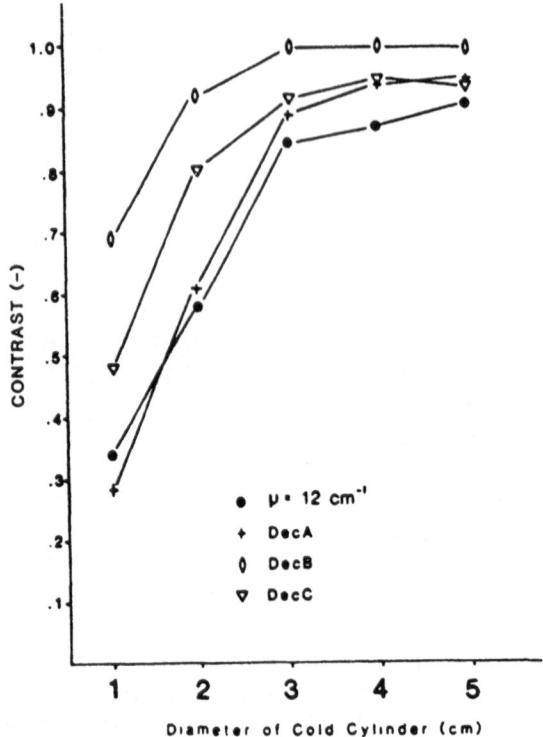

Figure 6: Image contrast vs
Diameter of cold cylinder in
phantom 2.  See Table 1 for
error estimates, and Figure 7
for transaxial images.

Table 1  Measured Values of Image Contrast and Mottle in Phantom 2

| | Contrast (Neg) Diameter of Cold Cylinder (cm) [ROI size (pixels)]* | | | | | Mottle (%) |
|---|---|---|---|---|---|---|
| | 1 [9] | 2 [25] | 3 [25] | 4 [49] | 5 [81] | |
| $\mu$=12cm$^{-1}$ | .35±.06 | .59±.04 | .83±.01 | .88±.02 | .88±.04 | 10.5 |
| DecA | .28±.04 | .63±.03 | .90±.01 | .95±.01 | .97±.01 | 5.8 |
| DecB | .70±.07 | .94±.08 | 1.00±.06 | 1.00±.06 | 1.00±.06 | 16.6 |
| DecC | .48±.03 | .81±.06 | .93±.02 | .96±.02 | .96±.02 | 8.7 |

* 128$^2$ resolution

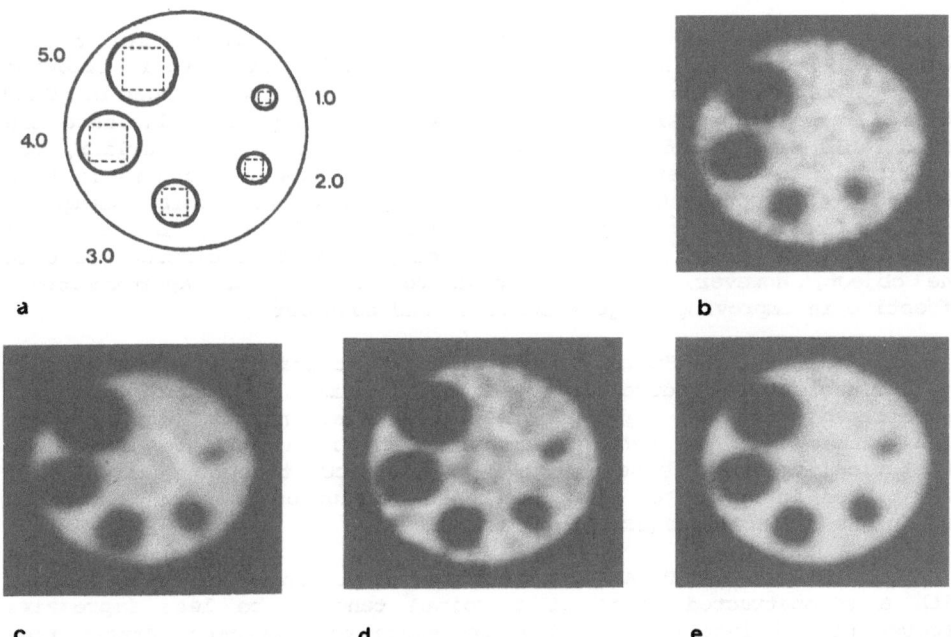

Figure 7: Results of scatter correction methods applied to data from phantom 2. a) schematic representation of a transaxial slice including ROI placement for contrast measurements and diameter of cold cylinders (cm), b) use of a reduced $\mu$ in attenuation correction, c) DecA, d) DecB, e) DecC.

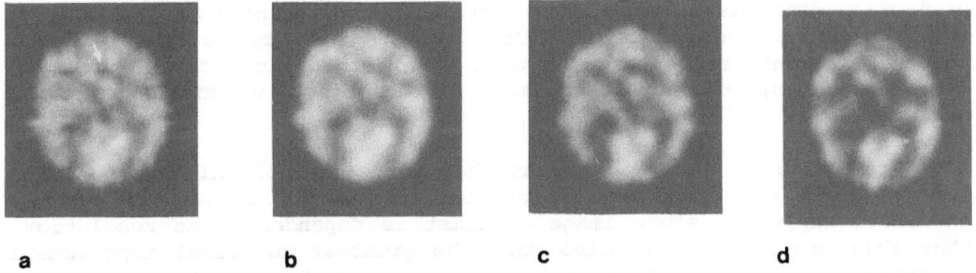

Figure 8: Results of scatter correction methods applied to data from patient 1. a) use of a reduced $\mu$ in attenuation correction (tumour indicated with arrow), b) DecA, c) DecB, d) DecC.

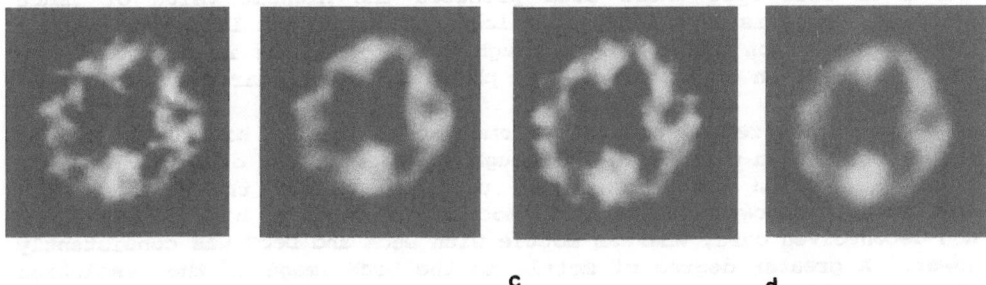

Figure 9: Results of scatter correction methods applied to data from patient 2. a) use of a reduced $\mu$ in attenuation correction (tumour indicated with arrow), b) DecA, c) DecB, d) DecC.

273

DISCUSSION AND CONCLUSIONS

The process of deconvolving the response of the imaging system to a point in a scattering medium has been shown to be effective in removing much of the resolution degradation caused by scattered photons in SPECT data. It is not possible for this process to entirely eliminate the undesirable effects of scatter because, as was mentioned earlier, the contribution of scatter to a particular point from all others is here assumed to be constant throughout the object volume. This assumption will not be strictly valid in practice. The use of an 'average' estimate of the contribution of scattered photons to a central point in the object, however, has been shown to be a useful approximation, effective in improving image resolution and contrast.

It is seen from Figure 6 and Table 1 that while all three methods of deconvolution produce improvements in image contrast over the non-deconvolved image, improvements with DecA are not as large as those with either DecB or DecC. Further, DecA is unable to match the resolution improvements seen with DecB and DecC; this is qualitatively illustrated in images of the pie-shaped resolution phantom (Figure 5) and in the clinical images, Figures 8 and 9.

The results for DecA (deconvolution of a single transaxial plane with a reconstructed image of a point) tend to be less impressive because of the inability of this procedure to eliminate scatter from adjacent planes. The long tails and shoulders of the scatter PSRF (Figure 1) illustrate how scattered photons generated at one position in the object can affect the image distribution at positions even centimeters away (Egbert and May, 1980). Deconvolution of only a single plane will not affect the presence of scatter created in planes nearby. Conversely, DecB and DecC are both able to remove the effects of scatter from other planes. DecB does this by eliminating scatter from projection data before backprojection, thereby sending improved data to the reconstruction process. DecC does this by deconvolving a three-dimensional reconstruction of a point containing scatter from the three-dimensional reconstructed image of the object, which also contains scatter.

From Figure 5 it would appear that three-dimensional deconvolution (DecC) gives the greatest improvement in image resolution. It was therefore expected, since image contrast is dependent upon resolution, that this procedure would also show the greatest numerical improvement in contrast. This, however, does not seem to hold true (see Table 1). Measurements of cold spot contrast with DecC consistently fall below those with DecB. Even though, for most cold spots, the DecC values are equal to those of DecB within ±1 standard error, this is not the case in the 1 cm cold spot where DecB produced the highest value of image contrast. This is a somewhat anomalous finding as the larger cold spots in the resolution phantom were roughly 1.0 - 1.5 cm in diameter. In visual inspection of images of that phantom, DecC appeared superior.

A possible reason for this anomaly could be the high estimates of image mottle seen with DecB. Although the measurement of mottle depends a great deal on the value of $\gamma$ used to produce the filter, DecB consistently showed values of mottle that were higher than the non-deconvolved case, whereas mottle with DecA and DecC was consistently lower. A greater degree of mottle in the DecB image of the resolution phantom would have affected the qualitative assessment of resolution.

It was mentioned above that the optimum filter shape (ie. choice of $\gamma$) is not markedly count-dependent. It is necessary to initially determine the filter shape separately for each of the three deconvolution procedures, but further change to the filter for the processing of subsequent images would not be required. This method of image processing would therefore be easy to implement on a routine basis.

It was previously not possible to carry out three-dimensional deconvolution due to limitations of time and workspace on the computing facilities available (Webb et al., 1985). Recent improvements in computing capability, however, have made it possible for each of the three methods discussed here to be completed in only a few minutes of central processor time, with the use of optimized computer programs. As DecA carries out only two 2-dimensional forward Fourier Transforms and one inverse FT, it can be completed very quickly. DecB performs this combination 64 times; computing time for this method can be reduced however, by storing the forward FT of only one view of the planar PSRF for use in all 64 deconvolutions, as all views of the point are theoretically identical. DecC, in carrying out three-dimensional deconvolution, requires a large work space on the computer and currently takes about twice as much time as DecB.

Three methods of applying constrained deconvolution of a point source response function to SPECT data containing scatter have been shown to be effective in improving image resolution and contrast in the final image. It is felt that the effectiveness comes from the ability of the deconvolution procedure to remove the degrading effects that scatter has on image resolution. Resolution improvements lead to increased image contrast and the detection of small structures with a higher degree of accuracy. The filter used to constrain the deconvolution is seen to be easily optimized and, once optimized, is useful for processing images containing a range of count densities.

REFERENCES

Andrews, H.C., and Hunt, B.R.,(1977). Digital Image Restoration, Prentice-Hall, Englewood Cliffs, NJ.

Axelsson, B., Msaki, P., and Israelsson, A.,(1984). Subtraction of Compton-scattered photons in single-photon emission computerized tomography, J Nucl Med., 25, 490-494.

Beck, R.N., Schuh M.W., Cohen, T.D., and Lembares, N.,(1969). Effects of scattered radiation on scintillation detector response, in: Medical Radioisotope Scintigraphy, IAEA, Vienna, (1969).

Beck, R.N., Jaszczak, R.J., Coleman, R.E., Starmer, C.F. and Loren, W.N.,(1982). Analysis of SPECT including scatter and attenuation using sophisticated Monte Carlo modelling methods, IEEE Trans Nucl. Sci, NS-29, 506-511.

Egbert, S.D., and May, R.S.(1980). An integral-transport method for Compton-scatter correction in emission computed tomography, IEEE Trans Nucl Sci., NS-27, 543-549.

Ehrhardt, J.C., Oberley, L.W., and Lensink, S.C.,(1974). Effect of a scattering medium on X-ray imaging, J Nucl Med., 15, 943-948.

Gonzalez, R.C., and Wintz, P.,(1977). Digital Image Processing, Addison-Wesley Publishing Company, Reading, Massachusetts.

Jaszczak, R.J., Coleman, R.E., and Whitehead, F.R.,(1981). Physical Factors affecting quantitative measurements using camera-based single-photon computed tomography (SPECT), IEEE Trans Nucl Sci., NS-28, 69-80.

Jaszczak, R.J., Greer, K.L., Floyd, C.E., Harris, C.C., and Coleman, R.E.,(1984). Improved SPECT quantification using compensation for scattered photons, J Nucl Med., 25, 893-900.

King, M.A., Doherty, P.W., and Schwinger, R.B.,(1983). A Wiener filter for nuclear medicine images, Med Phys., 10, 876–880.

King, M.A., Schwinger, R.B., and Penny, B.C.,(1986). Variation of the count–dependent Metz filter with imaging system modulation transfer function, Med Phys., 13, 139–149.

Lowry, C.A., and Taylor, D.N.,(1986). Improvements in image contrast and quantification using scatter subtraction in SPECT, Br J Radiol., 59, 728.

Metz, C.E., Atkins, F.B., and Beck, R.N.,(1980). The geometric transfer function component for scintillation camera collimators with straight parallel holes, Phys Med Biol., 25, 1059–1070.

Miller, T.R., and Sampathkumaran, K.S.,(1982). Design and application of finite impulse response digital filters, Eur J Nucl Med., 7, 22–27.

Miracle, S., Yzuel, M.J., and Milan, S.,(1979). A study of the point spread function in scintillation camera collimators based on Fourier analysis, Phys Med Biol., 24, 372–384.

Muehllehner, G,(1985). Effect of resolution improvement on required count density in ECT imaging: a computer simulation, Phys Med Biol., 30, 163–173.

Pang, S.C., and Genna, S.,(1979). The effect of Compton scattered photons on emission computerized transaxial tomography, IEEE Trans Nucl Sci NS–26, 2772–2774.

Todd–Pokropek, A.,(1980). Image Processing in Nuclear Medicine, IEEE Trans Nucl Sci., NS–27, 1080–1094.

Tsui, B.M.W., Gunter, D.L., and Beck, R.N.,(1982). Study of spatial resolution in single–photon ECT, J Nucl Med., 23, p45.

Waggett, D.J., and Wilson, B.C.,(1977). Improvement of scanner performance by subtraction of Compton scattering using multiple energy windows, Br J Radiol., 51, 1004–1010.

Webb, S., Long, A.P., Ott, R.J., Leach, M.O., and Flower, M.A.,(1985). Constrained deconvolution of SPECT liver tomograms by direct digital image restoration, Med Phys., 12, 53–58.

Ying-Lee, O.,(1983). An ECAT reconstruction method which corrects for attenuation and detector response, IEEE Trans Nucl Sci., NS–30, 632–635.

# NON-STATIONARY DECONVOLUTION USING A MULTI-RESOLUTION STACK

Andrew Todd-Pokropek

Dept of Medical Physics
University College London U.K.

ABSTRACT

Non-stationary deconvolution is of considerable importance is several areas of medical image processing. Quantitative errors occur in tomography as a result of the partial volume effect which has two components; the loss of 'recovery' due to the object being incomplete within the slice thickness, and loss due to sampling observed when the object is comparable in size to the resolution of the system. In SPECT, this second problem, in particular, is non-stationary since the resolution of the detecting system is a function of distance from the detector. This paper described a method for attacking such problems using a multi-resolution stack. A filter is chosen which generates successively the images of a multi-resolution stack, by successive blurring with a Gaussian filter function. The filter function chosen for this purpose should be a smoothing filter with only a slight blurring effect such that the sampling in the 'blurred direction' is reasonably fine. Prior to smoothing, a deconvolution filter is used, matched with the Gaussian blurring filters to give the range of deconvolutions required for different positions. Thus, after an initial stationary deconvolution a series of progressively smoother versions of this image are stored in a stack (S). The desired non-stationary filtered image can be shown to be an intersection of some given surface within the processed stack. In the case of the SPECT sampling problem, this intersection take the form of a simple radially symmetrical bowl shaped surface. The coordinates of this surface may be calculated in advance in terms of determining a k (scale space) coordinate in the processed stack corresponding each i,j coordinate in the original image. The third stage of the filtering operation is that of projecting this intersecting surface down to give a processed image I', such that I'(i,j)=S(i,j,k), where (i,j,k) is a point on the surface within the stack. In most cases this may be performed while only remembering one level of the stack at a time. The whole process then becomes highly efficient, and requires little storage space, being merely n times a compact linear filtering operation where n depends on the scale sampling chosen. It may be demonstrated that small values of n can be used with little distortion of the resulting image. Preliminary results, which could be of value in other types of tomographic instrumentation, have confirmed that such a technique can aid in eliminating non-stationary partial volume effects.

# 1. INTRODUCTION

Single photon emission computerized tomography (SPECT) reconstruction is normally handled by conventional tomographic reconstruction methods (see for example Natterer,1986). However, a basic assumption in the use of such methods is that properly formed line integrals have been measured, that is, for a point on the projection p at l,k (k depending on θ) then

$$p(l,k) = \iint f(x,y) \, \delta(l- x \sin\theta- y \cos\theta) \, dx \, dy \qquad (1)$$

where $f(x,y)$ is object being measured. However, as is well known, the data measured in SPECT is the weighted summation over a region of space as shown in Fig 1, and not the above delta function. A better approximation is

$$p(l,k) = \iint f(x,y) \, w(l-l',r) \, dx \, dy \qquad (2)$$

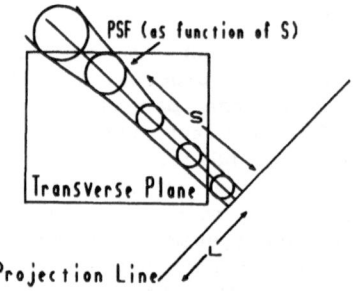

Fig 1. A diagram showing the change in point spread function of the system with increasing distance from the front surface of the detector.

where w is a weighting function, assumed to be stationary with respect to l, and which is effectively the point spread function (PSF) of the system, for all distances r along the line given in the usual from by $l=x \sin \theta + y \cos \theta$. For some given distance r, it is likely to take the form of the normal Gaussian like shape expected from the determination of static collimator PSF as a function of distance. The width (σ) of the Gaussian is presumably some function of r. It should therefore possible to set up a model for the SPECT tomographic acquisition in the form of Eq. (2). Several important assumptions have been made. Firstly, that w is independent of l the position on the detector where the measurement occurs, and secondly that w is independent of the object being measured.

Let **f** represent the activity distribution which is being estimated. This activity distribution is placed within some object **O** which encloses **f** but does not in any way have the same shape or characteristics.

A major problem in emission computerized tomography is that photons emitted from **f** may be attenuated or scattered. Two situations must be distinguished: a photon may be scattered and then detected at an incorrect position. Alternatively, a photon may be fail to be detected for a variety of reasons, all of which will be called here: attenuation. It is clear that both of these effects are dependent on both **f** and **O**. The system is of course three-dimensional. If the axes of a transaxial reconstruction are labelled x and y, then the axes perpendicular to this plane may be called z.

Three separate processes are occurring which affect the reconstruction: variations in PSF , variations in scatter, and variations in attenuation, all of which are interconnected. Note that the so-called partial volume effect (Hoffman et al., 1979) is a result of PSF variations and object size along the z axis.

2. AIM OF THE STUDY

The aim of this study was to attempt to quantitate data from SPECT studies. It was therefore not of interest as to whether the diagnostic quality of images was improved, nor was the detectability of small lesions as such an issue. The parameter considered to be critical was that of 'recovery'.

Recovery may be defined as the ratio of estimated activity within some region to true activity in the same region. For a perfect system this ratio should be unity. In practice, even with a perfect system, this ratio would be some constant value, to be determined, dependent on the efficiency of the system. However, unfortunately, recovery depends on many parameters, and, in particular, of the size of an object within which the activity is to be estimated, as shown in Fig 2. In addition, for Gaussian like response functions, which extend in theory to infinity, some truncation must be made limiting the spatial extent over which the integration is performed. Unfortunately, estimates of recovery are rather critical with respect to this choice, which is discussed later.

Other workers have attempted to resolve the problem of quantitation by determining the so-called recovery coefficient as a function of lesion size (Hoffman et al., 1979) such that, for the purposes of estimating true activity concentration, the observed activity within some lesion is scaled by this recovery coefficient, as a function of lesion size, for example as estimated from a curve such as given in Fig 2. However, this implies that the recovery coefficient must be stationary. Similarly it is difficult to know how to use such a technique for other than round (or regular) objects.

Thus in this (on-going) study, an attempt was made to render the system stationary, and to make pixel values independent of both $f$ and $O$ within certain limits, notably that the local activity distribution estimation was not made over very small region, i.e. for lesions much smaller than the FWHM of the system. Recently there have been a number of papers, for example Moore et al, (1987) and Zeeberg et al, (1987), which have discussed these problems of non- stationarity.

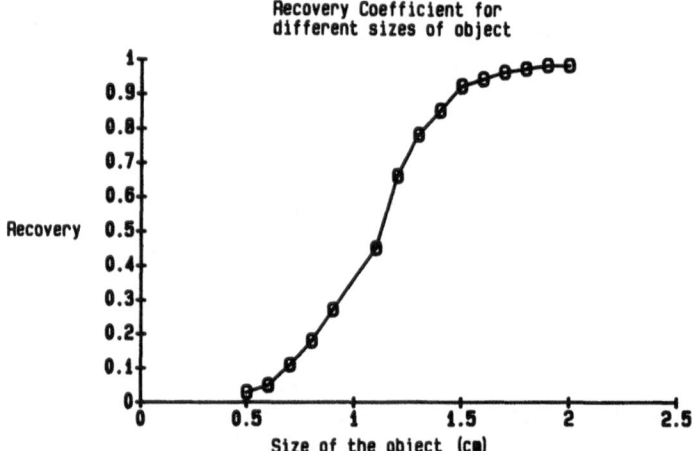

Fig 2. A plot of the recovery coefficient that might be expected for a normal SPECT system, as a function of the size of the object (cylindrical) being detected.

## 3. SCATTER CORRECTION: PREVIOUS WORK

A number of workers have proposed various methods for the correction of scatter in SPECT, in particular, Axelsson et al., (1984), Jaszczak et al., (1984) and Todd-Pokropek et al., (1984). Let $f'$ be the observed reconstructed image being an estimate of $f$ (the data without scatter) contaminated with scatter $s$. Essentially, what is being attempted to obtained a better estimate $\hat{f}$ of $f$ from

$$\hat{f} = f' - s \tag{3}$$

The main problem is how to estimate $s$. Axelsson et al., (1984), effectively assumes that $s$ can be obtained from

$$s = \alpha \ f' * a \tag{4}$$

where * is the convolution operator, **a** is an appropriate filter, and α is a subtraction coefficient. It remains to be seen how to estimate α and **a**. In fact Axelsson assumes that the form of **s** is Aexp(-Bx), where x is distance from the centre of the PSF, and then obtains fits for A and B.

Data can be acquired for other energy windows than the photopeak. Let **c** be the reconstruction of data obtained using a lower energy window, often called the Compton window. For Tc99m this might correspond to an energy window extending from say 100 to 120keV. Jaszczak et al., (1984) assumes that **s** equals **c**, and thus performs the operation

$$\hat{\mathbf{f}} = \mathbf{f}' - \alpha \, \mathbf{c} \; . \tag{5}$$

The technique which we have previously described (Todd-Pokropek et al., 1984) is similar, and assumes that **s** can be estimated from **c** but only after convolution with an appropriate filter. Thus if **p**' is the modified projection data from which $\hat{\mathbf{f}}$ is to be reconstructed, and $\mathbf{p_i}$ are the observed sets of projection data at various energies i, then it is assumed that

$$\mathbf{p}' = \sum_i \alpha_i \, \mathbf{p_i} * \mathbf{a_i} \tag{6}$$

where the $\alpha_i$ are appropriate weighting values, and $\mathbf{a_i}$ are appropriate filters. (In fact $\alpha_i$ and $\mathbf{a_i}$ can be folded together).

In Eq (6), it is possible to extend the definition from two dimensions, that is l,θ where l is a distance measured along a projection line, and θ is the angle at which the projection was obtained, into three dimensions, k,l,θ where k,l and the conventional cartesian coordinates of a point in a projection image obtained at angle θ. Thus the filtering extends between transverse slice planes. and out of plane scatter is also considered. This extension from two to three dimensions is essentially trivial, and only involves problems of implementation where memory size might be limited. The work described here was performed in two dimensions, but, it is believed, is equally applicable to three.

A further alternative method that has been employed is to solve the basic inverse problem,

$$\mathbf{p} = \mathbf{A} \, \mathbf{f} \tag{7}$$

where **p** are the observed projection data as usual, **f** is the required reconstruction and **A** is the transformation matrix, generating **p** from **f**. This problem can be solved in a variety of ways, and maximum likelihood (or possibly maximum entropy) iterative techniques can be used. The problem is of course how to determine **A**, for a real physical system. It is inadequate to model **A** in an analytic manner (e.g. to use the analytic inverse Radon transform) when attenuation and scatter are to be included in the model. A knowledge of the scattering medium is required. This can be obtained either by physical measurements of the object, or, in many cases, from the data themselves, for example by extracting a boundary contour. The matrix **A** can then be evaluated either by analytic methods (which has not been attempted so far) or by Monte Carlo simulations. The Monte Carlo method places a simulated point source at every point with the boundary of the scattering medium, and for each such point, determines by tracing the history of emitted photons, determines the probability of detection at each point in (what may be called) detector space. This method permits **A** to be determined for a given detector, scattering medium configuration, and, assuming that the system is linear in that it can be decomposed into the response to an ensemble of point sources, takes into account scatter and attenuation, within the accuracy of the Monte Carlo photon transport model. In practice, symmetries need to be exploited to reduce the computation size of the problem. This method has also been called the Inverse Monte Carlo (IMC) method (Floyd et al., 1985). It has the drawback of being computationally extremely expensive. It can also, in principle, be extended into 3-D.

In this last method, the variation of system response function, as a function of distance from the detector, is implicitly taken into account within the photon transport model. In all the other techniques described, it is excluded.

## 4. RESULTS USING STATIONARY SCATTER CORRECTION

In collaboration with workers at the University of Milan, an intercomparison has been made (Bettinardi et al., 1986) with respect to the accuracy of scatter correction using the three methods described in section 4, Eqs (4), (5) and (6), but excluding the Inverse Monte Carlo technique which was computationally impossible to implement and assess. These results have been published elsewhere (Bettinardi et al., 1986). In summary, they indicated that there was little difference between these three methods. All of them do a 'reasonable' job of correcting for scatter. All of them require weights (subtraction coefficients $\alpha$) to be determined. In general, for each method, the corresponding $\alpha$ is estimated by testing the method on a phantom with known activity distribution, and adjusting $\alpha$ such that the correct values are obtained.

This is fine, provided that $\alpha$, in each case, is independent of the object distribution. This is clearly not, true, as is shown in Fig 3, showing data obtained by the Milan group using the method of Eq. (4). This shows that the subtraction coefficient $\alpha$, (called 'A' by Axelsson) varies considerably when estimated using a hot source of fixed size at various distances from the centre of rotation of the system. Again, different values have been obtained when a cold source is substituted (Koral et al., 1987). Considerable variations in stationarity are observed.

Thus it is not surprising that all three methods tested gave similar results since their accuracy of scatter correction is dependent primarily on the accuracy of the estimation of the corresponding weight, which can, at best, only be an approximation for some range of object sizes and activity distributions. It is the basic hypothesis of this paper that account must be taken of such non-stationary effects.

## 5. THE MODEL.

The following basic model was assumed. The planar detector was assumed to move in a true circular orbit about the centre of rotation, with no offset between the centre of the projection and a perpendicular dropped from the axis of rotation. Thus the system was assumed to be circularly symmetrical about the centre of rotation in the transverse axial plane. The detector was assumed to be stationary, that is, for any point k,1 in the plane of the projection image, the PSF of the system was assumed to be strictly independent of k,1 but not of the distance perpendicular to the slice plane, which we will call s.

A Monte Carlo model originally developed by O Ying Lee, was considerably extended, and used to investigate the effect of scatter in SPECT. A·photon transport model was used for point sources at various positions within a scattering medium, and the PSF observed for projections at different angles, for different energy windows, recording, in addition, how many times the photon detected had been scattered. In fact the system binned the data into unscattered photons, single scattered photons, and multiple scattered photons. This data thus permits scattered and unscattered photons in the 'photopeak' window to be distinguished. Typically, a simulation for about 10M events was performed.

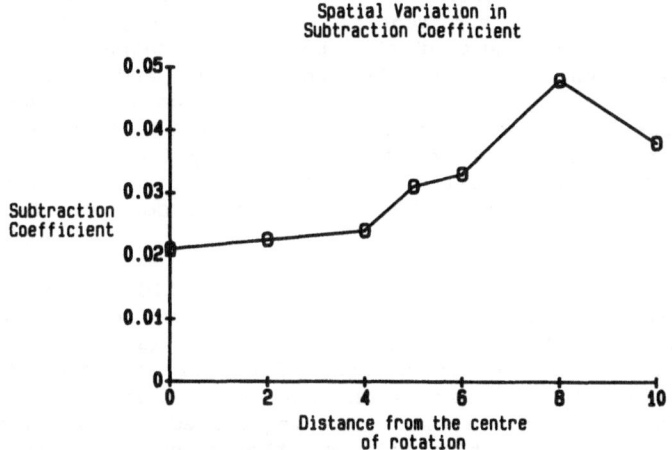

Fig 3. A plot of the subtraction coefficient (called A by Axelsson et al., 1984) as a function of distance form the centre of rotation, for a cylindrical hot object of constant size.

This simulation permitted the following model to be hypothesised for a SPECT system (O Ying Lee, 1985)  and suggested that

$$PSF(k',l',s) = A \exp(-Br^2) + C \exp(-Dr^2) \qquad (8)$$

where $r = \sqrt{((k-k')^2+(l-l')^2)}$ the radial distance from a point at k,l on the protection plane (the centre of the PSF being computed) for some perpendicular distance s away. This is the function which needs to be plugged into Eq. (2). A,B,C and D are appropriate coefficients for the particular value of s. Thus the point spread function is assumed to be the sum of two Gaussian functions. It is important to understand how the coefficients A-D depend, firstly, on the value of s, and secondly, on the form of the object. Let A and B describe a narrow function, while C and D describe a broader function (essentially the tails). By simulation it was found that A and B were largely independent of the object size and shape. This was not true for C and D. In essence, the shape of the central peak of the PSF is not strongly dependent on the shape of the object while the tails are, however, considerably modified. It was also observed that A could be reasonably matched by a $\exp(-\alpha s)$ function, while B could be fitted by $\beta/s^2$. Thus the height of the PSF decreased approximately exponentially with distance away from the detector, while the width of the PSF increased approximately linearly with increasing distance. These functions are essentially the same as those obtained for the conventional performance of parallel hole collimators as a function of depth in tissue. Note that this model should incorporate scatter within the detector, and not register only events arriving at the detector.

Using this model, it was possible to obtain estimates of the PSF as a function of distance s, for some pre-defined object size and shape. As an approximation, a circularly symmetrical cylinder of 20cm diameter was employed. The shape of the central PSF is largely independent of the precise diameter and shape of the object. The shape of the tails does vary to some extent. However, the chosen shape and size of object was felt to be a reasonable compromise. Information about the PSF can be determined for both unscattered, singly scattered and mixed events. The PSF for the multiply scattered events was very flat, and this component was treated as if it were a DC offset, which could be eliminated by a base-line shift, i.e. subtraction of a simple constant from the final reconstruction.

The data obtained using this model were validated, in as far as it was possible, by performing real measurements using a point source at various locations within a similar sized object (actually the so called Jaszczak phantom), making measurements for various energy windows. Such measurements could not distinguish scattered form unscattered events however. Also considerable error was introduced by non-uniformities in the detection system, particularly at other than photopeak energies. An attempt was also made to perform measurements using a Ge detector with very good energy resolution. However, when comparing such measurements to those obtained with a NaI detector, a correction must be made to take account of the different sizes of the detectors, and scatter within the detector, by no means a trivial exercise.

6. OBTAINING A CONSTANT PSF BY DECONVOLUTION

The data obtained using this model, plus the experimental data, permit a description of the PSF to be made at any point in the reconstructed field. When an object is similar in size, or has structures of the same size as the width of the PSF, then the response of the system to those structures would be excepted to decrease. In SPECT, this means that counts are lost for small structures. The basic hypothesis made was that much of the non-stationarity of the quantitative measurements in SPECT were a result of **differences** in the PSF at different positions, and it was these differences which made the use of the recovery coefficient inappropriate. However, if the PSF were the same at every position, these non-stationary effects could be eliminated. However, since the effective PSF is known at every position, a simple deconvolution process can achieve this, by convolving that data at some position i,j in the transverse slice plane with a filter f(i,j), or, after a Fourier transformation, F(u,v) in the frequency domain, described by

$$F(u,v) = H'(u,v)/H(u,v) \qquad (9)$$

where u and v are spatial frequency, H(u,v) is the observed PSF (in the frequency domain) for the position i,j, and H'(u,v) is the desired PSF which is now to result, which is, in effect, a window function. Such a window function is essential if the noise properties after the filtering operation are to be reasonable. H'(u,v) could be chosen to be an average value for the PSF, or, probably better, a lower limit on the PSF that could be expected, for example (in the space domain) a Gaussian of width about 5mm. The choice of H'(u,v) is rather dependent on the signal to noise ratio in the data. A process of deconvolution has also been proposed by O Ying Lee, (1983).

## 7. THE ASSUMPTION OF RADIAL SYMMETRY.

The **system** as described is to a reasonable approximation radially symmetric. The PSF at any distance $\xi$ from the centre of rotation will be independent of angle $\theta$. However, the **shape** of the PSF will not itself be radially symmetrical. It has a shape which will rotate with $\theta$. One can imagine the corresponding filter f(i,j) as always pointing towards the centre of rotation.

Since the aim of this work was to develop a computationally efficient algorithm, a further major approximation was therefore made. The shape of the PSF, for any radial distance $\xi$, was assumed to be rotationally symmetrical, and therefore the filter f(i,j) was only dependent on $\xi$ and not on $\theta$. This hypothesis was clearly not valid with respect to the tails of the PSF. However, these in their own right were much more dependent on the exact shape and form of the object. Since data were collected over $2\pi$, then the addition of all PSFs opposed by $\pi$ tended to reduce the asymmetry considerably. The largest asymmetric effects would be expected at the surface of a large object. Even there, the difference between radial and tangential width of the PSF was normally small and less than 10%. Thus this second order effect was not taken into consideration, and a circularly symmetrical PSF was determined as an average over angle.

## 8. IMPLEMENTATION: THE MULTI-RESOLUTION STACK.

Non-stationary deconvolution is computationally awkward. Initially an attempt was made to solve the problem by utilising the radial symmetry of the filtering operation. However, it was soon realised that a very simple and efficient algorithm could be derived using a multi-resolution stack.

Let the bottom level of such a stack be given by S(i,j,0). Then any level S(i,j,k+1) can be generated from the next lowest level S(i,j,k) by a rule such as

$$S(i,j,k+1) \quad = \quad \sum_{l,m=-n}^{+n} w(l,m) \ S(i-l,j-m,k) \tag{10}$$

where w(l,m) is some filter of size (2n+1)x(2n+1). Typically, Gaussian weights would be chosen such that each level of the stack is a Gaussian smoothed version of the next. This type of stack has well established well behaved properties (Koenderink, 1984). The set of data comprising the stack exists in i,j,k space, where i,j, are conventional Cartesian coordinates, and k is usually said to be a distance in scale space. Data only exists for integral values of k. However, in scale space, the distance between adjacent levels can be controlled by use of the weighting function w(l,m). If this function is very peaked, then there is little smoothing between adjacent levels. If it is very broad, then there is considerable smoothing between different levels.

Now, the deconvolution filtering operation that is to be designed is, in effect a family of filters, for different radial distances $\xi$. This family of filters is shown in Fig 4. Each filter for some value of $\xi=T$ is related to the filter for $\xi=T+1$, where T is an integer. It is possible to determine a smoothing filter which can applied to the sharper filter, will which generate the smoother filter. Since this filtering operation is strictly linear, there is no difference between using the smoother filter, or using the sharper filter and then smoothing the result. This notion leads to the idea of using the stack for performing the non-stationary deconvolution.

The original data is convolved with the sharpest filter of the set of filters, and then forms the bottom level of the stack. The Gaussian smoothing filter is then applied successively to generate further levels of the stack. ´Each level of the stack, then, has been convolved with some filter, from the set of filters, the precise filter having been used depending on the level in the stack. Thus, we can say that, for some radial distance $\xi$, a filter of a particular shape should have been used, and then determine which level in the stack corresponds to that filter. The corresponding data can then be extracted from that level in the stack, and placed in a matrix. Given that the stack is high enough so that the smoothest of the desired filters has also been 'generated', for every point in the original image, that is, for every value of $\xi$, there will be a corresponding point in the stack which contains the correctly filtered data. Thus the desired filtered image comprises a surface in the stack, and the final filtered image I'(i,j) is generated by a projection such that for each point i,j:

$$I'(i,j) = S(i,j,k), \quad k=f(\xi) \tag{11}$$

where S(i,j,n) is the three dimensional stack, and k, the distance in scale space, is some function of radial distance $\xi$.

Although this might sound complicated, in fact it becomes very simple in its implementation. The original data I(i,j) are filtered with the sharpest deconvolution filter desired, in fact in the frequency domain, after an FFT. This operation is linear and stationary, and the filter can have any desired shape. A second matrix is generated, which, for each point i,j records the appropriate value in n that should be used when employing Eq. (11). The lookup table $f(\xi)$ is pre-determined. The map determines which values of which level are to be stored in the result. It must be complete (determined for every point i,j), which usually implies that for any point i,j, the the value generated by $f(\xi)$ must be rounded to give the closest integral value for k. In fact, the method does not require the data to be in any way circularly symmetrical. Only the filters themselves must be rotationally symmetrical.

Thus S(i,j,0), the lowest level of the stack is generated using

$$S(i,j,0) = F^{-1}\{ \ F\{I(i,j)\}.F\{H'(i,j)/F\{H(i,j\} \ \} \tag{12}$$

where F{} is the Fourier transform and H and H' are the observed and desired PSF for the position of the broadest PSF (normally at the centre of rotation).

286

Looking at the map indicates whether any values for level 0 are to be retained. These are then transferred to the result image I'. The next level S(i,j,1) can then be generated, and the process repeated. It is not necessary, at any stage, to retain data from lower levels of the stack

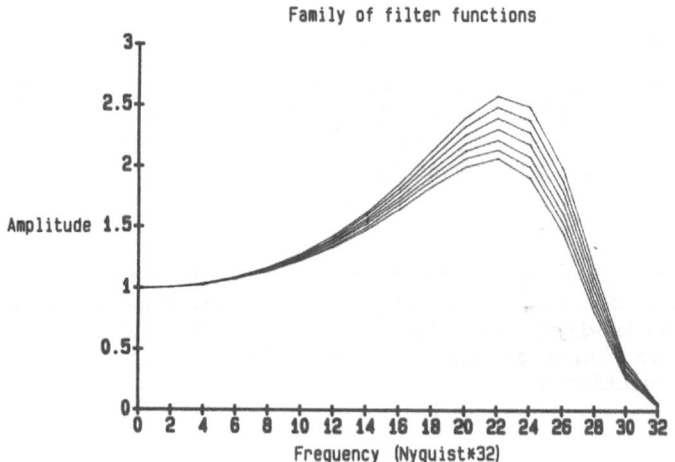

Fig 4. A family of filter functions, for various radial distances from the centre of rotation, plotted in the frequency domain. The sharpest filter is at the top. Each filter is systematically related by a smoothing filter to its neighbours.

The distance moved at each step in scale space is important. Too large a jump means that poor sampling in scale space will occur, and the approximations to the desired filters may cause undesirable effects. Too small a jump is scale space results in unnecessary computation. The sampling of scale space is determined, as previously mentioned by the values of w. The values actually used were

$$ w \; = \; 1/1024 \; \begin{vmatrix} 1 & 32 & 1 \\ 32 & 892 & 32 \\ 1 & 32 & 1 \end{vmatrix} \tag{13} $$

This filter is very flat (dropping to 0.92 at the Nyquist) and is of course orthogonally decomposable. Computationally, it is extremely efficient. Thus the whole deconvolution involved one filtering operation in the frequency domain, and n (tiny) convolutions in the space domain, where a suitable value for n, the number of levels in the stack, seems to be about 20. The actual value used will depend primarily on the size of the object, and the sampling in scale space. The storage space is required for three matrices of the same size as the reconstructed transverse plane, for the filtered data, for the map, and for the non-stationary filtered result.

This method can be extended to cover the three dimensional deconvolution process relatively easily, although more intermediate storage would then be required.

## 9. NON-STATIONARY SCATTER CORRECTION

A non-stationary scatter correction can employ a similar method, essentially a modification of Eqs. (4) and (5) given previously. A similar non-stationary deconvolution can be performed of the data obtained for all energy windows such that

$$\hat{f} = f' - \Sigma \alpha_i c'_i \tag{14}$$

where $\alpha_i$ is the subtraction coefficient for some window i and $c'_i$ is the non-stationary deconvolved image for the corresponding window. In this case the desired window function ($H'(i,j)$) of Eq. (12) is the PSF for the scatter in the photopeak window. The implementation is identical to the described in section 7.

## 10. RESULTS.

Only preliminary results have been obtained using the non-stationary deconvolution method as described. A test set of data was generated using the head phantom previously described (Todd-Pokropek et al., 1984). This head phantom comprised an aluminium wall, elliptical in shape, within which, cylinders and spheres of known size, and filled with activity on known concentration, - can be placed at various known positions. In collaboration with the University of Milan, a set of images for various configurations of sources were obtained, and analyzed. In addition, data from a cylinder of fixed size placed at various radial distances within a circularly symmetrical object, the Jaszczak phantom, were also assessed. The method was also tried out on simulated data.

It is not possible to remove the partial volume/ sampling effect completely. This could only be achieved if a complete deconvolution were performed, i.e. aiming to produce a system response which was a delta function. Noise generated by the deconvolution process does not permit this. However, the system can be rendered more stationary, and by an appropriate choice of window function (desired PSF), the recovery curve can be flattened for all but very small objects. The flatter the recovery curve for small objects, the greater the noise amplification. Fig 5 shows the recovery curve for a 1.2cm diameter cylinder at various radial distances, before and after non-stationary deconvolution.

The process of non-stationary deconvolution does not improve the signal to noise ratio, or rather, the contrast to noise ratio. The scatter subtraction whether stationary of non-stationary does improve the contrast to noise ratio, typically by a significant amount. The results for stationary scatter correction are to be reported in paper in preparation. The results reported here for non-stationary scatter correction are preliminary.

## 11. CONCLUSIONS

Obtaining quantitative estimates of activity concentration is important in SPECT. This requires that an attenuation correction is performed. However, attenuation correction cannot be performed satisfactory without a scatter correction. Although several stationary scatter correction methods have been proposed and tested, it appears that non-stationary effects are important, notably with respect to the observed values for recovery. In this paper, an efficient and effective non-stationary deconvolution method has been proposed, based on the use of a multi-resolution stack which, provided that the PSF at any point is assumed to be approximately radially symmetrical, can make the system behave in a much more stationary manner. It is anticipated that this non-stationary deconvolution technique should have wide applications for other types of medical images.

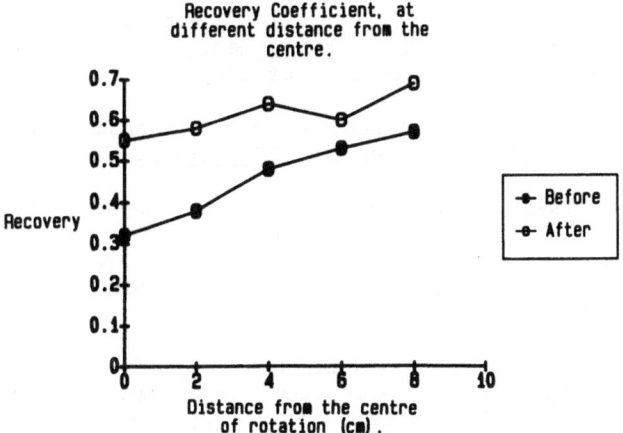

Fig 5. The recovery coefficient, plotted, for a cylindrical object of constant size, as a function of radial distance of the object from the centre.

ACKNOWLEDGEMENT

The author would like to acknowledge the advice and help given by the group form the University of Milan, notably M.C Gilardi and V. Bettinardi, and also from the assistance given by Dr O Ying Lee.

REFERENCES.

B. Axelsson, P. Masaki and A. Israelsson, (1984), Subtraction of Compton-scattered photons in single photon emission computerized tomography, J. Nucl. Med. 25:490-494.

V. Bettinardi, M.C. Gilardi, C. Pantalone, A. Todd-Pokropek, P. Gerundini and F. Fazio, (1986), Scatter correction techniques in SPECT, in "Proceedings. of the S.N.M.E. Annual Meeting", Goslar.

C.E. Floyd, R.J. Jaszczak and R.E. Coleman, (1984), Inverse Monte Carlo: a unified reconstruction algorithm for SPECT, IEEE Trans. Nucl. Sci. NS-32:779-785.

R.J. Jaszczak, K.L. Greer, C.E. Floyd, Jr., C.C. Harris and R.E. Coleman, (1984), Improved SPECT quantification using compensation for scattered photons, J. Nucl. Med. 25:893-900.

J.J. Koenderink, (1984), The structure of images, Biol. Cybern. 50:363-370.

K.F. Koral, S. Buchbinder, N.H. Clinthorne, W.L. Rogers, B.M.W. Tsui and E.R. Edgerton, (1987), Compensation for attenuation and Compton-scattering in absolute quantification of tumor activity, J. Nucl. Med. 28:577.

E.J. Hoffman, S-C. Huang, M.E. Phelps et al. (1979), Quantitation in positron emission computer tomography: 1. Effect of object size, J. Comput. Assist. Tomogr. 3:299-308.

S.C. Moore, M.F. Kijewski, S.P. Mueller and B.L. Holman, (1987), The noise power spectrum for SPECT: effects of non-stationary projection noise and attenuation correction, J. Nucl. Med. 28:630.

F. Natterer, (1986), "The mathematics of computerized tomography", Wiley, Stuttgart.

O. Ying Lee, (1983), An ECAT reconstruction method which corrects for attenuation and detector response, IEEE Trans. Nucl. Sci. NS-30:632-635.

O. Ying Lee, (1985), The mathematics and physics of computerized tomography. PhD Thesis, University of Delft.

A. Todd-Pokropek, G. Clarke, R. Marsh, (1984), Preprocessing of SPECT data as a precursor for attenuation correction, in "Information processing in medical imaging", F. Deconinck ed, Martinus Nijhoff, Boston, 130-150.

B.R. Zeeberg, A.N. Bice, S. Loncaric, H.N. Wagner and R.C, Reba, (1987), A theoretically-correct algorithm to compensate for a three-dimensional spatially-variant point spread function ion SPECT imaging, J. Nucl. Med. 28:662.

**Expert systems, Pacs, Image compression**

# DEVELOPMENTS TOWARDS AN EXPERT SYSTEM FOR THE

# QUANTITATIVE ANALYSIS OF THALLIUM-201 SCINTIGRAMS

E. Backer, J.J. Gerbrands, G. Bloom, J.H.C. Reiber (*),
A.E.M. Reijs (*), H.J. van den Herik (**)

Delft University of Technology
Department of Electrical Engineering
Delft, the Netherlands

(*) Erasmus University
Thoraxcenter
Rotterdam, the Netherlands

(**) Delft University of Technology
Department of Computer Science
Delft, the Netherlands

## INTRODUCTION

Sequential thallium-201 (Tℓ-201) scintigraphy has achieved widespread use for the assessment of exercise induced myocardial perfusion abnormalities (Pohost et al., 1977; Burrow et al., 1979; Simoons and Reiber, 1984). In this nuclear imaging technique, images of the myocard are acquired by means of a scintillation camera after intravenous administration of Tℓ-201. Thallium-201 is a radiopharmaceutical that distributes over the body as a function of distribution of cardiac output. Consequently, the Tℓ-201 accumulated in the myocard reflects regional myocardial blood flow. An area with reduced thallium-uptake early after exercise may be due to either transient uptake abnormalities (ischemia) or to previous myocardial infarction (scar). These possibilities can be distinguished by comparing the immediate post-exercise image with the late post-exercise or redistribution image taken between 3 and 4 hours later. An ischemic area is characterized by the fact that the thallium-uptake is reduced in the early image, but normal in the late post-exercise image. In the case of a scar, the uptake is low in both images. To minimize variations in the interpretation of the scintigrams and to quantify the perfusion abnormalities, the early and late post-exercise images must be compared in detail. This is only feasible by computer processing. Over the past years, we have developed an extensive software package for the quantitative analysis of thallium-201 scintigrams (Lie, et al., 1979; Lie, et al., 1981; Reiber et al., 1982).

In clinical practice, it has been observed that the cardiologists still rely heavily on the visual interpretation of the original images, in addition to interpretation of the quantitative results. Apparently, experience still plays an important role in the analysis of Tℓ-201 scintigrams. The existing software package may be described as a tool to obtain quantitative measurements from the scintigrams. The development of an expert *system as an* additional *software* tool aiming at the objective interpretation of scintigrams forms the central issue of this paper. The ultimate goal of such an enterprise does not aim to replace the cardiologist by any computer system, rather than to provide him with software tool both for quantitative measurements and objective interpretation in order to obtain more consistent and reproducable diagnoses.

The organization of the paper is as follows. First, we will outline the quantitative analysis and discuss how interpretation can be achieved on the basis of a comparison between computed circumferential profiles from the patient's images and normal profiles obtained from a group of normal subjects. Next we outline the global structure of ESATS, the Expert System for the Analysis of Thallium-201 Scintigrams, followed by a discussion of how the knowledge base is structured and implemented. Finally, we come to the way of reasoning towards a diagnosis and discuss some results which has been obtained from a set of test consultations of which catheterization results were known.

IMAGE ACQUISITION AND QUANTITATIVE ANALYSIS

The thallium scintigrams are acquired by using standard techniques. The patient performs a maximal or symptom limited exercise test on a bicycle ergometer. One minute prior to maximal exercise, 1.5 mCi Tℓ-201 is administered intravenously. Static thallium scintigrams are collected successively in three orientations: left-anterior-oblique under 45 degrees and 65 degrees (LAO45 and LAO65), and anterior (ANT). After four hours late post-exercise imaging is performed in the same sequence. The images are stored by the DEC gamma-11 computer system (PDP11-34) in matrices of size 64x64. After collection of all three views from the early and late post-exercise studies, the analysis is performed independently for each view.

The early and late images of a specific orientation are brought into registration automatically by means of some geometric calibration points. For this purpose, two external radioactive point sources are used, the images of which are acquired immediately preceding the actual data acquisition. Next, the center of the left ventricular activity structure in the early image is determined automatically on the basis of extrema in the row and column sum profiles of the image matrix (Lie et al., 1981). Subsequently, a closed myocardial contour is searched for by applying a sequential edge detection technique. For this purpose, the early image is transformed into a polar representation by resampling the image along 64 radii through the computed center position. In the polar domain, the contour is detected by means of an dynamic programming optimal path algorithm on the basis of cost coefficients. These coefficients are derived from gradient values along the radii. The detected contour is then transformed back to the image domain. This method of contour detection has proved to be very robust and succesful (Gerbrands et al., 1981; Gerbrands et al., 1986). The detected contour does not only define a region of interest for the quantitative analysis of myocardial perfusion, but partitions the image into an object region and a background region as well. This creates the possibility to obtain an estimate of the contribution of the background activity within the myocardial region. The background contribution is different for the early and late studies and distributed nonuniformly over the images. If one wants to compare the thallium uptake in the myocardium with normal values derived from a group of normal subjects, background subtraction is absolutely necessary. From each image, an estimated background image is computed by replacing the values within the detected myocardial contour by estimated background values. These values are obtained by bilinear interpolation of the background values just outside the detected contour. The computed background images are then subtracted from the original scintigrams, thus yielding images which are in a sense normalized and better suited for making comparisons.

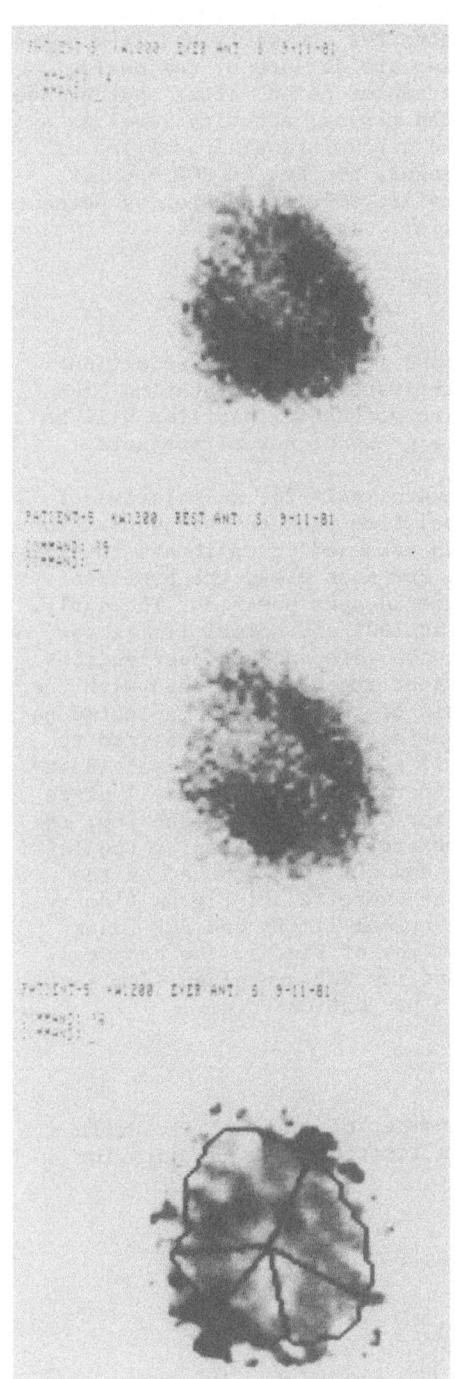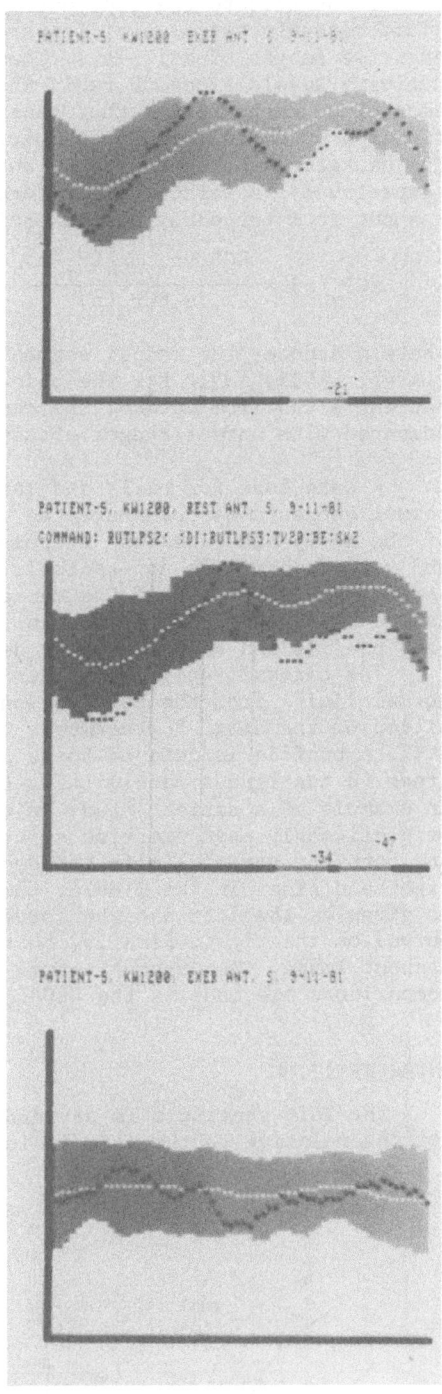

Fig. 1. Example of a patient study in the anterior view. On the top: left, the early post-exercise scintigram, right, the normal limits and the patient's ECP (dark curve). Middle: left, the late post-exercise scintigram, right, the normal limits and the patient's LCP (dark curve). Bottom: left, the washout image, right, the normal limits and the patient's WCP (dark curve).

CIRCUMFERENTIAL PROFILES

To quantitate the radionuclide activity distribution in the myocardium, circumferential profiles are calculated for the early and late post-exercise images of all views. These profiles are defined by the maximal activity levels along 60 radii through the center point, after appropriate smoothing. Each profile thus constitutes the maximal activity level as a function of radial segment number. From the circumferential profiles of the background corrected early and late images, denoted as ECP and LCP, respectively, a washout circumferential profile WCP is computed as percent washout from the early post-exercise profile:

$$WCP_i(n) = \frac{ECP_i(n) - LCP_i(n)}{ECP_i(n)} \times 100\%$$

where n denotes the radial segment number and i denotes the projection (LA045, LA065, ANT). For the objective quantitative interpretation of a patient's thallium uptake, the computed circumferential profiles will be compared with normal ranges obtained from a group of normal subjects.

A data base for early and late post-exercise $T\ell$-201 scintigrams of normal subjects has been created. The actual time between the acquisition of the early and late post-exercise studies was used to calibrate the late and washout profiles to precisely 4 hours. For each view, the profiles were aligned by means of the manually indicated apex position. The early, late and washout profiles were normalized at 100% and normal limits for each profile and each view were defined by the 10th and 90th percentiles.

The circumferential profiles of a patient study are aligned with the normal limits from the database on the basis of the manually indicated position of the apex. Furthermore, the patient's profile is normalized to 100%. A profile is defined to be abnormal if a segment of at least 18 degrees (3 contiguous radii) falls below the normal limits. Figure 1 gives an example of a patient study in the anterior projection. On the top, the original early post-exercise scintigram ('exercise') is given on the left, and both the normal limits (shaded region) and ECP (dark curve) on the righthand side. In the middle, the late post-exercise scintigram ('delayed') is given on the left and the corresponding normal limits and LCP (dark curve) on the right. Finally, on the bottom row of Fig. 1, the computed washout image, the washout normal limits and the WCP are given. Similar comparisons are made in the LA045 and LA065 projections.

INTERPRETATION

The left ventricle is divided into a number of anatomically defined regions relative to the user-indicated apex location. For the anterior

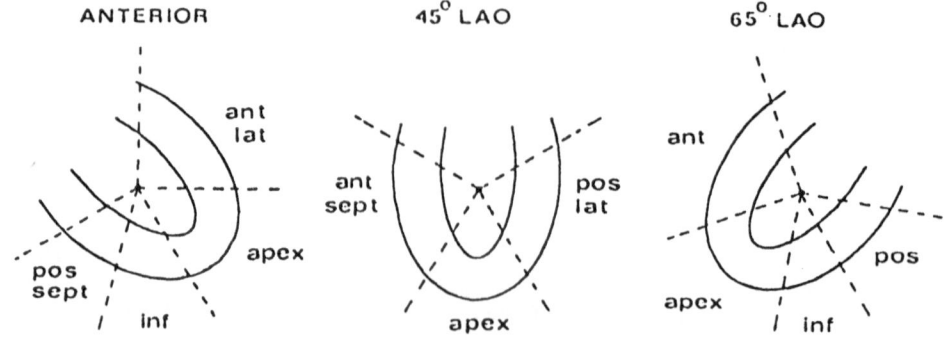

Fig. 2. Definition of anatomical regions

Table 1. Decision table on the type of abnormality
based on circumferential profiles
(N = normal  A = abnormal)

| ECP | LCP | WCP | Type of abnormality |
|-----|-----|-----|---------------------|
| N | N | N | normal |
| N | A | N | rapid washout |
| N | N | A | slow washout |
| N | A | A | undefined |
| A | N | N | ischemia |
| A | A | N | infarction |
| A | N | A | ischemia |
| A | A | A | partial redistribution |

view these regions are antero lateral, apex, inferior and postero septal,
as indicated in Fig. 2. Similarly, three regions are distinguished in
the LAO45-view and four in the LAO65-view.

    For each region, the areas of the abnormalities in the early and
late post-exercise and washout circumferential profiles are computed,
under the constraint of a minimum of three contiguous radii mentioned
above. Finally, the detected abnormalities are compared with the entries
of a decision table (Table 1), to define the kind of abnormality present.


THE GLOBAL STRUCTURE OF ESATS

    As it has been mentioned before, the ultimate goal is to provide the
cardiologists with a tool with the aid of which he is able to quantify reproducable the exact location, the extent, and the type of perfusion defect and to relate those observable defects to specific coronary insuffi-
ciencies. Figure 3 illustrates the impact of such a reasoning system.

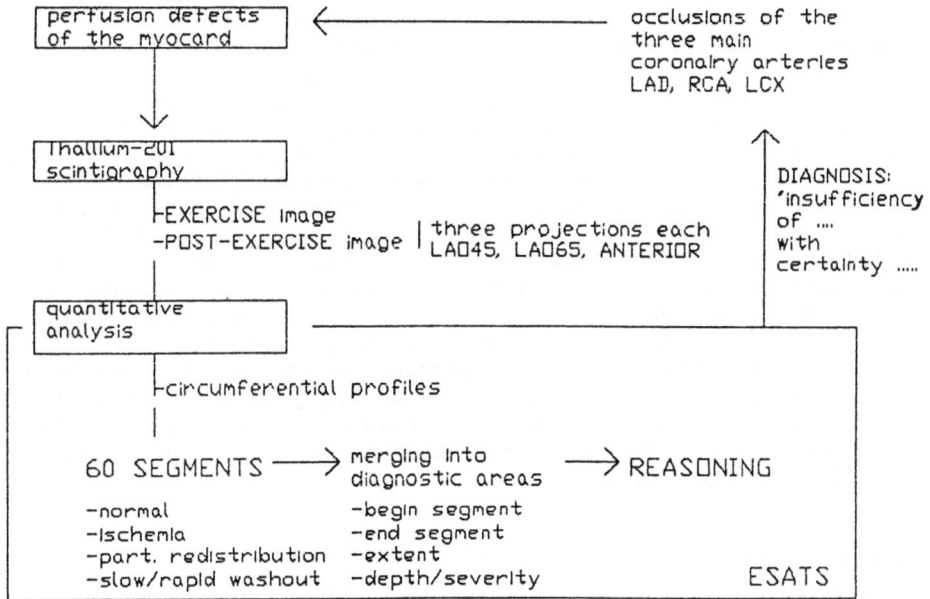

Figure 3. The impact of ESATS on the diagnosis about coronary insuffi-
          ciencies in relation to the observable thallium perfusion de-
          fects.

297

Thereby, problem-specific knowledge to be used for the inference problem as indicated, should be incorporated in the system under development. As this knowledge is often a more general kind of information then found in a conventional data base consisting of raw figures and measurements, sometimes incomplete and fuzzy as well, appearing as a collection of related facts, procedures, models and heuristics, a straight forward implementation in conventional computer programs is hardly feasible. In order to cope with that type of information a knowledge based (expert) system appears to be much more appropriate (Rich, 1983; Numao and Ishizuka, 1984).

As it has been mentioned before knowledge varies widely in both content and appearance. It may be specific, general, exact, fuzzy, procedural, declarative and so on. The representation of knowledge should be such that it can be easily used in reasoning, can be easily examined and updated, and can be easily judged as relevant or irrelevant to the problem at hand.

Production rules are a general method to represent knowledge that is particularly appropriate when knowledge is action-oriented. In many expert systems, as it is in ESATS, much of the knowledge is represented within production rules. The left hand side of a production rule (the condition part) expresses the characteristics of a situation in which it is appropriate to perform the action (the right hand side) of the rule. The production rules do not embody all the knowledge in a system. The structure of the knowledge base itself embodies part of the available (contextual) knowledge. Frames provide such an organizational scheme for knowledge bases. By providing the knowledge in modules (frames), the designer makes life easier for the algorithms that will access the knowledge. As such, a frame is a collection of knowledge relevant to a particular object, situation, or concept, providing a representation in terms of a set of attribute names and values for the attributes (declarative knowledge).

ESATS has been developed on the basis of production rules and frames in which the knowledge of scintigram-experts has been represented. Though the system is designed to be suitable for the analysis of scintigrams, it was kept in mind that the system should be flexible enough to allow for possible application to other tasks in the future.

The key parts of ESATS are a fact base, a knowledge base and a control mechanism which decides which reasoning step is to be taken. The control mechanism is able to perform a bottom up reasoning process as well as a top-down process. A rule agenda contains the numbers of rules which should be applied in the reasoning process. A rule agenda manager manages this agenda and decides which rule is to be applied next, removes its rule number from the agenda and sends the rule to a rule processor. The rule processor verifies the condition-part of the rule and if all conditions are satisfied, the action-part of the rule is carried out. Next, other rules, which become of interest by applying the previous rule, are placed on the rule agenda by the rule agenda manager. All declarative knowledge is represented in frames, while procedural knowledge is represented by production rules. External procedures are used extensively. In figure 4, the global structure of the system is illustrated, while figure 5 details the control mechanism of ESATS.


THE KNOWLEDGE BASE

As pointed out before, an expert will usually describe a specific problem area in terms of various objects, entities or concepts, and their interrelations. An attractive and widely-used structure to incorporate this kind of declarative knowledge into a knowledge base is the frame structure. A frame is similar to a record and consists of a predefined number of slots. Each slot contains a particular piece of information and together they completely define the object of interest. In ESATS a frame

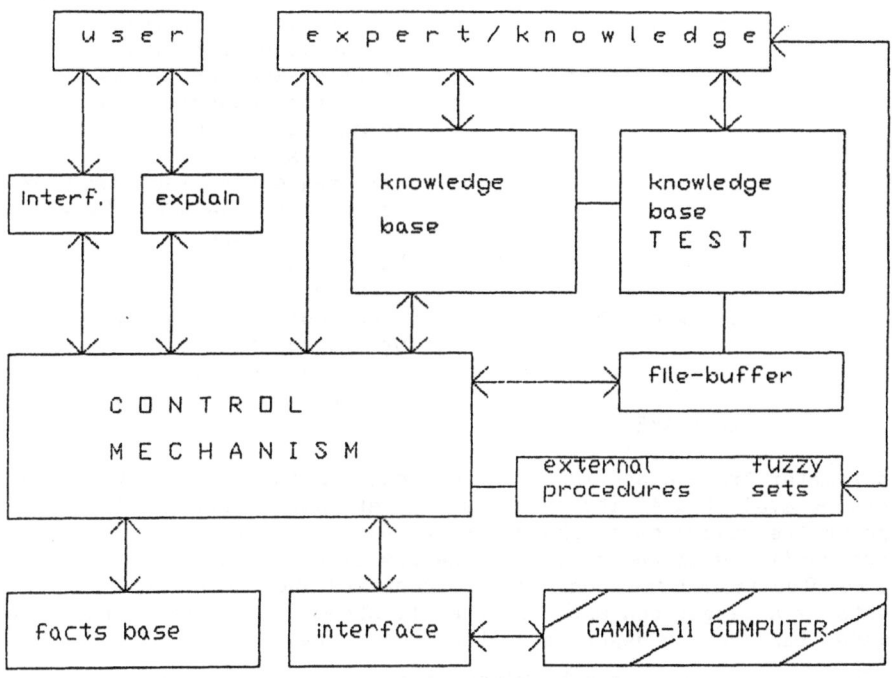

Figure 4. Global structure of ESATS

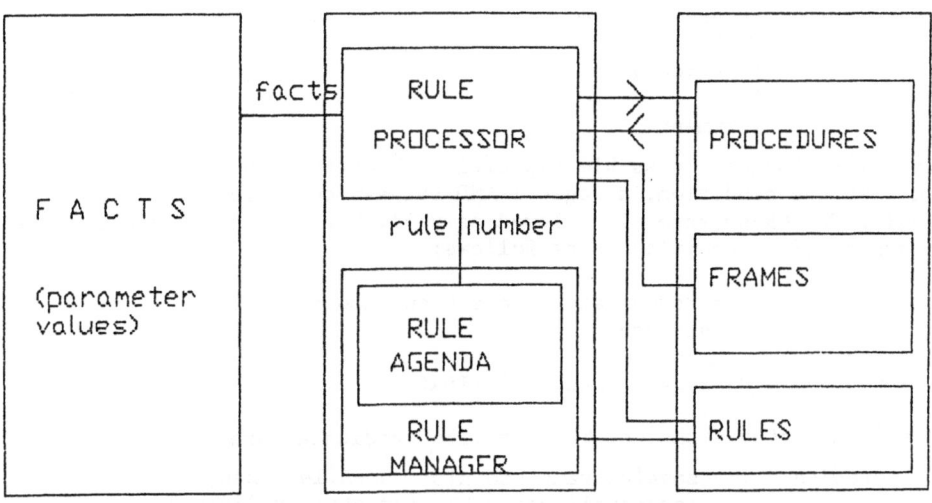

Figure 5. Control mechanism of ESATS

consists of the following slots:

```
<frame>::=FRAME <parameter name> ;
        <translation> ;              (important for the explain facility)
        <m/s valued> ;               (multi or single valued)
        <domain> ;                   (integer, float, boolean, string)
        (<pos value>;)0,1            (interval, legal values)
                                     (optional, 0 or 1 time)
        <trace class> ;              (goal: evaluation is the goal of
                                           this consultation
                                      normal: to be evaluated by expert
                                           system
                                      ask: request answer from user
                                      task: to be evaluated by external
                                           procedure
                                      key: value can be found in data
                                           base)
        (<argument> ;)0,1            (question: if ask parameter
                                      procedure: if task parameter
                                      data base: if key parameter)
                                     (optional, 0 or 1 time)
        ENDFRAME
```

The parameter trace class informs the control mechanism how this parameter can be evaluated if its value is not yet known. Additional information regarding the relevance of the rules for bottom-up or top-down processes is made available to the control mechanism of ESATS through a separate file. Related frames are combined into contexts and these contexts are subcontexts of a larger context. The overall structure of this part of the knowledge base can be described with a tree structure.

The second part of the knowledge base contains the domain expert's knowledge about how the presence of certain facts leads to conclusions about new facts, facts which were not yet known in this consultation. This type of knowledge, procedural knowledge, is incorporated in the knowledge base in the general form of IF-THEN rules:

    IF condition(s) THEN action(s)    cf.

The syntax of an IF-THEN rule in ESATS is

```
<rule>::= IF
          (<condition>)+
          THEN
          (<action>)+
          FI
          <comment>
```

where (.)+ denotes a possible repetition. When the condition part contains more than one condition, a logical AND between conditions is assumed by default. The OR-operator is allowed as well, but must be stated explicitly. The syntax of a condition is as follows:

```
<condition>::= <predicate><context><parameter><value>
<context>::= <string>
<parameter>::= <string>
<value>::= <string>|<integer>|<float>
```

where | indicates a choice. The possible predicates are

```
<predicate>::= same|notsame|known|notknown|lessthan|
               lessequal|greaterthan|greaterequal|equal
               notequal.
```

The first four predicates can only be used for textvalue or boolean parameters, the other predicates are restricted to integer or float parameter types. The action-part of an IF-THEN rule has the following syntax:

```
<action>::= (conclude<context><parameter><value><cf>|
             ask<context><parameter>|
             dotask<context><parameter>|
             execute<procedure>|
             write<message>|
             rule<rule nr>)+
<value>::= <integer>|<float>|<string>
<message>::= <string>'
<rule nr>::= <integer>
```

In 'conclude' the value of the context-parameter pair is established with a specific certainty factor. The action 'ask' indicates that the value of the context-parameter pair must be requested from the user. Obviously, the pair itself must have the parameter trace class 'ask' and the question to be asked will be found in the argument slot of the frame. The action 'dotask' indicates that the value of the context-parameter pair can be obtained by executing an external procedure. The pair must be declared as a task-parameter and the name of the procedure will be found in the argument slot. External procedures can also be executed directly by the 'execute' action.

An important feature of ESATS is the possibility to call external procedures, which form the third part of the knowledge base. There are three ways to accomplish this. First, it may occur that the value of a parameter is not known when this parameter appears in the condition part of the rule which is currently being processed. If the parameter is of trace class 'task', its value will be obtained by calling the procedure indicated in the argument slot of the frame. Second, a procedure may be called by a 'dotask'-action in a rule. Finally, a procedure may be called by the action part of a rule by means of 'execute'. In this case the procedure does not necessarily return the value of a context-parameter pair as is the case with the 'dotask' option. On the contrary, the procedure may return no data at all (e.g. just display an image) or return many data at once.

As we have seen, if a rule is processed, the condition part is evaluated and if all conditions are satisfied, the action part will be carried out. Examples of actions are the storage of a conclusion in the fact base, call an external procedure, activate another rule, etc. The certainty factor (cf) indicates the certainty with which the action part (conclusion) follows from the condition part. The certainty factors of conclusions are also stored in the fact base. When these facts are later used in the condition part of a rule, one must be aware of the fact that the conditions are only true with a limited certainty. As such, the certainty factors will play an important role in the reasoning process. The way how certainty factors propagate through the reasoning process is determined by a so called uncertainty calculus. In ESATS a slightly modified version of the Shortliffe-Buchanan model has been implemented. In many cases certainty factors are based upon pre-given fuzzy sets, for example, if we consider the following rule:

| IF | greaterequal | LA045-EXER DIFFERENCE | 80 |
|----|--------------|------------------------|-----|
|    | lessequal    | LA045-EXER DIFFERENCE | 100 |
| THEN | conclude   | LA045 DIAGNOSIS ISCHEMIE | 700 |

the relation between DIFFERENCE and the certainty factor is represented by a pre-given fuzzy set:

| DIFFERENCE | cf |
| --- | --- |
| 0 - 20 | 100 |
| 20 - 50 | 300 |
| 50 - 80 | 500 |
| 80 - 100 | 700 |
| 100 - ... | 1000 |

## THE FACT BASE

A frame forms a static, declarative description of a parameter. This parameter has no actual value in a frame. When the system obtains a value for the parameter, either by computation or by reasoning, this value is stored as a fact or instance. In essence, a fact is the dynamic part of a frame. It is, however, attractive to store frames and facts separately, much like the usual distinction between a long term memory and a short term memory.

## THE CONTROL MECHANISM

One of the most important requirements with respect to the control mechanism is the support of both bottom-up (forward chaining, data driven) and top-down (backward chaining, model driven) approaches. In the design of the controller for ESATS, many ideas were borrowed from HYDRA (Groen, et al., (1985), an expert system shell developed at the Department of Mathematics and Computer Science of Delft University. The basic idea is that there is a Rule Agenda (RA) containing the numbers of the rules to be processed. Each rule is assigned a priority. The priority assignment mechanism can be designed in such a way that both top-down and bottom-up analysis is supported. The agenda itself is controlled by the Rule Agenda Manager (RAM), and the rules are processed by the Rule Processor (RP). The RP receives from the RAM the number of the rule to be processed. It collects the rule from the rule base and verifies the condition part. If the condition part is TRUE the RP executes the action part. After verification of each subcondition a test is performed to decide whether further processing is useful. A condition is verified in the following way: if the value of the parameter is already known, it is collected from the fact base and tested. If the fact is now known it may be evaluated directly if it is an ask or task-parameter. In other cases, evaluation requires that other rules are processed first. The RP returns to the RAM the numbers of rules which have become of interest. These include the rules in the top-down and bottom-up slots of the frames. The manager assigns priorities to the rules to be processed and places the rules on the agenda. The rule agenda has been divided into two parts: an active rule agenda (ARA) and a not-active rule agenda (NARA). The ARA contains only rules within the current context, i.e. the context of the parameter which is currently being processed. All other rules appear on the NARA. The rules on the ARA are processed first, until the ARA is empty. The context with highest priority on the NARA defines the next context to be placed on the ARA. In this way we prevent the system from switching between contexts all the time. A problem which has not been investigated in all of its detail is the manipulation of the certainty factors (inexact reasoning) in relationship with the priorities to be assigned to the rules. Some common sense choices have been implemented in the present preliminary version of ESATS, but this complex problem is currently being investigated.

DIAGNOSIS

At the present state, the implementation of ESATS can be characterized by the following features:

a. The knowledge base consists of:
   - 511 frames
   - 135 rules
   - 12 external procedures
   - 51 fuzzy sets
   which are organized in a context-tree structure.
b. The forward and backward search strategy are modelled as 'breadth-
   first' strategies, while within a (sub)-context the strategy is
   'best-first'.

It has been pointed out that the basic quantitative evidence is provided by computing the differences between the computed circumferential
profiles and the 'normal' profiles. As a result we obtain labelled segments with respect to the type of defect. Segments which have the same
labels are merged into prediagnostic areas. Small areas are then merged
with larger neighbouring areas in accordance with some pre-given label-
priority scheme. Those priorities are based on existing clinical experience, and are at the moment given as follows:

| priority | label |
| --- | --- |
| 1 | ischemia |
| 2 | partial redistribution |
| 3 | infarct |
| 4 | slow washout |
| 5 | rapid washout |
| 6 | normal |
| 7 | undefined |

This relabelling proces continues until no small areas are left. As such,
we achieve the final diagnostic areas. Figure 6 illustrates the stages of
quantitative analysis before reasoning as indicated takes place.

Next, we compute three relevant parameters which characterizes the
resulting diagnostic areas. Those parameters are the depth (maximum difference), extent (the width of the diagnostic area) and the severity (the
total difference). Table 2 summarizes the resulting evidence obtained by
the quantitative analysis.

Table 2. Summary of quantitative findings

| begin | end | diagnosis | ext | dep | sev | anatomic regions |
| --- | --- | --- | --- | --- | --- | --- |
| 31 | 56 | normal | 26 | 0 | 0 | apical, outflow, postero-lateral |
| 57 | 14 | ischemia | 18 | 16 | 141 | outflow, antero-septal |
| 15 | 30 | infarct | 16 | 23 | 278 | antero-septal, apical |

Finally, based on the relationship between the anatomic regions on
the one hand, and the main coronary arteries which account for the supply
of blood of each of the anatomic regions on the other hand, the insufficiency of those coronary arteries is inferred by reasoning from the detected and labelled diagnostic areas. As a result, we may obtain a diagnosis like:

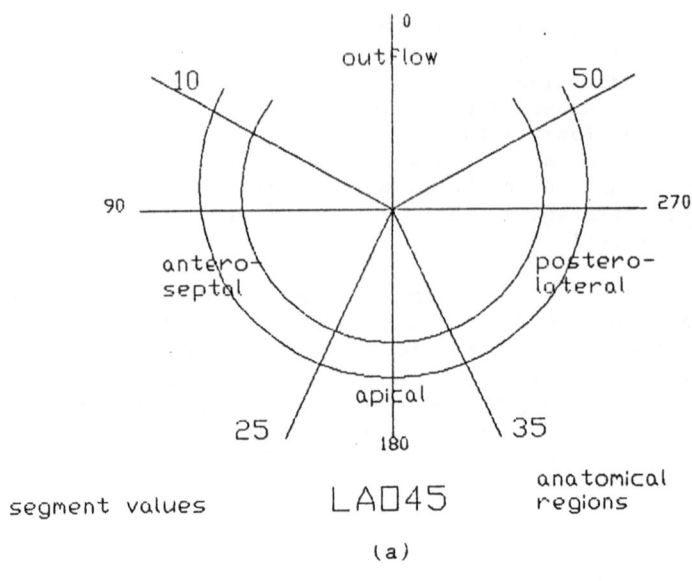

(a)

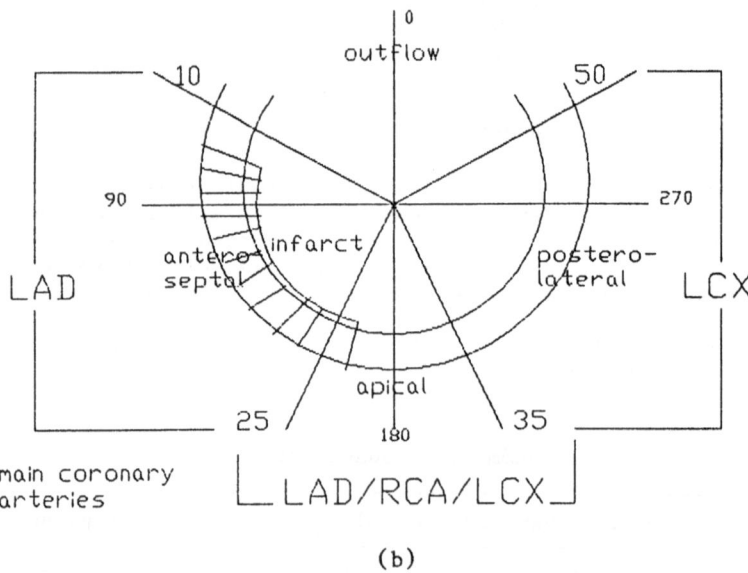

(b)

Fig. 6. Simplified illustration of the anatomical regions, the segment
values (a) and the detected diagnostic areas, the main coronary
arteries (b).

"due to a detected diagnostic 'infarct' area,
   insufficiency of the LAD ('left anterior descending artery') is
   concluded with certainty factor of 935;
   insufficiency of the RCA ('right coronary artery') is concluded
   with certainty factor of 134;
   insufficiency of the LCX ('left circumflex artery') is concluded
   with certainty factor of 134".

An example of a rule which might be responsible for such a diagnosis, can
be:
```
     IF    known diagnostic_area  area-i-anatomic_region
     THEN  conclude vessel_disease LAD
           fuzzy (diagnostic_area.area-i-view,
                   diagnostic_area.area-i-type_of_diagnosis,
                   diagnostic_area.area-i-anatomic_region,LAD)
           conclude vessel_disease RCA
           fuzzy (diagnostic_area.area-i-view,
                   diagnostic_area.area-i-type_of_diagnosis,
                   diagnostic_area.area-i-anatomic_region,RCA)
           conclude vessel_disease LCX
           fuzzy (diagnostic_area.area-i-view,
                   diagnostic_area.area-i-type_of_diagnosis,
                   diagnostic_area.area-i-anatomic_region,LCX)
```

Note that calling a fuzzy set is in essence calling an external procedure
with the only difference that a fuzzy set returns a certainty factor.


RESULTS

   Sofar, nothing really has been said about the knowledge acquisition
process although the question where knowledge comes from is an appropriate
one to begin with. The thallium-201 knowledge base, as developed sofar, is
based on discussions with scintigram-experts, case studies and so on, un-
doubtedly incomplete and possibly still naive. As a fact, the process of
knowledge acquisition has just begun (Hayes-Roth, et al., 1983).

   A more or less controlled experiment has been performed to validate
the developments up to now. A set of 12 patients has been considered of
which it is known that they suffered a single-vessel disease with severe
coronary insufficiency and for which catheterization results were available. Table 3 presents the resulting confusion matrix when comparing the
maximum certainty factor results of ESATS with the catheterization evidence. Even if these results should be considered very preliminary, they
are encouraging in the light of the modest efforts spent to knowledge acquisition.

Table 3. Confusion matrix of ESATS versus
         catheterization results

|                          |     | ESATS: |     |     |
|--------------------------|-----|--------|-----|-----|
|                          |     | LAD    | RCA | LCX |
|                          | LAD | 6      |     |     |
| Catheterization results: | RCA | 2      | 2   |     |
|                          | LCX |        | 1   | 1   |

## CONCLUSIONS

The basic structure of the expert system ESATS has proven to be adequate and flexible in combination with the existing method for quantitative analysis of Thallium-201 scintigrams. Rule-priority, uncertainty calculus, external procedures and fuzzy sets are still elements under development and further research. Likewise, an appropriate explain facility needs also further research. But, most important, many clinical studies with 'well defined' patients will be needed to achieve a scintigram knowledge base which incorporates 'high level' scintigram-expert knowledge and which will lead to robust and reliable performance.

## REFERENCES

Burow, R.D., Pond, M., Schafer, A.W. and Becker, L., Circumferential Profiles: A new method for computer analysis of thallium-201 myocardial perfusion images, Journal of Nuclear Medicin, 20, 771-777 (1979).

Gerbrands, J.J., Hoek, C., Reiber, J.H.C., Lie, S.P. and Simoons, M.L., Automated left ventricular boundary extraction from technetium-99m gated blood pool scintigrams with fixed or moving regions of interest, Proceedings IEEE 2nd International Conference on Visual Psychophysics and Medical Imaging, 155-159, Brussels (1981).

Gerbrands, J.J., Backer, E. and Van der Hoeven, W.A.G., Quantitative evaluation of edge detection by dynamic programming, in: Pattern Recognition in Practice II, E.S. Gelsema and L.N. Kanal, eds., North-Holland/Elsevier (1986).

Groen, A., Van den Herik, H.J., Hofland, A.G., Kerckhoffs, E.J.H., Koppelaar, H., Stoop, J.C. and Varkevisser, P.R., Performance model of a parallel knowledge-based system, in: Systemica, Delft University Press (1985).

Hayes-Roth, F., Waterman, D.A. and Lenat, D.B., in: Building expert systems, Addison-Wesley (1983).

Lie, S.P., Reiber, J.H.C., Simoons, M.L., Withagen, A.L.A., and Gerbrands, J.J., Quantification of the location and extent of defects in thallium-201 uptake and redistribution patterns, Proceedings IEEE Conference on Computers in Cardiology, 307-310, Geneva (1979).

Lie, S.P., Reiber, J.H.C., Simoons, M.L. and Gerbrands, J.J., Computer processing of thallium-201 myocardial scintigrams, Proceedings IEEE 2nd International Conference on Visual Psychophysics and Medical Imaging, 19-25, Brussels (1981).

Numao, M, and Ishizuka, M., A frame-like knowledge representation system for computer vision, Proceedings 7th IAPR International Conference on Pattern Recognition, 1128-1130, Montreal (1984).

Pohost, G.M., Zir, L.M., Moore, R.H., McKusick, K.A., Guinay, T.E. and Beller, G.A., Differentiation of transiently ischemic from infarcted myocardium by serial imaging after a single dose of thallium-201, Circulation, 55, 294-302 (1977).

Reiber, J.H.C., Lie, S.P., Simoons, M.L., Wijns, W. and Gerbrands, J.J., Computer quantitation location, extent and type of thallium-201 myocardial perfusion abnormalities, Proceedings IEEE 1st International Symposium Medical Imaging and Image Interprettion ISMIII'82, 123-128, Berlin (1982).

Rich, E., Artificial Intelligence, Mcgraw-Hill (1983).

Simoons, M.L. and Reiber, J.H.C., in: Nuclear imaging in clinical cardiology, Martinus Nijhoff/Kluwer Academic (1984).

# KNOWLEDGE-BASED SEGMENTATION OF SUBTRACTION ANGIOGRAMS

J. Van Cleynenbreugel, F. Fierens, C. Smets, P. Suetens, and
A. Oosterlinck

ESAT-MI2, Katholieke Universiteit Leuven
de Croylaan 52B
B-3030    Heverlee (Belgium)

## ABSTRACT

Work in progress on knowledge-based blood vessel segmentation of
subtraction angiograms is reported.  The proposed approach is centered
around different modular stages which are linked through the concept of a
multi-layered image representation.  At the bottom level classical image
processing techniques are used to extract edges, center lines and bars.
At the intermediate stage, low-level geometrical knowledge has been encoded
to construct blood vessel segments.  The higher levels will contain general
blood vessel knowledge and application domain-dependent knowledge in order
to create a final representation of the blood vessels.  Although the system
is only partly implemented, a result already of practical use will be discussed.

## INTRODUCTION

Blood vessel segmentation is an essential part of solving practical
applications in medical imaging-based diagnosis (detection of stenoses and
malformations, flow studies, 3-D reconstruction from a stereoscopic view).
As large inter- and intra-observer variations in human interpretation of
stenotic lesions are reported in clinical practice, the need for a reliable
analysis tool emerges.  It has been shown that angiography-based determination of blood vessel narrowing can be done more precisely using a computer-assisted system (Reiber et al., 1984).  A three-dimensional reconstruction of the blood vessel centerline is important for the evaluation of
carotid and coronary arteries and the cerebral vessel tree.  In this case,
abnormalities in relative position and orientation of a vessel and abnormal
variations of the cross-section can easily be visualized.  Hence, an exact
description of the position of the blood vessels is required.

Commercial semi-automatic systems performing stenosis evaluation are
available.  However, they are strongly interactive and require that the
radiologist enters an approximate center line of the blood vessel to be
evaluated.  Subsequently, an edge following procedure searches for the
edges of the specified blood vessel segment by means of a dynamic programming
algorithm (van Ommeren et al., 1986 and Reiber et al., 1986) and measures
the diameter of the blood vessel along this segment.  Of course, this method

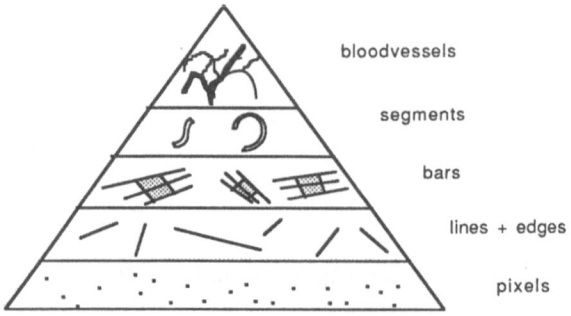

Fig. 1. Multi-layered image representation

of working can not be followed to obtain a structural description of a
complex cerebral blood vessel tree. A knowledge-based approach which has
the necessary flexibility to handle the complexity of the subtraction image,
seems to be more appropriate.

Blood vessel segmentation on DSA-images is well suited to be
solved by an expert analysis system for two reasons. First, perceptual
experts – i.e. radiologists –, who are able to outline the blood vessels
unambiguously, do exist in this field. The knowledge they use, is partly
heuristic and often cannot be immediately described. Thus, an exploratory
design method seems appropriate. Second, traditional image segmentation
methods suffer from several shortcomings : e.g. some edges are missing,
while others are irrelevant. Using heuristic knowledge may be valuable to
guide the process of segmentation.

A major characteristic of our approach is its multi-layered image representation. Using this paradigm (Fig. 1) the image segmentation gradually
moves from the raw image data towards a structured description of the relevant anatomical elements. At the bottom level a primal sketch-like structure
is obtained by using classical image processing techniques. A knowledge-
based system – structured in three modular stages –, is used to refine and
extend this primal representation.

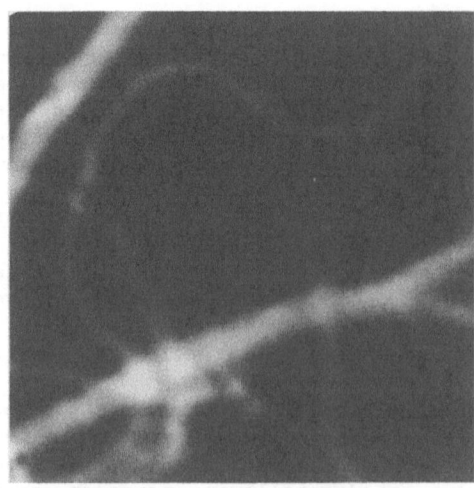

Fig. 2. Original subtraction angiogram

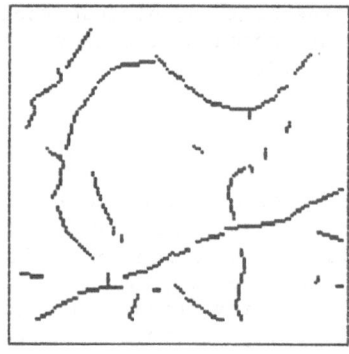

Fig. 3. Detected center lines          Fig. 4. Detected edges


A practical result of the current implementation is mentioned.
Conclusions and future work are discussed in the last section.


A LOW LEVEL IMAGE REPRESENTATION

Three different information levels are handled in the low level
processing stage : pixels, lines/edges and bars. Of course, pixels can
only be characterized by their position and greyvalue. Line and edge information is extracted by modified versions of well-known image processing
techniques. Blood vessel edges are detected by a Nevatia-Babu edge operator
(Nevatia & Babu, 1980). Blood vessel center lines are obtained by an improved maximum intensity detector (Fischler and Wolf, 1983 and Smets et al.,
1987). The combined use of these techniques offers some advantages. This
is mainly due to their complementary character in extracting important
information from the image : the edge detector is very well suited to find
broad, high contrast blood vessels, while the intensity detection algorithm
performs better on thin, low contrast ones. After thresholding, thinning
and linking, this edge and center line information is approximated by a
series of piecewise linear segments. For that purpose the line finding
approximation technique explained in Nevatia and Babu (1980) was slightly
adapted. Figure 2 shows an original subtraction angiogram. Center lines
and edges found by the discussed algorithms are shown in figures 3 and 4.

At a third stage in our model, bar-like primitives are constructed.
Bars are defined as a set of two almost parallel straight edges with a
center line in between. As such, they are characterized by ten points,
a width and a length (Fig. 5). Bars obtained by our method accumulate
more evidence than the ones defined in Ritchings et al., 1985.

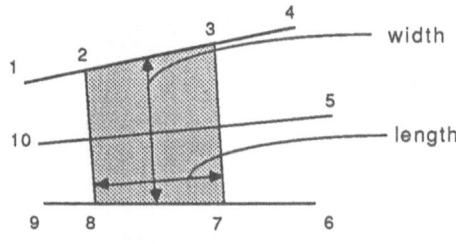

Fig. 5. Representation of a bar

In our opinion, bars are a natural primal representation, because their local approximation of a blood vessel takes into account directional information. This aspect has been ignored in Stansfield, 1986.

KNOWLEDGE-BASED SEGMENTATION

The system's knowledge-based part will consist of three modular sections. The first phase uses only geometrical and topological knowledge in order to improve the primal image representation. The second part should exploit general blood vessel knowledge (e.g. that the width of a normal blood vessel gradually decreases or that the intensity strongly increases where vessels cross). The third phase will be built around domain specific knowledge, available from radiologists : the type of the angiogram (e.g. carotid or coronary), important regions in the image, the medical history of the patient, the probability of a certain disease.

The main purpose of the first phase is to verify and improve the primal description. As a result the segmentation will move one step higher in the multi-layered representation as it attempts to build up segments. A segment is a representation of a (part of a) blood vessel and will be derived by extending bar primitives using heuristic knowledge.

The knowledge-based derivation of these segments is written in OPS5, a rule-based expert system tool, which was mainly chosen for practical reasons. The system runs on a VAX-750 computer and contains at the moment some 70 production rules. These rules describe the geometrical and topological reasoning knowledge needed to connect the bar primitives to larger segments. So far, the geometrical part of the rule-base is able to delineate most parts of the bloodvessels where no crossing or branching occurs. Even with only one third of the rule-base implemented the results can already be useful in a practical application (Section 4).

Initially, the working memory (WM) - the part of OPS5 where the data resides - contains only bar primitives, free edges and free center lines. These free edges and free lines were derived during the preprocessing but were not used to construct bars. The production rules that reason on this data are structured into a number of sequential phases, i.e. clusters of rules in which the order of evaluation is irrelevant.
The first set of rules tries to establish "primitive relations" between the WM elements of type "bar". No use is made of the free edges and free center lines. A typical situation handled in this phase is shown in figure 6. It will trigger the following production rule :

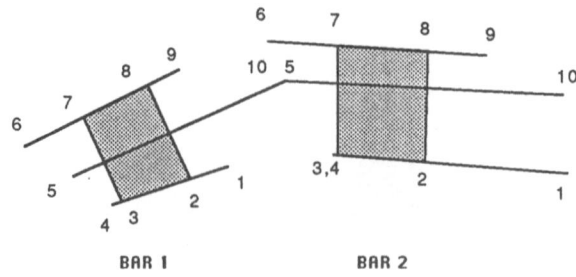

Fig. 6. Example of a primitive relation

```
IF      there is a bar BAR1
   AND  there is a bar BAR2
   AND  the coordinates of point 10 of BAR1 and point 5 of BAR2
        are almost identical
```

THEN make a primitive relation TOUCHING-CENTER-LINES between
     BAR1 and BAR2

When all primitive relations between pairs of bars have been established,
the second phase, called "build relations", becomes active. This set of
rules tries to combine all primitive relations that have been established
between a pair of bars, into a higher order relation. The example rule
pictured below will clarify this.

```
IF      there is a primitive relation SAME-SIDE between BAR1 and BAR2
   AND  there is a primitive relation TOUCHING-CENTER-LINES between
        BAR1 and BAR2
```

THEN make a relation SAME-SIDE-TOUCHING-CENTER-LINES between BAR1 and
     BAR2

Besides combining already established primitive relations, the rules also
build hypotheses for primitive relations that were not detected although
the situation shows strong evidence for them. An example of such a hypothesis generating rule is the following :

```
IF      there is a primitive relation SAME-SIDE between BAR1 and BAR2
   AND  there is a primitive relation TOUCHING-CENTER-LINES between
        BAR1 and BAR2
   AND  there are NO primitive relations TOUCHING-SIDE or SAME-SIDE
        between BAR1 and BAR2 on the other side

THEN    make a relation ONE-MISSING-LINK
        between BAR1 and BAR2
```

The third phase of the geometrical rule-base is concerned with the connection of bars into segments. Bar elements of which the established relations
are considered to give sufficient confidence, are connected first. In a
next step, verification of the hypotheses takes place. Conceptually, this
is accomplished by moving downward in the multi-layered representation.
So, free edges or free center lines are looked for to solve the missing
link relations. When such edges or center lines are not available, a local
resegmentation on the original image will be performed.

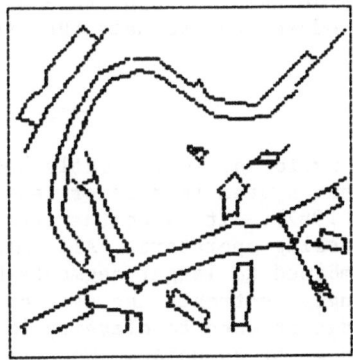

Fig. 7. Segments from Figure 2

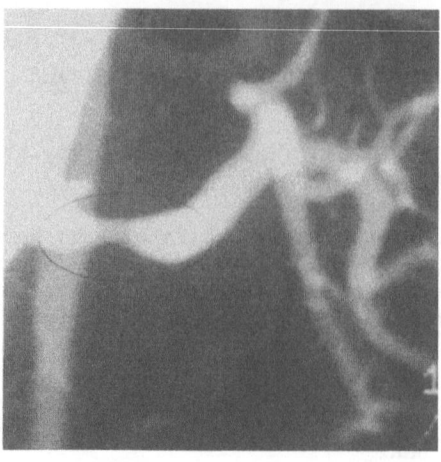

Fig. 8. Angiogram, containing a stenosis

This resegmentation can be done by relaxing the parameters of the initial edge or line finding algorithm or by using a different detection method. At present, the threshold value in the original algorithms is decreased until an edge is found or until a prespecified lower bound is reached. The resegmentation step creates new free edges or center lines that will automatically trigger rules within this third phase.
The segments obtained from Fig. 2 are shown in Figure 7.


A PRACTICAL RESULT

Although our general approach to blood vessel segmentation is partly implemented, the results obtained so far are stimulating and even of practical use. As an illustration of the latter, an example will be given to show the applicability of our concept in the area of diagnosing stenoses.

In order to relieve the task of the radiologist, our system can, in its current state, automatically describe a blood vessel in the neighborhood of the stenosis. Figure 8 shows an example of an angiogram, where a radiologist has indicated a region of interest. By concentrating on this region, primitives are derived (Figure 9). The result of applying our knowledge-based technique on this primal sketch is shown in Figure 10. This result can immediately be used as input to a dynamic programming algorithm as to refine the edges and evaluate the stenosis.


CONCLUSIONS

The approach we have developed, is basically bottom-up. As a result this segmentation-improvement system is more or less domain independent (Van Cleynenbreugel et al. 1987). It is neither very sensitive to the choice of basic image processing operators. All image primitives extracted by the low level can be combined to larger segments by using geometrical reasoning. This fact strongly contrasts the system proposed in Stansfield (1986), where model knowledge is used to classify image primitives, either as belonging to a blood vessel or as noise. We note however, that it will be difficult to outline blood vessel segments which are completely absent in the primal representation, using our current implementation.

Anatomical model knowledge will at least simplify their recognition. Work is under way to implement such general blood vessel knowledge. The use of a multi-resolution approach is also being investigated. Segmenting a blurred image yields a first rough description of the wide blood vessels. This information can be used to guide the segmentation of the full resolution image.

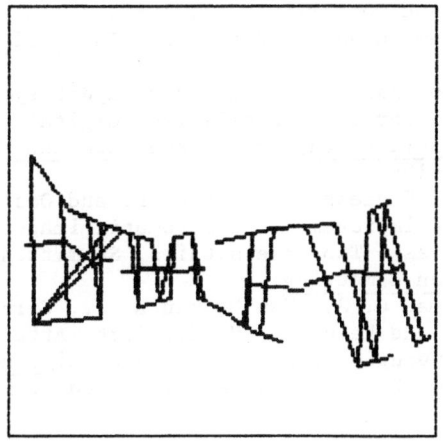

Fig. 9. Bar primitives from Figure 8

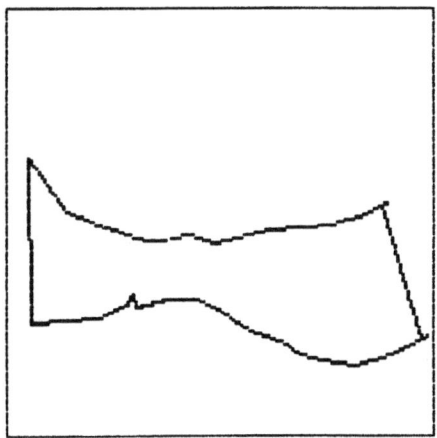

Fig. 10. Segmentation of Figure 8

REFERENCES

Fischler M. and Wolf H., 1983, A general approach to machine perception of linear structure in imaged data, SRI Technical Report 276.
Nevatia R. and Babu K., 1980, Linear feature extraction and description, Computer Graphics and Image Description, 13, 257-269.
Reiber J. H. C., Kooijman C. J., Slager C. J., Gerbrands J. J., Schuurbiers J. H. C., den Boer A., Wijns W., Serruys P. W. and Hugen-

313

holtz P. W., 1984, Coronary Artery dimensions from cineangiograms;
methodology and validation of a computer-assisted analysis procedure,
I.E.E.E. Trans. Med. Imaging MI-3, 131-141.

Reiber J. H. C., Serruys P. W. and Slager C. J., 1986, Quantitative Coronary
and Left Ventricular Cineangiography, 190-201, Martinus Nijhoff
Publishers.

Ritchings R. T., Colchester A. C. F. and Wang H. Q., 1985, Knowledge-based
analysis of carotid angiograms, Image and Vision Computing, 3, 4,
217-222.

Smets C., Suetens P. and Oosterlinck A., 1987, A line segmentation technique
based on maximum intensity detection, Internal report ESAT/MI2
K.U.LEUVEN.

Stansfield S. A., 1986, ANGY : A rule-based expert system for automatic
segmentation of coronary vessels from digital subtracted angiograms,
I.E.E.E. Transactions on Pattern Analysis and Machine Intelligence,
PAMI-8, 2, 188-199.

Van Cleynenbreugel J., Fierens F., Suetens P. and Oosterlinck A., 1987,
Knowledge-based improvement of automatic image interpretation for
restricted scenes ; Two case studies, Submitted for publication in
Image and Vision Computing.

Van Ommeren J., Kooijman C. J., Van Meenen R. J., Gerbrands J. J., Schulte
A. V. M. C. L. and Reiber J. H. C., 1986, Artery detection and
analysis in cineangiograms, Pattern Recognition in Practice II,
331-343, Gelsema E. S. and Kanal L. N., eds., North Holland.

# INTRODUCTION TO PACS FOR THOSE INTERESTED IN IMAGE PROCESSING

G. Q. Maguire Jr.

M. E. Noz

Department of Computer Science
Columbia University
500 West 120th Street
New York, NY 10027 USA

Department of Radiology
New York University
550 First Avenue
New York, NY 10016 USA

A. Bakker, K. Bijl, H. Didden, and J. P. J. de Valk

Leiden University Hospital
Rijnsburgweg 10
2333 AA Leiden, The Netherlands

## Abstract

This paper gives a brief overview of PACS, including the basic components of a PACS system and what operations are or should be provided by it. This includes as well, a discussion of desired response time.

Current designs and simulations emphasize the requirements of physicians. The requirements of those interested in image processing may be different. For example, prefetching algorithms are being designed to provide images to a human, primarily a diagnostician. The requirements for a program which involves retrospective analysis of a series of studies and/or patients, may require a much different approach.

Use of PACS by those wishing to digitally analyze images has received little attention. Now is the time for this group of "users" to formulate and communicate their needs - before the system designs have been cast in code (and standards!).

## Introduction

The need to provide more interactive clinical consultations as well as retrieve images quickly and control the flow of image information has promoted the idea of incorporating a **local area network** (LAN) into imaging departments. This need was fueled by the observation that the full capabilities of digital image-producing modalities were rarely utilized routinely and by the proliferation of imaging techniques and clinical specialists participating in the generation and interpretation of them.

For a discussion of the technical details associated with local area networks and a summary of the status of many of the PACS implementations the reader is referred to (Noz, 1986).

### Overview of PACS

PACS stands for **Picture Archiving and Communication Systems**. This acronym comes from the Society of Photo-Optical Engineers (SPIE) conference: *First International Conference and Workshop on Picture Archiving and Communication Systems (PACS) for Medical*

*Applications*, held in January, 1982 at Newport Beach, California. To provide a foundation for this talk I would like to quote from the introduction to the conference proceedings written by André Duerinckx, the chairman of the conference and editor of the proceedings: (Duerinckx, 1982)

> The purpose of this new series of conferences and workshops on Picture Archiving and Communication Systems (PACS) is to help physicians, medical physicists, and equipment manufacturers plan future medical imaging departments. Medical specialties affected include: diagnostic radiology, radiation therapy, and clinical pathology.
>
> The 1982 PACS Conference, which is the first in the PACS Conference series, will cover the picture archiving and picture communication aspects of medical imaging. Image acquisition, image display, image processing, computerized patient record keeping, and management information system aspects have been dealt with in various other conferences and will not be discussed here.
>
> Most PACS use analog and/or digital (on-line and/or off-line) PACS subsystems. Digital electronic PACS are a first step towards a ''filmless'' medical imaging department. Digital PACS might influence the clinical operation of medical imaging departments by providing: (1) a fast access digital electronic storage medium for pictures, rather than a film copy; (2) a fast image communication link between imaging systems and viewing stations scattered over the different medical departments; and potentially (3) a link between imaging systems, image processors and patient record management information systems.

From this introduction we can see that the original emphasis of PACS was primarily to provide a filmless imaging department (item (1) above). That is, the goal was an electronic replacement for film and the clients were chiefly radiologists and pathologists. I will refer to these systems as first generation PACS systems.

Since this initial effort, a second generation of PACS is beginning to be defined; its goal is to regard images as just another data type in an office automation system and its clients are anyone who deals with images. The emphasis in second generation PACS is a system which integrates image generation, display and analysis, storage (both short term and archival), production of hardcopy, communication between all of the subsystems and between systems, and management of both the images and the system. This is very similar to the development of the **Manufacturing Automation Protocol** (MAP) which tries to tie all manufacturing systems together. However, in medical imaging there is no major ''consumer'' with the size of General Motors. Thus, although the number of medical imaging procedures is enormous, they are performed by a very large number of independent organizations (much like the automobile industry used to be). The result is that PACS progress has been much slower than that of MAP. An interesting aspect of second generation systems is that most of the things which the 1982 PACS conference specifically excluded are components of second generation systems! Thus just as MAP has caused the development of the **Technical and Office Protocol** (TOP) to interconnect the front office operations associated with manufacturing to the manufacturing systems, a development of second generation PACS will be an analogous system to allow **Hospital Information Systems** (HIS) and PACS to talk to each other. As we will see later this interaction is essential.

## Basic Components of a PACS

There are five basic components of a PACS: input, output, storage, communication, and control. Like many schemes for classification, not all of these components are completely separate entities.

Input components — digital image sources, digitizers (for input of data produced by analog sources), digital media (tape, floppies, etc.)

Output components — viewing stations, hardcopy devices, and digital media (for output)

Storage — file servers, local disk drives, archiving systems

Communication — local area networks, wide area networks, buses, and interfaces

Control — protocols used in the interaction between the subsystems, network management systems, interaction with the hospital (or other management) information system, and user commands.

While it is possible to view these as components of a single system due to the changes in the price performance of the components it has become feasible to treat these five components as simply the components of a distributed system. The nature of the objects which this system must manipulate and the constraints which are imposed on the operation of this system makes PACS a very challenging system problem[1]. In the next section we will address the problem of the objects which a PACS must manipulate. The following sections will address the operations to be performed and the constraints upon the system.

This evolution from centralized system to distributed systems can be seen as a direct result of the changes in the cost/performance of many of the subsystems which have occurred since 1981. Thus, many readers will recognize the same basic functions in the distributed systems as are in centralized image processing architectures (see for example (Gordon, 1981)) but with the internal buses replaced by networks.

## Objects in the PACS Environment

While most people who do image analysis realize that images consist of a large number of pixels and associated data - very few PACS efforts have made appropriate provisions for this associated data. Rather, most of the efforts have predefined the attributes which an image may have (for example the ACR/NEMA Standard 300 (NEMA, 1986) image format). This mirrors the fixed formats which were commonly used for storing images on magnetic tape for image exchange (Jaffe, 1981, Billingsley, 1982). In addition, many formats have restricted images to only two dimensions (NEMA, 1986) rather than allow higher (or lower) dimensionality (Haney, 1982, Baxter, 1982a, Maguire, 1982a, Baxter, 1982b).

A notable exception is the **Computer Assisted Radio-Therapy** (CART) (CART, 1984) project in scandinavia which has developed a CART standard **database** (DB) which users can query to find out the meaning of any attribute, the standard units for this attribute, preferred coordinate system, etc. With this database, CART has made it very easy for users to determine (by consulting an on-line database) if there is an existing entry for the attribute which they wish to describe for an image, if there is not they can register a new attribute (the DB even keeps the name of the person who introduced the attribute) (CART, 1986). One of the characteristics of the CART project has been to apply the computer to all of the details in the entire chain from treatment plans based on CT (or other digital image) data to verification of the therapy - for this process to be successful all of the different subsystem must agree on the meaning of each of the attributes and the value and interpretation of the pixels. The development of a PACS standard database for attributes of images which provides for easy extension by users is essential for future PACS developments and has not been addressed by ACR/NEMA (NEMA, 1986).

In order for applications running on different types of processors to exchange data, standards for PACS will have to address the translation into and out of whatever external data representation is used by the communication system(s). There are a number of interesting problems concerning the conversions of some representations such as floating point numbers, particularly in conjunction with process migration (which is mentioned later) (Smith, 1987).

In addition to the pixel data and descriptions in the form of, for example, key-value pairs (e.g. attributes and values) there is a need to be able to associate free text descriptions with images. The provision for free text allows the inclusion of descriptions which do not fit into the standard keys, but which are important for describing the image. A detailed description of the considerations for these three component databases can be found in (Zeleznik, 1983a).

Thus we see that an image really consists of three components: structured/formatted data, free text, and pixels. To estimate the minimum storage requirements for an image we have used data derived from the radiology department at New York University Medical Center (in 1981) (Maguire, 1982b) of approximately 54 bytes of formatted text data and 1200 bytes of free text.

This same study indicated that based on conservative estimates of the resolution required for digitizing images from film that the storage requirements for a 700 bed hospital with 100,000 exams per year over a 10 year period would be:

---

[1]It is the nature of the objects and the constraints which makes PACS interesting from a computer science point of view

| Type | Data Volume | Number of Items |
|---|---|---|
| Formatted text data | $5.4 \times 10^7$ bytes | $10^6$ items |
| Free textual data | $2.4 \times 10^9$ bytes | $4 \times 10^6$ documents |
| Image data | $1.4 \times 10^{13}$ bytes | $5 \times 10^7$ images |
| Total | $10^{14}$ bytes | $\sim 10^7$ |

## what operations are or should be provided by a PACS

There are many possible functional levels within which a PACS may exist. These range from the simplest system, which may do nothing more than retrieve images when given a patient's identification, to implementation of intelligent query systems (Bharg, 1980) or 'expert systems' (Thomas, 1982). Fundamentally, a PACS must provide a minimum of three services: archive image data, retrieve image data, and display image data. In fact, a useful PACS must provide additional services, if it is to be well accepted and fully utilized. The following is a minimal set of operation classes which a working PACS must support. (Zeleznik, 1983b)

Data archiving    Provides acquisition, permanent archival of, and access to, all patient data including images and text.

Data retrieval    Provides highly selective retrieval, based on user queries, of all patient data in the archive.

Interactive data display
    Provides convenient methods of interactive display of all patient data.

Image processing/analysis
    Provides processing capabilities for enhancement of image data along with access to the data for retrospective and statistical analysis, which may utilize the pixel as well as the ancillary data. In addition, the results of these analyses may be stored as new ancillary data.

Data output    Provides methods of outputting patient data, in forms suitable both for human use and use by other digital equipment.

Personal workspace environment
    Provides the user with his/her own personal environment for interactive analysis of data.

Electronic mail    Provides a means of communication between users and the system, in all directions.

User help    Provides a highly sophisticated, on-line user help system.

Data security    Provides both read and write access control mechanisms to protect against misuse of the database.

## Constraints

As was mentioned earlier PACS would be simply yet another distributed system, however the nature of the objects which it must manipulate and the response time constraints make the problem much different than that of previously studied distributed systems. In order to achieve the responsiveness that users have indicated they want requires the use of caching and prefetching. By using caching techniques the system moves the objects which are being referenced to faster storage systems. Prefetching involves anticipatory transfer of objects prior to their first reference. The ability to prefetch is predicated on the ability to predict which objects will be referenced and when they will be referenced. See (Bakker, 1986) for a discussion of an initial set of rules to use for prefetching and deletion.

### Response time

If the image is available local to where the reference is being made the desired response time ranges from several seconds for the display of the image (if it is on a local disk) to milliseconds for switching between the display of images already loaded into memory. Intermediate between these is the desire for the next *block*[2] of data which an image processing program needs. Given the size of images in common use within medical imaging, 8 kbytes $\cdots$ 16 Mbytes, this implies transfer rates ranging from 4 kbytes/second to 8 Mbytes/second for static images! Sequences of dynamic images can have even higher data rates. These high data rates are presently only possible with parallel head transfer disks. These disks have recently begun to appear as standard products rather than special purpose devices.

If the desired data is not available locally, some amount of time will be required to locate the closest copy of the data and then time will be required to transfer the data to the local system. The transfer will occur over some type of local area network for transfers of more than a few meters or via a bus for very local transfers - present local area networks are limited to signaling rates of 100 Mbits/second using fiber-optic networks such as ANSI X3T9.5 **Fiber Distributed Data Interface** (FDDI) (Joshi, 1984) and ~ 128 Mbytes/second for electrical buses. Future fiber-optic networks are being viewed as both LANs and micro-buses and are expected to have data rates of 500 to 1000 Mbits/second.

While the data rates of future fiber-optic networks may help by increasing the transfer rate of the network there still remain two major problems:

1. disk transfer rates have increased very slowly, although capacities have increased more rapidly[3]; and

2. the processing requirements of protocols used for networks has limited their effective data transfer rate to very low rates.

The overhead which the communication protocol imposes has lead to proposals for simpler protocols for bulk transfer of data, such as *NETBLT: A Bulk Data Transfer Protocol* proposed in RFC-998 (Clark, ??). With standard transport level protocols - it is not uncommon to have a transfer rate at the transport level of 1.8 Mbit/second over a 10 Mbit/second network. (Strauss, 1987) Thus, although the ACR/NEMA Standard 300 protocol was designed to allow transfers at up to 8 Mbytes/second the combination of small packets with a software implementation of the protocol on a 1 MIPS processor resulted in a 6 kbytes/second transfer rate (as stated during the presentation of (Hemminger, 1986)). With a 1 MIPS processor, an 8 kbyte/second transfer rate would allow for approximately 500 instructions to be executed per byte transferred, while an 8 Mbytes/second transfer rate would only allow 1/2 an instruction per byte processed! Unspecialized input/output routines often have an overhead of several hundred instructions per byte (for byte mode I/O) thus limiting rates to approximately 16 kbytes/second for 1 MIPS processors. Utilizing separate processors and additional hardware support for protocol processing allows much higher performance, such as the 1/8 Mbyte/second performance of some recent Ethernet controllers — this is roughly 16 instructions per byte transferred. The advent of RISC processors with very high speed processing of a simple instruction set has produced single chip processors capable of greater than 8 MIPS — utilizing these processors in network interfaces in conjunction with protocols which have been optimized for local area networks with very low error rates should allow networks to have performance comparable to SMD disks. For even higher data rates see section .

Given the transfer rates of most archiving devices (~ 200 kbytes/second), the time required to mount optical disk platters or other media (~ 30 seconds), and the probability of subsequent references after the initial reference - there is a need for buffers between the archive and the produces/consumes of images. This would seem to suggest a standard hierarchical storage system with caching such as has been extensively studied in computer systems. However, while objects in both situations poses high *locality of reference* within objects we do not yet understand the reference properties between images for PACS. Although much work has been done on caching (Smith, 1985, Clark, 1985, Stamos, 1984, Strecker, 1983, Clark, 1983), and there have been many simulations of caching in systems, the previous caching studies involved many small objects (typically each was less than 1 kilobyte in size with a new object being generated roughly every 10 instructions in systems such as SMALLTALK). Unfortunately, this is very different from the problems which occur in PACS systems where the objects are typically $10^5$ bytes in size and there

---

[2]This block is the next logical quanta of data which the algorithm needs and need not be related to the physical organization of data on a secondary storage device.

[3]See (McKusick, 1984) for a description of the throughput for disk systems as a function of the bus, block size, and processor.

are only thousands of these objects generated per day.

One constraint of the image objects which we can take advantage of is that they are by and large write once, in that once they are transferred from the system where they were created they are not modified in place, but rather any processing produces a new version. This is very similar to the situation in engineering and business databases (see (Bernstein, 1987)). The advantage of this type of objects is that you do not have the problems of consistency which occur in databases which allow updates in place (and therefore avoid spending time executing locking protocols).

Storage Capacities

The storage capacities for both local disks and archives is technically feasible[4] and, due to the change in the cost/performance of magnetic and optical media and drives, subsystems which meet the needs of PACS are becoming available at attractive prices.

# Compression

One important issue with regard to PACS consists of whether or not a lossy compression algorithm should be used to enhance system response time. While it may be ultimately decided that this is acceptable when simply viewing images, this may **not** be acceptable when image processing is to be performed on these images. It should be the job of the designer of the PACS system to ensure that it is obvious to the user whether the image has been compressed and how to recover as much as possible of the original data if compression has been used. If the archived data is to be used retrospectively for image processing we should avoid lossy compression of the stored data.

# Requirements - who sets them and what are they

Current designs and simulations (massar, 1985) primarily emphasize the requirements of physicians. The requirements of those interested in image processing may be different. For example, prefetching algorithms are being designed to provide images to a human, primarily a diagnostician. The requirements for a program which involves retrospective analysis of a series of studies and/or patients, may require a much different approach.

These requirements might be typified by:

- Image processing tasks might benefit by migrating the process performing the analysis nearer to the archive.

- Images retrieved for analysis purposes, might **not** necessarily have to be preserved in the on-line buffer for ''current'' patients.

- It would be beneficial to assign ''background'' priority to these analyses so that the processing and retrievals can be done when the interactive demand is low. See (Romney, 1986) for a study which details the number of images generated as a function of the time of day.

# Optical networks

In order to achieve transfer rates comparable to or better than parallel head transfer disk will require the use of optical networks with electro-optic network interfaces. Let us assume an optical ring network with very high data rates and the size of the network, i.e. the number of bits which could be stored on the network itself, equal to the size of the buffer – then a user could simply wait for the data that they were interested in to go by! This design is reminiscent of the mercury delay lines used in the 1950s. Is this feasible? If we were able to achieve a signaling rate of $10^{15}$ bits/second (roughly $10^{14}$ bytes per second) one light second of cable would be able to store all of the data in the archive. This would eliminate the need for intermediate buffers, local disks, etc. If the velocity of propagation were 0.8c, one light second of cable would be $0.8 \times 10^5$ km of cable. To compare this to geographic scales, the distance across the U. S. from east coast to west coast is ~5 $\times 10^3$ km, therefore this would be about 16 x the U. S. coast-to-coast distance.

---

[4]Although previously only organizations such as the U.S. National Center for Atmospheric Research (NCAR) or Livermore National Laboratory could afford to archive $10^{13}$ bits/year (Kaisler, 1984).

Let us consider instead keeping only the working set of images, which would otherwise require storage in the on-line buffer. Since roughly $5 \times 10^9$ bytes/day of new data is acquired, combining this with a factor of 16 for the additional archival data required for comparison purposes and scaling by a factor of 10 for two weeks worth of data - the resulting buffer requires about $6 \times 10^{12}$ bits. Thus it is about 1/1000 of the size of the archive; this corresponds to 80 km of cable. Is this an unrealistic amount of cable? If we consider the 12 bundles of 12 fibers each which are installed between the two campuses of Duke University (as described by AT&T at PACS IV), and assume that the two campuses are 1 km apart, this would be 144 km of fiber. Clearly 80 km of fiber is thus not unreasonable.

What is wrong with the above argument for a fiber optic implementation of the network, local disk, and buffer? The first problem is that $10^{15}$ bits/second is much higher than the practical signaling rates which we are currently able to achieve by roughly a factor of $10^6$. The second problem is that this data rate is roughly a factor of $10^6$ faster than any electronics we have to interface to this network! The first problem means that using a 100 Mbit/second network such as FDDI would require more than $4 \times 10^7$ km of cable, which is clearly impractical. Perhaps technology will be able to support faster modulation of optical signals. The second problem can be solved by using optical finite state machines (Husain, 1986) to simply take every millionth bit as part of a packet, thus bringing the data rate to the level which GaAs processors might be able to handle.

## Conclusion

First generation PACS are being developed and are reaching the product stage, while second generation PACS is still in the research stage.

Use of PACS by those wishing to digitally analyze images has received little attention. As D. Meyer-Ebrecht observed at the first PACS conference: "The discussion equally involves the medical community in bringing forward their requirements, and the technical disciplines in reporting on the development of system architectures and device technologies." (Meyer-Ebrecht, 1982). While the second generation systems are still in the requirements analysis phase it is time, for those interested in using the digital data which PACS can provide, to formulate and communicate their needs. If they wait, system designs will continue to be installed which digitize the video signal sent to the CRTs of various imaging systems. In addition, the standards which will describe what data is kept and how it is kept will have gathered so much inertia, due to capital expenditures, they will be nearly impossible to change over the next decade.

## Acknowledgments

One of us, (GQM), wishes to thank the U.S. National Science Foundation and the Netherlands Organization for Pure Research-National Informatics Facility for having provided the funds to spend spring semester 1986 at Leiden University Hospital working with A. Bakker, K. Bijl, H. Didden, and J. P. J. de Valk. This stay provided both time to think about PACS and the stimulation of encountering different viewpoints regarding PACS and PACS implementation schemes. I had previously thought about having an expert system for generating PACS configurations, however, the Leiden group's simulation work has forced me to think about simulation as the means which the expert should use to evaluate a given configuration. One of us (GQM) would like to thank IBM for Faculty Development Award, and Hewlett-Packard for an equipment grant.

## References

Bakker, A.; Didden, H.; de Valk, J. P. J. and A. D. A. Massar. *Considerations on an algorithm for activation of images in a multi-layer storage within a PACS.* Society of Photo-Optical Engineers, February, 1986.

Baxter, B. S.; Hitchner, L. E.; and Maguire Jr., G. Q. *Characteristics of a protocol for the exchange of digital image information,* pages 273-277. Society of Photo-Optical Engineers, January, 1982.

Baxter, B, S.; Hitchner, L. E.; and Maguire Jr., G. Q. A Standard Format for Digital Image Exchange. American Association of Physicists in Medicine Series, Report number 10. American Institute of Physics, N.Y., N.Y., 1982. 11 pages.

Bernstein, P. A Practical Theory of Concurrency Control for Replicated Data. Computer Science Department Colloquium, Columbia University.

Bhargava, B. Design of Intelligent Query Systems for Large Databases. In S.K Chang, K.S. Fu, eds (Ed.), *Pictorial Information Systems*, New York, Berlin: Springer-Verlag, 1980.

Billingsley, F. C. *Landsat computer-compatible tape family*. Society of Photo-Optical Engineers, January, 1982.

Dahlin, H. and Hamren, M. CART - Computer Aided Radio Therapy - Presentation of an Integrated Information System in Radiotherapy. Medical Computer Physics/UDAC. Akademiska sjukhuset, S-751 85 Uppsala, Sweden, 1984. 73 pages.

Moeller, T. CART NEWS: CART standard database.

Clark, D. Cache Performance in the VAX-11/780. *ACM Transactions on Computing Systems*, February 1983, *1*, *(1)*, 24-37.

Clark, D. and J. S. Emer. Performance of the VAX-11/780 Translation Buffer: Simulation and Measurement. *ACM Transactions on Computing Systems*, February 1985, *3*, *(1)*, 31-62.

Clark, D. D.; Lambert, M. L. and L. Zhang. NETBLT: A Bulk Data Transfer Protocol. Network Working Group, Request for Comments: 998.

Duerinckx, A. J. *Introduction*. Society of Photo-Optical Engineers, January, 1982.

Gordon, B. G. *Transportability of image processing system architectures*, pages 105-111. Society of Photo-Optical Engineers, August, 1981.

Haney, M. J.; Johnston, R. L.; and W. D. O'Brien, Jr. *On standards for the storage of images and data*. Society of Photo-Optical Engineers, January, 1982.

Hemminger, B. M.; Thompson, B. G. and S. M. Pizer. *Ongoing implementation of a prototype medical communications system at the University of North Carolina*. Society of Photo-Optical Engineers, February, 1986.

Husain, A. Optical Processing for Future Computer Networks. *Optical Engineering*, January 1986, *25*, *(1)*, 108-116.

Jaffe, R. S. *Standard format for the transmission of digital images*, pages 405-411. Society of Photo-Optical Engineers, September, 1981.

Joshi, S. and Iyer, V. New standards for local networks push upper limits for lightwave data. *Data Communications*, July 1984, *13*, *(7)*, 127-138. Description of ANSI X3T9.5 Fiber Distributed Data Interface and 100 Mbit/s fiber optic networks.

Kaisler, S. H. Fifth IEEE Symposium on Mass Storage Systems. *IEEE Computer Architecture Technical Committee Newsletter*, June 1984, , 1-1 to 1-58.

Maguire Jr., G. Q.; Baxter, B. S.; and Hitchner, L. E. *An AAPM standard magnetic tape format for digital image exchange*, pages 284-293. Society of Photo-Optical Engineers, 1982.

Maguire Jr., G. Q.; Zeleznik, M. P.; Horii, S. C.; Schimpf, J. H.; and Noz, M. E. *Image processing requirements in hospitals and an integrated systems approach*, pages 206-213. Society of Photo-Optical Engineers, January, 1982.

Massar, A.D.A. Simulation of a Communication System for Medical Images. In *Laboratorium voor schakelterchieu en techniek dor informatieverwerkende machines*, Univeristy of Delft, The Netherlands: Master's Thesis, 1985.

McKusick, M. K. et al. A Fast File System for UNIX. *ACM Transactions on Computing Systems*, August 1984, *2*, *(3)*, 181-197.

Meyer-Ebrecht, D. *Introduction to PACS*. Society of Photo-Optical Engineers, January, 1982.

National Electrical Manufacturers Association (NEMA) and the American College of Radiology (ACR). ACR-NEMA 300-1985 Digital Imaging and Communication Standard.

Noz, M. E., Maguire Jr, G. Q. and Erdman, W. A. Local Area Networks in an Imaging Environment. *CRC Critical Reviews in Medical Informatics*, April 1986, *1, (1)*, 81-133. Invited Review Paper.

ter Haar Romney, B. M. ; Meijwaard, J.; ten Hertog, A.; de Graaf, C. N.; and P. P. van Rijk. *Radiological information flow between departments and out-clinics in the Utrecht University Hospital in the Netherlands.* Society of Photo-Optical Engineers, February, 1986.

Smith, A. J. Disk Cache - Miss Ratio Analysis and Design Considerations. *ACM Transactions on Computing Systems*, August 1985, *3, (3)*, 161-203.

Maguire Jr., G. Q. and J. M. Smith. A Survey of Process Migration Mechanisms. Unpublished - draft.

Stamos, J. Static Grouping of Small Objects to Enhance Performance in a Paged Virtual Memory System. *ACM Transactions on Computing Systems*, May 1984, *2, (2)*, 155-180.

Strauss, P. OSI throughput performance: Breakthrough or bottleneck? *Data Communications*, May 1987, *16, (5)*, 53-56.

Strecker, W. Transient Behavior of Cache Memories. *ACM Transactions on Computing Systems*, November 1983, *1, (4)*, 281-295.

Thomas, A. J. *Pictorial Information System Architectures for Diagnostic Imaging.* Society of Photo-Optical Engineers, January, 1982.

Zeleznik, M. P.; Maguire Jr., G. Q.; and Baxter, B. S. . *PACS data base design*, pages 287-295. Society of Photo-Optical Engineers, May, 1983.

Zeleznik, M. P.; Maguire Jr., G. Q.; Baxter, B. S.; Noz, M. E.; Schimpf, J. H.; and Horii, S. C. . *PACS user level requirements*, pages 172-177. Society of Photo-Optical Engineers, May, 1983.

ERROR-FREE DATA COMPRESSION METHODS APPLICABLE TO PACS

C. Robert Appledorn

Department of Radiology

Indiana University Medical Center
Indianapolis, Indiana 46223  USA

Andrew E. Todd-Pokropek

Department of Medical Physics

University College
London, WC1, UK

## INTRODUCTION

Digital imaging procedures are characterized by the large volumes of data that can be produced. With routine nuclear medicine studies, a single patient procedure will quickly exceed a one megabyte (Mbyte) storage requirement. Even with the introduction of economical large capacity disk drives allowing for on-line storage, these data continue to pose a significant impediment to the development of PACS (picture archiving and communication) systems. This is because the required storage (space) becomes too large for the available storage and, more significantly, the transmission rate (time) between locations can become too slow to be acceptable in a clinical environment.

To attack these two problems of space and time, one must examine data compression methods if one is to effectively reduce the storage requirements and transmission times associated with these digital imaging procedures. Our primary investigative goal is the development of error-free compression methods in which the recovered study is exactly identical to the original study prior to the archival/compression of the study.

## IMAGE ENTROPY

The storage required of a study is directly related to the distribution or total variation of data values within the study. The distribution can be described with the histogram of those values or, as we approach expected value, the probability density function (pdf) associated with those values. This histogram can be a one-dimensional, a co-occurrence, and/or a multidimensional description of the data values. However, we are not particularly interested in the explicit structure of the histogram at this time; hence, we assume a one-dimensional description for simplicity. This restriction will be relaxed later.

The total variation often is described in terms of entropy which leads to a convenient description of storage requirements. The entropy H(x) associated with a random variable x with known probability density function p(x) is given conventionally by

$$H(x) = -\, \Sigma \; p(x) \; \log \, p(x)$$

where logarithms are base two, allowing one to interpret entropy values in terms of storage (bits/pixel). Conditional and joint probability density functions allow the introduction of higher order entropy descriptions as easily leading to

$$H(z,x) = H(z/x) + H(x).$$

If one assumes that the data value can be described with an additive noise model

$$z = x + n$$

where z is the measurement, x is the signal component, and n is the additive noise component, then the entropy description can be extended. In this case, measurement entropy H(z) will consist of two components: signal entropy H(x) and noise entropy H(n),

$$H(z) = H(x) + H(n).$$

The measurement entropy H(z) can be identified with the joint entropy H(x,n) of signal and noise combined, the signal entropy H(x) with signal alone, and the noise entropy H(n) with the conditional entropy H(z/x) of the measurement given the signal value.

Signal entropy has strongly correlated image elements and, hence, represents reduceable/compressible data – the object of our investigation. Noise entropy has un/weakly-correlated image elements and represents irreduceable data. For a data compression scheme to qualify as error-free, it must be capable of recovering both the signal variation and the noise variation without distortion.

IMAGE ENTROPY – SIGNAL AND NOISE

In order to gain some insights into the compression problem, we initially explore four cases involving the variational structure of the image to be archived. These problems represent differing variances of signal and other/noise that contribute to the total image entropy.

Case I: no signal variance, no noise variance.
This is the trivial or degenerate case in which the image consists of a single constant value everywhere and all image elements are (clearly) correlated with each other. The image entropy is zero. The compression algorithm is to store that single constant value (one number) along with some overhead information regarding image size, etc.

Case II: no signal variance, noise variance.
This situation occurs when the image element data are distributed about a constant mean value. If the data values are Poisson distributed with pdf parameter m, the mean value, then one can show that the entropy

of this case is given asymptotically by

$$H = 1/2 \; \log(2\pi e m)$$

for large m ( > 10 ). This is a useful result because it provides a lower bound on the storage requirements associated with the other/noise variation. As such, it is a measure of the "cost" of error-free compression methods.

Case III: signal variance, no noise variance

This situation describes a signal with correlated data in which this correlated redundancy can be removed using, for example, predictive coding. Predictive coding describes a data element in terms of its previous neighbors. The coefficients of the predictive equation can be stored to yield high compression ratios. To illustrate this process, we consider three brief examples.

Case IIIa: no prediction

The signal consists of a ramp and the probability density function is uniform; $p(x_i) = p(x_j)$. This is the maximum entropy condition that results in maximum storage requirements. This is the usual clinical situation when compression methods are not employed and images are stored according to "word-mode" or "byte-mode".

Case IIIb: perfect prediction

Again, the signal consists of a ramp; however, a simple linear predictor is employed:

$$x_i = x_j + \Delta x$$

where $\Delta x$ is the incremental value between neighboring image elements. The predictions are exact. For this (trivial) situation, only $\Delta x$ need be stored and this case degenerates to Case I: no signal variance and no noise variance.

Case IIIc: imperfect prediction

The signal contains a more complex structure and the predictive equation is not perfect. Given a set of previous element values $x_j$, a prediction is calculated:

$$x_i = f(x_j)$$

Typically, the predictor equation is linear and the coefficients of this equation can be stored. In addition, because the prediction is not perfect, we must also compute and store the residual difference between the actual value and the predicted value, namely,

$$r_i = x_i - x_i$$

The resulting residuals will ideally be randomly distributed with "other" variance $\sigma_r^2$. The entropy associated with gaussian distributed residuals

327

$$H(r) = 1/2 \log(2\pi e \sigma_r^2)$$

determines the required storage for the image.

The selection of the predictor equation is influenced by the resulting residual entropy. One wishes to minimize H(r) with respect to an appropriate choice of predictor equation.

Case IV: signal variance, other/noise variance

In this real-life problem, one has an image that has both signal and noise. The total entropy for this case is given, to a first approximation, by

$$H(image) = H(signal) + H(noise)$$

This is actually Case IIIc -- the variance of the signal can be reduced using predictive equations and the resulting residuals and the measurement noise combine to determine the other/noise variance. The entropy for this residual variance determines the image storage.

## CODE LENGTH

In order to achieve a reduction in the storage requirements and the transmission times for digital images, it is necessary to encode the data values in some manner that results in less space being occupied by the image. In the parlance of information theory, one wishes to encode a source alphabet $X = \{x_1, x_2, \ldots, x_M\}$ with a code alphabet $A = \{a_1, a_2, \ldots, a_D\}$. Each symbol of the source X is encoded with a sequence of symbols of the code A. If the code alphabet contains only two symbols (D = 2), it is referred to as a binary code. We restrict this discussion to binary codes for obvious reasons.

The process of encoding the source image data values consists of associating the source symbols $x_i$ with a given code word, which is simply a sequence of $a_j$'s. Frequently, the source symbols are of fixed length (e.g., 8-bits for "byte" mode and 16-bits for "word" mode storage) while the encoded sequences of code symbols will be variable in length. If shorter code sequences are assigned to more frequently occurring source symbols, then an overall reduction in space/time requirements can be achieved.

A few restrictions are necessary if the encoding is to be useful. It will be assumed that each code word is distinct and corresponds to one source word. In Table 1, it can be seen that Code A is not uniquely decipherable whereas Codes B, C, and D can be deciphered. Of these three codes, Codes B and D are said to be instantaneous; i.e., no code symbol contains a previous symbol as a prefix as does Code C. The instantaneous property is desirable although not necessary. Codes C and D are referred to as comma codes because the symbol 0 acts as a separator between encoded words; however, Code C does not have the instantaneous property.

The aim of error-free coding is to obtain codes that have the following two properties: 1) unique decipherability and 2) minimum average length L.
Codes with both properties are called optimal. It can be shown that if a code is optimal among instantaneous codes, then it is optimal among all uniquely decipherable codes. Hence, it is sufficient to consider instantaneous codes only.

328

Table 1. Four Binary Coding Schemes

| Source Symbols | Code A | Code B | Code C | Code D |
|---|---|---|---|---|
| $x_1$ | 0 | 0 | 0 | 0 |
| $x_2$ | 1 | 10 | 01 | 10 |
| $x_3$ | 00 | 110 | 011 | 110 |
| $x_4$ | 11 | 111 | 0111 | 1110 |

Table 2. Multiple – Symbol Encoding

| Source Symbols | Probability $p(x_i)$ | Code E |
|---|---|---|
| $x_1$ | 1/3 | 0 |
| $x_2$ | 1/3 | 10 |
| $x_3$ | 1/6 | 110 |
| $x_4$ | 1/6 | 111 |

$$H(x) = 1.918 \text{ bits/symbol}$$
$$L_1 = 2.000 : 1.918 \leq L_1 \leq 2.918$$
$$L_2 = 1.944 : 1.918 \leq L_2 \leq L_1 \leq 2.918$$

Table 3. Medical Image Entropy

| Study Type | Matrix Size | Image Entropy |
|---|---|---|
| HIPDM SPECT | $64^2$ | $4.40 \pm 0.41$ |
| "Rotating" MUGA | $64^2$ | $6.21 \pm 0.70$ |
| Ventricular DSA | $128^2$ | $4.19 \pm 0.96$ |
| NMRI Brain | $256^2$ | $3.49 \pm 1.24$ |

The noiseless coding theorem states

$$H(x) \leq L \leq H(x) + 1.$$

Simply stated, the resulting encoded data values will result in an average code length L that is within one bit of the image entropy H(x). (Refer to Table 2.) If the left-hand equality is strictly satisfied, then the code is referred to as absolutely optimal.

Actually, the average code length L can become arbitrarily close to the image entropy H(x) if sequences of the source symbols are encoded. If pairs of source symbols are encoded resulting in an average code length $L_2$, then $L_2 < L_1$ where $L_1$ is the resulting single symbol code length. (Refer to Table 2.) Similarly, triples of source symbols results in an average code length $L_3 \leq L_2 < L_1$. In general, with encoding n symbols at a time, one obtains an extended coding theorem:

$$H(x) \leq L_n \leq H(x) + 1/n.$$

This property leads to a multiplicity of adaptive algorithms that seek to minimize space/time requirements by extending the encoded source word length.

This entropy associated with a number of classes of medical images was examined to determine if encoding methods would lead to useful results. (Refer to Table 3.) The table illustrates that for diverse image sets that is a degree of redundancy and that between 2:1 to 4:1 compression should be achievable with medical images. Thus one concludes that the entropy results indicate that signal compression followed by residual/noise encoding should be pursued.

Of course, nothing has been stated regarding the means or methods for signal encoding. This is the topic of the next section.

DYNAMIC STOCHASTIC MODELS

We reject at the onset a predictor equation that is deterministic in nature; e.g., Fourier series expansions. Although deterministic models may satisfy a criterion such as least-squares, there is no relationship between this and the ability to predict. Thus we turn to dynamic stochastic models of the form

$$x(t) = f(z(t-1),\theta) + w(t)$$

where $z(t-1)$ is the observation history for $x(t)$, $\theta$ is a finite vector of parameters for the predictor equation $f(-)$, and $w(t)$ is a zero mean IID sequence.

In practice, one needs to determine $\theta$ (the predictor equation coefficients) and $w(t)$ (the other/noise residuals) and store them. For ease and speed of implementation, it is necessary to restrict the functions that be considered to a finite set of candidates. The problem of determining of the predictor function reduces to selecting a "best" candidate according to some optimality criterion. The criterion we employ reflects parsimonious behavior (minimum number of parameters, $\theta$) for a minimum prediction error (residual variance). Currently, only linear autoregressive predictors are considered.

As an initial investigative tool, a univariate output difference equation in terms of the scalar variable x is employed as the linear predictor equation:

$$x(t) = z^T(t-1)\theta + w(t)$$

$$z(t-1) = [x(t-1),\ldots, x(t-m)]^T$$

$z(t-1)$ is the vector of past values of $x(t)$, $\theta$ is an m-vector, and $w(t)$ is a zero mean sequence of residuals with variance $\sigma_r^2$. Parameter estimation techniques are used to identify values for $\theta$; however, the order m is not known a priori and must be determined.

The importance of the selection of an appropriate class order m cannot be over emphasized. An arbitrary choice of m will yield least-squares estimates for the parameter vector $\theta$; however, this arbitrary choice of m will not yield minimum prediction error, i.e.,

$$R_m = E\{[\ x(t) - x(t\backslash t-1)]^2\},$$

where $x(t)$ is the actual image value and $x(t\backslash t-1)$ is the predicted value in terms of its previous neighbors. One can show that for a redundant model with n extra and unnecessary parameters in the coefficient vector $\theta$, the prediction mean-square error increases. If m is the correct order, then $R_{m+n} > R_m$.

One decision rule for class selection that is derived from likelihood methods is to choose the order m that minimizes

$$L_m = \frac{[\ \text{number of measurements}\ ]}{2} \log(\ \text{residual variance}\ ) +$$

$$+ \text{ number of estimated parameters .}$$

ENCODING METHODS

There are a number of approaches available for constructing codes that are uniquely decipherable and minimum length. In this section, we examine three illustrative methods and, later, compare their performance with clinical digital data. The methods examined include

1. Huffman
2. Shannon - Fano
3. Lempel - Ziv

The most widely known optimal encoding method is due to Huffman and, hence, is known as Huffman coding. In its simplest form, it analyzes the histogram of values associated with the image and assigns variable length codes to each datum value. The shortest length codes represent the most frequently occurring values resulting in the minimum length property.

Shannon-Fano encoding also relies upon the generation of the code from the histogram of data values. Here, the histogram is sorted in order of decreasing probabilities and partitioned into two equiprobable groups. The symbol "zero" ($a_1$) is assigned to the "left-hand" group and the symbol "one" ($a_2$) to the "right-hand" group. This partitioning and symbol assignment is repeated until code sequences have been constructed for each source data value. The resulting code is instantaneous and, under certain conditions, can be absolutely optimal. Ambiguity occurs when a decision regarding the selection of the equiprobable partition must be made when the two groups are not distributed exactly equally (i.e., 50:50). Hence, the Huffman algorithm is usually selected over Shannon-Fano methods.

The Lempel-Ziv algorithm is a more recent development and represents a minor departure from the previous "historical" code generation/encoding techniques. Here, initial code assignments are made without analysis of the image histogram; therefore, one would expect an inefficient non-optimal code at this point, which is true. The optimality is recovered as the data values are because a history of sequences of source symbols is generated. As previously occurring sequences are subsequently encountered, a new code is generated to represent that source sequence. Thus a block encoding of the data is performed that is initially inefficient and non-optimal but becomes increasingly optimal as the source data are processed. Of course, if histogram analysis in multiple dimensions were added to the basic algorithm, its performance properties would be improved, but its on-line capability would be lost.

The Lempel-Ziv algorithm represents further an on-line adaptive method whereby source data sequences are detected during the encoding process. This adaption leads to a minimization of the resulting average code lengths to near optimal performance. The concept of adaption can also be introduced into the Huffman encoding procedure in a variety of ways. Whereas the usual Huffman code construction algorithm is implemented on a byte-by-byte basis, an easy adaptive extension is to examine both single-byte and two-byte combinations. This results in a compromise algorithm based upon the single dimension histogram and portions of the two-dimensional histogram. This concept can be extended to higher dimensions, but the user must be wary of space considerations of algorithm implementation.

The performance of these encoding methods for the residuals was measured over the medical image classes presented in Table 1. (Refer to Table 4.) Here, image sequences of fixed file length (here,128 kilobytes/file) were compressed/encoded. The resulting file length as a percentage of the initial file length was recorded as well as the encode/decode time. The encoding procedures were implemented in software; thus, the timing information should be regarded as suspect.

Table 4. Encoding Algorithms

| Algorithm | Resulting File Size | Timing (sec) Encode | Decode |
|---|---|---|---|
| Huffman (single byte) | 38.0% | 2.3 | 3.4 |
| Huffman (Adaptive) | 38.0% | 23.6 | 16.8 |
| Lempel-Ziv | 31.0% | 2.9 | 1.9 |

## DISCUSSION AND CONCLUSIONS

For a typical SPECT brain study (I-123 HIPDM, 120 images, 64 x 64 x 16 bits, 5.5 million counts total), direct Huffman encoding achieved an average storage of 4.37 bits/pixel. Autoregressive reduction of the signal variance reduced this storage requirement to less than 3.5 bits/pixel. This value essentially represents the noise entropy and cannot be reduced further without abandoning error-free coding methods.

If a not-quite-error-free coding method is desirable, then several approaches are available to the investigator. Rebinning the histogram of residuals appears to be a natural approach; however, we have not explored this method fully at this time. We are doing so currently.

## REFERENCES

Gallagher RG, "A simple derivation of the coding theorem and some applications", IEEE Trans Inform. Theory, IT-11:3-18, 1965
Gallagher RG, "Variations on a theme of Huffman", IEEE Trans Inform Theory, IT-24:668-674, 1978
Huffman DA, "A method for the construction of minimum redundancy codes", Proc. IRE, 40:1098-1101, 1952

Kashyap RL and Rao AR, <u>Dynamic Stochastic Models from Empirical Data</u>, Academic Press, New York, (chapter VIII), 1976

Thomas JB, <u>Statistical Communication Theory</u>, John Wiley and Sons, New York, (chapter 8), 1969

Todd-Polropek AE, Chan C and Appledorn CR, "Image data compression techniques applicable to image networks", In <u>Information Processing in Medical Imaging</u>. S. L. Bacharach (ed.), Martinus Nijhoff Publishers, Dordrecht/Boston, pp. 522-536, 1986

Welch TA, "A technique for high performance data compression", <u>IEEE Computer</u>, 17:8-19, 1984

# LOSS-LESS IMAGE COMPRESSION IN DIGITAL ANGIOGRAPHY

J.H Peters[1], P. Roos[1,2], M.C.A. van Dijke[1,2], and M.A. Viergever[2]

1. Philips Medical Systems Division, Best, The Netherlands
2. Delft University of Technology, The Netherlands

ABSTRACT.

In this paper the performance of several data compression techniques on angiographic images is investigated. Data compression is restricted to loss-less intraframe algorithms. Data compression involves two subsequent steps, decorrelation and coding.

Various decorrelation methods are described and their performances are measured in terms of entropy. Because Huffman coding in general approaches these entropy numbers to within a few percent, coding is not investigated seperately. It is shown that a hierarchical decorrelation method based on interpolation outperforms all other methods considered.

## INTRODUCTION

Digital angiography is a tool for imaging blood vessels and cardiac chambers. Because vessels provide no contrast with X-rays, contrast media (usually iodinated solutions) are injected to opacify the vessels under study. Historically, all recordings were made on large area film ( typically 30x40 cm). Because of its limited dynamic range and restricted potential for image manipulation, film is rather ineffective in displaying poorly opacified vessels (Verhoeven, 1981).

Digital angiography systems as they are now manufactured are basically a conventional image-intensifier television chain interfaced to a digital video processor. As an example of processing, a pre-injection image can be subtracted to remove disturbing overlaying tissue and bone structures.

Current DSA systems can process and store up to 3 images/second of $512^2$ x 10 bit resolution for a total of 1000 images, sufficient for one day or about 10 patients. At the end of each day, hard copies (typically on 20x25 cm films) of selected subtraction images are made from each patient study and retained with the patient file. In some studies, for instance of the heart, a higher acquisition rate is needed and images are stored in subtracted form on an analogue disk (up to 30 images/second, total of 500 images). These may be transferred to 35 mm film for archival.

Three important aspects to improve future equipment are:
- higher resolution; this involves many parameters, including an upgrade of the image matrix size, e.g. $1024^2$ pixels/image.
- higher acquisition rates; some applications may desire even 100 images/second,
- full digital archiving.

Straightforward multiplication would require either 3 optical disks or 19 IBM 3480 cartridges per patient with a recording time of about 4 hours or 20 minutes respectively! The need for compression in order to improve storage capacity and speed may be obvious.

The present research project seeks to investigate the applicability of various data compression algorithms to digital angiography. The scope of the research project is limited by two constraints:

1. Compression should be loss-less. In this way, discussion with radiologists on the subject to what degree lossy coding is acceptable can be prevented. It enables an objective comparison of compression algorithms on the basis of their efficiency only. Although objective criteria also exist in lossy coding (e.g. Mean-Square-Error distortion), opinions diverge about the relevance of such measures to image quality. Since image quality arguments do not apply to loss-less coding, they cannot possibly delay the implementation of these compression algorithms in future equipment.

   A second reason for this restriction is that the images are submitted to some post-processing such as enhancement and subtraction which tend to enlarge degradation.

2. Compression is applied at the interface to the storage medium. This implies intraframe compression of 'raw' digital image data, which is completely defined within the present DSA equipment.

How To Compress Data?

A common characteristic of digital images is that neighbouring pixels are highly correlated. To store the image straightforwardly is therefore inefficient: most of the encoded data are redundant. Data compression aims to reduce this redundancy by a two step-procedure. The first step is to transform the correlated raw data into a set of approximately decorrelated data.

In the second step the data are coded with a Variable Length Coder (VLC), for instance a Huffmann code. Such a VLC exploits the 'peaked-ness' of the histogram by assigning short code words to frequently occuring amplitudes and longer code words to others. Optimally the codelength distribution must be inversely proportional to the logarithm of the histogram sequences.

In this paper we concentrate ourselves on the comparison of different reversible decorrelation methods.

336

## DECORRELATION METHODS

In this section we discuss methods to decorrelate digital images, with emphasis on their reversibility. The methods are divided into three classes: transform coding, predictive coding, and hierarchical coding.

### Transform Coding

A block transform can be represented as a matrix multiplication, $F = T.f.T^t$, where f is a block of the original input image, F a block of the decorrelated image and T the transformation matrix. The Karhunen-Loeve decorrelation transform (see Rosenfeld and Kak, 1982) is optimal in the sense that it generates transform coefficients that are completely uncorrelated. This KL-transform however, has the disadvantage that for every image the autocovariance matrix has to be evaluated together with its eigenvalues and eigenvectors. In this section several other transforms that require less computational effort are discussed.

**Walsh-Hadamard Transform.** The classical one-dimensional Walsh-Hadamard transform (WHT) and its inverse can be built up from the matrix $H = \frac{1}{\sqrt{2}} \cdot \begin{pmatrix} 1 & 1 \\ 1 & -1 \end{pmatrix}$.
A loss-less transformation can only be obtained if the normalisation coefficient $\frac{1}{\sqrt{2}}$ is shifted to the inverse transform.
The matrix transform reads in simple equations: $y_0 = x_0 + x_1$, $y_1 = x_0 - x_1$ where $x_0$ and $x_1$ are integer input values. Since $y_0$ and $y_1$ are both odd or both even, one of the Least Significant Bits (LSB) can be deleted. This results in a maximal gain of one bit per two coefficients $y_0$ and $y_1$.
In practice this principle is applied to two dimensional blocks of 4x4, 8x8 and 16x16 pixels.

**Discrete Cosine Transform.** The Discrete Cosine Transform is known in the literature as an efficient transform which closely approximates the KL-transform in its energy compaction properties (decorrelation). The DCT is defined as

$$F(u,v) = \frac{2}{N} C(u,v) \sum_{i=0}^{N-1} \sum_{j=0}^{N-1} f(i,j) \cos\left(\frac{(2i+1)u\pi}{2N}\right) \cos\left(\frac{(2j+1)v\pi}{2N}\right)$$

where $c(u,v) = \frac{1}{2}$     $u = v = 0$

$$= \frac{1}{\sqrt{2}} \quad u = 0, \quad v = 1, 2.....N-1$$
$$v = 0, \quad u = 1, 2.....N-1$$

$$= 1 \quad u = 1, 2....N-1$$
$$v = 1, 2....N-1$$

The transform produces real-valued coefficients which have to be quantised (rounded off) first before coding. This quantisation introduces errors in the reconstruction process. These errors can be

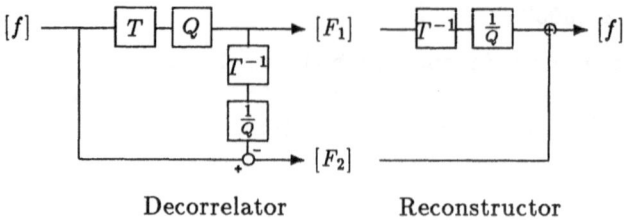

Decorrelator                Reconstructor

Fig.1. The reversible DCT; $T$ is the DCT,
$Q$ is the scaling and rounding off operator

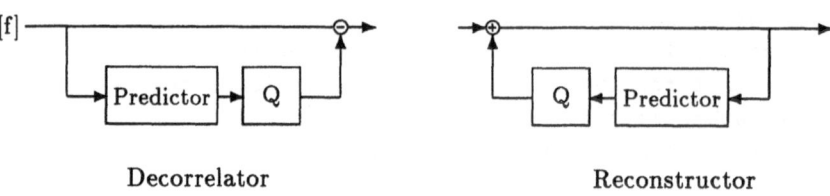

Decorrelator                Reconstructor

Fig.2. Construction and reconstruction of the reversible DPCM

made arbitrary small by increasing the quantisation accuracy. However long before reaching an almost loss-less condition the compression efficiency will have dropped severely. A solution to this problem is adopted here in additionally transmitting the transformation errors, see Fig.1. The entropy of this error signal increases if the quantisation accuracy is reduced. An optimum can be found as will be shown later on.

Predictive Coding

Differential Pulse Code Modulation. An easy to implement and often used data compression technique is Differential Pulse Code Modulation (DPCM) (See Biemond, 1982). The two dimensional DPCM equations are:

Predictor:    $\hat{f}(i,j) = \sum_{p,q \in \Omega} a(p,q).f(i-p,j-q)$

Differential signal:    $F(i,j) = f(i,j) - \hat{f}(i,j)$

where $\Omega$ is the window from which the real coefficients $a(p,q)$ are taken from the two dimensional image plane ($X$ is the position of the pixel to be predicted):
$$\left( \begin{array}{ccc} a(i-1,j-1) & a(i-1,j) & a(i-1,j+1) \\ a(i,j-1) & X & \end{array} \right).$$

A block diagram of the DPCM technique that realises the decorrelation is presented in Fig.2.

Minimising the variance of the differential signal $F(i,j)$ by varying the weighting coefficients $a(p,q)$ results in a set of orthonormal equations: Yule-Walker equations. The solution of this set of equations can be obtained assuming the image has an exponentially decaying autocovariance function with correlation coefficent $\rho$ (See Biemond, 1982). For a three point window (obtained by setting

338

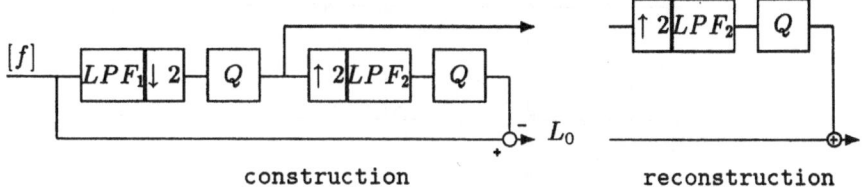

construction                    reconstruction

Fig.4. Construction and reconstruction of the lower level
of the Laplacian Pyramid.

## Hierarchical Coding

Hierarchical coding is a class of decorrelation methods in which the
decorrelation is built up in several steps. Each step generates a
higher level with a lower resolution. This decomposition allows
progressive transmission and reconstruction: first the lowest
resolution image is received (highest level) and subsequently the next
levels of the hierarchical datastructure (pyramid) add finer detail to
the image.

Laplacian Pyramid. The Laplacian Pyramid is a hierarchical
datastructure with many applications, for instance in pattern
recognition and texture analysis ( Burt and Adelson, 1983). The
pyramid is based on splitting the frequencies of the input image into
several bands. Consider Fig.4 which represents the construction of the
lower level of the pyramid.

By means of low-pass filter LPF1, the high frequencies are
suppressed and subsequently sampling is decreased by a factor of 2 in
each direction ($\downarrow 2$). On one end this signal is used to re-estimate the
original image by means of upsampling and interpolation. The
difference to the original can be coded directly. On the other end
this signal is used as an input for the next stage of filtering and
subsampling, and so on. The high frequencies, naturally corresponding
to high resolutions, are stored in the lower levels of the pyramid and
the lower frequencies in the higher levels.

Hierarchical Interpolation. In Hierarchical Interpolation (HINT)
(See Endoh and Yamazaki (1986), first a subsampled version of the
original image is transmitted (see in Fig.5 :  $\odot$ ).

The decorrelation is hierarchical: in the second step the
intermediate pixels (the $\bigcirc$'s) are estimated by interpolation of 4
surrounding $\odot$ pixels. This estimation is subtracted from the actual
pixel value, and the difference which will usually be very small is
subsequently coded. Now the X pixels can be estimated using $\odot$ and $\bigcirc$,
and so on for $\square$ and · successively.

S-transform. The Sequential-transform is an extension of the WHT.
The first level consists of a WHT with blocksize 2x2. In the second
level the DC-coefficients (DC-coefficient is the first coefficient of
each block) are processed again with the same WHT, in the third level

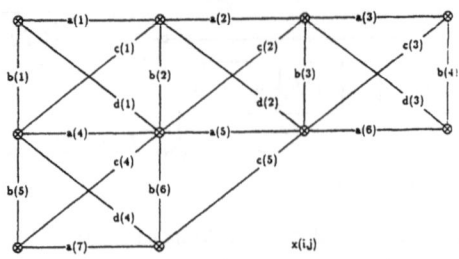

Fig.3 Window with contour directions,
where a(r),b(r),c(r),d(r) are
the differences in corresponding directions.

$a(i-1, j+1) = 0)$, this gives the following class of predictors:

$$\hat{f}(i,j) = \rho.f(i, j-1) + \rho.f(i-1, j) - \rho^2.f(i-1, j-1)$$

In this class of predictors the correlation coefficient $\rho$ is a parameter, which usually has a value around 0.95. The predictor can be symbolically denoted by $\begin{pmatrix} -\rho^2 & \rho \\ \rho & f(i,j) \end{pmatrix}$

Adaptive DPCM. By adapting the coefficients $a(p,q)$ in the prediction equation in DPCM to changing local statistics, it is possible to exploit the presence of potential contours in the image. Determination of the variable coefficients is based on the previously coded information, See Heiss (1986) and Zschunke (1986). We try to locate the presence of possible contours by calculating, in several directions, the differences in pixel greyvalues. If the differences in a certain direction are large, a contour in this direction can be assumed. Having detected such a contour, the corresponding coefficient $s_k$ is diminished. From the window as shown in Fig.3 the differences in four directions can be calculated : a is the east-west direction (-), b the north-south (|), c the southwest-northeast (/) and d the southeast-northwest (\).

The adaptive prediction coefficients are calculated from the differences as follows:

$$s_k = \sum_r \frac{1}{k^3(r) + \Delta} \qquad k = a, b, c, d$$

The coefficients $s_k$ are normalised such that $s_a + s_b + s_c + s_d = 1$ (no energy is removed or added). The estimation now becomes:

$$\hat{f}(i,j) = s_a.f(i, j-1) + s_b.f(i-1, j) + s_c.f(i-1, j+1) + s_d.f(i-1, j-1)$$

Analogously with DPCM the difference $f(i,j) - \hat{f}(i,j)$ is transmitted/stored. The purpose of $\Delta$ is to avoid 'division by zero' in the algorithm. The choice of the value of $\Delta$ effects the compression efficiency.

340

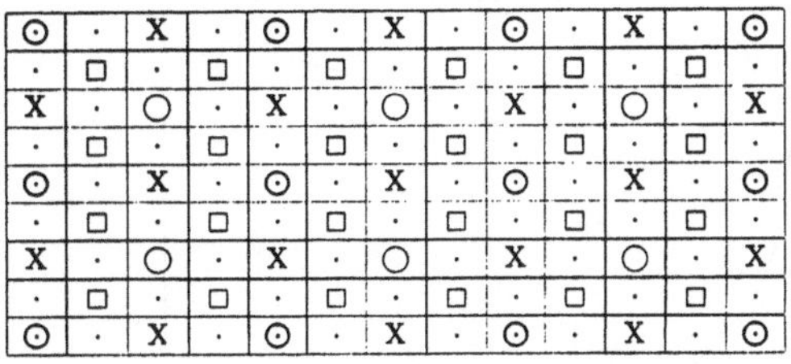

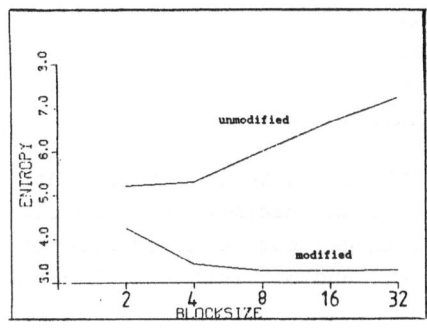

Fig.5 Classification of the pixels in
Hierarchical Interpolation.

Fig.6

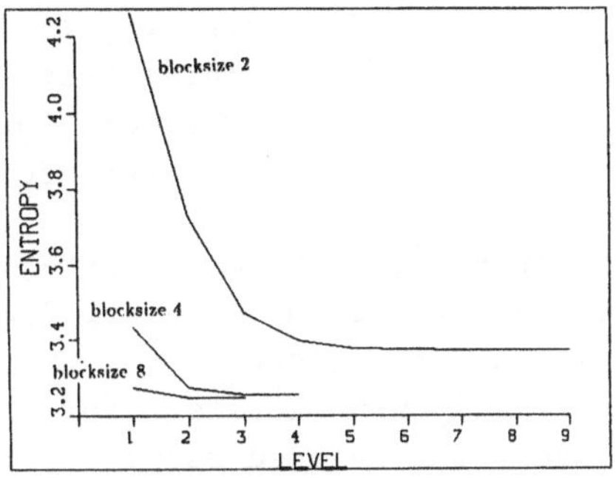

Fig.7

Fig.6 Entropy of series B-images decorrelated using the WHT with
and without modification.

Fig.7 Entropy of series B-images decorrelated using the WH/S transform,
blocksize 2,4,8

the DC-coefficients of the second level are processed, and so on. The
S-transform can be further extended using any NxN WH-matrix.

RESULTS

The above described decorrelation methods are tested on two
different series of angiographic images of the heart. The images all
have a size of 512x512 and are digitised into 8 (series A) and 9
(series B) bits per pixel (bpp), respectively. The next sections
contain the results of the tests on series B (averaged) where in the
conclusions the optimal results of both series are presented.

Walsh-Hadamard- and S-Transform

To show what influence deleting one of the two LSB's of the WHT has
on the decorrelation performance, the entropy for different blocksizes
is plotted in Fig.6.

In the WHT presented here, modified or not modified, the blocksize
dependent scaling coefficient which is normally divided over the
forward and inverse transform, is put only in the inverse transform.
It is therefore that the entropy of the unmodified WHT increases for
large blocks.

The WHT can be regarded as an S-transform with only one level. The

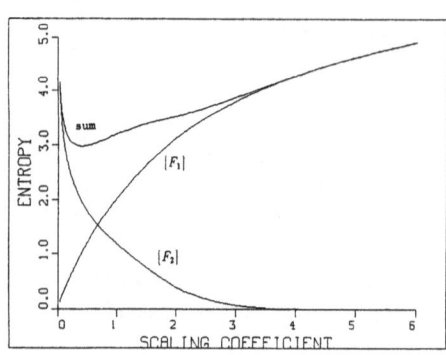

Fig.8 Entropy of the image decorre-
lated using the loss-less
Discrete Cosine Transform.
See text for further details.

influence of further decorrelation of the DC coefficients for various
blocksizes is shown in Fig.7 as a function of the decomposition level.
With a basic blocksize of 2x2, our 512x512 images can be decomposed in
maximally nine levels.  For blocksizes of 4x4 and 8x8 four and three
levels can be used respectively.

Discrete Cosine Transform

In Fig.8 the entropy of the DCT transform itself ($[F_1]$) as well as
the difference signal ($[F_2]$) are given as a function of the transform
quantisation accuracy.  $q = 1$ corresponds to the usual normalisation
practice wherein forward and backward transforms are equally normalised
and coefficients are rounded off to integer values.

The entropy of the DCT signal increases with increasing quantisation
accuracy while the difference signal will diminish.  At $q = 4$ the
difference entropy has almost become zero, however actual measurements
demanded $q = 8$ to obtain fully loss-less compression!  The 'sum' entropy
for $q = 8$ is however much larger than the optimum of 2.97 bit.

A problem for this DCT occurs when the signals $[F_1]$ and $[F_2]$ have to
be Huffman coded.  Because code words are assigned with integer
lenghts, coding inefficiency is large for small entropy signals
(usually below 2 bits coding efficiency drops very fast).  The entropy
numbers may therefore be somewhat misleading.

Differential Pulse Code Modulation

In the literature (Biemond, 1982), a particular class of predictors
incorporating only one parameter $\rho$ is defined as follows:
$$a_1 = -\rho^2 \quad a_2 = \rho \quad a_3 = 0 \quad a_4 = \rho \text{ where } \Omega : \begin{pmatrix} a_1 & a_2 & a_3 \\ a_4 & x & . \end{pmatrix}.$$
These predictors are known as solutions of Yule-Walker equations.  The
entropy is minimal for $\rho$ around 0.95, but it varies only slightly.
Also a number of arbitrary other predictors is tested.  It appeared
that $\begin{pmatrix} -0.5 & 0.5 & 0.25 \\ 0.75 & x & . \end{pmatrix}$ is better then the best Yule-Walker predictor.
This predictor however can be approximated by a YW predictor with

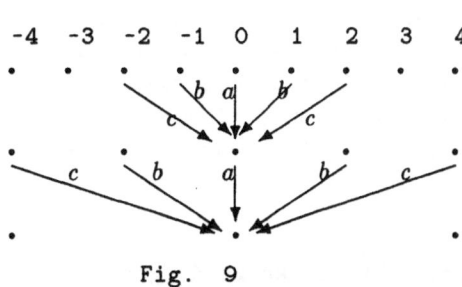

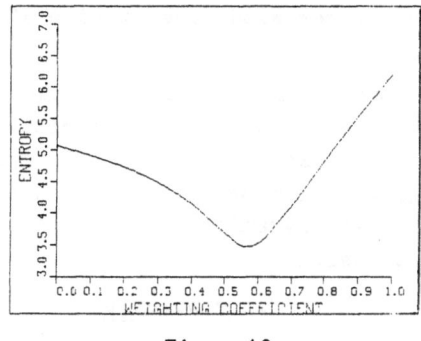

Fig. 9                                    Fig. 10

Fig.9 One-dimensional low-pass filter used in the Laplacian Pyramid.
Fig.10 Entropy results of varying the weighting coefficient in the
       Laplacian Pyramid.

$\rho = 0.75$ which is scaled such that the total sum equals 1:
$\begin{pmatrix} -0.6 & 0.8 & 0 \\ 0.8 & x & . \end{pmatrix}$ This predictor gave an entropy of 2.75, e.g. better
then all other YW-equations with $\rho$ around 0.95 but is worse then the
former predictor by 0.003 bit. The assumption that the image
autocorrelation function fitted the exponential model for $\rho \approx 0.95$
appears to be justified. Therefore the exponential model itself seems
not optimal for this kind of images.

Adaptive DPCM

    The effect of changing the parameter $\Delta$ around its optimal value (=
8) in ADPCM is negligible: the method turns out to be rather
insensitive to $\Delta$, for $4 \leq \Delta \leq 12$. For the first series of images,
non-adaptive DPCM with optimal correlation coefficients in the
YW-equation is slightly better then adaptive DPCM. For the other series
which incorporates more noise, however, adaptive DPCM is substantially
better: DPCM does not perform well on noisy images. Adaptive DPCM has
a more globale prediction scheme and can therefore compensate for this
noise by increasing $\Delta$.

    The way in wich the coeficents a,b,c and d are calculated can be
changed. Also the power of $k(r)$ can be changed. All these
modifications appeared to have no significant (positive nor negative)
effect on the entropy.

Laplacian Pyramid

    In implementing the Laplacian Pyramid a separable two dimensional
low-pass filter is used. In Fig.9 this filter is shown in one
dimension only. This low-pass filter w(n) contains one degree of
freedom: $w(0) = a$, $w(\pm 1) = b = \frac{1}{4}$, $w(\pm 2) = c = \frac{1}{4} - \frac{a}{2}$. In the following
plot (Fig.10) the entropy is given as a function of $a$.
    Since the Laplacian Pyramid did not perform well on the angiographic
images in contradiction to our expectations, it has been further
investigated. Optimising the low-pass filters by using sinc-functions

with proper windowing of size 128x128 did not lead to a considerable decrease in entropy.

The algorithm increases the number of samples by a factor of $\frac{4}{3}$, which turns out to be prohibitive to reach a high compression factor. Therefore we changed the subsample factor from 2 to 3, but results were negative also because of a decrease in decorrelation performance. The Laplacian Pyramid seems therefore not well suited for loss-less data compression.

## Hierarchical Interpolation

The HINT algorithm as presented above, with blocksize 4, gave an entropy of 2.74 bit. The method can be extended by enlarging the blocksize. This modification resulted in an entropy gain of 0.1 bit.

## CHOICE OF THE BLOCKSIZE

In transform compression the image is divided into blocks and each block is transformed separately because of simplicity and calculation time. The transform coefficients are VLC coded according to their statistics. These coding tables must be stored together with the coded transformed coeffients. The number of coding look-up tables equals the number of pixels within one block. For large blocks this implies a lot of histograms and therefore a lot of code tables. For large blocksizes, the extra decorrelation as a consequence of enlarging the blocksize is offset by the storage of the extra code tables.

Experiments have shown that the storage of the code tables dominates the extra decorrelation for blocksize 32 and larger. Presenting entropy numbers where blocks of 32 or larger are used in the decorrelation is therefore not relevant. In general, blocksize 8x8 is sufficient; larger blocksizes do not add to the decorrelation significantly.

## CONCLUSIONS

## Comparison of Decorrelation Methods

In Fig.11 all the decorrelation methods presented in this paper are compared with respect to their (optimal) performances. The lowest curve represents the entropy of the decorrelation methods with optimal parameters applied to the images from series B (9 bits, low noise). The upper curve represents the entropy numbers for series A (8 bits, noisy). For the DCT results for series A can be improved slightly by optimising the scaling coefficient $q$ towards $q = 0.1$ (see point x in Fig.11).

Taking into account other important aspects of decorrelation methods, besides the compression factors, we draw the following conclusions.

- The Laplacian Pyramid is not useful in reversible data compression of angiographic images; it cannot make up for the additional storage needed for the low-pass images.

344

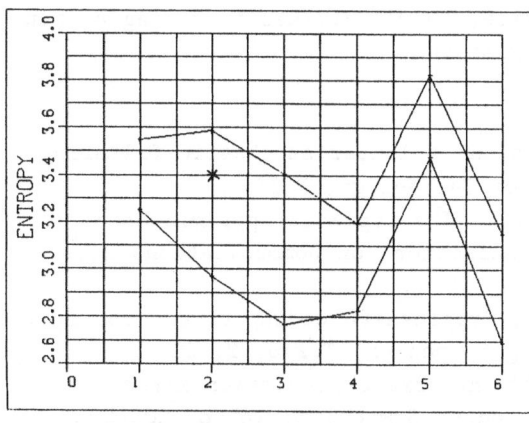

Fig.11 Overview of decorrelation results

1:   S-transform
     (blocksize 4x4, 4 levels)
2:   DCT (blocksize 8x8, q=0.4)
3:   DPCM ( $\rho$ = 0.95)
4:   ADPCM
5:   Laplacian Pyramid (a=0.6)
6:   HINT

- The WHT and S-transforms decorrelate insufficiently, even if the LSB dependency, created by the butterfly structure, is eliminated.

- The error-free DCT decorrelates well and results in low entropies, divided over two signals.  Actually coding the two signals requires another type of coding algorithm than a VLC since a VLC is inefficient for coding low entropy signals.  The DCT must be adapted to the image statistics to reach optimal results.

- DPCM methods approximate the decorrelation of the reversible DCT, there is however the major disadvantage of its sensitivity to channel errors.

- HINT appears to decorrelate best.  Other advantages of this algorithm are its simplicity, the absence of parameters and its low sensitivity to noise.

    Loss-less intraframe compression has turned out to be, despite the restrictions, a useful tool in storing and transmitting angiographic images.  For our two series of medical images loss-less compression restricts to a factor of about 3.

Future Investigations

    The experiments have been performed on angiographic images only. The performance on other kinds of images, e.g.  from Magnetic Resonance or Computer Tomography equipment will be investigated subsequently. For those applications demanding a substantially higher compression factor, the loss-less requirement must be dropped.

    Another interesting extension to the procedure is to consider not just single images but sets of images, either in three dimensions or in time.  No significant improvements can be expected if loss-less compression is required due to uncorrelated image noise but a large gain may be expected for lossy coding.

    For low-entropy signals, for instance the DCT transmission components, Huffman coding is not very efficient, so other coding

techniques such as Rice coding (Rice, 1979), arithmetic coding or run
length coding may be worthwhile examining.

REFERENCES

Biemond, J. (1982), Image restoration; a linear stochastic filtering
    approach, Delft University of Technology, Delft.
Burt, P.J. and Adelson, E.H. (1983).  The Laplacian pyramid as a
    compact image code, IEEE Transactions on Communications 31,
    532-540.
Endoh, T. and Yamazaki, Y. (1986), Progressive coding scheme for multi
    level images, Picture Coding Symposium, Tokyo, 21-22.
Heiss, R. (1986), An adaptive DPCM intraframe prediction method
    without switching, Picture Coding Symposium, Tokyo, 202-203.
Rice, R.F. (1979), Practical universal noiseless coding, SPIE
    vol.  207, Applications of Digital Image Processing III.
Rosenfeld, A. and Kak, A.C. (1982), Digital picture processing,
    2nd edition, Academic Press, Vol.1 Chapter 5, New York.
Verhoeven, L. (1981), Comparison of enhancement capabilities of film
    subtraction and digital subtraction methods, SPIE vol.  314,
    Digital Radiography.
Zschunke, W. (1986), Private discussions at Picture Coding Symposium,
    Tokyo.

# Display & Workstations

# A NETWORKED WORKSTATION APPROACH TO MULTI-DIMENSIONAL BIOMEDICAL IMAGE ANALYSIS

R. A. Robb, M. C. Stacy, and C. N. McEwan

Biodynamics Research Unit
Mayo Foundation
Rochester, MN  55905

## INTRODUCTION

The capability to extract objective and quantitatively accurate information from multi-dimensional biomedical images has not kept pace with the capabilities to produce the images themselves. This is a paradox, since on the one hand the new 3-D and 4-D imaging capabilities promise significant potential for providing greater specificity and sensitivity (i.e., precise objective discrimination and accurate quantitative measurement of body tissue characteristics and function) in clinical diagnostic and basic investigative imaging procedures than ever possible before, but on the other hand, the momentous advances in computer and associated electronic imaging technology which have made these 3-D imaging modalities possible have not been concomitantly developed for full exploitation of their capabilities. We have developed a network approach which integrates powerful new microcomputer-based systems and permits detailed investigations and evaluation of 3-D and 4-D (dynamic 3-D) biomedical images. The network features an "intelligent" manager for efficient allocation of resources and ready access to all the information in a large 3-D image data base for rapid display, manipulation, and measurement. The system software provides important capabilities for displaying, manipulating and quantitatively analyzing both structural and functional data and their relationships in various organs of the body. Although the overall power of the system comes from the synergistic integration and utilization of networked components, the architecture permits and has fostered development of advanced image processing software which is transportable to a variety of stand-alone workstations.

## BACKGROUND

Multi-dimensional imaging has become widely used in both biomedical research and clinical applications (Robb, 1985). At the microscopic level, 2-D images of cells and tissues are produced by both manual and computerized microscopes. Optical and electron microscopy allow the scanning of adjacent slices so that a 3-D image may be obtained (Jimenez et al., 1986). X-ray diffraction crystallography results in 2-D images which may be used to deduce 3-D structures (Durbin et al., 1986). On a larger scale, several diagnostic and research modalities used in medicine provide various types of multi-dimensional images. Positron Emission Tomography (PET) produces volume images of the distribution of a radioisotope within the body (Kehtarnavaz et al., 1984). Thermography obtains 2-D images of the temperature distribution at the surface of the body (Rao and Shah, 1984). Projection angiography collects 2-D slices which integrate the information from a volume, so that isolated 3-D structures such as vessels can be identified by the use of a small number of different views of the volume (Barillot et al., 1985). Magnetic Resonance Imaging (MRI) allows the direct collection of 3-D images or sequences of 2-D slices through an organ (Herman et al., 1982). Conventional B-mode ultrasound provides 2-D reflection images of tissue interfaces. Time sequential images are routinely used clinically for observing moving structures such as the heart. With appropriate positional information, a 3-D volume can also be obtained by sweeping the volume with the transducer (Harris et al., 1980; Matsumoto et al., 1981). X-ray Computed Tomography (CT) is also routinely used for collecting 2-D images of the body. This modality also lends itself to the collection of serial parallel sections which span a region of interest (Bloch and Udupa, 1983). The head and neck are routinely studied in 3-D by CT for the planning of cranio-facial surgery (Marsh and Vannier, 1983; Jackson and Bite, 1986). The physiology of the brain and eye have been studied in 3-D from serial sections (Toga and Arnicar, 1985; Schwartz and Merker, 1986). Bony structures such as the spine (Rhodes et al., 1984), and limbs (Rhodes et al., 1985) have been developed using conventional serial slice CT. Such studies facilitate the design of implantable prostheses. Conventional CT is also used for radiotherapy treatment planning (Bloch and Udupa, 1983).

Clinical applications have generally been limited to the study of stationary organs. However, the increasing use of fast CT is spurring the study of dynamic objects, such as musculo-skeletal interactions in the limbs (Robbin et al., 1986), and the physiology of the lungs (Hoffman and Heffernan, 1985), heart (Hoffman and Ritman, 1985), and stomach (Seide and Ritman, 1984).

Most approaches for displaying and analyzing 2-D, 3-D, and 4-D images aim to provide interactive viewing of both 2-D and 3-D images in a unified environment (Fuchs and Pizer, 1984). One of the simplest tasks, and often the most useful approach, is to display isolated 2-D slices from a 3-D or 4-D data-set on a conventional 2-D display. There has been much work on the faithful presentation of 2-D images (Pizer et al., 1984). In addition, software approaches for displaying and analyzing 3-D images present to the user some sort of 2-D representation of the volume. As yet, there are few techniques particularly designed to handle 3-D or 4-D images directly. The usual approach has been to consider such images as a sequence of separate 2-D images. Both hardware and software techniques have been developed for displaying 3-D volumes, but generally have not provided full quantitative analysis capabilities (such as editing and mensuration).

Some hardware approaches for presenting 3-D images include rotating an array of LEDs (Jansson and Kosowsky, 1984), and use of a spinning mirror (Simon, 1977). Hardware for presenting stereo displays has also been developed (Lipton, 1984). Several groups have developed space-filling 3-D displays which are based on a vibrating mirror. The mirrors display either a large number of isolated points throughout the volume (Fuchs et al., 1982; Sher, 1986), or a true 3-D raster (Baxter et al., 1982; Harris and Camp, 1984). Some novel computer hardware has also been designed and built for presenting 3-D images (Fuchs and Pizer, 1984; Hunter, 1984; Goldwasser, 1984). Such hardware is generally optimized for a particular object representation and display algorithm.

Software approaches to the analysis of images have the advantage of independence from a particular hardware configuration. This allows them to be reused on different systems. They may also be implemented in a shorter time and with less effort and cost than a dedicated hardware system. The main disadvantage to software approaches, particularly for large 3-D and 4-D data-sets, is the difficulty in obtaining rapid performance. One of the simplest techniques is to extract 2-D slices from the volume image. These may be oriented along the major body axes (Glenn et al., 1975), or obliquely through the volume (Rhodes et al., 1980; Harris et al., 1978a). Software techniques for conveying 3-D information include integrated projections of the volume onto the display screen, sometimes with prior dissolution of structures from the volume (Harris et al., 1978b), stereo displays generated from projection images (Harris et al., 1978a), and shaded surface display (Hodges and McAllister, 1985; Herman, 1986). One of the most popular techniques for presenting

3-D structures is to use depth-shading of object surfaces. An important precursor to shaded surface display is the extraction of a 3-D surface description from a raw 3-D volume image. This segmentation step is often required not only for display but for measurement as well. However, the segmentation step is an area which is in need of improved algorithms (Heffernan and Robb, 1985b; Pizer et al., 1986), particularly for the extraction of soft tissue structures, and for images such as those produced by MRI and ultrasound. Shaded surface display algorithms for medical applications have been based on conventional polygonal models (Fellingham et al., 1986), a cuberille model for the surface (Herman and Liu, 1977), a contour model for the surface (Heffernan and Robb, 1985a; Fellingham et al., 1986), and an octtree model of the 3-D object (Hunter, 1984).

Integrated systems (workstations) for the analysis of 2-D, 3-D, and 4-D images are beginning to emerge in the commercial and research markets. As yet, there has not appeared any system which has satisfied the needs of both biomedical research and clinical diagnostic applications. The reason for this may be that the focuses of the two areas have been different. The medical imaging systems and hence the commercial image analysis workstations have been targeted at the practice of radiology where it may be sufficient to simply visualize structures within the body. This philosophy has spawned the development of so-called PACS (Picture Archiving and Communications System) (Gray and Rutherford, 1984). Such systems aim to duplicate the capabilities of a film-based radiology department, but without the use of film (Birkner, 1984; News, 1985; Grewer et al., 1985; Risser, 1984). This limited focus has diluted general enthusiasm for such systems, particularly in view of the high cost required to achieve the desired performance. There are now some systems available which are aimed at medical specialties other than radiology. For example, several companies sell workstations or services which are designed for surgery planning (Rhodes et al., 1984; Fuchs and Pizer, 1984; Fellingham et al., 1986). A variety of image analysis workstations have been developed for a range of research applications. These systems vary widely in their goals and capabilities. some of the systems have been designed to handle volume images from a variety of sources, and so could find application in a variety of medical circumstances (Lenz, 1984; Scharnweber and Tonnies, 1984; Oswald, 1985; Goldwasser et al., 1985).

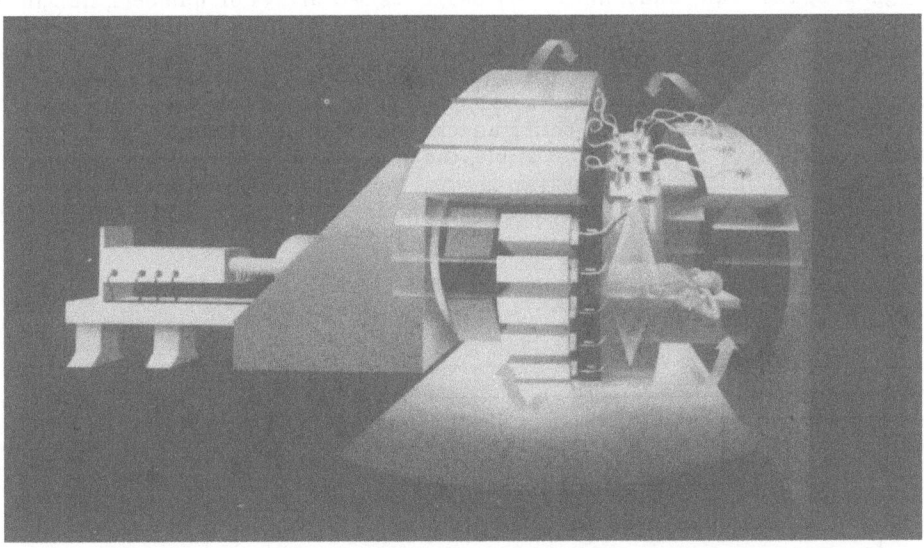

Fig. 1.  Artistic depiction of Dynamic Spatial Reconstructor (DSR), a 4-D image scanner at the Mayo Clinic. (From Raytheon Company. With permission.)

The Biodynamics Research Unit (BRU) at the Mayo Clinic has been involved in the analysis of 3-D and 4-D images since the early 1970's. The successful development of the Dynamic Spatial Reconstructor (Robb, 1983; Ritman et al., 1980), shown diagrammatically in Figure 1, has provided a ready source of 3-D and 4-D imagery from a variety of biomedical investigative and clinical studies which use this device. During this time, several unique and useful analysis techniques have been developed in the BRU. These include projection/dissolution display (Harris et al., 1978b), stereo displays (Harris et al., 1978a), interactive oblique sectioning algorithms (Harris, 1981), shaded surface display algorithms (Heffernan and Robb, 1985a), and space-filling virtual 3-D display using a vibrating mirror system (Harris et al., 1986; Camp et al., (In Press)). Many of these capabilities have been developed on different computer systems as the need for them arose. Recently, these established tools and several new important capabilities have been made applicable to a wide variety of multi-dimensional biomedical images (e.g., CT, MRI, PET, ultrasound, etc.) and integrated into a single comprehensive software package which runs on a dedicated, powerful image analysis workstation (Robb et al., 1986).

SOME PHILOSOPHY

The effective extraction of accurate quantitative information from 3-D and 4-D images requires new-conceptual approaches and methodologies in image processing. As indicated in Figure 2, there are essentially three major tasks associated with any analysis of biomedical imagery: 1) display, 2) editing, and 3) measurement. These tasks are interrelated, often overlapping, and co-exist in a rather classical channel of feed-back, feed-forward information passing. The capabilities of a multi-dimensional image analysis computer system should be fine-tuned to effectively facilitate these tasks and to provide adroit exploration of all relationships (i.e., structural and functional) existing within the data.

The traditional sequential approach to interactive image analysis is illustrated in Panel A of Figure 3. The general purpose of such analysis is to optimize the parameters of some "image transformation", Ti, so that the observer (who applies his own mental transform) can "understand" the image. The critical element of such a concept in both 2-D and 3-D image processing is interactive feedback, allowing the human operator to control some or all of the transformation parameters.

Panel B in Figure 3 includes the image transformation produced by the display. Although computers can "understand" 3-D images as 3-D arrays of numbers, humans cannot usefully understand numerical representations as images. In order to present this numerical information meaningfully to humans, a "display transformation", Td, is introduced into the system. This transformation (which includes both a conceptual and a physical element) may often be as complex as the image transformation, but is in general a better-behaved and better-understood function. Nonetheless, if this transformation is to be as useful as possible, the operator must have control of its parameters as well. The observer evaluates what the transformation has accomplished and if it helps convey and/or elucidate the information desired. This implies

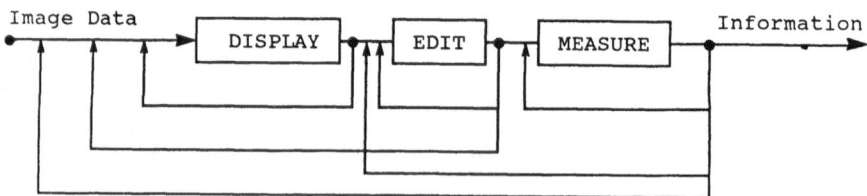

Fig. 2.    Diagram of major processes involved in multi-dimensional image analysis and their feedback relationships.

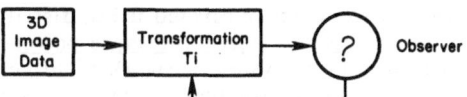

**A. Sequential Single Transformation Model**

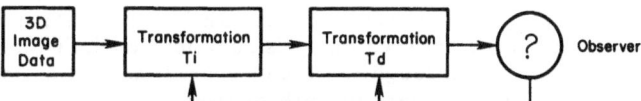

**B. Sequential Multiple Transformation Model**

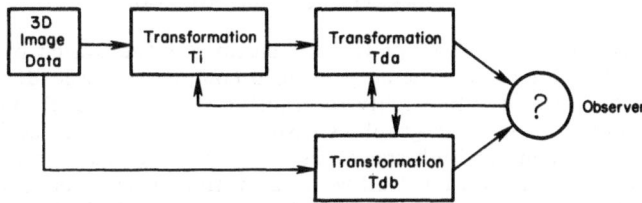

**C. Parallel Multiple Transformation Model**

Fig. 3.    Three conceptual models for interactive display and analysis of 3-D image data. (From Robb et al., 1986. With permission.)

not only that the observer knows what he wants to happen, but that he understands what the transformation actually has done to the original data. In the traditional sequential approach applied to a 3-D medical image, this task is analogous to understanding the three-dimensional structure of an organ by sequentially viewing parallel adjacent slices through the organ, such as is often done in CT imaging. Not only must the observer "know what he wants" (i.e., that these slices together represent an organ with which he is familiar), but he must also mentally reconstruct the separate sectional views of the structure into its complete continuous form.

Panel C of Figure 3 introduces the parallel version of interactive image analysis. In this framework, the importance of understanding the transformation Ti is explicitly addressed by presenting the operator simultaneous "before and after" views of the image. The difference between the sequential and parallel methods may be compared to the difference between driving an automobile toward a given destination with and without a roadmap. Not knowing the route results in a random, time-consuming exercise to get from here to there, while using a roadmap to select the optimal route results in saving of time and reasonable assurance of accuracy in reaching the goal.

The parallel image analysis method includes a divergent case - where Tda and Tdb are conceptually and physically separate. However, conceptually different display methods may be combined on the same physical display device and still fit the model. The central concept is that <u>3-D image analysis is largely an editing task,</u> and efficient tools for permitting data exploration, transformation, and reduction are critical to the effective performance of this task. The important mechanism associated with this concept is that the observer is allowed to interactively modify the image (and display) transformation and be presented a "before and after" view of its effects.

Turning from conceptual to practical considerations, one must recognize that the large volume of data to be processed in multi-modal, multi-dimensional biomedical image analysis requires simultaneous and efficient management of I/O and computation. This may be accomplished through the use of large expansion mainframe systems, but it can, in fact, also be accomplished using distributed processing

frame systems, but it can, in fact, also be accomplished using distributed processing approaches which are concomitantly <u>less expensive and more powerful</u> than single mainframe systems. Attention to design of system network architecture and utilization of current state-of-the-art microprocessor technology, makes this possible. A multi-dimensional image data base can be very large, especially when extended to 4-D (e.g., sets of 3-D images related through time). Therefore, movement of data in the system must take place as efficiently as possible, and data information structures need to be shared between analysis functions to limit the frequency of transfers. This can be done through the use of shared memory segments large enough to hold the entire 3-D image or with software which performs efficient image memory paging. Interactive manipulation of large 3-D images also requires an efficient method for archival image storage and retrieval.

Efficient computation of image transformations is facilitated by maintaining the entire 3-D image in the system memory. Rapid computation and display of the multi-dimensional data permits highly interactive visual feedback mechanisms to guide the analysis process. The graphics display system needs to be integrally interfaced to the system for high-speed transfers of image data and graphics functions. The display resolution must allow, at a minimum, one image at full size to be displayed, along with some other graphics and text, and ideally should allow for multiple image display at full image size with related graphics and/or text included.

Rapid, multi-format image display and highly interactive graphics are crucial to and should be included in all aspects of multi-dimensional image analysis. For this reason, the design of the user interface is extremely important to the success of the system. The user interface should be friendly and intuitive and should be supported by a well-designed (ergonomic) station with conveniently arranged display and input device(s).

BRUNET

The Biodynamics Research Unit (BRU) at the Mayo Clinic conducts basic research in biological structure and function relationships and in computer technology and algorithms for multi-dimensional biomedical image processing, display and analysis. A variety of collaborative research projects within Mayo and with other institutions is carried out. To support these projects, an integrated network of small but powerful computers has recently replaced a central mainframe computer system. Figure 4 is a diagram of this architecture, which is called BRUNET. Three major divisions of a variety of workstations are respectively focused on ultrasound, DSR, and advanced algorithm research. The systems include powerful workstations from SUN Microsystems, Silicon Graphics, and Charles River Data Systems, as well as advanced image procssing systems from Pixar and Kontron Electronics and a robust number cruncher from Masscomp.

An extensive evaluation of computing systems which could be configured into an integrated network to meet the current and projected needs of multi-dimensional image analysis in the BRU was undertaken. This evaluation involved "hands-on" testing and comparison of a variety of state-of-the-art microprocessor-based workstations. The investigation of various vendors products resulted in a configuration of a variety of microprocessor-based systems integrated into a standard network determined to best meet current and projected multi-dimensional image and analysis needs. The SUN 3 computer series from Sun Microsystems was determined to provide the best overall combination of capabilities for both routine data processing and software development. The SUN product line offers excellent software development and maintenance tools. In addition, the SUN systems provide one of the best current UNIX standards to facilitate import/export of software.

All components in the computer network run under the UNIX operating system, and have compatible network file communication protocols (TCP/IP). The overall system can readily grow or shrink simply by adding or deleting components to and from the network as appropriate. Workstations are configured so as to function independently of the network if desired, but can benefit from availability of other resources on the network if connected to it. The file servers can be readily expanded to support an increased number of users and/or programmers. The primary language used is "C", in which all Resource programmers are proficient, but Fortran, Pascal, Lisp, Basic, Forth, and Assembly languages are available and used as required and appropriate.

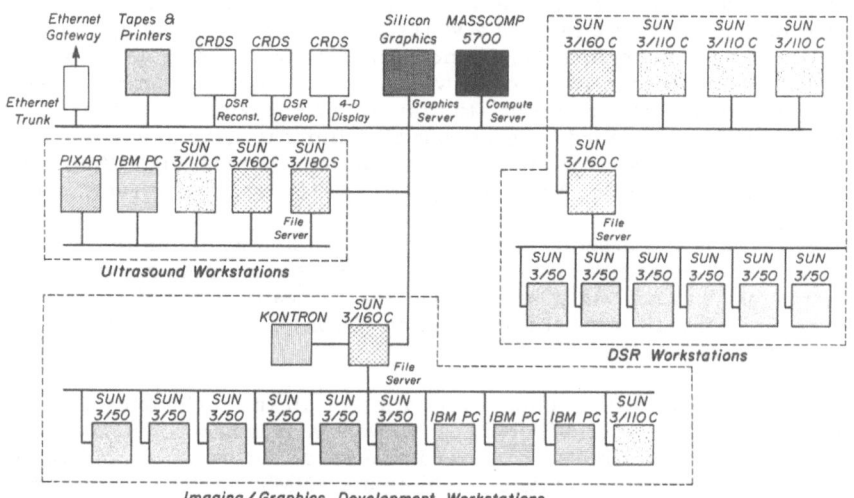

Fig. 4.    Network of multi-dimensional image analysis systems in the Biodynamics Research Unit.

The networking and distributed processiong concepts provide several advantages over even large stand-alone systems:

1.  Software development takes place in an optimized environment.
2.  Dedicated image analysis computers provide high bandwidth between the cpu and the display, a requirement for real-time image processing interactivity.
3.  Compute intensive tasks can be queued and batched on separate processors, avoiding interruption of interactive tasks.
4.  Expensive hardware which has intermittent usage can be shared by all users (examples are printers and array processors).
5.  Redundant software in the network is reduced by shared copies of operating systems and applications code.
6.  System maintenance time is reduced.
7.  All users of the network have "electronic" access to each other, allowing for sharing of data, programs, and even ideas (mail).

The BRUNET system is inter-connected by 10 Mb per second Ethernet cable. There are three separate Ethernet LANs (local area networks) connected together through gateways, allowing all systems to communicate with each other. The network protocol used is TCP/IP, and the workstations use Sun's Network File System (NFS) to provide rapid access to disk files throughout the network.

The SUN 3/50 systems throughout the network are used primarily for software development, providing programmers with multiple windows to view data and programs. In addition, they offer a prototyping capability for images and graphics developed for analysis on the production workstations. The image analysis systems, SUN 3/110s and 3/160s, share identical architectural design, except for color capability, with the 3/50s to permit compilation of application software on software

capability, with the 3/50s to permit compilation of application software on software developer's systems, reducing the cpu load on the analysis system. Software development on the Masscomp and Silicon Graphics systems can also be accomplished on SUN 3/50s through windows logged into those systems.

The Masscomp 5700 system has been designated a compute server in BRUNET. It features dual 68020 processors, each having a high-speed floating point accelerator, a separate 13 Megaflop Vector Accelerator (array processor), and a 380 Mb disk drive. This system performs like a large computer mainframe to accommodate the compute-intensive tasks in the BRU. Jobs which require large disk capacity can be handled in much less time than on a workstation. The Masscomp also serves as a batch processor for the systems on the network, through a "compute daemon" facility. A network daemon is a process which runs continuously on a processor, waiting for requests from the network to provide some service. A compute daemon on the Masscomp can be loaded with various algorithms to serve any of the other tasks on the other systems. Workstation users who require these algorithms are transparently connected to the Masscomp system to efficiently perform the work.

Other functions and programs may be explicitly requested from the compute server. Users working at a workstation can call an interface program to specify a set of parameters, and have them transported automatically to the Masscomp for lengthy computations, allowing the workstation to continue uninterrupted with interactive analysis tasks.

To provide optimal utilization and allocation of all the compute cycles and memory capacity available on BRUNET, a Network Management System (NMS) has been designed. The network may be viewed as a set of common user interfaces connected to a large parallel processor architecture. NMS enables each system in the network to share tasks with any other system in an efficient, transparent way. The scheme is illustrated in Figure 5. Systems requiring service will broadcast requests, indicating the requirements of the service desired, such as memory allocation and cpu time. Any other system in the network which has the required resources and/or services available may respond with a status packet. The calling system may then assign the job to the system which best fulfills the requirements

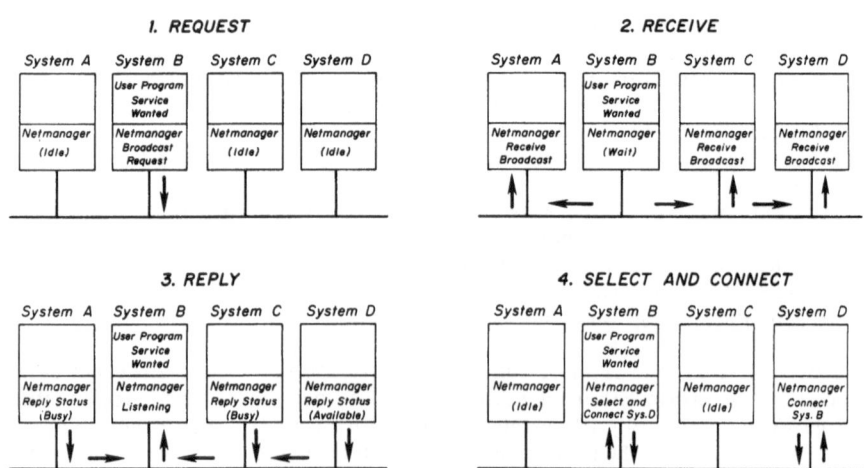

Fig. 5.    Diagram of typical operator cycle of network manager software system: 1) a non-directed request for service is made by one of the systems (system B); 2) the request is received by all systems; 3) a status reply of availability is returned to the requesting system; 4) the system available (system D) is selected and connected to provide the requested service.

of the job. Through careful software design, functions which require intense computation can be distributed throughout the network, and the data then collected back into the calling system. Busy systems have the right to reject jobs, and load changes in any "usurped" system's status cause NMS to "dump" the job back onto the network for another system to handle. In the worst case, if no system resources are available to handle the request, the calling system would compute the task itself.

In summary, the BRUNET configuration is designed to efficiently and cost effectively meet current and projected computing needs in multi-dimensional image processing, with built-in flexibility to accommodate change.

ANALYZE

A variety of multi-dimensional image analysis software modules have been integrated into a comprehensive, highly-interactive and intuitive software system called ANALYZE. This software is written in "C", is well-documented, will run on most standard workstation systems supported by UNIX, and is available from the BRU. The ANALYZE system consists of a hierarchial set of processes, each process representing a particular analysis task, as indicated in Figure 6. The modules share image memory segments and communicate with each other to pass related image information. The integration of these subprocesses allows for multiple analyses where the output of one process may be in the input to another. Image data is input to the system using the *TAPE* and *DISK* processes. Once the data is loaded, *MIRAGE, DISPLAY* and *OBLIQUE* are used to select and orient the data to be analyzed. The *EDIT* and *MANIP* processes allow the user to select, modify, and manipulate (e.g., combine) particular objects or regions of itnerest in the image data. Quantitative measurements and statistical analyses and graphics are made and recorded using the *BIOPSY* module. The results of image editing, manipulation, and measurement can be displayed in various formats including projection display in *PROJECT*, shaded surface display in *SURFACE*, and in a movie formate using the *MOVIE* module.

Several software libraries to support the graphics functions, user interface, image file management, image memory management, and interprocess communication have been developed and are common to all of the ANALYZE modules. A "pop-down" menu structure is used for the operator interface, where only keywords are displayed at the top of the screen with underlying menus displayed when a keyword is selected (using a mouse or tracing tablet).

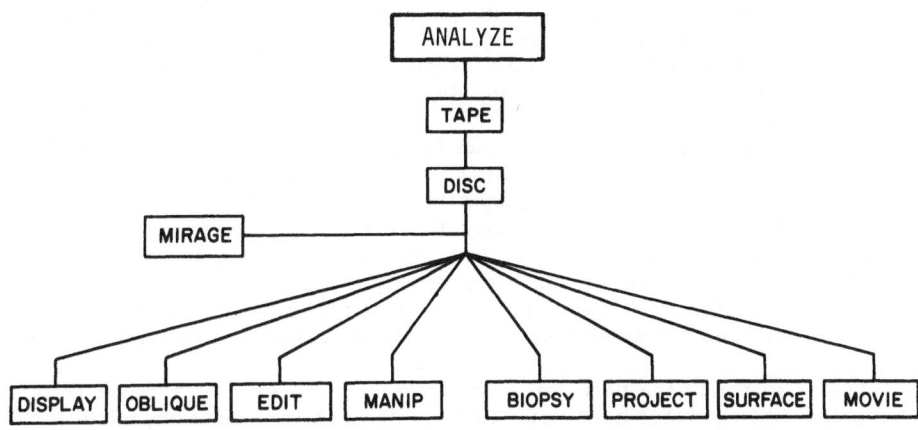

Fig. 6.    Diagram of ANALYZE software system implemented on workstations. (From Robb et al., 1986. With permission.)

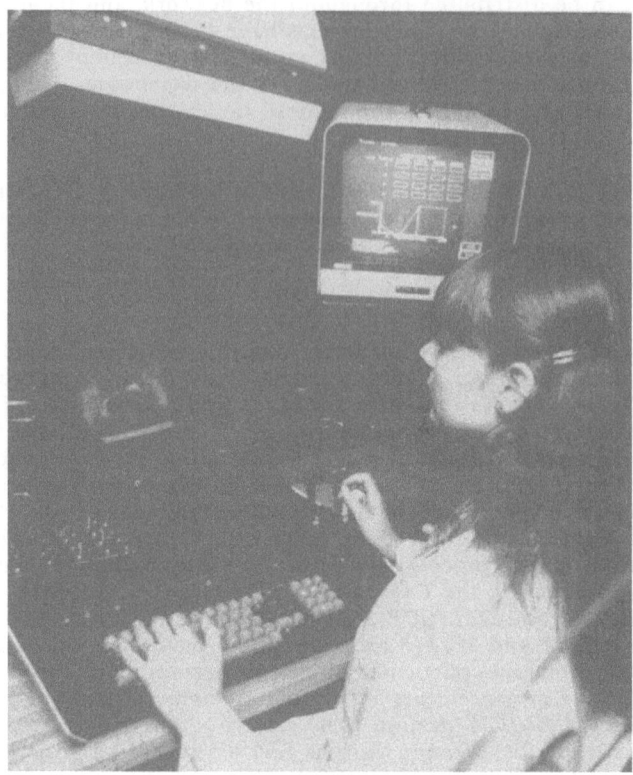

Fig. 7.    Photograph of 3-D image display workstation. (From Robb,
R. A., Proc. CAR '87, pp. 642-656. With permission.)


<u>3-D Display Workstations</u>

The varifocal mirror display system (see Figure 7) attached to the network is
unique in that it is specifically designed to provide high resolution in the 3-D
raster mode (Harris et al., 1986) and is most comparable with the nature of 3-D CT
image data (most other mirror systems are designed for more general "point-
plotting" operations (Fuchs et al., 1982; Sher, 1986; Baxter et al., 1982)). The
system can display a "stack" of 32 CT images every 1/30 sec, providing a true 3-D
representation of the object under study. A look-up table provides interactive
intensity mapping (windowing), and an "overlay volume" permits non-destructive
imposition of graphic constructs into the display.

Several independent software modules for controlling the vari-focal mirror
display are known collectively as *MIRAGE*, which are functionally linked to
ANALYZE. Current 3-D mirror display software provides for the display and/or
erasure of image data in any selected region and from any arbitrary viewpoint, the
interactive control of simultaneous multiple intensity windows (Figure 8), the
selection of oblique sections via plane cursor (Figure 9, left), the extraction of
single-point coordinates or "branching tree" coordinate sets via a point/line cursor
(Figure 9, right), and the non-destructive erasure of image data in arbitrary regions.

One task in which the varifocal mirror system has proven of value is for pre-
viewing and editing image data, prior to more detailed investigation, including
surgical procedures. As an example, Figure 10 shows a montage of 3-D CT scans of
the head displayed in the mirror (of course, the 3-D effect is lost in photography),
including a "zoom" view of an acoustic neuroma.


358

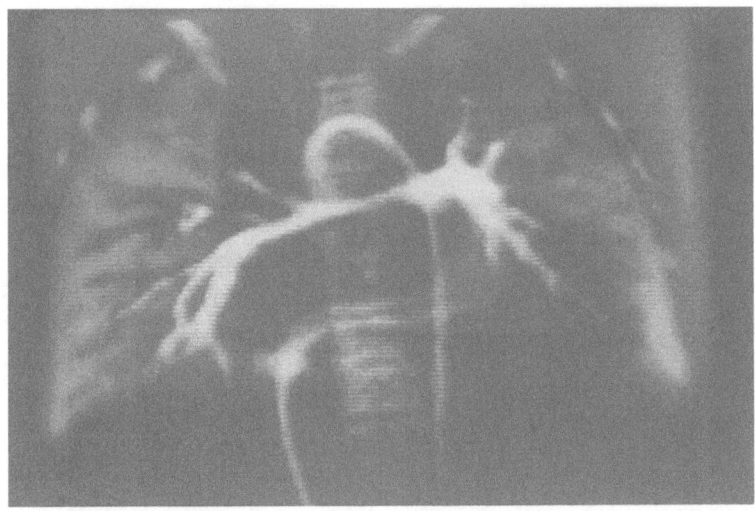

Fig. 8.    Simultaneous display of contrast-filled pulmonary arteries and air content of lungs as displayed in varifocal mirror. 3-D scan data is from Mayo DSR. (From Camp et al., Proc. 20th Annual Hawaii Intl. Conf. System Sciences, 1987, pp 23-36. With permission.)

Although the true three-dimensional nature of the display is perhaps its most useful feature, the power of the system also lies in its capabilities for dynamic interaction, permitting one to "explore" the data. Often serendipitous findings of significant interest result from such explorations, which either augment the original analysis objectives or provide impetus for changing or expanding the initial objectives.

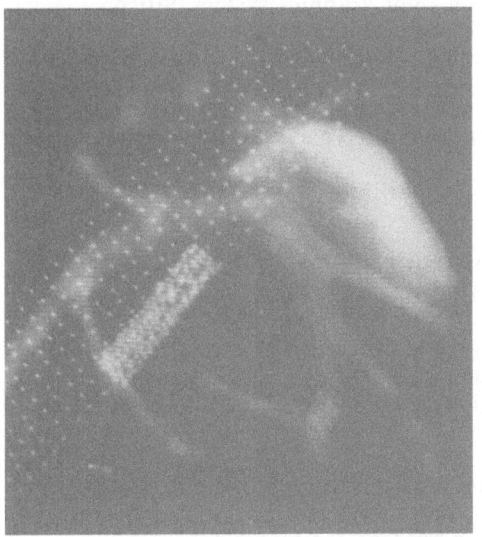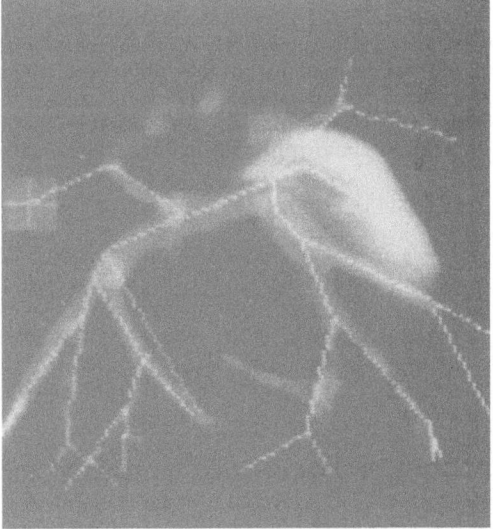

Fig. 9.    Left - Photograph of varifocal mirror display with plane-cursor imposed. The orientation of the described plane is under interactive control.
Right - Photograph of varifocal mirror display of pulmonary arteries with "stick-figure" graphic imposed. Trace coordinates are recorded in a format which maintains the branching relationship between points. (From Robb et al., 1986. With permission.)

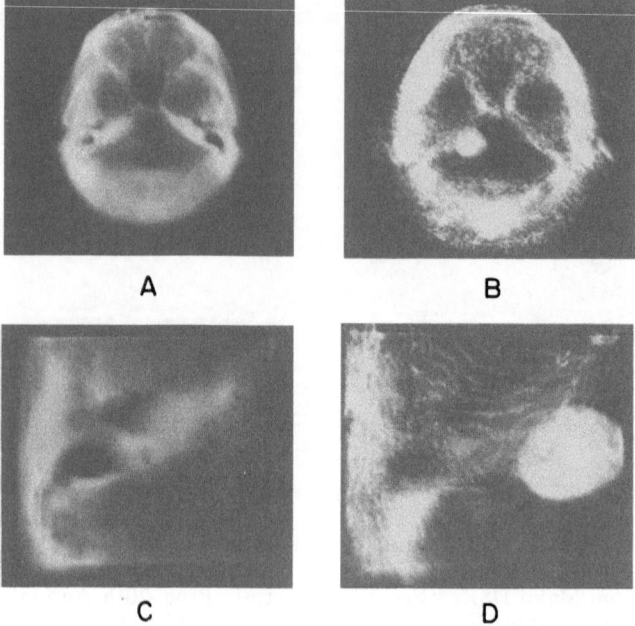

Fig. 10.   Images photographed from mirror 3-D display of head scanned by
serial section CT.  Top left panel shows original data; top right
is windowed to show tumor; bottom left is zoom view showing petrous
bone and air in internal auditory meatus; and bottom right is zoom
view showing acoustic neuroma wrapped around ridge of petrous bone.

Three-dimensional display capability is also provided by a liquid crystal stereo
shutter (Tektronix) attached to a high resolution color graphics system (Silicon
Graphics IRIS 3030W) on the network.  This device provides very useful multi-
observer 3-D viewing of static or rotational sequences of images by simply wearing
a pair of passive circularly polarized glasses.  The geometry engines of the Silicon
Graphics system permit rapid computation of new views (3-D floating point coordinate transformations at rates up to 100,000 per second).  This capability permits
interactive manipulation of the stereo views.

2-D Display Workstations

Figure 11 is a photograph of one of the BRUNET workstations, featuring a SUN
3/160 system with color display, keyboard and mouse.  This configuration is typical
of a standard workstation area which uses the ANALYZE multi-dimensional image
analysis software.  With reference to the software architecture illustrated in Figure
6, several examples of typical multi-dimensional image display, editing and measurement capabilities possible with these workstations and the ANALYZE software will
next be described and illustrated.

The *DISPLAY* process in ANALYZE allows for the manipulation and multi-format
display of 2-D sections extracted from the 3-D image data set.  Images can be
arbitrarily sized and rapidly formatted and displayed on the screen by selection of a
starting position and automatic display increments.  Since the entire volume image
resides in memory, images can be displayed at rates between 5 and 20 images per
second, depending on size.  Variable image orientations can be selected.  Figure 12
shows a display of twelve sections from a CT head scan displayed with this module.
Each row of sections is a different slice orientation.  The sections can be selected

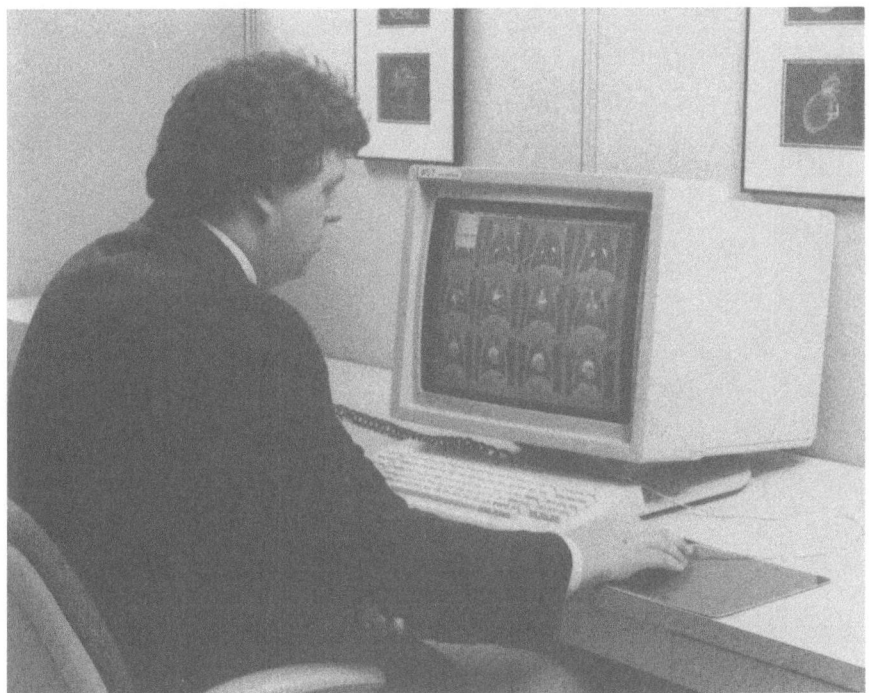

Fig. 11.    SUN 3 color workstation running ANALYZE software.

orthogonal to any major-axis and displayed with arbitrary increments between sections. The image(s) can be processed before display using any of several transforms, including windowing, thresholding, smoothing, inverting, contouring, and
rotating; none of which alters the original data set. This module is used to review,
select, and non-destructively process image data prior to further analysis.

An important part of multi-dimensional image analysis is the selection of the
optimal viewing orientation for the image data. Most of the ANALYZE processes
allow the user to select one of the three orthogonal viewpoints of the current 3-D
image data. The *OBLIQUE* process provides an interactive method for entirely arbitrary viewpoint selection by providing the user with pictorial feedback cues to
indicate the current orientation of the volume image data. The user can rapidly
"fly" an image plane through the image data using standard aeronautical terms like
pitch (nose up/down), roll (right/left), yaw (rotate on plane), elevate (raise or lower
level), and slide (translate) with variable increments for each of the maneuvers. As
the orientation of the plane (viewpoint) changes, the resulting oblique image is
rapidly (less than 1 sec) calculated and displayed along with reference information.
The graphic reference data includes the intersection of the current oblique plane on
three mutually perpendicular, orthogonal planes of the image, and a diagrammatic
representation of the volume in the form of a cube, showing the orientation of the
current plane within the cube. Figure 13 depicts a typical screen in the *OBLIQUE*
process using a full DSR volume scan of the chest for display. The upper three
images are orthogonal central sections of the 3-D image volume (sagittal, coronal,
and transverse), with the intersection of the current selected oblique image
indicated by the line drawn on each reference image. The current thin oblique
image is displayed in the center of the screen, with a "thickened" image consisting
of 10 parallel oblique sections summed together at the left. Any sequence of
parallel oblique sections can be selectively added together to produce thicker
sections. The viewing orientation selected may be used to generate a stack of

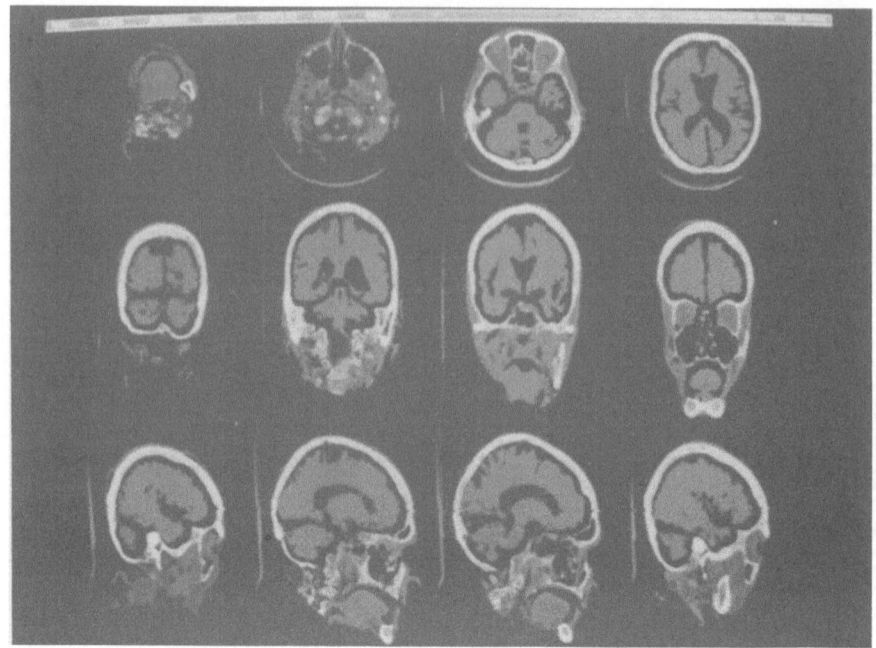

Fig. 12.   A montage produced by the *DISPLAY* module which illustrates a set of intensity windowed transverse, coronal and sagittal x-ray CT slices through a head.

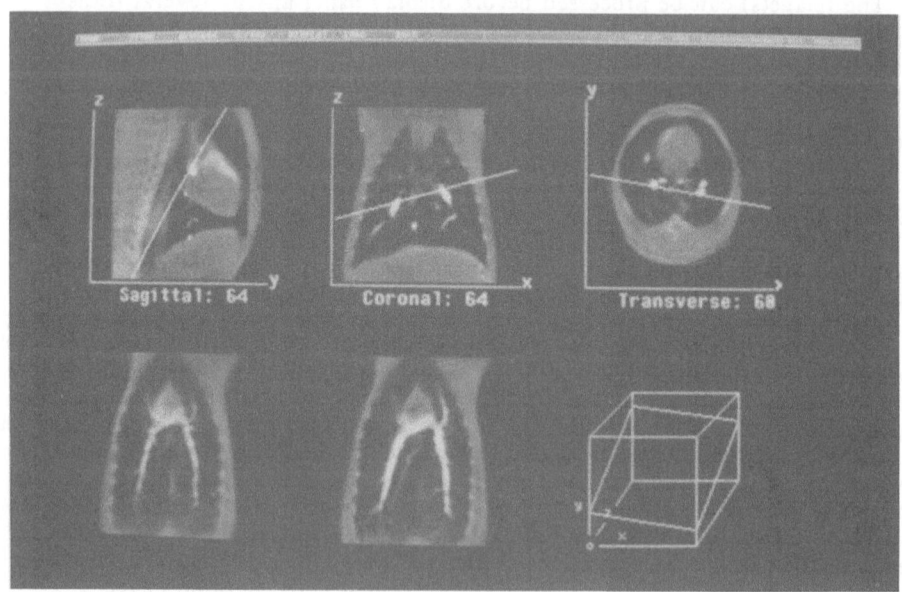

Fig. 13.   A typical screen in the *OBLIQUE* module during selection of arbitrary oblique slices through a 3-D chest image.  Bottom center image is oblique slice computed through volume at orientation indicated by lines on orthogonal reference images (top row).  Image at lower left is "thickened" oblique slice.

adjacent sections parallel to the oblique section chosen. This new oriented 3-D image can then be stored in the data base for subsequent analysis.

The *EDIT* process allows the user to modify the image data in memory using a set of interactive editing tools. The editing tools include interactive global and regional windowing, intensity thresholding, erasing, painting, and cut-and-paste operations. These tools are used extensively for segmenting a volume image into binary objects, and for outlining or tracing features of interest. Figure 14 shows a screen of the workstation during interactive thresholding of several CT head slices simultaneously to segment the skull from the brain (hard tissue vs. soft tissue).

The *MANIP* module is a collection of operations that provide the user with a set of tools to analytically manipulate image data. Addition, subtraction, multiplication, and division can be performed on sets of volume image data. Binary image data sets created through the *EDIT* module can be used as "masks" (by multiplying) to filter out information in a given image data set. Other applications of these processes include normalization of image data sets with control images, correction for a non-linear distribution of image densities, and selected enhancement of objects in the image data. Figure 15 shows a sequence of CT head slices in which a tumor has been visually enhanced by processing with the *MANIP* module. The original data was windowed, thresholded and scaled to obtain just a tumor image, which was then added back to the original data. Another feature of the *MANIP* module is the capability to selectively modify spatial relationships within the image data. Interpolation, sizing, and partitioning on the image data can be performed. *MANIP* also contains some special purpose analysis techniques, including warping algorithms and multinominal fits of functional data for image mapping, and corrections for physiological parameters (e.g., percent air content in the lungs).

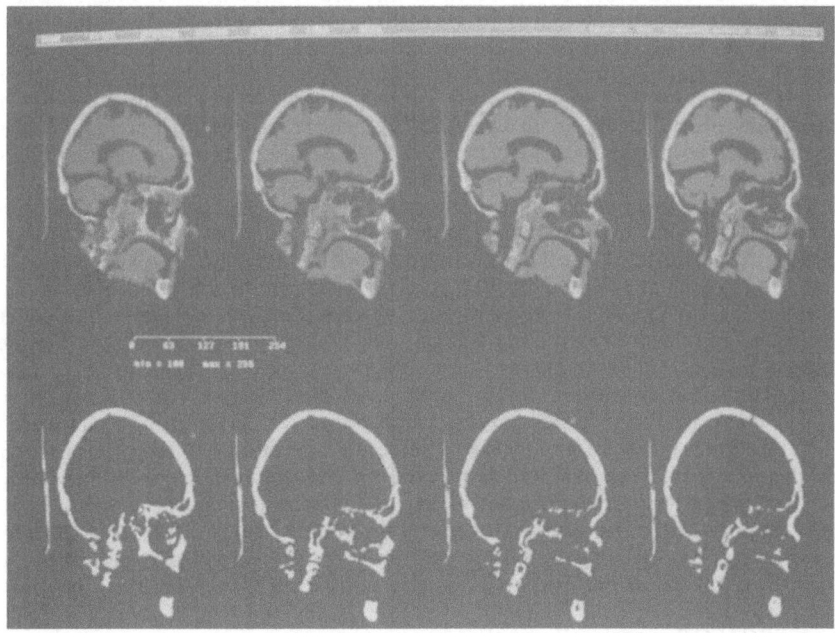

Fig. 14.    Multiple slices through volume scan of head, showing original data (top) and simultaneously thresholded data (bottom) using *EDIT* module to segment bone from soft tissue.

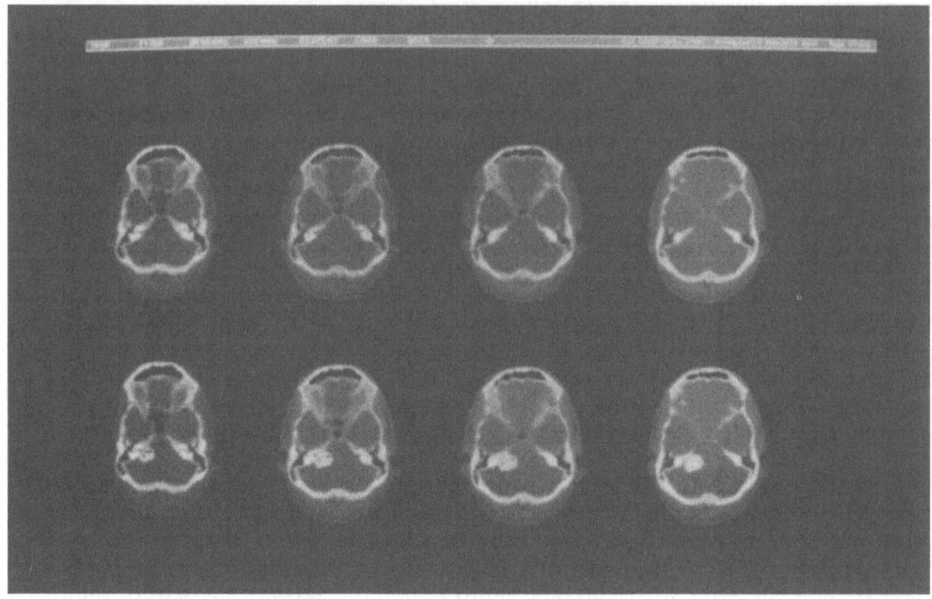

Fig. 15.   Volume image processed with *MANIP* module.  Bottom row shows
enhanced tumor (acoustic neuroma) obtained by adding a filtered
tumor mask to original data shown in top row.


Once the data has been selected and manipulated to the point where region-of-
interest (ROI) measurements or specific parametric information about the image data
is desired, the *BIOPSY* process is selected.  This process displays a set of serial 2-D
sections upon which measurements can be made.  These serial 2-D sections can be
interactively selected from any portion of the multi-dimensional image data set
using a variable increment factor to scan through the sections.  Repeated measurements through the multi-dimensional image data set can be performed by specifying
a range of image slices to process.  The screen shown in Figure 16 is an example
of the use of the *BIOPSY* module on a CT head scan.  Three basic types of "numerical samples" can be specified in the *BIOPSY* process to provide image data
measurements:  point samples, line samples, and area samples.  A sampling threshold
may be set to specify a range of information to include in the sampling functions.
The information generated from a point sample consists of the multi-dimensional
coordinate of the point (3-D or 4-D) and the image pixel value (e.g., density) at
that point.  Line profiles can be generated and displayed along any arbitrarily
oriented line which is selected by interactively specifying its endpoints in an image.
Sampling areas can be specified as regular shapes, namely rectangles and ellipses, or
by tracing a free-form area on the image.  Multiple sampling areas can be specified
on a single image.  Information provided by area sampling includes the area, maximum and minimum values within the area, area coordinates, the sum, standard deviation, and mean of image pixel values, brightness-area product, and the number of
image data elements above and below a selected threshold.  A histogram of the data
within the specified area sampled is plotted on the display screen.  Areas can be
automatically sampled through a set of serial sections to provide a volumetric
sampling function.  Individually traced area samples can be summed together to provide an arbitrarily shaped volumetric sample through the multi-dimensional image
data.  Traces may be saved and recalled for future reference or use.

The *PROJECT* process allows the user to interactively create projection images
of a 3-D image, with the capability to vary the angle of projection, dissolution
range, and dissection parameters.  This algorithm is analogous to the conventional

x-ray process, with the significant advantages that x-ray-like images can be produced from any arbitrary viewpoint without using more x-ray, and the numbers representing the structure to be projected can be modified to effect desired enhancements, such as transparency, in the projection. The user can specify the axis of rotation, angle of projection, sub-volume to project, range and percentage of dissolution (dissolution means selective reduction in value of selected pixels in the 3-D volume to effect transparent viewing through certain structures within the projection image). The interpolation method used for projecting the ray paths can be selected from three types: nearest neighbor, linear, and bi-linear interpolation. Figure 17 is a montage of projection images of the chest from a DSR volume scan, showing successive steps in transparency. Such displays can also be effective in a movie loop when a rotational sequence helps convey the three-dimensionality of the structures.

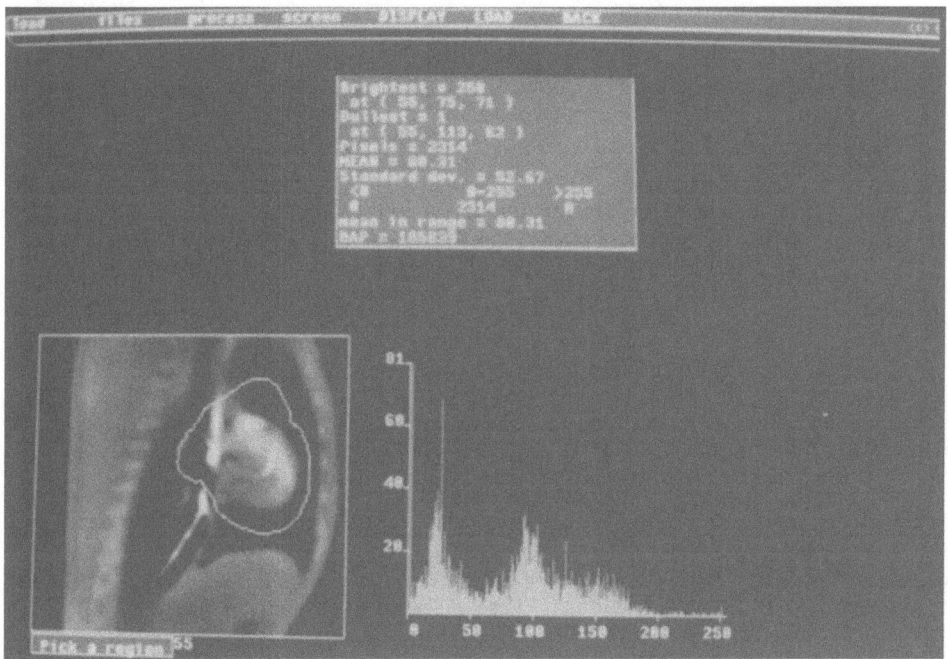

Fig. 16.  Example of the statistics and histogram computed by the *BIOPSY* module for a selected region-of-interest in a 3-D volume image of the chest.

Display of the surface of 3-D objects is often useful for conveying shape and relative dimensions, and for verifying that a given object has been properly identified. Thus, several tools are provided in the *SURFACE* module for processing object surfaces. The task of identifying and extracting a surface from a volume image is performed by segmentation algorithms. The first stage in this process generally involves manual interaction with the images in the volume in order to erase connections between structures with the same greyscale value. The next step is to form a binary volume by thresholding the greyscale volume to a user-specified window. At this stage, a 3-D connectivity algorithm may optimally be used to ensure that spurious objects are separated from the structure(s) of interest. The final step is the extraction of the surface description from the binary volume image. The surface model employed for display has been described elsewhere (Heffernan and Robb, 1985a). The algorithm is fast and produces realistic images.

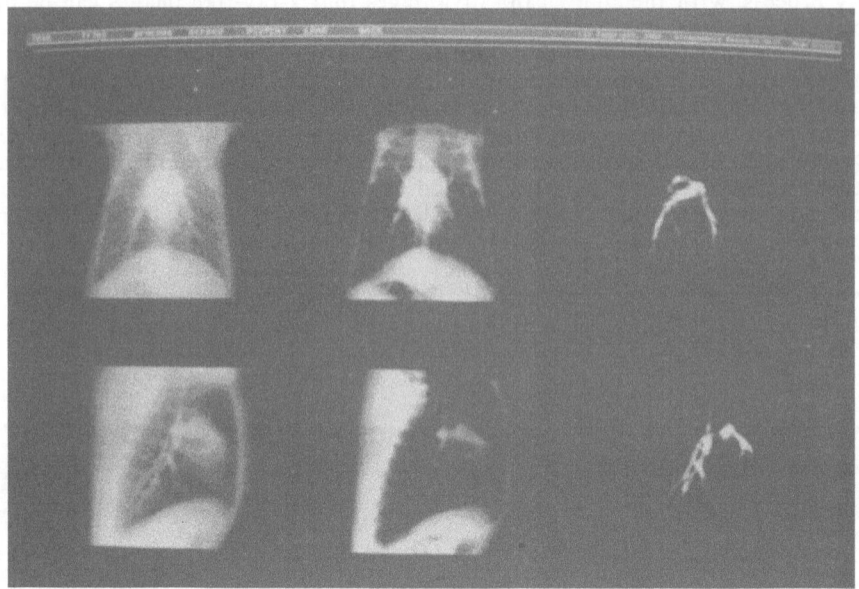

Fig. 17.    Sequence of projection images of chest determined from DSR volume
scan showing successive dissolution of soft tissue to enhance visualization of intra-thoracic pulmonary structures.  Top row shows
coronal images and bottom row shows sagittal images.


Figure 18 shows the realism achievable with the surface display algorithm.  The
top row shows skin (soft-tissue) images of a full head CT scan of a cadaver from
different viewpoints.  The bottom row shows bone (hard-tissue) images of the skull,
with missing lower and upper left mandible.  All images were segmented by thresholding using the *EDIT* module, as previously illustrated in Figure 14.

Figure 19 shows two rows of the same cadaver head for which prosthetic
implants for the upper and lower mandible were determined and inserted by the
computer.  Figure 20 shows a summary of clinical cranio-facial surgery case plans
processed on the BRU workstations.  These cases all involved computer generation
of prosthetic implants by matching and filtering a mirror image computed from the
contralateral side of the skull.

Figure 21 illustrates capabilities for editing shaded surface displays of the skull
to facilitate surgery planning.  Illustrated is a view of the screen during an interactive cranio-facial surgical simulation session using the *SURFACE* module.  The
frontal bone flap is in the process of being repositioned and the orbital "osteotomy"
has been performed and repositioned inferiorly.  The workstation and ANALYZE
software are being used to plan and simulate such surgical procedures.  The main
emphasis has been on cranio-facial surgery planning because of the three-dimensional space analysis difficulties in the cases.  As with conventional cranio-facial
surgical planning, computer assisted planning relies on observation and measurement
of the normal and pathological antomy.  Detailed measurement of linear and angular
relationships, volumes of the orbit, anterior cranial fossae or of regional bone
content are made.  Surgical simulation is the application of the therapeutic ideas
evolved using ANALYZE to simulate most of the surgical steps in an interactive,
freelance, fashion.

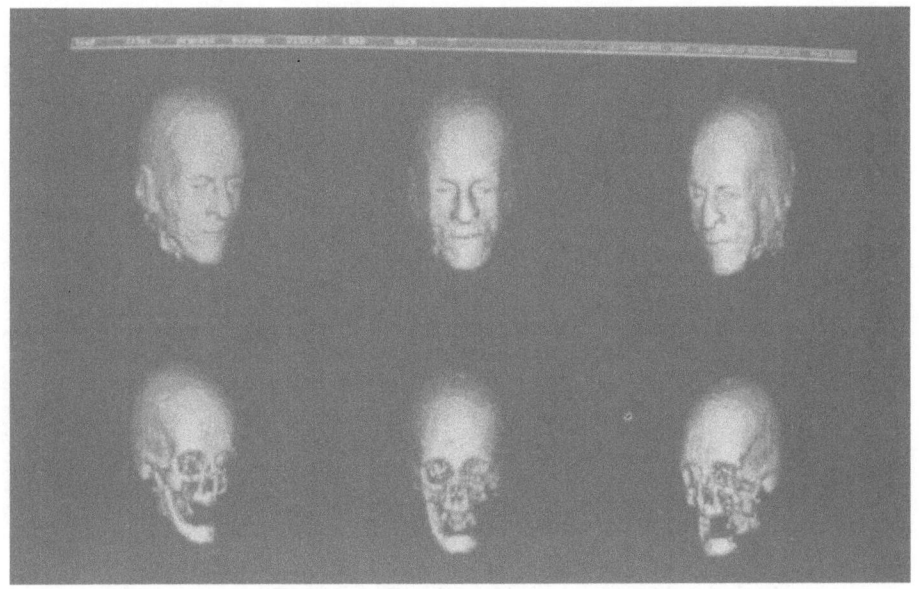

Fig. 18.    Shaded surface display of cadaver head produced by *SURFACE* module
showing soft-tissue (top row) and hard-tissue (bottom row) displays
of skin and skull, respectively.

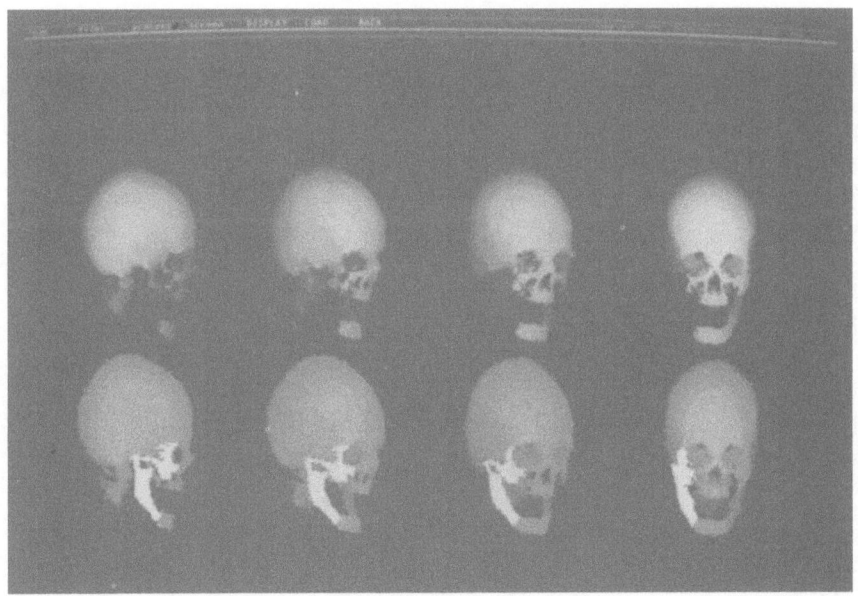

Fig. 19.    Top row shows original volume scan from different views.  Bottom
row shows volume imaged after prosthetics have been computed and
inserted for display by computer.

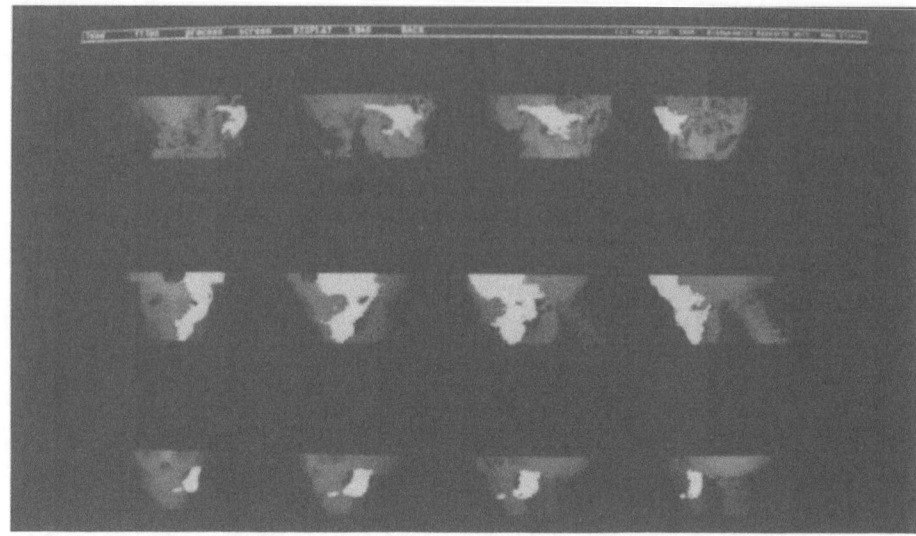

Fig. 20.  Examples of three cases of cranio-facial surgery planning and prosthetic implant computation using ANALYZE software. Each row shows slightly rotated views of three different studies. Highlighted portion of each image is computed implant.

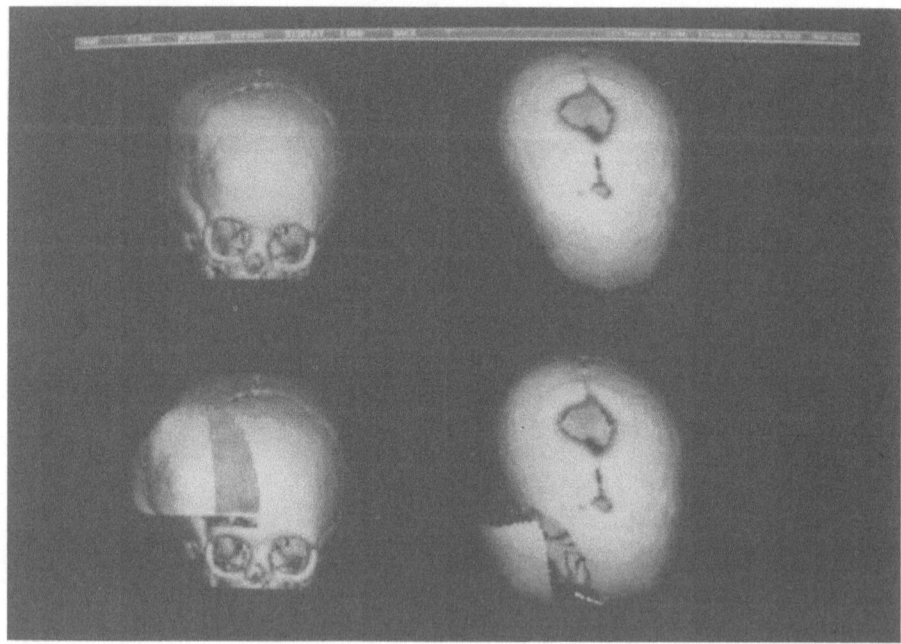

Fig. 21.  Example of the workstation screen in the *SURFACE* module showing shaded surfaces of bone from two views (top row) emphasizing the particular clinical problem (plagiocephaly). Surgical simulation of the osteotomies required to correct the deformity is shown in the bottom row. The right orbit has been repositioned and the right frontal bone flap has been "resected", prior to final positioning.

Figures 22 and 23 further illustrate how the shaded surface display process can be used to visualize and understand spatial relationships of intra-cranial structures in 3-D. Figure 22 shows a sequence of six surface displays of a slab "cut-away" through the head revealing a large (2-3 cm) right acoustic neuroma. (These images are normally displayed in full color on the actual workstation.) The top row shows superior views, looking down into the skull at different tilt angles to reveal a cut through the brain with the tumor nestled against the ridge of the petrous bone. The bottom row shows inferior views of the head slab, showing more of the bony cranial structures and portions of the caudal brain, but obscuring the tumor. Figure 23 is the same volume image but shows some examples of "computer surgery". First the skull and brain were removed, leaving only the outer skin and muscle and the tumor as if suspended in space (top row). Second, the skin, muscle, and brain have been eliminated, leaving only the skull and tumor (bottom row). And Figure 24 shows elimination of the outer soft tissue and skull, leaving only the brain and tumor, for the same six views as shown in Figure 22.

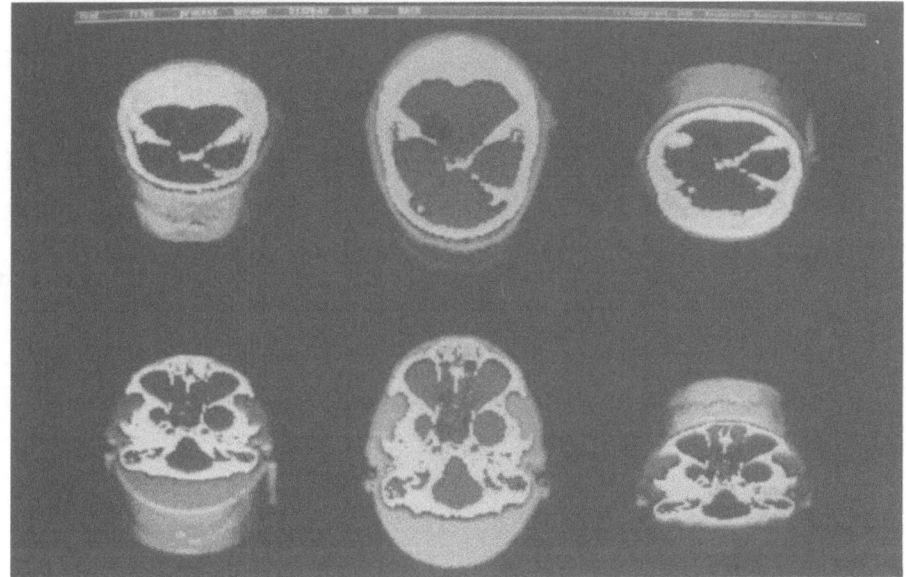

Fig. 22.    3-D shaded surface displays of "slab" through patient head, showing all structures from superior view (top row) and inferior view (bottom row). Large acoustic neuroma near ridge of petrous bone can be seen in superior views.

Figure 25 illustrates a useful combination of display techniques wherein CT grey-scale projection images are superimposed on the surface displays. Projection images, partially transparent if desired, may be mapped onto shaded surface displays to provide simultaneously both 3-D spatial orientation and tissue density information in an anatomic region of interest. This may potentially enhance in a single display the diagnostic and/or treatment information available in the data.

A *MOVIE* module provides the user with the capability to rapidly display a sequence of images like any of those shown in this paper. The images can be sets of 2-D or edited 3-D images, serial sections, projection/dissolution images, rotating 3-D shaded surface displays, oblique sections generated through time, etc. Control of a video recording disk is provided for making hardcopy video sequences. The *MOVIE* module includes a feature to create titles and labels which are displayed with the images to help annotate particular segments of the movie.

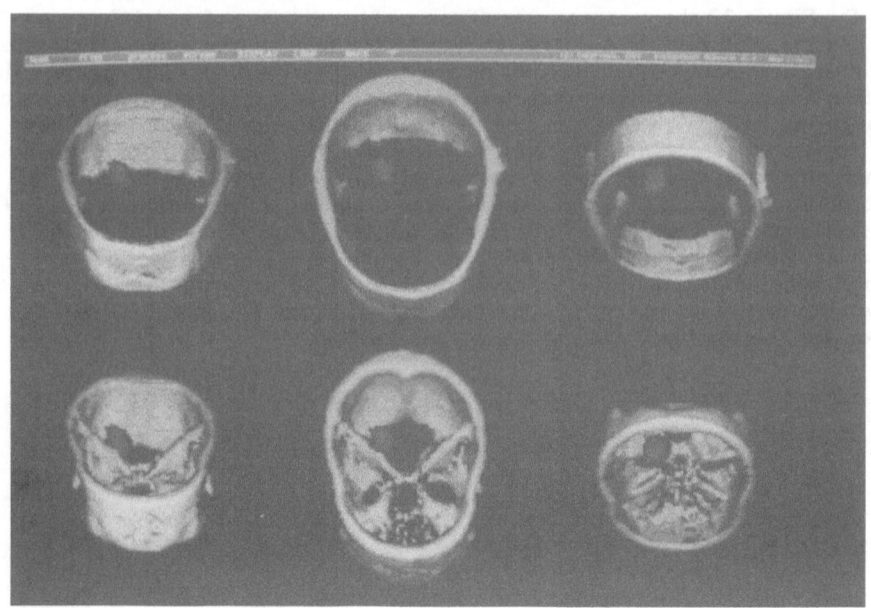

Fig. 23.    Same data as in Figure 22, but with various editing of surfaces
before display.  Top row shows superior views in which skull and
brain have been removed, leaving outer soft tissue and tumor.
Bottom row shows only skull and tumor.

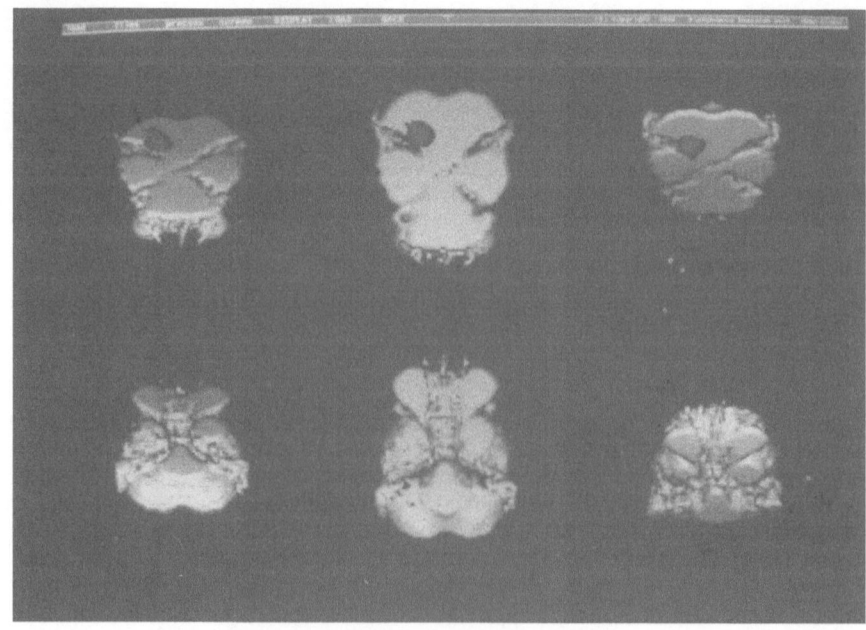

Fig. 24.    Same data and views as in Figure 22 showing only the brain and
tumor.

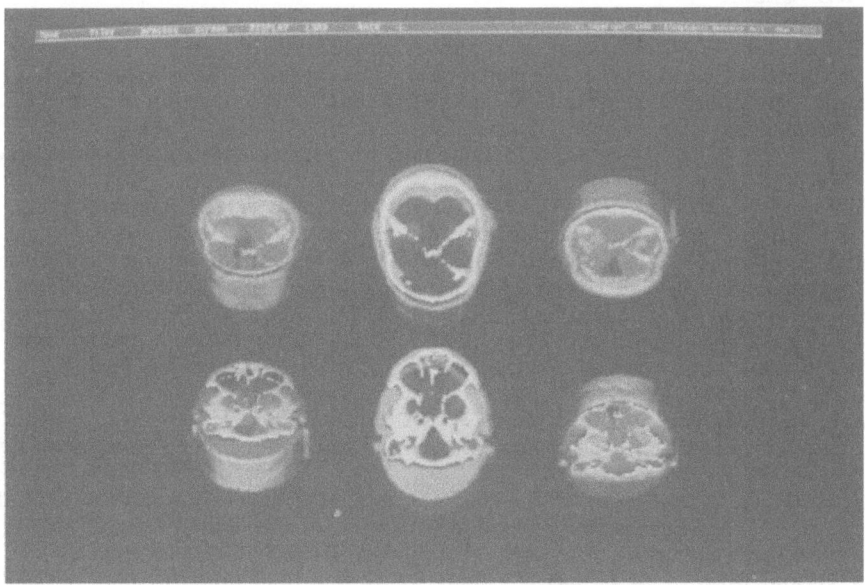

Fig. 25.    Six cut-away views of head displayed as combination of shaded surfaces and projection images mapped onto surface at selected level of
cut through head.  Outer tissue and skull are rendered as surface
displays, brain and tumor are superimposed as x-ray projections.


SUMMARY

The advances in medical imaging capabilities over the last decade have been
developed, applied, and accepted at an unprecedented volume and pace.  The continuing evolution promises even greater capabilities for accurate non-invasive diagnoses, as well as for quantitative biological investigations, based on new high-
speed, high-resolution, full three- and four-dimensional imaging systems.  The
"ideal" three- or four-dimensional imaging system would provide simultaneously and
rapidly all of the advantages and eliminate all of the limitations of the different
imaging modalities presently available.  Certainly at the crux of such a system will
be an integrated computer-based workstation which facilitates full exploitation of
the imaging system.  We have developed advanced multi-dimensional image display
and analysis software on several current workstation architectures using standard
languages and operating systems, with both stand-alone and network capabilities.
These implementations provide comprehensive capabilities for multi-dimensional image
display, editing, and measurement in a readily transportable product.

ACKNOWLEDGEMENTS

The authors express appreciation to their colleagues in the Biodynamics
Research Unit whose dedicated efforts have made this work possible.  Special recog-
nition is given to Jon Camp, Dennis Hanson, and Ron Karwoski for their contribu-
tions to the system hardware and software.  Image data was provided by Drs. David
Reese and Glenn Forbes of the Mayo Department of Radiology, Drs. Peter Kay and
Ian Jackson of the Mayo Section of Plastic Surgery, and Dr. Eric Hoffman of the
Mayo Department of Physiology and Biophysics.  Appreciation is also extended to
Marge C. Fynbo and Steve Orwoll for preparation of this manuscript.  This work is
supported by grants RR-02540 and HL-04664 from the National Institutes of Health.

# REFERENCES

Barillot, C., Gibaud, B., Scarabin, J. M., and Coatrieux, J. L. (1985). 3-D reconstruction of cerebral blood vessels, IEEE CG&A, 5,13-19.

Baxter, B., Hitchner, L. E., and Anderson, R. E. (1982). Application of a three-dimensional display in diagnostic imaging, JCAT, 6,1000-1005.

Birkner, D. A. (1984). Design considerations for a user oriented PACS, Proc. ISMII '84, 89-101

Bloch, P. and Udupa, J. K. (1983). Application of computerized tomography to radiation therapy and surgical planning, Proc. IEEE, 71,351-355.

Camp, J. J., Stacy, M. C., and Robb, R. A. (1987), A system for interactive volume analysis (SIVA) of 4-D biomedical images, J. Med. Sys., (In Press).

Durbin, R. M., Burns, R., Moulai, J., Metcalf, P., Freymann, D., Blum, M., Anderson, J. E., Harrison, S. C., and Wiley, D. C. (1986). Protein, DNA, and virus crystallography with a focused imaging proportional counter, Science, 232:1127-1132.

Fellingham, L. L., Vogel, J. H., Lau, C., and Dev, P. (1986). Interactive graphics and 3-D modelling for surgical planning and prosthesis and implant design, Proc. NCGA '86, 3,132-142.

Fuchs, H., Pizer, S. M., Heinz, E. R., Bloomberg, S. H., Tsai, L. C., and Strickland, D. C. (1982). Design of and image editing with a space-filling 3-D display based on a standard raster graphics system, Proc. SPIE, 367:117-127.

Fuchs, H. and Pizer, S. M. (1984). Systems for three-dimensional display of medical images, Proc. 1984 Intl. Joint Alpine Symp., 1-6.

Glenn, W. V., Jr., Johnson, R. J., Morton, P. E. and Dwyer, S. J., III (1975). Image generation and display techniques for CT scan data: Thin transverse and reconstructed coronal and sagittal planes, Invest. Radiol., 10:403-416.

Goldwasser, S. M., Reynolds, R. A., Bapty, T., Baraff, D., Summers, J., Talton, D., and Walsh, E. (1985). Physician's workstation with real-time performance, IEEE NC&A, 5:44-57.

Goldwasser, S. M. (1984). A generalized object display processor architecture, IEEE CG&A, 4:43-55.

Gray, M. J. and Rutherford, H. (1984). Functional specifications of a useful digital multi-modality image workstation, Proc. ISMII '84, 8-12.

Grewer, R., Monnich, K. J., Schmidt, J., Svensson, H., and Wendler, Th. (1985). Design of interactive workstations for the interpretation of medical images in pictorial information systems, Proc. Intl. Symp. CAR '85, 679686.

Harris, L. D., Robb, R. A., Yuen, T. S., and Ritman, E. L. (1978a). Non-invasive numerical dissection and display of anatomic structure using computerized x-ray tomography, Proc. SPIE, 152,10-18.

Harris, L. D., Camp, J. J., Ritman, E. L., and Robb, R. A. (1986). Three-dimensional display and analysis of tomographic volume images utilizing a varifocal mirror, IEEE Trans. Med. Imag., 5:67-72.

Harris, L. D. (1981). Identification of the optimal orientation of oblique sections through multiple parallel CT images, JCAT, 5:881-887.

Harris, L. D. and Camp, J. J. (1984). Display and analysis of tomographic volumetric images utilizing a vari-focal mirror, Proc. SPIE, 507:38-45.

Harris, L. D., Robb, R. A., Johnson, S. A., and Khalafalla, A. S. (1978b). Stereo display of computed tomographic data, in: "Challenges and Prospects for Advanced Medical Systems," H. E. Emlet, Jr., ed., Symposia Specialists, Inc., Miami, FL, pp. 127-135.

Harris, L. D., Evans, T. C., and Greenleaf, J. F. (1980). Display of 3-D ultrasonic images, in: "Acoustical Imaging", K. Y. Wang, ed., pp. 227-237.

Heffernan, P. B. and Robb, R. A. (1985a). A new method for shaded surfaced display of biological and medical images, IEEE Trans. Med. Imag., 4:26-38.

Heffernan, P. B. and Robb, R. A. (1985b). Display and analysis of 4-D medical images, Proc. Intl. Symp. CAR '85, 583-592.

Herman, G. T., Udupa, J. K., Kramer, D. M., Lauterbur, P. C., Rudin, A. M., and Schneider, J. S. (1982). Three-dimensional display of nuclear magnetic resonance images, Opt. Eng., 21:923-926.

Herman, G. T. and Liu, H. K. (1977). Display of three-dimensional information in computed tomography, JCAT, 1:155-160.

Herman, G. T. (1986). Computer produced stereoscopic display in radiology, Proc. NCGA '86, 3:71-79.

Hodges, L. F. and McAllister, D. F. (1985). Stereo and alternating-pair techniques for display of computer-generated images, IEEE CG&A, 5:38-45.

Hoffman, E. A. and Heffernan, P. B. (1985a). A computer graphics-aided 3-D analysis of heart-lung interaction reconstructed via DSR scanning, Proc. NCGA, 3:81-92.

Hoffman, E. A. and Ritman, E. L. (1985b). Invariant total heart volume in the intact thorax, Am. J. Physiol.: Heart & Circ. Physiol., 249:H883-H890.

Hunter, G. M. (1984). 3-D frame buffers for interactive analysis of 3-D data, Proc. SPIE, 507:178-182.

Jackson, I. T. and Bite, U. (1986). Three-dimensional CT scanning and major reconstructive surgery of head.and neck, Mayo Clinic Proc., 61:546-555.

Jansson, D. G. and Kosowsky, R. P. (1984). Display of moving volumetric images, Proc. SPIE, 507:82-92.

Jimenez, J., Santisteban, A., Carazo, J. M., and Carrascosa, J. L. (1986). Computer graphic display method for visualizing three-dimensional biological structures, Science, 232:1113-1115.

Kehtarnavaz, N., Philippe, E. A., and de Figueiredo, R. J. P. (1984). A novel surface reconstruction and display method for cardiac PET imaging, IEEE Trans. Med. Imag., 3:108-115.

Lenz, R. (1984). Processing and presentation of 3-D images, Proc. ISMII '84, 298-303.

Lipton, L. (1984). Binocular symmetries as criteria for the successful transmission of images in the stereo-dimensional (TM) brand stereoscopic video system, Proc. SPIE, 507,108-113.

Marsh, J. L. and Vannier, M. W. (1983). The "third" dimension in craniofacial surgery, Plas. Recon. Surg., 71,759-767.

Matsumoto, M., Inoue, M., Tamura, S., Tanaka, K., and Abe, H. (1981). Three-dimensional echocardiography for spatial visualization and volume calculation of cardiac structures, J. Clin. Ultrasound, 9,157-165.

News (1985). AT&T ventures into radiology market with DIM system, Diag. Imag., 7,45.

Oswald, H. (1985). A medical workstation for three-dimensional display of computed tomogram images, Proc. Intl. Symp. CAR '85, 565-577.

Pizer, S. M., Zimmerman, J. B., and Staab, E. V. (1984). Adaptive grey level assignment in CT scan display, JCAT, 8,300-305.

Pizer, S. M., Fuchs, H., Mosher, C., Lifshitz, L., Abram, G. D., Ramanathan, S.,
Whitney, B. T., Rosenman, J. G., Staab, E. V., Chaney, E. L., and Sherouse, G. (1986). 3-D shaded graphics in radiotherapy and diagnostic imaging, Proc. NCGA '86, 3,107-113.

Rao, K. H. S. and Shas, A. V. (1984). Computer assisted thermography and its application in ovulation detection, Proc. ISMII '84, 459-464.

Rhodes, M. L., Azzawi, Y. M., Chu, E. S., Pang, A. T., Glenn, W. V., and Rothman, S. L. G. (1985). A network solution for structure models and custom prostheses manufacturing from CT data, Proc. Intl. Symp. CAR '85, 403-412.

Rhodes, M. L., Glenn, W. V., Rothman, S. L. G., Azzawi, Y. M., and Quinn, J. F. (1984). CT image processing using commercial digital networks, Proc. 1984 Intl. Joint Alpine Symp., 37-43.

Rhodes, M. L., Glenn, W. V., Jr., and Azzawi, Y. M. (1980). Extracting oblique planes from serial CT sections, JCAT, 4,649-654.

Risser, T. (1984). Processing and presentation of 3-D images, Proc. ISMII '84, 61-65.

Ritman, E. L., Kinsey, J. H., Robb, R. A., Gilbert, B. K., Harris, L. D., and Wood, E. H. (1980). Three-dimensional imaging of heart, lungs, and circulation, Science, 210,273-280.

Robb, R. A. (1983). High-speed three-dimensional x-ray computed tomography: The Dynamic Spatial Reconstructor, Proc. IEEE, 71,308-319.

Robb, R. A., Heffernan, P. B., Camp, J. J., and Hanson, D. P. (1986). A workstation for interactive display and quantitative analysis of 3-D and 4-D biomedical images, Proc. 10th Annual Symp. Computer Appl. Med. Care, IEEE Cat. No. 84CH2341-6,240-256.

Robb, R. A. (1985). "Three-Dimensional Biomedical Imaging," Volumes I and II, CRC Press, Boca Raton, FL.

Robbin, M. L., An, K. N., Linscheid, R. L., and Ritman, E. L. (1986). Anatomic and kinematic analysis of the human forearm using high-speed computed tomography, Med. & Biol. Eng. & Comput., 24,164-168.

Scharnweber, H. and Tonnie, K. D. (1984). Three-dimensional reconstruction and display of complex anatomical objects, Proc. 1984 Intl. Joint Alpine Symp., 7-11.

Schwartz, E. L. and Merker, B. (1986). Computer-aided neuroanatomy: Differential geometry of cortical surfaces and an optimal flattening algorithm, IEEE CG&A, 6,36-44.

Seide, K. and Ritman, E. L. (1984). Three-dimensional dynamic x-ray computed tomography imaging of stomach motility, 1984, Am. Physiol. Society, G574-G581.

Sher, L. D. (1986). Graphics in space: See it now, Proc. NCGA, 3,101-106.

Simon, W. (1977). A spinning mirror auto-stereoscopic display, Proc. SPIE, 120,180-183.

Toga, A. W. and Arnicar, T. L. (1985). Image analysis of brain physiology, IEEE CG&A, 5,20-25.

# A MULTIPROCESSOR
# ADAPTIVE HISTOGRAM EQUALIZATION MACHINE

John D. Austin[1] and Stephen M. Pizer[1,2]

Department of Computer Science[1]
Department of Radiology[2]
The University of North Carolina at Chapel Hill
Chapel Hill, NC 27514

## ABSTRACT

Contrast Limited Adaptive Histogram Equalization (clahe) provides excellent contrast enhancement of medical images, but may be too slow for regular use in a clinical setting. The essential properties of real clahe and artifacts that may be present in an interpolated clahe algorithm are discussed. An alternate form of the clahe algorithm that can be computed quickly on special purpose parallel hardware is described, as well as the architecture for such a machine.

## INTRODUCTION

Contrast Limited Adaptive Histogram Equalization (clahe) is a powerful contrast enhancement technique used for the display of images where different spatial regions of the images have different contrast enhancement requirements. Extremely effective results (Figure 1) have been produced from several medical imaging modalities including Computed Tomography (CT), Magnetic Resonance Imaging (MRI), Digital Radiography, and Radiotherapy Treatment (RT) portal and localization films.

Clahe has evolved from Adaptive Histogram Equalization (ahe), which was invented independently by Ketcham (1976), Hummel (1977), and Pizer (1981a; 1981c). It involves applying to each pixel a histogram equalization mapping based on the pixels in a region surrounding that pixel. Clahe and ahe have the advantages that they are reproducible, automatic, and simultaneously present contrast in all contrast ranges in all image regions.

An excellent description of ahe, other adaptive techniques, and an observer study comparing ahe to intensity windowing can be found in Zimmerman (1985). A detailed description of ahe can be found in Pizer et. al. (1984), and of clahe and variations in Pizer et. al. (1986) and Pizer et. al. (1987). Observer studies by Zimmerman and Pizer (1985) and ter Haar Romeny et. al. (1985) indicate that for certain image classes, intensity windowing has no significant advantages over ahe in local contrast presentation in any contrast range. Observer studies on CT data comparing clahe and ahe are currently being conducted by Zimmerman at

Washington University, and comparing clahe and intensity windowing by Perry at the University of North Carolina. Use of clahe with a wide variety of examples over many imaging modalities has suggested that clahe is preferable to ahe and will become the method of choice. In an informal comparison of enhanced RT portal films conducted at the Workshop on Megavoltage Imaging and Image Enhancement at UNC in February, 1987, clahe was judged superior to other filtering and contrast enhancement techniques.

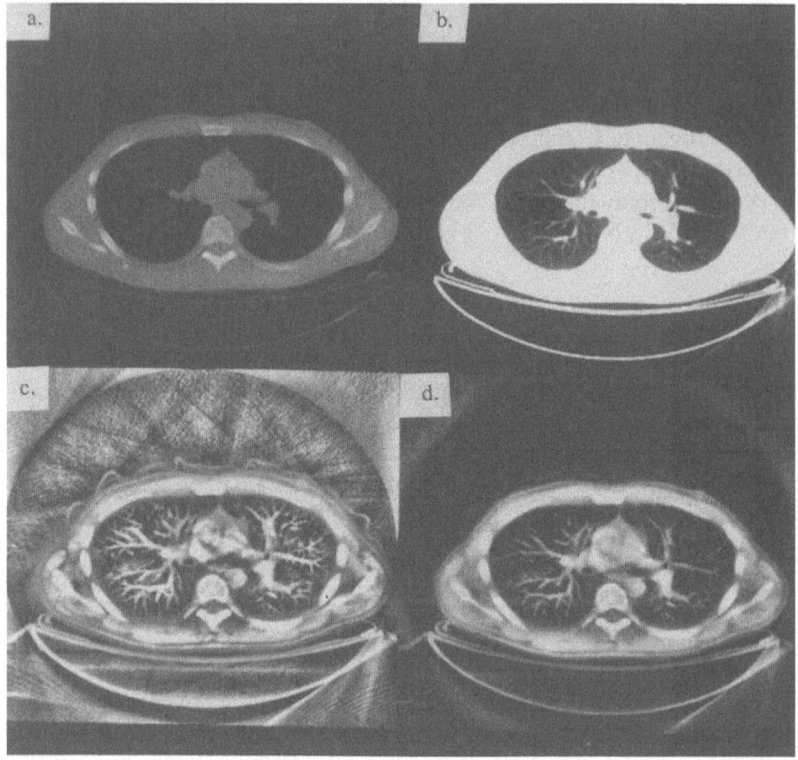

Figure 1: 512 x 512 chest CT. a) original; b) interactively windowed for the lungs; c) real, unclipped ahe with a 64 x 64 pixel region size; and d) real, clahe with a 64 x 64 pixel region size

If clahe is to be clinically useful for application to a wide variety of medical images, it must be computable in a few seconds per 2d image or slice. The goal of the research described in this paper is computation of a clahe image at this speed on a small, inexpensive, special purpose computing machine. We describe in detail an algorithm for clahe and an alternate algorithm that produces a nearly identical result but designed for implementation on such a machine. The architecture of a Multiprocessor Adaptive Histogram Equalization Machine (mahem) is described, and estimates for computation time and implementation size are given. Finally, we show how this particular architecture allows yet another algorithm speedup, successively refined clahe.

376

# CONTRAST LIMITED ADAPTIVE HISTOGRAM EQUALIZATION

Ahe uses local histogram equalization in an attempt to maximize the information transfer from an image to an observer (Zimmerman 1985). Equalizing the histogram is identical to mapping the output intensity at a pixel in proportion to its rank within the histogram. Within regions of relatively homogeneous intensities, there can be some overenhancement. Clahe (Pizer, 1987) limits the amount of enhancement in these regions.

Real clahe requires the computation of a local histogram at every pixel in the image, clipping the histogram, renormalizing the histogram, and mapping the output pixel to an intensity proportional to its rank in this modified histogram. On a MicroVAX GPX II this requires about 3 hours (with clever programming) for a 512 x 512 image. An alternate method, interpolated clahe computes local histograms at a grid (8 x 8, typically, in a 512 x 512 image) of sample points and uses a linear interpolation scheme to approximate the mapping at the other pixels. On a MicroVAX GPX II this requires about 3 minutes for a 512 x 512 image. Because of the much faster speed, interpolated clahe is the method generally used in practice. However, it can produce undesired artifacts (to be described), so it is desired to find a fast method for real clahe.

Since real clahe requires the computation of the entire local histogram at each pixel, an implementation on a special purpose machine will be expensive in either time or space. We are motivated to investigate the essential properties of the clahe algorithm in an attempt to find a simpler algorithm that can produce equivalent results. We describe in detail real clahe, emphasizing a real time implementation, and conclude this section with a discussion of the artifacts that can be produced by interpolated clahe.

An Algorithm for Real Clahe

In clahe, each pixel in the image is mapped to an output intensity proportional to its rank in a contrast limited local histogram (described below) in an m x m region of pixels surrounding the pixel. This region, called the contextual region, is typically 1/16 to 1/64 the area of the entire image. To compute real clahe, for each pixel at location x,y in the image:

1. The m x m contextual region centered at x,y is chosen, and a histogram of recorded intensities in this region is computed.
2. For all histogram bins that exceed a pre-specified clip limit:
    a. Reduce the number of pixels in the bin to the clip limit.
    b. Redistribute all clipped pixels equally into all bins in the histogram.
3. In this contrast limited histogram, the rank of the recorded intensity $i_{in}$ at x,y is determined, and scaled to produce a fractional rank, r, $0.0 \leq r \leq 1.0$.
4. This rank is used to compute an output intensity level, $i_{out}$, in some grey scale ranging between $i_1$ and $i_2$, that is:
    $$i_{out} = i_1 + r * (i_2 - i_1).$$

Figure 2a is a sample histogram of intensities from some region of an image. The clipping operation described in step 2 of the algorithm transforms this histogram to the contrast limited histogram shown in Figure 2b. The cumulative histogram gives the rank of a pixel within the contextual region directly, and is shown for the unclipped case in Figure 2c and for the clipped case in Figure 2d.

If the cumulative histogram is scaled to have the same input and output ranges, the slope indicates the amount of contrast enhancement produced by clahe. A slope of 1 corresponds to

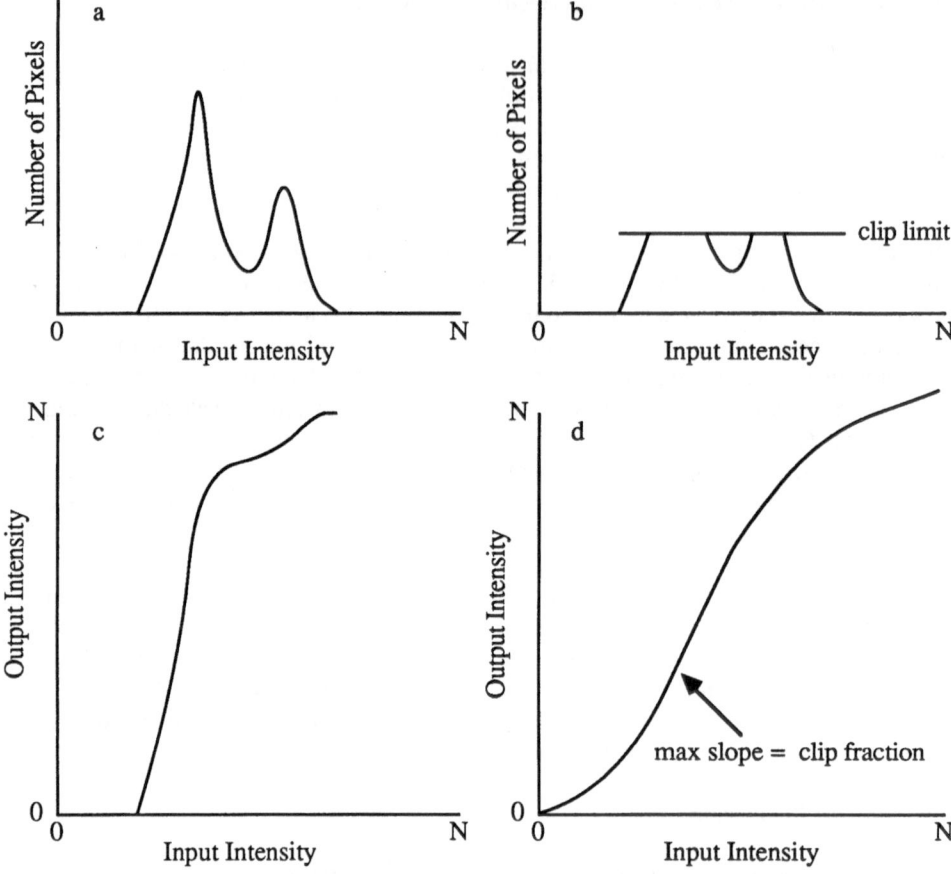

Figure 2: a) Original histogram from sample region of an image; b) contrast limited histogram; c) cumulative original histogram; and d) cumulative contrast limited histogram.

no enhancement, and increasing slopes give increasingly higher enhancement. The histogram is the derivative of the cumulative histogram, and thus the height of a histogram bin is also proportional to the amount of contrast enhancement. Contrast limitation can be defined either as limiting the slope of the cumulative histogram (Figure 2d) or limiting the bin height of the histogram (Figure 2b). We define the clip fraction as the maximum slope allowed in the scaled cumulative histogram, and the clip limit as the maximum height of a histogram bin. The clip fraction is typically between 5 and 20, and predictable for a given image class (e.g., chest CT, abdomen MRI, RT implant localization).

Essential Properties of Clahe

The output mapping function for a particular region should allow a pixel chosen from the generally limited range of intensities within the region to map to a much broader range of pixel values allowed in the display. Furthermore, a better output mapping function should be produced if more input data in the local region of the image is used to produce the mapping. Unfortunatly, the use of more data will require more computational resources, which we are trying to minimize. This section discusses in general terms the essential properties of clahe that must be preserved in any alternate algorithm: local adaptation of the contrast enhancement mapping, the use of all pixels to determine the output mapping, and limitation of the amount of contrast enhancement.

Histogram equalization attempts to use the available display levels as well as possible by distributing pixels evenly among them. In global (non-adaptive) histogram equalization a large number of pixels in a certain intensity range at any spatial location in the image (e.g. the background) will have a strong affect on the mapping of all pixels. The use of local pixels only in clahe allows for greater contrast enhancement because spatially distant pixels are ignored. However, since the local range of intensities is much less than the range in the image, if the histogram was equalized only within the small intensity range in the region, there would be little affect on the output mapping. The full range of intensities must be used, which results in a modification of the output range of each particular region.

Thus, we find two factors adaptively contribute to the contrast enhancement found in clahe. In regions where the range of intensities is relatively large, most of the contrast enhancement is provided by the equalization of the histogram. In regions where most pixels fall in a narrow range, most of the contrast enhancement is provided by modification of the output range. Region histograms examined from CT images and RT portal film images typically have an intensity range from 25% to 75% of the full image range. The method used to modify the output range is extremely critical.

The mapping of a limited local range to the full range available in the display has been used in adaptive linear min-max windowing techniques. For example, with Local Range Modification (Fahnestock and Schowengerdt, 1983), at each pixel in the image, the minimum and maximum intensities within the m x m contextual region are determined, and the output intensity is mapped linearly from this range to the full scale range. This mapping will produce progressively smaller amounts of contrast enhancement as the range of intensities in the region increases, and when the full range is present in the region, there is no contrast enhancement.

This technique can also produce severe ringing around image edges. The ringing is due to the fact that the mapping is dependent on only three pixels, the minimum, maximum, and pixel of interest. Consider two horizontally adjacent pixels that have the same intensity in the input image. Their mappings in the output image will differ only if the minimum or maximum pixel intensity in each contextual region is different, which occurs if the minimum or maximum for the left pixel is in the extreme left column of its contextual region. If this is the case, there is virtually no limit to the difference in output intensities of the two equal input intensity pixels.

With clahe, since the mapping in the modified output range is dependent on all pixels in the contextual region, ringing artifacts are only present with extremely small contextual region sizes that are not used in practice. If we again consider the two horizontally adjacent equal intensity pixels, the difference in their output intensities with clahe (their ranks) depends on all pixels in the two columns of their contextual regions that do not overlap. The worst case difference occurs if all pixels in the replaced column of the left pixel are less (or greater) than the given pixel intensity and all of the pixels in the new column are greater (or less) than the given pixel intensity. The difference in the ranks of the adjacent, equal input pixels can be no more than m and the difference in output intensities is now limited to 1/m * full display scale. With 512 x 512 images, a 64 x 64 contextual region is typically used, so even in the unusual worst case where the pixel intensities are as described, the difference is less than 15%. More importantly, since a single pixel cannot affect the mapping, it adapts gracefully from region to region.

While clahe enhances noise in the same proportion to signal, in relatively homogeneous regions or regions where the signal to noise ratio is small, there can be distracting levels of noise in the output image (Figure 1c). Contrast limitation has two affects on the output mapping: it places a maximum on the output intensity difference of of two input intensities, and it reduces the output range available to the local region.

Consider an image that has been scaled so that the input and output ranges are equal. If two pixels here input intensities p and q with t pixels in each intensity bin of the histogram between p and q, without contrast limitation, in the output image, these pixels would be separated by an intensity proportional to (p-q)*t. In clahe, with a clip fraction of, for example, 5 (assumed to be less than t) they would be separated by an intensity of only (p-q) * 5. In addition, the redistribution of pixels to all intensity bins in the image limits the effective output range to which the actual pixels in the region can be mapped. Without contrast limitation, the full range is available.

We have examined contrast limited histograms of CT images and RT portal film images and found typically a small number of histogram peaks (usually 1, 2, or 3) are clipped while the number of clipped pixels varies widely; approximately 25% to 75% of the pixels are clipped in regions requiring contrast limitation. Because of these large region to region differences, ahe with global contrast limitation is quite ineffective.

We conclude that any approximations to the clahe algorithm must be locally adaptive, the mapping should not depend on a single or small number of pixels, and there must be a locally adaptive means of limiting contrast in certain image regions.

A Mathematical Description of the Clahe Algorithm

If the image is scaled such that the number of intensities (N) is equal to the number of pixels in the contextual region (m*m), the calculation of the rank for a pixel with intensity n can be expressed as

$$
r_n = \frac{\displaystyle\sum_{i=0}^{n} \min(\text{cliplimit}, h_i) + \sum_{j=0}^{n} \dfrac{\displaystyle\sum_{k=0}^{N} \max(0, h_k - \text{cliplimit})}{m * m}}{m * m}
$$

where $h_i$ is a histogram bin. The summation in i represents the rank of a pixel given that a maximum of clip limit pixels at any single intensity in the local histogram may contribute to its rank. Since each region will have a different number of clipped pixels, redistribution is required to normalize the ranks computed in different regions. The normalization is provided by the summation in j, which is the contribution of all clipped pixels in the region redistributed equally into all intensity bins in the full range of the image. Finally, the rank is scaled to the range 0 to 1 by dividing by the region size. In simplified terms,

$$
r_n = \frac{\text{rank in a clipped histogram + redistributed clipped pixels}}{\text{region size}}
$$

In regions where there is a wide range of well distributed intensities, little or no clipping will occur. If no clipping occurs,

$\min(\text{cliplimit}, h_i) = h_i$,  and
$\max(0, h_i - \text{cliplimit}) = 0$,

and the equation reduces to that for unclipped ahe,

$$r_n = \sum_{i=0}^{n} h_i$$

In regions where all of the intensity bins are clipped (which rarely occurs in practice), the equation reduces to the sum of two linear terms:

$$r_n = \frac{n*cliplimit + n*(m*m-n*cliplimit)}{m*m}$$

Modifying the Clahe Algorithm

It is useful to consider separately the contributions of the contrast limited rank and of the redistributed clipped pixels.

The rather complicated expression for redistribution of clipped pixels in the clahe equation is easily simplified. The image is offset so the minimum intensity is 0. For a given region R, let $\alpha_R$ be the amount redistributed to each intensity bin. Since the region size m*m is fixed across the entire image and we redistribute into all intensity bins in the image, $\alpha_R$ depends only on C, the number of clipped pixels in region R,

$$\alpha_R = \frac{m*m - C}{N}$$

The contribution by the redistribution to the rank of a pixel with intensity $i_{in}$ in a contrast limited histogram is

$$redistribution = \alpha_R * i_{in}$$

This expression allows a much simplified approach to the redistribution. Only the total number of clippped pixels and the original intensity are required to compute this term.

The original clahe equation specifies a straightforward way to compute the contribution of the contrast limited rank given the complete histogram. Again, we wish to avoid computation of the complete histogram at each pixel, so we will introduce a factor $\beta_{R,I}$ to specify the contribution of a pixel at intensity I to the rank of any one pixel in the contextual region. $\beta_{R,I}$ depends on both the region R and the intensity I of the contributing pixel. If there is no clipping in the given bin, $\beta_{R,I} = 1$. If there is clipping, $\beta_{R,I}$ * the number of pixels in the bin will equal the clip limit.

The resulting equation for the contribution of the clipped histogram bins is

$$clipped\ rank = \sum_{i=0}^{n} \beta_{R,i} * h_i$$

The resulting complete equation for clahe,

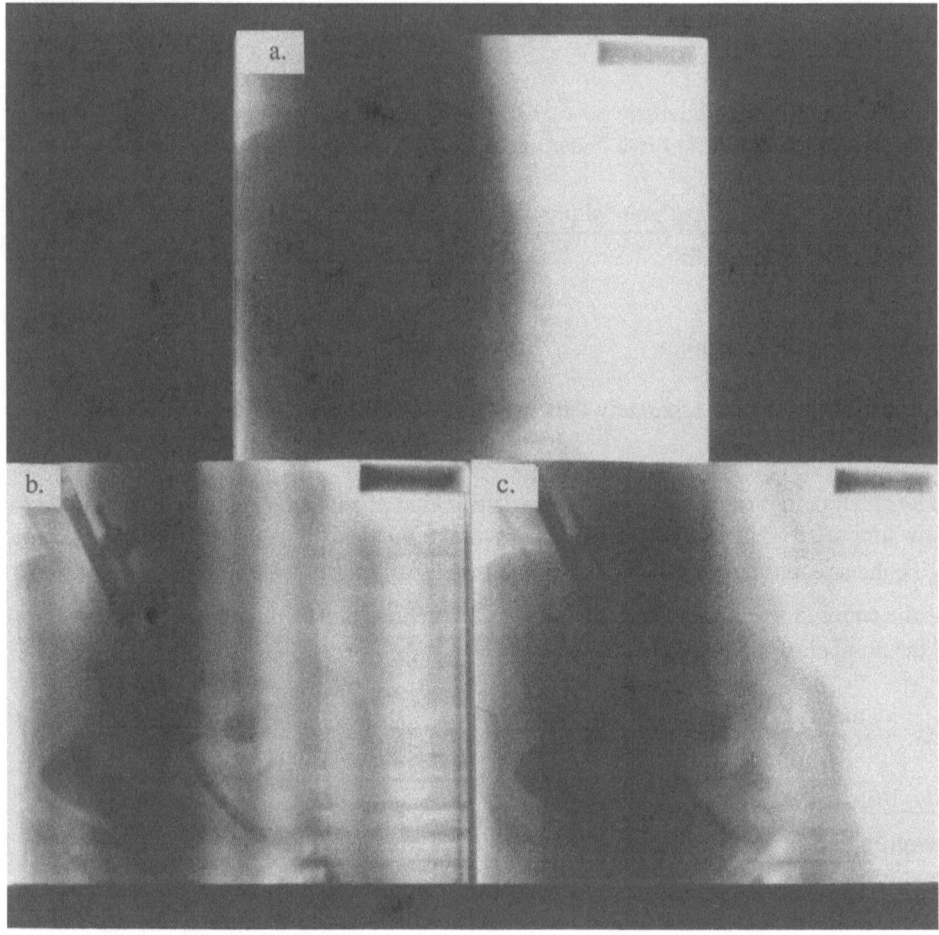

Figure 3: 512 x 512 radiotherapy gynecological implant localization film.
a) original; b) interpolated clahe; and c) uninterpolated clahe, both with 64 x 64
contextual region sizes and clip fractions of 10.

$$r_n = \sum_{i=0}^{n} \beta_{R,i} * h_i + \alpha_R * i_{in}$$

will be easy to implement if $\beta$ and $\alpha$ can be easily determined or accurately approximated. If
an approximation is used, the previously discussed essential properties of clahe must be
preserved. Before describing the implementation of the algorithm, we digress briefly to
discuss interpolated clahe.

Interpolated Clahe

Interpolated clahe usually produces very satisfactory results, but there are occasional
undesired artifacts not produced by real clahe. Figure 3 is an RT gynecological implant
localization film. There is a left to right monotonic intensity increase across the right half of the
original image (Figure 3a) that is not seen in the original. The interpolated clahe image (Figure
3b) displays a wavelike intensity variation across the right half of the image that is the same
period as the sampling grid. This artifact is not present in the real clahe image (Figure 3c).
The source of this variation is the interpolation between two mappings produced from

histograms of pixels in two quite different intensity ranges.

We have only observed this artifact with RT portal film images and radiographs and have not observed them with CT or MRI. This result persuades us to implement real clahe and not the interpolated version. A direct implementation of the interpolated clahe algorithm would require about one-third the hardware of the approach described below, and compute clahe about three times as fast.

## A MULTIPROCESSOR ADAPTIVE HISTOGRAM EQUALIZATION MACHINE

### The Mahem Algorithm

The mahem implementation closely approximates the clahe algorithm in two passes. During the first pass, the number of pixels in a contextual region equal to the center pixel $E_{i,j}$, that is, the number of pixels in histogram bin, is computed. The total is then used in the second pass to find $\beta_{R,I}$ in a lookup table. During the second pass, the contrast limited rank $R_{i,j}$ and the total number of clipped pixels $C_{i,j}$ in the region are computed. Finally, $\alpha_R$ is computed from $C_{i,j}$, multiplied times the original intensity and added to the contrast limited rank, and stored in memory. The algorithm proceeds as follows:

```
for all pixels p_{k,l} in the image {
        for all pixels p_{m,n} in the contextual region of p_{k,l} {
                if (p_{k,l} == p_{m,n})
                        E_{k,l} = E_{k,l} + 1
                }
        }
for all pixels p_{k,l} in the image {
        for all pixels p_{m,n} in the contextual region of p_{k,l} {
                if (p_{m,n} < p_{k,l})
                        R_{k,l} = R_{k,l} + β[E_{m,n}]
                C_{k,l} = C_{k,l} + β[E_{m,n}]
                }
        R_{k,l} = R_{k,l} + α[C_{k,l}] * p_{k,l}
        }
```

On a serial computer this algorithm is extremely slow. However, each pixel requires only three storage locations, and the only operations required in the inner loop of each pass are a comparison and an addition, both shown above in bold. Since pixel $p_{m,n}$ is in the contextual region of many pixels $p_{k,l}$, the comparison and and then the addition can be computed at many pixels simultaneously with only a small amount of hardware required at each pixel. The result is that a small part of the rank of many pixels is computed simultaneously. We have found that enough processors to compute one column (or one row) of the contextual region is a reasonable compromise between speed and size.

This algorithm contains two approximations. For implementation ease, we have chosen to use scaled integer arithmetic rather than floating point computation. In the floating point case, we would add one to the rank counter if the given histogram bin was less than the clip limit, and a fraction less than one determined by the ratio of the bin height to the clip limit otherwise.

Using integers, we instead use three bits to quantize the fraction to one of eight values between 1 and 8. A bin height less than the clip limit will be incremented by 8, and those bins above the clip limit by a value between 1 and 7. This quanitization results in a small amount of error in the computation.

The value that should be used to look up the increment is the number of pixels within the contextual region of pixel k,l equal to the given pixel. Instead, the first pass counts the number of pixels equal to the given pixel within its own contextual region. Depending on the relative positions of the two pixels, as few as one-fourth of the pixels are included in both of the regions. The remaining pixels are, however, adjacent to the proper region. Use of the proper region would require computation of the complete histogram for each region, and the amount of hardware required prohibits this method.

Fortunately, neither of these approximations has a great deal of affect on the image. Figure 4a is an original abdomen CT scan and the image in Figure 4b has been processed with real clahe. The image in Figure 4c has used discrete values to increment the rank instead of the proper fraction, and there is little difference. The use of the incorrect region, illustrated in Figure 4d, results in considerably less clipping than the correct region, but selection of a smaller clip fraction compensates for this. Figure 4e is the image that will be computed by mahem using this algorithm and shows the result of both approximations, and Figure 4f the mahem algorithm with a smaller clip fraction.

Mahem Architecture

Mahem (Figure 5) has three basic components: an interface to the host computer, memory to store the original, processed, intermediate, and displayed image data, and processors that perform the clahe computation. The host interface allows communication of data and commands via a DMA interface (or PACS in a clinical setting) with a host computer. From the interface, data is transferred via the main system data bus to memories which are implemented with video RAMs. These devices are 256K bit dynamic RAMs augmented with a shift register that allows high speed access to a selected row of stored data. In typical frame buffer memory applications, this shift register is used to output data at video rates to the analog circuits. In mahem, this shift register transfers data between the memories and clahe processors, which allows computation to proceed at speeds not limited by the slower memory random access time.

Consider first a machine with a single clahe processor. After the original image data has been transferred to memory, a clahe execute command is sent from the host computer to the clahe controller. The controller transfers a pixel value from original image memory to the clahe processor (Figure 6), where it is stored in a register. During the first pass, those pixels that are in the contextual region of the pixel stored in the register are sequentially shifted from image memory into the comparator logic in the clahe processor. Each pixel is compared to the original, and if they are equal, the adder logic increments the equal value. After all pixels in the contextual region have been compared, the equal count is stored in memory, where it will be used during the second pass to look up in a table the value that will be added to the contrast limited rank. During the second pass, all pixels in the contextual region are again compared to the original, and if less than the original, the value from the lookup table is added to the rank value. The lookup value is also added to the clip counter value regardless of the result of the comparison. After all pixels in the contextual region have shifted through the clahe processor, the final rank value and final clip value are used to compute the actual clahe'd image value for the pixel, which is transferred from the processor to the rank memory. This process is repeated for all pixels in the image.

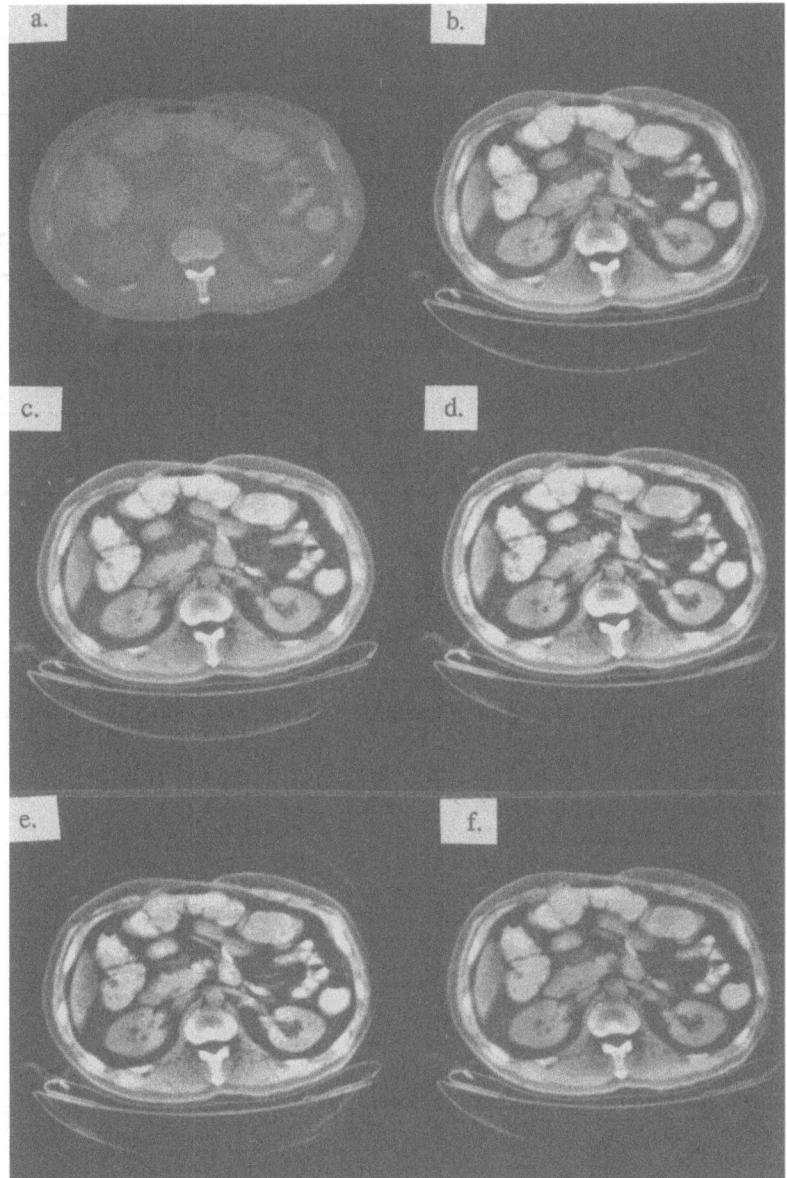

Figure 4: 512 x 512 abdomen CT, all real clahe'd versions processed
with a 64 x 64 contextual region, b-e with a clip fraction of 10.
a) original; b) real clahe; c) discrete increments; d) wrong region for
equal count; e) both discrete increments and wrong region; and
f) both discrete increments and wrong region with clip fraction of 5.

This method is very inefficient for a single processor. However, the individual processors
are very small, and the controller can be common to many clahe processors. Additional
processors can be added that simultaneously compute ranks for pixels that have adjacent
contextual regions. In mahem, these processors are allocated to compute pixels in adjacent
rows. The next section discusses the timing analysis for a single processor and multiple
processor systems.

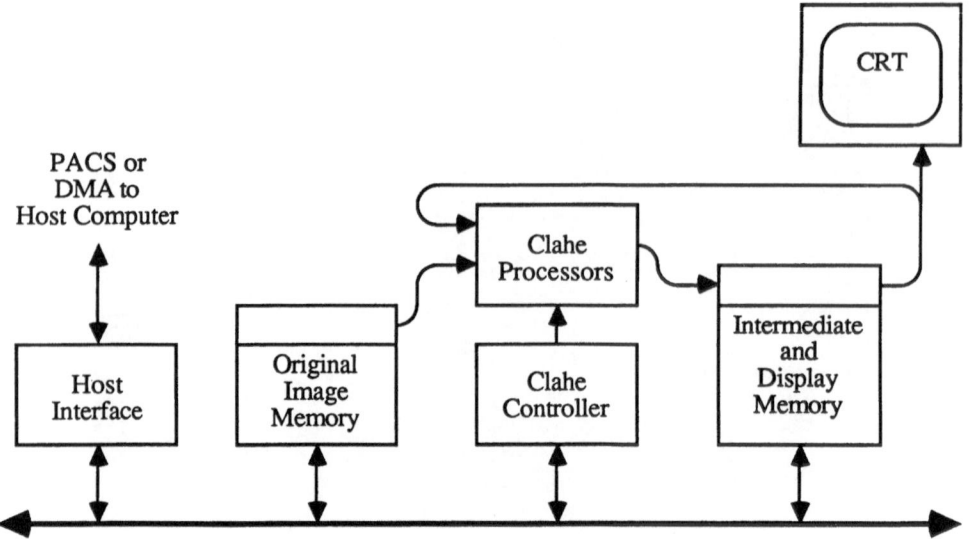

Figure 5: Block diagram of the mahem system.

Timing Analysis

The parameters that determine the computation speed of the mahem algorithm are:

| Parameter | Symbol | Typical Value |
|---|---|---|
| VRAM shift speed | $t_s$ | 100 nsec |
| VRAM random access time | $t_a$ | 250 nsec |
| Image size | $n_x \times n_y$ | 512 x 512 |
| Contextual region size | $m_x \times m_y$ | 64 x 64 |
| Number of Processors | $p$ | 64 |

The typical VRAM values in the table are very conservative estimates.

One Processor System. For the one processor system, the following steps must be computed for every pixel:

Step 1. The original pixel data is transferred to the clahe processor via the random access port, which depends on the access time to the memory

$$t_{step1} = t_a$$
$$= 250 \text{ nanoseconds}$$

Step 2. For every row in the contextual region, pixel data is loaded into the shift register and shifted to the clahe processor for counting the number of equal pixels in the region, which requires

$$t_{step2} = m_y * (t_a + t_s * m_x)$$
$$= 64 * (250 \text{ nsec} + 100 \text{ nsec} * 64) = 0.43 \text{ milliseconds}$$

Step 3. The total number of equal pixels are stored in the equal memory via the random

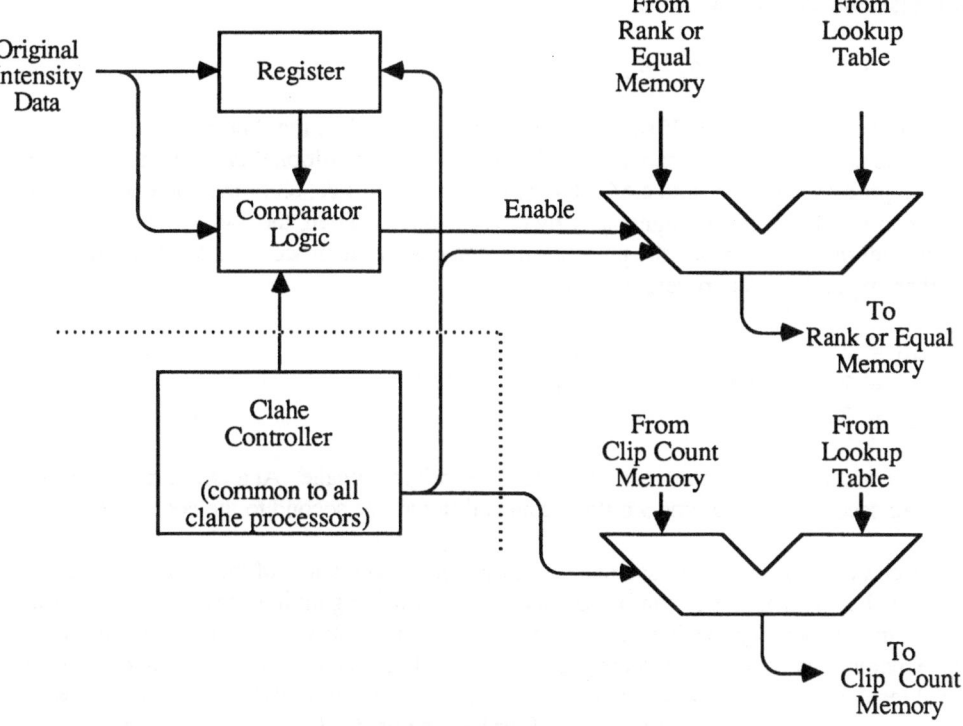

Figure 6: Block diagram of the clahe processor.

access port, which again depends on the memory access time,

$$t_{step3} = t_a = 250 \text{ nsec}$$

Step 4. For every row in the contextual region, pixel data is loaded into the shift register and shifted to the clahe processor for computation of the rank and counting the total number of clipped pixels,

$$t_{step4} = m_y * (t_a + t_s * m_x)$$
$$= 64 * (250 \text{ nsec} + 100 \text{ nsec} * 64 ) = 0.43 \text{ milliseconds}$$

Step 5. Compute the final value from the rank and total number of clipped pixels and write the data via the random access port into the rank memory.

$$t_{step5} = t_a = 250 \text{ nsec}$$

The actual computation of the final value may require additional time, but this can be overlapped with the computation of the next pixel value.

The total time to compute the image is therefore
$$t_{total} = n_x * n_y * (t_{step1} + t_{step2} + t_{step3} + t_{step4} + t_{step5})$$
$$= 512 * 512 * (250 \text{ nsec} + 0.43 \text{ msec} + 250 \text{ nsec} + 0.43 \text{ msec} + 250 \text{ nsec})$$
$$= 22.5 \text{ seconds}$$

If we neglect the negligible time required for steps 1, 3, and 5, we can rewrite the equation

387

for the general case of one processor as:

$$t_{total} = 2 * (n_x * n_y * m_y * m_x) * t_s$$

Multiprocessor System. If additional processors are added, the time required for the comparisons in step 2 above can be done in parallel by the additional processors. For example, in a two processor system with a 64 x 64 contextual region size, 63 of the context affecting pixels can be compared simultaneously by the processors. Then, the 64th pixel will also affect a new pixel that must replace the previous pixel in one of the processors. With p processors, p less than $m_y$, and the 64 processor system,

$$
\begin{aligned}
t_{total} &= 2 * (n_x * n_y * m_x * m_y * t_s) / p \\
&= 2 * (512 * 512 * 64 * 64 * 100 \text{ nsec}) / 64 \\
&= 3.2 \text{ sec}
\end{aligned}
$$

This does not include the time required to load the original image. At a DMA rate of 500K bytes per second, the load time would add an additional one second to the computation.

Once the number of processors exceeds the region size, some of the processors have no data to which their intensity can be compared, so no further gain in speed is realized. If the original image memory size is smaller than the image, data must be transferred to and from the image memory as computation proceeds. The computation can be organized such that some partial results and some complete results are computed each time part of the image is loaded. If a system has only enough storage for one-fourth of the original image, the computation time would increase by a factor of four. However, this assumes that the host can have new data immediately upon request, so realistically this time will be somewhat more. If both the image size and the contextual region size are larger than the memory and number of processors available, the computation slows drastically. Each time data is shifted into the clahe processors, new image data must be transferred from the host, so the computation time is determined by the much slower data transfer rate.

Size Estimates

The entire display and processing system could be realized using approximately twelve double-height MULTIBUS (12 inches by 12 inches) boards. Approximately 100 ICs can be placed on each board.

The 512 x 512 x 16 bit data memories will each require 16-256K VRAMs. Along with support chips, these memories would fit on two boards. The display memory is only 8 bits wide, so 8 memory chips are required. A small amount of circuitry must be provided to process the data coming from the rank counter memory to the display memory, and could reside along with the display memory and analog circuits on the video board. A DMA controller requires no more than 50 ICs. Allowing for the complexity of a 64 processor system, the controller should require no more than 100 TTL chips and reside on one board. Each clahe processor requires about 10 ICs, so 10 clahe processors would fit on each board.

SUCCESSIVELY REFINED CLAHE

The mahem algorithm computes many output pixels in parallel, with each pixel from the contextual region input sequentially to the clahe processors. The computation time is therefore proportional to the number of pixels in each contextual region. With successively refined clahe, we use only a small sample of pixels in the contextual region each pixel to approximate its output value (as opposed to interpolated clahe where all pixels in the contextual region of a sample set of pixels is used). While the image will contain artifacts of this sampling, the sampled image is only displayed until fully computed image is displayed.

For successively refined clahe, the pixels are selected from a uniformly sampled grid and the final image computed in successive passes, each sampled at a finer resolution than the previous pass. For example, if we sample every eighth pixel in every eighth row, a sampled result could be presented 64 times as fast as the final image. While computing the image at the next finer sampling, the previous image is displayed to allow the user to adjust the contextual region size or clip levels. If no adjustments are made, computation proceeds and successively better images are presented until the final image is displayed.

A successively refined version of ahe has been implemented on the Pixel-planes raster graphics engine (Poulton, et. al. 1984; Fuchs, et. al., 1985). The sampled image is first displayed in 70 milliseconds, and the final image is produced in less than 5 seconds. This demonstration of near real time ahe on Pixel-planes has excited physicians and stimulated the mahem research. Unfortunately, the Pixel-planes architecture requires custom VLSI components and is a large and expensive machine for this one application.

In the mahem implementation random x-y pixel access is much slower than serial access via the shift register port. Uniform sampling is not practical, so we will instead sample at a very coarse grid in the y direction and use every pixel in the x direction. While this image is not as high quality as the grid sampled image, it is still useful to present while waiting for the final image to be computed.

Figure 7 shows several processed chest radiographs. The images in the top row are the original, fully processed ahe, and fully processed clahe. The images in the second row have been processed with ahe using 8 x 8 sampling, 4 x 4 sampling, and 2 x 2 sampling, as is done on Pixel-planes. The images in the bottom row have been processed with ahe using 1 x 64 sampling, 1 x 32 sampling, and 1 x 4 sampling, as will be done on mahem. Figure 8a shows the percentage of pixels that were within 10%, 5%, and 1% of their fully processed value after each of 4 passes when sampled equally in x and y. Figure 8b shows the same data for sampling in the y direction only.

In mahem only region sizes of $2^R$ pixels are used so that the range of possible ranks is 0 to $2^{R-1}$. This allows a simple shift operation to scale the rank value to the typical display range of 0 to 255. Because not all pixels are compared in successively refined clahe, it can produce a rank in the range of 0 to $2^R$ and cannot easily be scaled. The number of pixels at the maximum value is usually small, and since this image is only displayed until the fully sampled version is computed we will allow the overflow value to be displayed as 0.


DISCUSSION

Mahem satisfies the need for a fast implementation of clahe. For single-image studies, it will allow interactive region size and clip limit selection by the user. For multi-image studies it can serve as a computing resource, allowing the full study to be processed in a short time.

While the algorithm is quite fast, we would much prefer a solution that would allow computation in one pass instead of two. Regular ahe can be computed in one pass, but the

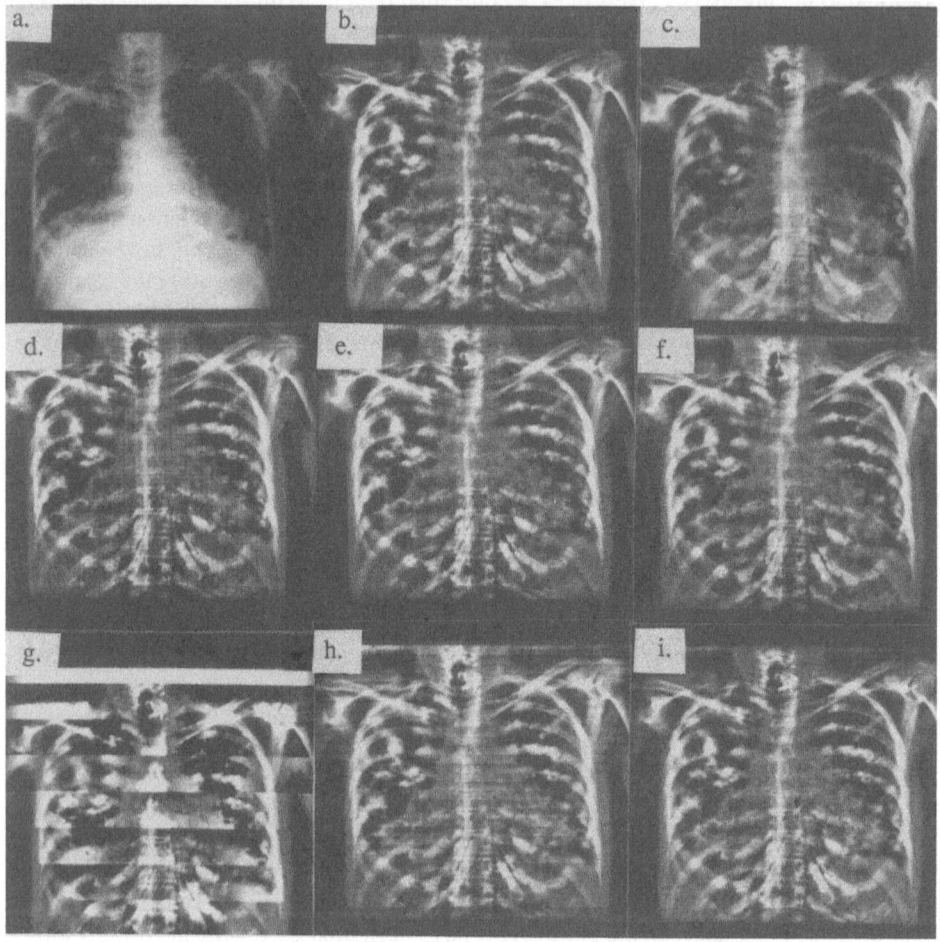

Figure 7: 512 x 512 chest radiograph. a) original; b) real ahe; c) real clahe with clip fraction of 10; d) real ahe sampled 8 x 8; e) real ahe sampled 4 x 4; f) real ahe sampled 2 x 2; g) real ahe sampled 64 x 1; h) real ahe sampled 16 x 1; and i) real ahe sampled 4 x 1.

clipping operation requires information from the entire region before beginning the rank calculation. We believe the requirements established for a contrast enhancement method (local adaptation, no dependence on a small number of pixels, and locally adaptive contrast limitation) preclude the use of a single pass algorithm.

Algorithm development is complete and we will finalize the mahem architecture during the summer of 1987. Design and implementation of the system will follow, and we expect to have a working prototype complete in late 1988. This machine will become available in the UNC Radiology department for use by radiologists and radiotherapists.

ACKNOWLEDGEMENTS

We thank Henry Fuchs for suggesting the successive refinement algorithm, John Zimmerman for technical discussions and comments on this paper, Sharon Core and Sharon Laney for typing and production assistance, Michael McGuffey for software assistance, and

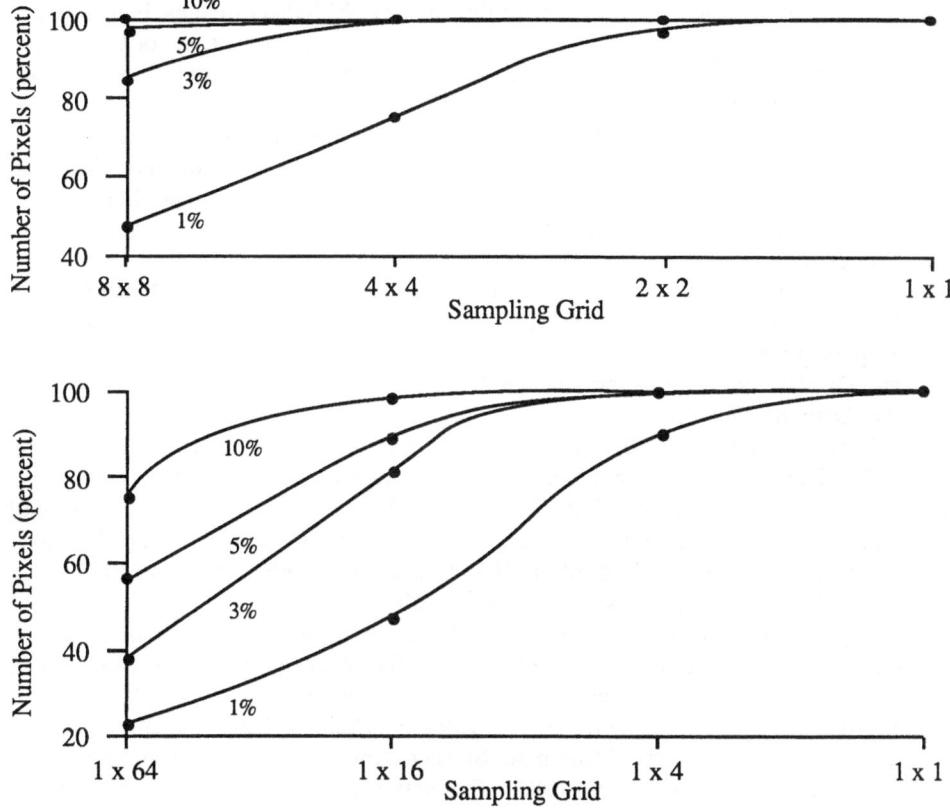

Figure 8: Number of pixels within a given percent of final value, composite of three 512 x 512 CT images, real ahe with a 128 x 128 region size. top) Sampled in x and y; bottom) sampled in y only.

Bo Strain and Karen Curran for photography. This research has been partially supported by NIH Grant # 1 R01 CA 44060-01.

REFERENCES

Fahnestock, J.D., and Schowengerdt, R.A. (1983). Spatially Variant Contrast Enhancement Using Local Range Modification, Optical Engineering, 22(3), 378-381.

Fuchs, H., Goldfeather, J., Hultquist, J.P., Spach, S., Austin, J.D., Brooks, F.P., Eyles, J.G., and Poulton, J. (1985). Fast Spheres, Shadows, Textures, Transparencies, and Image Enhancements in Pixel-planes, Computer Graphics, 19(3), (Proceedings of SIGGRAPH '85), 111-120.

Hummel, R.A. (1977). Image Enhancement by Histogram Transformation, Computer Graphics and Image Processing, 6, 184-195.

Ketcham, D.J., Lowe, R.W., and Weber, J.W. (1976). Real-time Image Enhancement Techniques, Seminar on Image Processing, Pacific Grove California, Hughes Aircraft Company, 1-6.

Pizer, S.M. (1981). An Automatic Intensity Mapping for the Display of CT Scans and Other Images, Medical Image Processing: Proceedings of the VIIth International Meeting on Information Processing in Medical Imaging, Stanford, California, Stanford University, 276-309.

Pizer, S.M. (1981). Intensity Mapping for the Display of Medical Images, Functional Mapping of Organ Systems: 11th Annual Symposium on the Sharing of Computer Programs and Technology in Nuclear Medicine, New Orleans, Louisiana, P.D. Esser (ed.), Society of Nuclear Medicine, 205-218.

Pizer, S.M., Amburn, E.P., Austin, J.D., Cromartie, R., Geselowitz, A., Greer, T., ter Haar Romeny, B.H., Zimmerman, J.B., and Zuiderveld, K. (1987). Adaptive Histogram Equalization and Its Variations, Technical Report, Depart. of Computer Science, University of North Carolina, to appear in Computer Vision, Graphics, and Image Processing.

Pizer, S.M., Austin, J.D., Perry, J.R., Safrit, H.D., and Zimmerman, J.B.(1986). Adaptive Histogram Equalization for Automatic Contrast Enhancement of Medical Images, Application of Optical Instrumentation in Medicine, XIV: Medical Imaging, Processing, and Display and Picture Archiving and Communication Systems (PACS IV) for Medical Applications, 242- 250.

Pizer, S. M., Zimmerman, J. B., and Staab, E. V. (1984). Adaptive Grey Level Assignment in CT Scan Display, Journal of Computer Assisted Tomography, 8(2), 300 - 305.

Poulton, J., Fuchs, H., Austin, J.D., Eyles, J.G., Heinecke, J., Hsieh, C-H, Goldfeather,J., Hultquist, J.P., and Spach, S. (1985). PIXEL-PLANES: Building a VLSI-Based Graphic System, Proceedings of the 1985 Chapel Hill Conference on VLSI, Rockville,MD, Computer Science Press, 35-60.

ter Haar Romeny, B., Pizer, S.M., Zuiderveld, K. Zimmerman, J.B., Amburn, P., Geselowitz, A., van Waess, P.F.G.M., de Goffau, A.. (1985). Recent Developments in Adaptive Histogram Equalization, Radiology, 157(P), 396.

Zimmerman, J.B., (1985). Effectiveness of Adaptive Contrast Enhancement, Ph.D. Dissertation, Department of Computer Science, University of North Carolina.

Zimmerman, J.B., and Pizer, S.M. (1985). Evaluation of the Effectiveness of Adaptive Histogram Equalization, Proceedings of 25th Fall Symposia - Imaging, Society of Photographic Scientists and Engineers, 189-190.

# A GRAPHICS WORKSTATION FOR PET DATA ACQUISITION AND DISPLAY

A.Geissbühler[1], D.Townsend[1], and S.Kuijk[2]

[1] Division of Nuclear Medicine, Geneva University
Hospital, Geneva, Switzerland
[2] Division of Nuclear Medicine, VUB, Brussels,
Belgium

## INTRODUCTION

Positron Emission Tomography (PET) is a quantitative
imaging modality that enables human physiology and metabolism to
be measured *in vivo* for a number of important clinical
applications (Phelps et al., 1986). The necessary measurements
are obtained from the set of reconstructed tomographic images
resulting from a PET scan. The important stages in this
measurement procedure are therefore positron data acquisition,
tomographic reconstruction including normalisation and
correction for physical effects such as photon attenuation and
scatter, display and manipulation of the reconstructed images
and the definition of suitable regions of interest. Physiologic
parameters are obtained by modelling the variations of the count
densities in the regions of interest as a function of, for
example, time.

It is obviously important that these procedures, which are
an essential aspect of PET, should be carried out in a
simple-to-use and flexible computing environment. To date, most
of this work has been performed on DEC VAX computers, or
equivalent, equipped with a separate display system. However,
the new generation of high performance computer workstations
offer an integrated solution to PET data analysis by providing a
powerful CPU, large memory capacity and a high resolution colour
graphics display screen within a single package. Accelerators
are usually available for high performance, three-dimensional
graphics with almost real-time rotation of complex shaded
surfaces. The workstations offer the power and flexibility of a
general-purpose computer (including high-level language
support), combined with performance (for some applications)
normally associated with special-purpose hardware.

The major drawback to the use of these workstations for
PET, or medical imaging in general, is the unavailability of
adequate software. Although the workstation operating system
usually includes a wide range of sophisticated and flexible
software tools, the provision of an easy to use, high-level

software interface still requires considerable programming effort (Robb et al., 1986; Robb et al, 1987). This paper will describe the development of, and features available with, such a software package. Even though the development has been carried out within the APOLLO DOMAIN environment, most of the principles and features implemented are common to any workstation solution to the PET data analysis problem.

THE HIDAC CAMERA

The High Density Avalanche Chamber (HIDAC) positron camera is a large area, high spatial resolution PET imaging system (Townsend et al., 1987a). The current design consists of dual HIDAC detectors mounted on a gantry which rotates around the patient during the PET scan. Positron data is acquired from a very large number of possible angular directions (typically, $2^{21}$). The PET image is reconstructed directly in three dimensions rather than as a set of independent slices, the alternative approach of commercial, multi-ring cameras. Details of the detector design (Jeavons et al, 1983), the reconstruction algorithm (Schorr et al, 1983) and the camera performance (Townsend et al, 1987b) may be found elsewhere.

The software system to be described in this paper must provide the facilities for positron data acquisition, three-dimensional tomographic reconstruction, and manipulation and display of three dimensional image matrices. The software interface to the system must be friendly and simple to use for medical technicians and clinicians.

COMPUTER CONFIGURATION

As previously explained, PET data require many computational resources for both data processing and for image generation. Although it is possible to use a single workstation for both calculations and display, the decision was taken to use

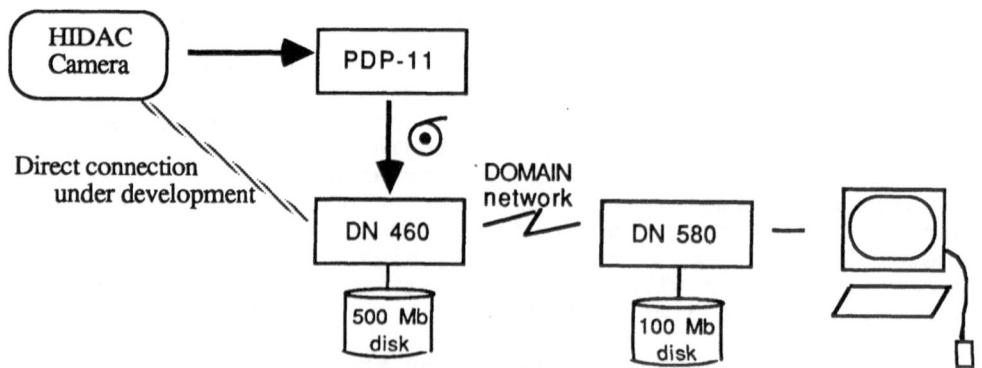

Fig.1  Computer configuration

two workstations so as to provide adequate response time for the image display. One system (the diagnostic workstation) is dedicated to handle the user interface, and to display menus and images. In this implementation it is an APOLLO DN580 configured with a 1280x1024x8 bits deep, high resolution display, 3.5 Mb of memory, a 100 Mbyte disk and a mouse. The second system (the computational server), which has to perform intensive calculations is an APOLLO DN460, with 8 Mb of memory, a 500 Mbyte Winchester disk and a 1600 bpi magnetic tape unit. The workstations are linked by the high-speed DOMAIN network (fig.1).

Currently, data from the HIDAC camera are acquired on a DEC PDP11/44 and stored on disk in list mode, i.e. the coordinates of the individual positron events are recorded. However, the APOLLO computer system will eventually be connected directly to the HIDAC camera by an interface that has been developed at the Vrije University in Brussels. At the present time, data are transferred from the PDP11/44 to the APOLLO on 1600 bpi magnetic tape.

SOFTWARE CONFIGURATION

The software configuration was designed to optimize the use of the networked environment and to minimize the amount of data being transferred between the computers. To avoid concurrent access to the data files and to improve memory utilisation, it was decided that only the computational server would access data, communicating the results of the calculations (usually bitmaps) to the diagnostic workstation.

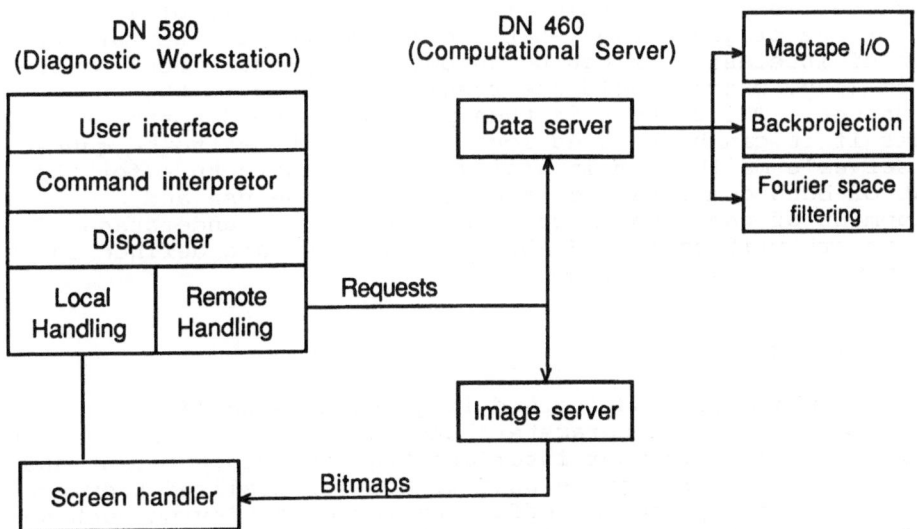

Fig.2   Software configuration

The DN580 operates as the master (graphics) node, communicating with the DN460 (the computational node) through a mailbox system. Servers on the computational node initiate tasks at the request of the graphics node, thereby leaving that node free to service other user requests. As soon as the task on the computational node has completed, the graphics node is informed and receives the results of the calculations, usually in the form of a status code (the request failed or succeeded), or as a bitmap (see fig.2).

Two different servers run on the computational node:

- the data server activates the modules for magnetic tape I/O, data conversion (to APOLLO format) and tomographic reconstruction (backprojection and Fourier space filtering).
- the image server uses the files created by the data server modules to prepare 2-D or 3-D images that will be displayed on the graphics node. It also performs various image processing functions such as 2-D and 3-D filters, arithmetic operations, thresholding and contouring.

Since the two servers run independently, it is possible for the user to initiate tomographic reconstructions and view images simultaneously. The modular approach facilitates the maintenance and development of the program by separating the user interface from the numerical data processing. The integration of new features in the program is simplified by the use of an internal language defining, for each function, the parameters which are necessary, how they are to be defined and the corresponding prompt message to be shown.

A command interpreter, called by the interface-handling module, uses these definitions to collect all the information necessary to build a request. This information can be provided by the user (e.g. which slice is to be processed), or is already known by the program (e.g. what are the bounds of the current region of interest), or can be automatically calculated by the program (e.g. where should the result be placed in the spreadsheet). The request is then passed to the dispatcher which decides if it can be handled locally or if it has to be queued in a server's mailbox. Maintaining the same structure for the format of both commands and requests makes the use and development of the program coherent and easy to understand. The programs are written in PASCAL, and the menus are defined in the menu compiler language DIALOG.


USER INTERFACE

Since the data handling and image processing of PET scans require many different parameters and functions, it is important to develop a friendly user interface that is both coherent and intuitive, so that it can be used without specialised knowledge of the operating system. An efficient way of achieving such an interface is to use pop-up menus so that the user is not overloaded with unnecessary information. These menus can also be used as check-lists, allowing the operator to verify all the parameters and options, before initiating time-consuming data

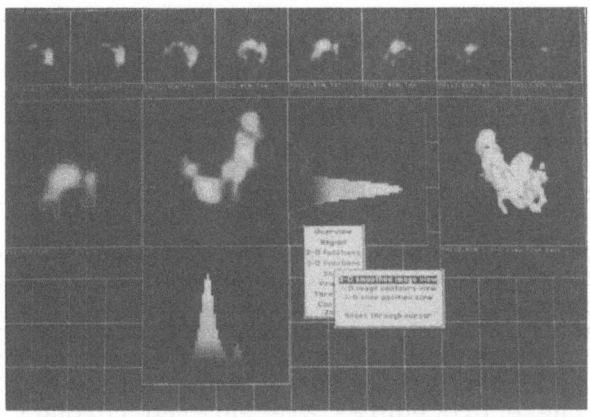

Fig.3 Spreadsheet layout showing images of various sizes,
profiles, a three-dimensional view and pop-up menus.


analyses.

The presentation chosen for the image handling module
resembles a spreadsheet in which numbers are replaced by images
(fig.3). Each cell or group of cells in the spreadsheet contains
an image, together with a description of the contents and the
history (i.e., how it was created and modified). Operations can
be applied to one or several cells, modifying them or creating
new cells. The user can delete, copy, move, zoom, add text and
hardcopy parts of the spreadsheet. Such an approach enables the
user to, for example, compare data from different files, to view
images before and after they have been modified, to view
transverse, frontal and sagittal slices, and to view the data in
the form of shaded 3-D surfaces. Since all functions operate in
the same way, it is rather easy to implement new features;
this is an important aspect since the software is used for both
clinical and research purposes. It is also possible to combine
commands into pipelines, or more complicated scripts, that can
be used to perform repetitive sequences, as ,for example, the
creation of a standard clinical report following a routine
examination. Other useful features include a prompt window
(which explains to the user what he is expected to do), a status
window, and a journal which keeps track of the main events.
Online help is available at any time.

The sections which follow will provide more details on the
facilities which are available at each stage in the data
analysis.


DATA ACQUISITION

As explained above, the data is currently acquired on a DEC
PDP11/44, and then transferred on magnetic tape to the APOLLO
DN460. After format conversion, the list-mode data, patient
information and acquisition parameters are stored in the
database. In the future, an APOLLO interface will be available

which will allow a direct connection between the HIDAC camera
and the APOLLO computer system. At that time, the PET data will
be collected on the APOLLO disk and the workstations will
control the camera. This configuration will also considerably
increase the potential data acquisition rate.


DATA RECONSTRUCTION

The theoretical principles and practical implementation of
the image reconstruction procedure have been described in detail
elsewhere (Schorr et al, 1983; Townsend et al, 1983). A two-step
process is used: back-projection of the photon event lines,
followed by a three-dimensional Fourier space deconvolution of
the positron camera point response function. All the parameters
required for these procedures are entered through the
appropriate pop-up menus prior to initiation of the
reconstruction. The options and parameter values selected are
immediately displayed on the screen for operator verification.
The software also offers the possibility to re-run all or part
of the reconstruction with different parameter values. The
output files are automatically renamed to avoid inadvertant loss
of previously-reconstructed images.

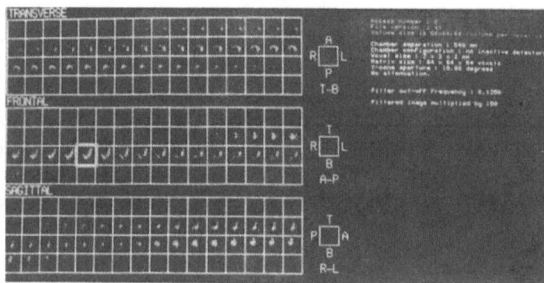

Fig.4   Overview of a thyroid scan showing 64 transverse,
        frontal and sagittal slices and the parameters used
        for the image reconstruction.


IMAGE HANDLING

## The image overview

Following tomographic reconstruction, an overview of the
image is created. This overview consists of a bitmap showing the
transverse, frontal and sagittal slices and information about
the patient and the parameters used in the reconstruction. The
overview, an example of which is shown in fig.4, is displayed
whenever a file is selected from the database for image
handling. It provides the operator or clinician with an initial
impression of the shape, size and image quality of the scanned
organ. The user then selects the appropriate slices to be
studied which are transferred into the spreadsheet for
subsequent manipulation.

## Spreadsheet functions

The spreadsheet functions can be divided into three main groups: spreadsheet editing functions, functions operating on 2-D images (slices), and functions operating on 3-D images (volumes). Spreadsheet editing functions allow the user to move, copy, delete, zoom, and hardcopy parts of the spreadsheet, and to change the colour scale. As these functions do not require any knowledge of the numerical data, they can be performed directly on the graphics workstation.

The functions operating on 2-D images are applied to the slices of 3-D volume images. They include median, linear and interactively defined filters. Arithmetical operations combine either two different slices, or a slice and an operator-selected constant value. Slice profiles or statistics can also be obtained. These operations require data from the image file and are therefore performed by the image server on the DN460.

The functions operating on 3-D images, which are also performed on the DN460, include thresholding, contouring, panelling and 3-D display. The threshold is a numerical value separating two regions of the image, e.g.the background and the signal. The threshold value cannot always be automatically determined from the image and must often be chosen by operator interaction. It may depend on many different parameters such as the size and shape of the organ, the level of background and the image statistics. A number of facilities are provided to help the user choose the correct threshold by calculating density histograms, profiles, or by using special colour scales. Once the threshold has been chosen, the program estimates the corresponding organ volume.

## Three-dimensional image display

The boundaries of the organ corresponding to a particular choice of threshold may be linked into a 3-D surface by stacking the contours from adjacent slices. This is the panelling operation. These surfaces can be displayed after hidden-surface removal with different shadings. Three-dimensional images can be observed from any direction, rotated interactively, and put in the spreadsheet. Two modes of display can be selected (fig.5): wireframe or shaded surface. Wireframe images can be calculated rapidly and rotated in real time. It is also possible to create simple stereoscopic views of the organ by overlaying two wireframe views of the same image, calculated from slightly different eye position with each drawn in a different colour (usually red and green). The stereoscopic effect is achieved by viewing the screen through special glasses. This display mode is useful in order to highlight errors or mismatches in the contours, which can then be corrected using the contour editor. Currently, it requires about one minute for the computer to create a shaded surface image, and thus it is not possible to rotate them in real time (see later). The software used at the present time to create such images is MOVIE.BYU (Brigham-Young University, Provo, Utah).

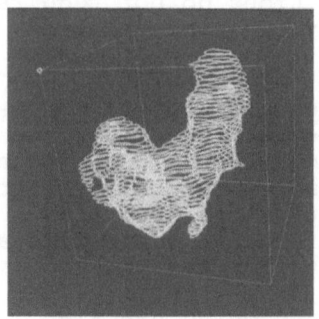
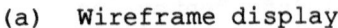
(a)  Wireframe display

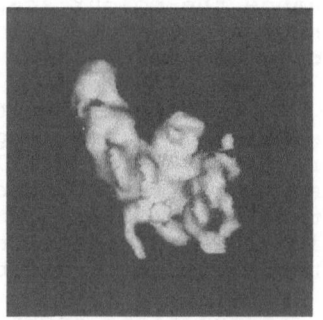
(b)  Shaded surface

Fig.5 Three-dimensional display modalities.

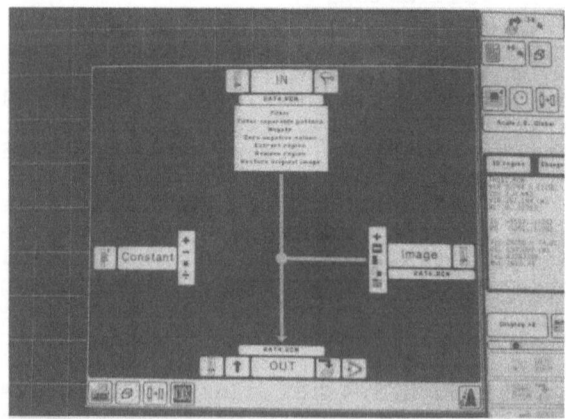

Fig.6 Image calculator showing the flow and combination of
data. Possible combinations include (image + image),
(image + constant), extraction of 3-D regions of
interest, and 3-D filtering. The 3-D filters can be
defined interactively. The results can be viewed either
by displaying stacked slices or by putting slices in the
spreadsheet. The results of numerical calculations are
displayed in the window on the right.

## Image calculator

Certain applications require three-dimensional manipulations that cannot be performed in the spreadsheet (e.g. merging two different files, using special 3-D filters, extracting specific regions of the image or calculating statistics about the activity in a region of the image). These functions are provided by the image calculator (fig.6). The 3-D image resulting from these calculations can be manipulated as any image from the database, e.g. sliced in a particular orientation, or entered into either the spreadsheet or the database.

## FUTURE DEVELOPMENTS

The software system described in this paper, although still under development, is currently operational and is actually used for data processing and display of images from the HIDAC positron camera for both clinical and research applications. A number of developments of the software are planned for the future. These will include:

- the provision of data acquisition software on the DN460 to allow the positron list-mode data to be collected directly onto the APOLLO disk. This step awaits the availability of the hardware interface for the camera.
- the use of the specialised APOLLO hardware for the display of three-dimensional surfaces. This will replace MOVIE.BYU and will allow more rapid display of such surfaces. Almost real-time display would be possible with the use of the APOLLO graphics accelerator, although the rate of display depends strongly on the actual number of panels composing the surface.
- as mentioned previously, PET is a quantitative imaging modality which requires not only image display facilities but also analyses based on local count densities in the image. The current software has provision to extract these densities from arbitrary three-dimensional regions-of-interest. As a future development, it will be necessary to include the models of flow and metabolism that enable measurements related to human physiology to be extracted from the image data.

## ACKNOWLEDGEMENTS

This work is supported by the Fonds National suisse under grant request 3.853-0.85. S.K. is a Research Assistent of the Belgium National Foundation for Scientific Research. The authors also acknowledge the financial help from the DeReuter Foundation of Geneva.

## REFERENCES

Jeavons, A.P., Hood, K., Herlin, G., Parkman, C., Townsend, D.W., Magnanini, R., Frey, P.E., Donath, A., (1983). The high-density avalanche chamber for positron emission tomography, IEEE Trans. Nucl. Sci., NS-30(1), 640-645.

Phelps, M.E., Mazziotta, J.C., Shelbert, H.R., (Eds) (1986).
    Positron Emission Tomography and Autoradiography, Raven
    Press, New York.
Robb, R.A., Heffernan, P.B., Camp, J.J., Hanson, D.P., (1986). A
    workstation for interactive display and quantitative
    analysis of 3-D and 4-D biomedical images, in: Proceedings
    of Computer Applications in Medical Care, Washington, D.C.
Robb, R.A., Stacy, M.C., McEwan, C.N., (1987). A networked
    workstation approach to multi-dimensional biomedical image
    analysis, in: Proceedings of this meeting.
Schorr, B., Townsend, D.W., Clack, R., (1983). A general method
    for three-dimensional filter computation, Phys. Med.
    Biol.,28, 305-312.
Townsend, D.W., Clack, R., Magnanini, R., Frey, P., Donath, A.,
    Schorr, B., Jeavons, A.P., Froidevaux, A., (1983). Image
    reconstruction for a rotating positron tomograph, IEEE
    Trans. Nucl. Sci., NS-30(1), 594-600.
Townsend, D.W., Frey, P.E., Jeavons, A.P., Reich, G.,
    Tochon-Danguy, H-J., Donath, A., Christin, A., Schaller,
    G., (1987a). The HIDAC positron camera, To appear in J.
    Nucl. Med.
Townsend, D.W., Clack, R., Defrise, M., Tochon-Danguy, H-J.,
    Frey, P., Kuijk, S., Deconinck, F., (1987b). Quantitation
    with the HIDAC positron camera, in: Proceedings of this
    meeting.

# VOLUME RENDERING OF 3D-TOMOGRAPHIC IMAGERY

K. H. Hohne, M. Riemer, U. Tiede, and Bomans

Institute of Mathematics and Computer Science in
Medicine (IMDM),
University Hospital Eppendorf, Hamburg, F.R.G.

## SUMMARY

Radiological examinations are increasingly based on sequences of cross-sectional images. In current clinical applications, the three-dimensional (3D) relationships contained in these examinations must be inferred by the observer through analysis of multiple two-dimensional (2D) images. In this paper, methods for the direct display of 3D gray level data are investigated. In the chosen approach, the 3D presentation of bone and skin surface serves to orient the viewer, while planar reformation and/or transparent projections can be applied for the assessment of soft tissue structures in regions of interest. The resulting images represent the original image data in a way that is more suitable for observation of 3D relationships than the conventional cross-sectional viewing mode. This may facilitate the diagnostic process and enhance the interpretability of the images. Routine clinical application of this technique requires special computer hardware.

## INTRODUCTION

An ever-increasing number of medical diagnostic images are obtained from X-ray Computed Tomography (CT), Magnetic Resonance Imaging (MRI), and Positron Emission Tomography (PET), which produce sequences of two-dimensional (2D) cross-sectional slices. The current predominant method of analyzing these images is by sequential observation of individual 2D slices and the viewer's subsequent 'mental reconstruction' of three-dimensional (3D) relationships. Computerized reformations of CT scans have produced 3D perspective display of bony anatomy that have proved clinically useful in craniofacial surgery and orthopedics (Boecker et al, 1985; Chen et al., 1985; Hemmy et al., 1983); Herman et al., 1985; Lineweaver et al.; Templeton et al., 1984; Vannier et al., 1984; Vannier et al.; Witte et al., 1986). A general application of this procedure in diagnostic radiology is limited by the fact that only predefined surfaces (mostly bone) can be visualized and that all other information is not used or lost in the reformation process. The classic approach requires a-priori knowledge of the gray scale properties of the lesion in order that a restricted region for 3D display be selected. In diagnostic radiology , however, the aim of the diagnostic process is precisely to find and define such regions. It is thus generally not possible to produce a 3D presentation of structures other than bone or skin surface prior to viewing the original gray scale images. General diagnostic application of 3D display techniques therefore requires presentation of the gray scale range for analysis. A few recent investigations have dealt with the software and hardware problems of displaying 3D tomographic volumes that preserve the entire original gray scale data (Goldwasser et al., 1985; Jackel, 1985; Lenz et al., 1986; Lenz et al., 1986; Höhne et al., 1987). It is the objective of this paper to evaluate viewing operations that allow the exploration of gray level volumes.

MATERIAL

The viewing operations are demonstrated with five data sets as shown in table 1.

Table 1: Data used for the 3D-presentation

| case | modality | matrix size | slices | device |
|------|----------|-------------|--------|--------|
| 1 | CT | 512 x 512 | 123 | Siemens Somatom DR 3 |
| 2 | MRI | 256 x 256 | 128 | Siemens Magnetom |
| 3 | MRI | 256 x 256 | 128 | Siemens Magnetom |
| 4 | MRI | 256 x 256 | 26 | Philips Gyroscan |

The images were produced with the program system VOXEL-MAN-8 (8 stands for eight bit gray scale resolution), that we have developed in our institute during the past two years. It is the extension of VOXEL-MAN-1 which works on binary data only. VOXEL-MAN-8 is written in PASCAL and implemented on a VAX-11/780 computer. The resulting images are displayed on a VTE Picturecom or a Comtal-Vision-One display system.

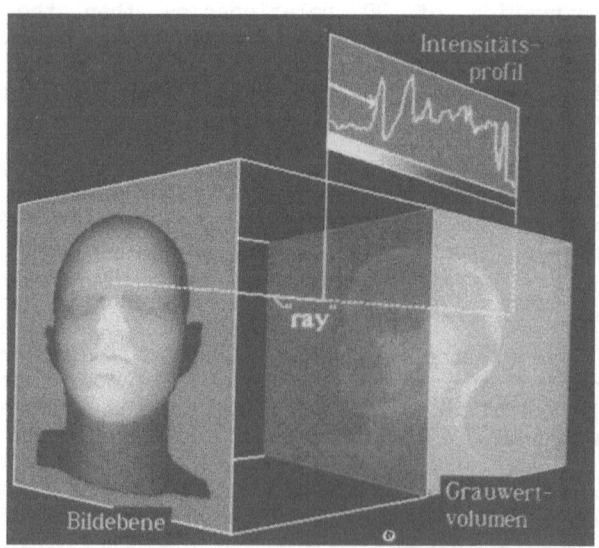

Fig. 1. Principle of the ray tracing algorithm. In the shown example a simple distance image is produced from the intensity profile.

METHOD AND RESULTS

### Preprocessing

To save storage space we compressed the CT values to a dynamic range of 256 gray values. To achieve cubic volume elements ('voxels') a linear interpolation of the intensity values between the original slices is performed. In order to produce a view from a desired perspective the entire image volume is rotated in the computer memory by resampling the data. Trilinear interpolation is used for the assignment of the gray scale values in the resampled volume.

### Generalized projections

The rotated volume can now be viewed by a set of simple 'projections', as shown in fig. 1. The intensity profile along rays through the volume are analyzed and the computed parameters are written onto the image plane. One simple parameter is the distance of the skin surface (as shown in fig. 1), which produces a simple surface image when the distance is mapped into an inverse gray scale. There are various other parameters. The images obtained this way can be considered as generalized projections of the object onto the image plane. The following basic projections have been implemented and tested:

### Projection of a surface

The computationally least expensive way of projecting a surface onto an image plane is distance shading, the computation of the inverse of the distance to each surface voxel. For a more realistic impression of the surface, shading methods (gradient shading) that take the surface inclination into account have been developed (Chen et al., 1985): In our implementation, gray scale data is utilized to produce surface shading based on the partial volume averaging effect. Here the gray values in the neighborhood of the surface voxel are used as a measure of the

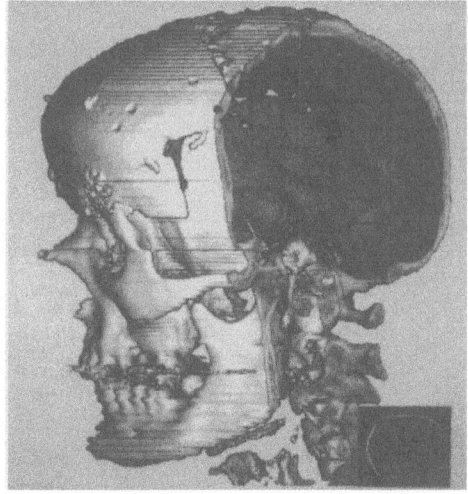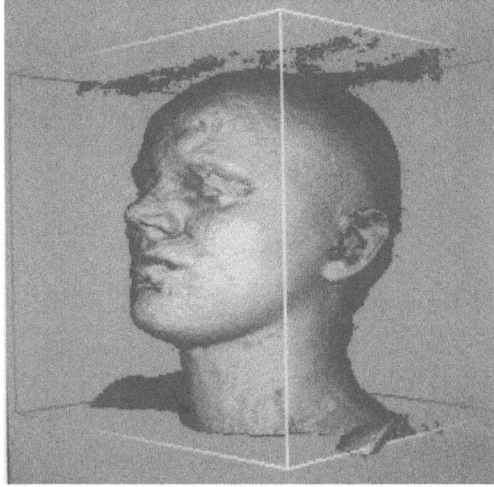

Fig. 2. Surface images. Left: Bone surface of a skull with an oblique cut (CT, case 1). Right: Skin surface of a head (MRI, case 2).

relative volume of adjacent tissue types (air/skin, soft tissue/bone) within the voxel. These relative volumes are related to the surface inclination. Thus the <u>gray level gradient</u> can be considered as a measure for surface inclination. This method ('gray level gradient shading') has been used in this study. It is described in greater detail elsewhere (Höhne et al, 1986; Tiede et al., 1987). Examples of a bone and a skin surface are shown in fig. 2.

## Projection of cut planes

Here only the gray values in the chosen plane are used to produce a new tomographic image. This is in principle the same as conventional reformatting. When, however, the cuts are displayed together with the remaining skin surface, the orientation of the cut plane becomes apparent immediately. This is demonstrated fig. 4.

## Transparent projections

In cases where the region of interest is not within a single plane, we can use an imaging mode similar to the classic X-ray projection. Here the intensity value in the image plane is computed simply by summing up the gray values in a certain range of the projection ray. In contrast to the classic X-ray technique, we can here choose which spatial range (depth) and/or intensity range is to be included in the projection. Fig. 3 shows as an example a look-through-projection of a layer of 2 cm along the skin surface of a human knee. As an advantage of this procedure vessels not being in one plane become visible in a single image. The same result is achieved when the same operation is applied to a human head.

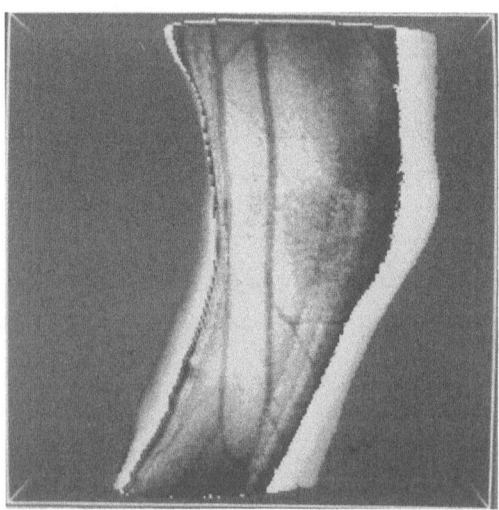 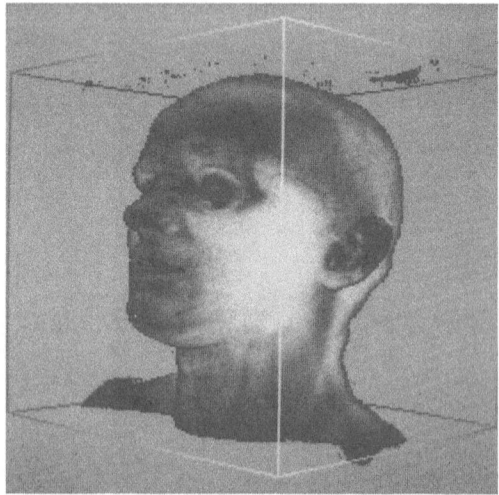

Fig. 3. Selective transparent projection. Left: Layer of 1 cm along a knee (MRI, case 4). Right: Layer of 0.5 cm along the surface of a head (MRI, case 2).

The described procedure is unique in enabling us to produce new images by combining these projections in a variety of ways: Skin or bone surfaces are displayed primarily for the <u>orientation</u> of the viewer in 3D space. The <u>diagnostic assessment</u>, however, can be performed on gray level planes and/or transparent projections that can be variously combined into this coordinate system, according to the viewer's decision. Fig. 5 shows as an example of multiple surfaces a head where bone and skin have been peeled off thus opening up the view to the brain. The surface structure of the brain is different in both hemispheres. Views containing multiple cuts enable the "dissection" of the brain uncovering a tumor in the right hemisphere.

For the exploration of the correlation of different kinds of objects such as soft tissue and bone structures "selective reformatting" has turned out to be a useful tool (fig. 6). As an example reformatting is performed only for soft tissue with exception of a tumor. In a further example the bones around a temporomandibular joint (TMJ) are excluded from reformation and presented as surfaces. This procedure allows the assessment of the soft tissue structure around the TMJ.

## Use of color

The described procedure differs from classic tomography in that a single image can contain more than one kind of pictorial representation. If this representation is displayed only in gray scale, image ambiguities may occur. For example the meaning of a certain shade of gray depends upon its location within the image. The assignment of a unique color to the different constituents of the image, such as cut planes or object surfaces, helps to ensure an unambiguous perception of the image.

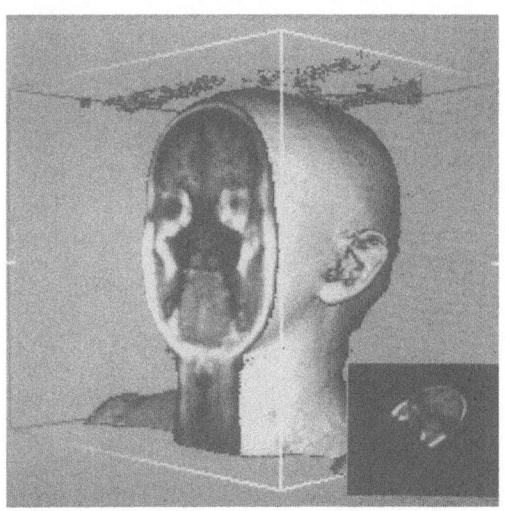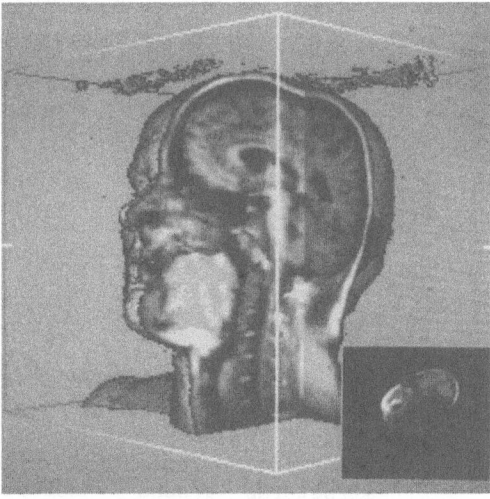

Fig. 4. Combined surface and cross-sectional images (MRI, case 2). The location of the MRI slice becomes immediately apparent (left). Multiple cross-sections allow the 3D-exploration of the gray level volume (right).

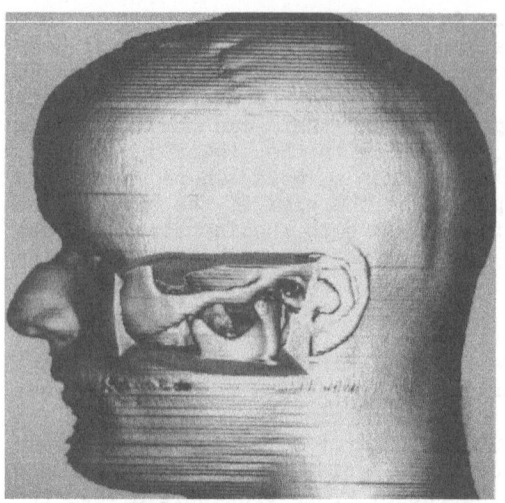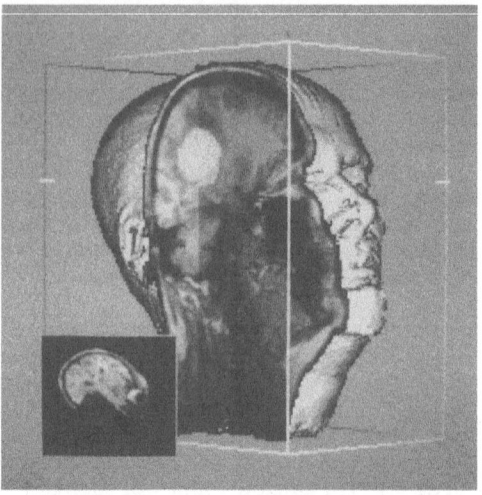

Fig. 5. Imaging a brain tumor (MRI, case 3). Left: A multiple surface image shows that the appearance of the brain is different in both hemispheres. Right: A dissection uncovers the tumor in the right hemisphere an allows the measurement of its location.

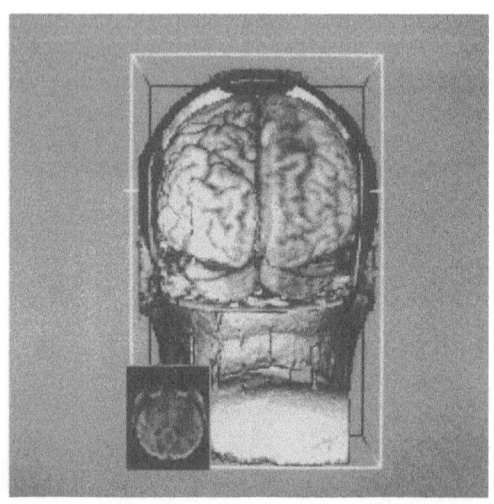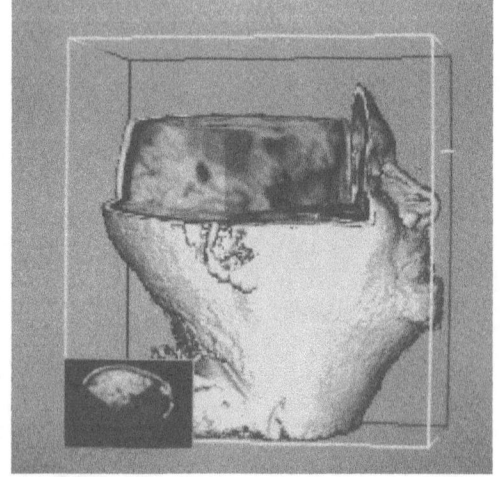

Fig. 6. Selective reformatting allows the exploration of tissue structures around interesting 3D-objects. Left: Reformation around a tumor (MRI, case 3). Right: Reformation around a temporomadibular joint (CT, case 1)

# DISCUSSION

## Relevance for radiology

Until recently, radiology was restricted to planar images of three-dimensional objects. This restriction was due to technical limitations rather than to radiologic needs. In the past few years, we have become able to generate 3D images of bony structures, a technique that is increasingly used in craniofacial surgery and orthopedics. The methods presented in this paper extends the existing technology, applying it to diagnostic radiology so that we can view cross-sectional gray level image sequences in three dimensions. Once the three dimensional context of the outer surface and/or bone is available for orientation we can "navigate" visually within the object without having to rely upon a mental 3D-reconstruction.

## Technical approach

For a clinical application the major technical problem involves the achievement of sufficiently high speed for an interactive operation. In pure surface display a variety of data structures can be used for the fast manipulation of 3D objects (Boecker et al., 1985; Hemmy et al., 1983; Vannier et al., 1984; Meagher, 1982). If we want to rotate a gray scale object for inspection without knowing its structure (e. g. surfaces), we have basically the choice between two ways of implementation: 1) to compute the intensity values in the image plane from the original data whenever we make a projection, or 2) to rotate the CT volume once and simply scan lines or columns of the rotated matrices for the projections. The first technique is used effectively in most methods displaying surfaces only, since the original data are generally compressed to binary data describing a surface only. In some cases even further compression is applied (Boecker et al., 1985). When we deal with gray level data we are confronted with at least 8 times more information (8 bits instead of one bit/voxel). In such cases the second approach has proved more effective in our study. It turned out that for inspecting the gray level information inside the object, a small number of viewing directions (three or less) are sufficient. The object can then be explored through simple variation of the projections. It is, however, decisive that <u>perspective projection</u> is used for the generation of the images. Otherwise cuts and windows do not look three-dimensional.

In the experimental environment the rotation of a volume of $256^3$ voxels took between 15 and 30 CPU-minutes. The projections took between 10 and 60 seconds each. Such times are certainly not sufficient for daily clinical work, but could be tolerated in a research environment. For routine clinical applications, more powerful hardware is definitely necessary. We are, however, convinced that hardware solutions should not be implemented until studies such as the present one have determined which operations are really useful. Otherwise it is possible that trivial properties, which the user might find useful, could not be included in the system.

# FURTHER DEVELOPMENTS

The program VOXEL-MAN-8 can be considered as one step within an evolution from pure surface visualisation to an object oriented exploration of volume data (see fig. 7). In a further advanced state then projections such as 'show pathological regions of gray matter with transparent brain surface' could be possible. A prerequisite is an

| Program | Object representation | "Projection" |
|---|---|---|
| VOXEL-MAN-1 | 1 bit: object/non object (binary voxel model) | surface of the object |
| VOXEL-MAN-8 | 8 bit: intensity parameters (gray scale voxel model) | surfaces, reformatted planes, look-through projections according to specification of spatial and/or gray scale window conditions |
| VOXEL-MAN-N | N bit: intensity parameters + semantic attributes (generalized voxel model) | surfaces, reformatted planes, look-through projections of <u>objects</u> according to the specification of conditions for the <u>objects</u> |

Fig. 7. Evolution of the voxel model

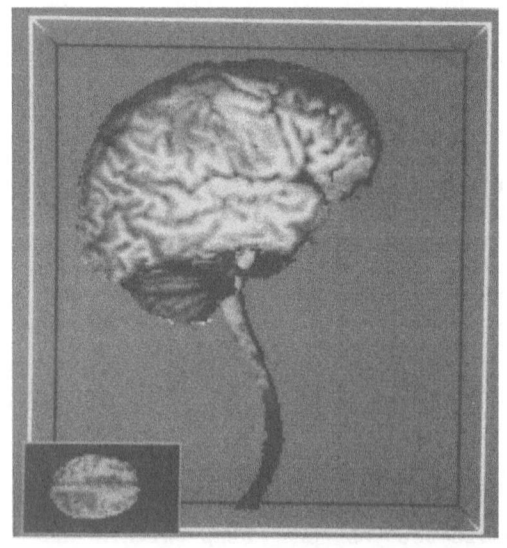 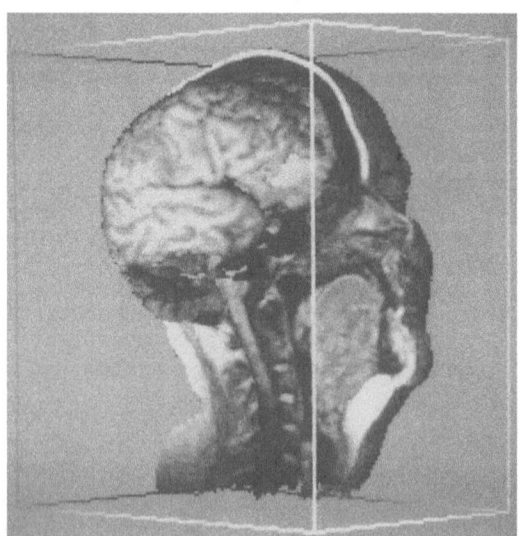

Fig. 8. 3D-display of a brain (MRI, case 3) based on a segmentation using the Marr-Hildreth operator. Left: The isolated brain. Right: Brain together with surrounding structures

object representation, that also contains semantical attributes in each voxel (membership to a certain organ, normal abnormal etc.). The automatic determination of such attributes is nontrivial, but at least in the case of MRI not hopeless. As a first step towards the realisation of such a _generalized voxel model_ within a system VOXEL-MAN-N, we have implemented a second volume ('attribute volume') that may contain attributes which presently are determined in a semiautomatic way. In a first experiment we determined the brain volume of case 3. Using a 3D-version ov the Marr-Hildreth operator (Bomans et al., 1987) we performed a presegmentation. By interactive removing nonmeaningful bridges between the obtained segments could be generated to a well described volume. By application of the previously described algorithms to this volume only the images of fig. 8 were computed.


CONCLUSION

We have demonstrated a method of viewing 3D tomographic data that uses 3D skin and bone surface display for the viewers orientation, while planar reformation and/or transparent projections can be applied for the assessment of soft tissue structures in regions of interest. Instead of being constrained to parallel planar images, we can 'navigate' within the three-dimensional surface and bone anatomy and choose optimum viewing conditions according to the anatomic environment. The described software solution is certainly not yet fast enough for routine clinical application. For research application, however, the processing time (10 - 60 sec/view) with computers found in radiological research environments seems to be tolerable. For a final specification of clinical hardware solutions further research work of the described kind has to be done.


ACKNOWLEDGEMENTS

The authors would like to thank Drs. G. Witte and M. Heller (Dept. of Radiology) for many discussions, and Dipl.-Inform. M. Bomans for assistance in preparing the paper. We are also grateful to Siemens (Erlangen) for providing the MRI-volume data of the head.


REFERENCES

Boecker,F.R.P., Tiede,U., and Höhne,K.H. (1985). Combined use of different algorithms for interactive surgical planning, in: Computer assisted radiology, Lemke,U. (ed.). Berlin New York Tokyo, Springer, 572-577.

Bomans,M., Riemer,M., Tiede,U., Höhne,K.H. (1987). 3-D Segmentation von Kernspintomogrammen, 9. DAGM-Tagung Braunschweig, in: Informatik Fachberichte, Springer, in press.

Chen,L.S., Herman,G.T., Reynolds,R.A., and Udupa,J.K. (1985). Surface shading in the cuberille environment, Computer Graphics and Applications 5, 33-43.

Goldwasser,S.M., Reynolds,R.A., Bapty,T., Baraff,D., Summers,J., TaltonD.A., and Walsh,E. (1985). Physicians workstation with real time performance, Computer Graphics and Appplications 5, 44-57 .

Hemmy,D.C., David,D.J., and Herman,G.T. (1983). Three-dimensional reconstruction of craniofacial deformity using computed tomography, Neurosurgery 13, 534-541.

Herman,G.T., Vose,W.F., GomoriJ.M., and Gefter,W.B. (1985). Stereoscopic computed threedimensional surface displays, RadioGraphics 5, 825-852.

Höhne,K.H., DeLaPaz,R.L., BernsteinR., and Taylor,R.C. (1987). Combined Surface Display and Reformatting for the 3D-Analysis of Tomographic Data, Investigative Radiology, in press.

Höhne,K.H., and Bernstein,R. (1986). Shading 3D images from CT using gray level gradients, IEEE Transactions on Medical Imaging 5, 45-47.

Jackel,D. (1985). The graphics PARCUM system: A 3D memory based computer architecture for processing and display of solid objects, Computer Graphics Forum 4, 21-32.

Lenz,R., Danielsson,P.E., Cronstroem,S., and Gudmundson,B. (1986). Interactive display of 3D medical objects, in: Pictorial information systems in medicine, Höhne,K.H. (ed.). Berlin New York Tokyo, Springer 449-468.

Lineweaver,W., DeLaPaz,R.L., Federle,M., Cann,C., Barton,R., and Trengrove-Jones,G. Threedimensional Tomography of Facial Fractures, Submitted to Annals of plastic surgery.

Meagher,D. (1982). Geometric modelling using octree encoding, Computer Graphics and Image Processing 19, 129-147.

Templeton,A.W., Johnson,J.A., and Anderson,W.H. (1985). Computer graphics for digitally formatted images, Radiology 152, 527-528.

Tiede,U., Höhne,K.H., and Riemer,M. (1987). Comparison of Surface Rendering Techniques for 3D Tomographic Objects, in: Computer Assisted Radiology, Lemke,U. (ed.). Berlin New York Tokyo, Springer 599-610.

Vannier,M.W., Gado,M.H., and Marsh,J.L.. Threedimensional display of intracranial soft tissue structures, American Journal of Neuroradiology 4, 520-521

Vannier,M.W., Marsh,J.L., and Warren,J. (1984). Threedimensional CT reconstruction images for craniofacial surgical plannning, Radiology 150, 179-184.

Witte,G., Hoeltje,W., Tiede,U., and Riemer,M. (1986). Die dreidimensionale Darstellung computertomographischer Untersuchungen kraniofacialer Anomalien, Fortschr. Roentgenstr. 144,4, 24-29.

Yasuda,T., Toriwaki,J., Yokoi,S., and Katada,K. (1984). Threedimensional display system of CT images for surgical planning, Int. Symposium on Medical Images and Icons. Silver Spring MD: IEEE Computer Society 322-327.

# Applications 1: DSA, Ultrasound, NMR

A SYSTEM FOR IMAGE REGISTRATION IN

DIGITAL SUBTRACTION ANGIOGRAPHY

J. Michael Fitzpatrick*, John J. Grefenstette*, David R. Pickens†, Murray Mazer†, and James M. Perry‡

*Department of Computer Science, Vanderbilt University, Nashville, Tennessee 37235

†Department of Radiology and Radiological Sciences, Vanderbilt University Medical Center, Nashville, Tennessee 37232

‡Department of Cardiology, Vanderbilt University Medical Center, Nashville, Tennessee 37232

## 1. INTRODUCTION

In the diagnosis of coronary atherosclerosis radio-opaque dye is injected into the interior of the coronary arteries to make them visible in X-ray images. Because of the confusing presence of overlying or underlying soft tissue and bone and because of the small size of the coronary arteries, large dye concentrations are required to render the arteries sufficiently visible for diagnosis. Because of its increased contrast sensitivity, digital subtraction angiography (DSA) has the potential for providing diagnostic images of the coronary arteries with significantly reduced dye concentrations (Levin, 1984; Tobis et al., 1983; Riederer and Kruger, 1983). In DSA a series of images is acquired during the time period which begins before the injection of dye and continues until the arteries are opacified. These images are then combined into a final processed image in which the change in opacity of the arteries leads to enhanced arterial contrast. A particularly useful and commonly applied DSA technique, "temporal subtraction", involves the subtraction of a "mask" image, acquired before opacification, from a "contrast" image, acquired after opacification. Ideally, temporal subtraction produces an image in which nothing appears except those arteries in which the amount of dye present has changed, but its usefulness in practice is limited by the image degradation caused by patient motion during image acquisition. The rigid motion of bones and the elastic motion of soft tissue in the field of view cause changes in X-ray opacity which are unrelated to the influx of contrast material. When the two images are subtracted these changes appear as ghost-like artifacts which obscure the arteries to be examined.

Many techniques have been developed to solve the problem of motion artifacts in DSA including remasking (Oung, 1984), pixel shifting (Levin, 1984), temporal filtering (Kruger, 1981; Riederer et al., 1983; Miller et al., 1984), dual energy subtraction (Pfeiler et al., 1984; Brody, 1984), hybrid subtraction (Van-Lysel et al.,1983), tomosynthesis (Kruger et al., 1984; deVries et al., 1985), and K-edge subtraction (Hughes et al., 1985; Akisada et al., 1986). K-edge subtraction is essentially immune to motion artifacts but, because it requires a synchrotron to produce the required mono-energetic X-ray beams, it is currently not a practical solution to the problem. None of the other techniques has been shown to improve substantially the diagnostic quality of DSA in the presence of motion artifacts (Levin, 1984; Kruger and Riederer, 1984; deVries et al., 1985).

Another technique for dealing with this problem is to reduce the degradation arising in temporal subtraction by means of image registration. The registration is carried out by performing a geometrical transformation of the mask image so that it is in registration with the contrast image. After the registration, because of the realignment of soft tissue and bone in the two images, the motion artifacts disappear from the difference image, leaving a diagnostically useful image of the arteries. This technique, which was applied as early as 1975 to the comparison of images of the lung (Kinsey and Vannellii, 1975; Price et al., 1975), has until recently remained largely unsuccessful. Recent work on this technique is, however, showing renewed promise toward solving the motion artifact problem in DSA (Fitzpatrick et al., 1984; Yanagisawa et al., 1984; Venot and Leclerc, 1984).

This paper describes our current approach to the removal of DSA motion artifacts by means of X-ray image registration. In Section 2 we present some of the theoretical considerations with respect to image registration in DSA. In Section 3 we describe our registration system, and in Sections 4, 5, and 6 we describe some experiments, present the results, and discuss their implications.

## 2. IMAGE REGISTRATION IN DSA

The technique of image registration for the removal of motion artifacts in DSA is illustrated schematically in Fig. 1. A mask image and a contrast image serve as the input to the process; the output is a subtraction image. A region of interest (ROI) is selected, presumably containing an artery or arteries which are to be examined. These arteries, invisible in the mask image, are opacified in the contrast image, but only faintly visible because of the presence of overlying soft tissue and bone. The primary and principal image processing step is the geometrical transformation, or "warping" of the mask image to bring it into registration with the contrast image at all points within the ROI. Once the warped mask image has been produced, the secondary step is performed: the formation of a difference image by means of the subtraction of the warped mask from the contrast image to remove the image signal arising from the registered soft tissue and bone. Ideally, the result, within the ROI at least, is an image in which only the opacified arteries are visible. This image may contribute to the diagnosis of arterial disease.

### The Existence of Suitable Transformations

There are several difficulties associated with this technique which must be addressed. The most fundamental of these is the question of the existence of an appropriate geometrical transformation to bring the mask and contrast images into registration throughout the ROI. If such a transformation is applied to the mask image before subtraction, then the difference image will be zero everywhere except for those positions at which dye has appeared. The transformation could be, in fact, be described as one which would produce a zero difference image if there were no influx of dye. Unless such a transformation exists, motion artifacts cannot, in general, be removed by this technique. Such a transformation will not be possible if parts of objects which are completely out of the field of view when the mask image is acquired have moved into the ROI when the contrast image is acquired. Except for ROI's very near the image boundary, this effect should not present a serious problem. A more serious aspect of this question arises because of the projective nature of the X-ray images. Each image is a two dimensional projection of a three dimensional space. The objects in the space, tissue and bone, undergo elastic three dimensional motion, but the warping used in the registration technique is a two dimensional transformation of the two dimensional projection images.

If all points in all objects in the space (with the exception of the inflowing contrast medium) move such that points which lie on the same X-ray trajectory in the mask image remain so in the contrast image regardless of their motion along that trajectory, then the motion is equivalent to two dimensional motion. It is simple to see that a two dimensional mapping of the image exists which corresponds to this special case of three dimensional motion. For more general motion, it is necessary to consider carefully the physics both of the imaging process and of the motion of the imaged medium in order to determine whether an appropriate image transformation exists. In the appendix to this paper, we provide a proof that, subject to mild restrictions, there exists a two dimensional transformation of the image which will produce a change which is identical to the change produced by any three dimensional motion. The proof applies to a special class of images which we call "projected density" images, for which the image value at each point in the image is proportional to the line-integral of the density of some conserved quantity.

As described in the appendix, the image produced by a suitably calibrated X-ray image formation system approximates a projected density image, wherein the linear X-ray attenuation coefficient serves as the density of a conserved quantity. Thus, registration does have the potential for solving the problem of motion artifacts. This proof reveals two important facts concerning the two dimensional transformation: (a) it is one-to-one, meaning that each point in the untransformed image is mapped into a single point in the transformed image, and (b) it must include a factor to account for the change in image intensity which accompanies the thickening or thinning of the imaged medium when it suffers compression or expansion. With the vector $\mathbf{x}$ representing the coordinates, $x, y$, of a point in image space, the first fact reveals that each point, $\mathbf{x}_1$, in the untransformed mask image, $p(\mathbf{x}_1, t_1)$, acquired at time $t_1$, gives rise to exactly one point, $\mathbf{x}_2$, in the transformed image, $p(\mathbf{x}_2, t_2)$, acquired at $t_2$, and thus drastically reduces the size

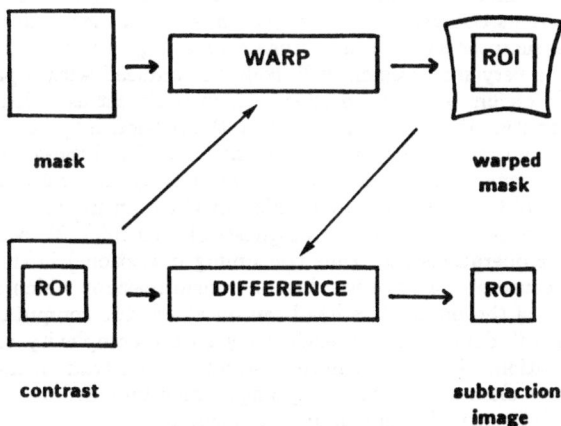

Fig. 1.   Schematic illustration of image registration in DSA. The boxes marked WARP and DIFFERENCE represent image processing. The ROI is a user-selected region of interest. The arrows indicate the direction of data flow.

of the class of transformations which must be considered when searching for an optimal one. The second fact reveals that a simple mapping of image intensity values from the untransformed image into the transformed image cannot in the general case produce a satisfactory registration. Image values should not only be moved around, but, in order to compensate for changes in intensity due to expansion and contraction, should also be multiplied by the Jacobian of the transformation, which is defined for the two dimensional mapping $\mathbf{x}_1(\mathbf{x}_2)$, as

$$J(\mathbf{x}_1(\mathbf{x}_2)) \equiv \frac{\partial x_1}{\partial x_2}\frac{\partial y_1}{\partial y_2} - \frac{\partial x_1}{\partial y_2}\frac{\partial y_1}{\partial x_2}.$$

The image transformation should have the form

$$p(\mathbf{x}_2, t_2) = J(\mathbf{x}_1(\mathbf{x}_2))\, p(\mathbf{x}_1(\mathbf{x}_2), t_1). \tag{1}$$

The function $\mathbf{x}_1(\mathbf{x}_2)$, which represents the mapping from $\mathbf{x}_2$ to $\mathbf{x}_1$, is the inverse of the one-to-one mapping from $\mathbf{x}_1$ to $\mathbf{x}_2$, and it gives rise by Equation (1) to the image transformation from $p(\mathbf{x}_1)$ to $p(\mathbf{x}_2)$. The Jacobian in Equation (1) will be greater than zero for all transformations corresponding to physical motion. It will be less than one, reducing the transformed image intensity, at those positions for which the transformation from $\mathbf{x}_1$ to $\mathbf{x}_2$ represents a local expansion and will be greater than one, increasing the transformed image intensity, at a local contraction. It will be equal to one, having no effect, when the local motion corresponds to rigid body motion, i.e., some combination of (two dimensional) translation and rotation.

417

## Suitable Mappings

An appropriate transformation for the types of motion which can be expected to be present in images of a moving patient will require a mapping for which the target image coordinates are allowed to be nonlinear functions of the original coordinates (Kruger and Riederer, 1984). We will refer to such mappings, and their associated image transformations, as being nonlinear with the understanding that the set of nonlinear functions includes the set of linear ones, which in turn includes translations (pixel shifting), rotations, scaling, and skewing. Nonlinear transformations often suffer from three problems: (a) they may produce non-one-to-one mappings, (b) they may be discontinuous or have discontinuous derivatives, and (c) they may be computationally complex. The effects of these problems are, respectively, that there may be "folds" apparent in the transformed image, there may be discontinuous contours apparent in the images where the transformation undergoes a sudden change, and the determination of the best warp may take too long to be practical. The first effect, image folding due to non-one-to-one mapping of pixels, is likely to be the most serious because it can produce an image artifact where none existed. When considering images of structures such as the coronary arteries, a sudden large density change in the image, even if over a very small region, will likely be confused with a pathological condition or could hide a stenotic region. The second effect, which is almost as serious, may also produce sudden changes in intensity. It can act in two ways: the motion may be discontinuous and, because of the presence of the Jacobian factor, discontinuous brightness changes may be produced where there were none. The third effect appears during the search for appropriate settings for the parameters of the transformation which produce an improved registration. Because of the large number of pixels involved in any diagnostically useful ROI, because of the necessity of performing arithmetic operations (i.e., time consuming operations) in the computation of each target position, and because of the large number of transformations which must be considered before a suitable setting of the parameters has been obtained, the computational complexity of the registration process will depend almost exclusively on the complexity of the computation of an individual target position. Thus, to achieve a successful registration, the coordinate mapping should be selected from a class of nonlinear mappings which includes only one-to-one functions which are continuous, differentiable, and simple to calculate.

## The Evaluation Function

The goal of the optimal registration system is to produce a difference image in which the interfering background misregistration has been reduced to the point at which the dye-filled arteries are clearly visible to the human observer. The system must have some measure of the success of the registration to guide its search for a suitable geometrical transformation which achieves this goal. Because of the large number of such evaluations which must be made during the search, it is infeasible to use a human observer for this purpose. Thus, it is necessary to define an evaluation function whose value can be calculated automatically. Since success is entirely a function of the difference image, the automatic evaluation should be a function of the pixel values of the difference image. Examples of such a function are the sum of the pixel values (not a good choice), the mean of the absolute values of the pixels, the sum of the squares of their values, the area of the image within which the absolute values are insignificant, the inverses of any of these quantities, etc. A common measure of similarity between two images, the cross correlation, is not a function of the difference image, but is in some cases approximately so (Rosenfeld and Kak, volume 2, p. 37, 1982).

An ideal function should be monotonically related to the human observer's estimate of the success of the registration, so that improvement based on the function corresponds to improvement in the eyes of the observer. The construction of such a function would require detailed knowledge of the observer's judgement process, and would probably require a complex calculation. Some functions are clearly not ideal in this respect. The sum of pixel values, for example, could be made arbitrarily large or small without improving the registration simply by adding the same constant to each pixel. Because the cross correlation is a function of the two images to be subtracted, as opposed to the difference image itself, it does not appear to be an ideal choice. It is particularly unreliable when the image brightness averaged over an area the size of the ROI varies from location to location within the mask image, but can be improved by normalization or by means of high-pass filtering of the images being compared (Svedlow et al., 1978; Frei et al., 1980). Functions which are intuitively appealing, such as the others mentioned above, should ultimately be experimentally compared with human observation to determine their usefulness.

A problem with any such function is that the ideal difference image is not zero. The inherent changes due to the influx of dye must remain while the changes due to motion are removed. While such a registration always exists (see Appendix), it is not always possible, even for a human observer, to distinguish between the changes due to motion and the changes due to the influx of dye. A priori information about the inherent changes may be used to reduce the effect on the evaluation function. Venot and Leclerc, for example, (Venot and Leclerc, 1984; Venot et al., 1986a; Venot et al. 1986b) have designed an evaluation function which stochastically estimates the area of the image within which the absolute values are insignificant in comparison to the noise of the acquisition system. This function is relatively insensitive to small areas of large inherent change in the image. The mean of the absolute values and the sum of squares, on the other hand, are characterized by relatively less sensitivity to large areas of small inherent change. The function of choice will depend on the characteristics of the inherent image changes for a given clinical application. Whether automatic registrations in the face of such changes in the image can in fact be successful will depend on a complex interaction between the evaluation function chosen and the character of the images to be registered, and can only be decided on the basis of experience with clinical images.

Finding a Successful Mapping

Once a class of suitable mappings and an evaluation function have been chosen, it is necessary to select a mapping which optimizes the evaluation function. The selection of a mapping will involve choosing values for some set of parameters to specify the desired mapping within the class. If the function increases with image similarity, its value should be maximized; if it increases with image difference, then it should be minimized. Thus, the problem of image registration is reduced to the problem of function optimization. Because of the complex nature of the images and of the motion, the number of parameters is necessarily large and the evaluation function is likely to exhibit a highly nonlinear and multimodal dependence on the parameters. The multimodal nature of the problem, that is, the presence of multiple hills and valleys in the functional variation, means that simple hill climbing techniques are inappropriate, since such techniques are likely to find only a local, as opposed to a global, optimum unless the starting point happens to be well placed (Frei et al., 1980; Horn and Bachman, 1979). The large number of parameters eliminates exhaustive search from consideration and reduces the likelihood of improvement in hill climbing through repetition from many starting points. Without incorporating specific knowledge about the two dimensional projection of the physical motion or making use of information from images acquired at other times or from other perspectives, the success of the registration depends on the use of a robust optimization procedure which is capable of finding a global optimum, or near-optimum, of a highly nonlinear, multimodal function in a large parameter space in a reasonable length of time.

3. THE SYSTEM

We refer to our method for reducing motion artifacts as "optimal registration". We choose this terminology because we use image registration to reduce the artifacts and we treat the determination of the image transformation which produces the desired registration as a problem in function optimization. The registration is optimal only within constraints which we impose: that the transformation belong to the class of two dimensional geometrical transformations which we specify, that the quality of registration be measured by a difference function which we specify, and that the search for the best transformation be effected by means of the search algorithms which we specify (the genetic algorithms, described below). The method involves several manual steps followed by a series of automatic calculations which lead to a mask image which has been registered with a contrast image. The manual steps include the selection of the image pair to be registered, one mask image and one contrast image, and the selection of an ROI on the contrast image. The mask image is then automatically transformed geometrically so that the subimage corresponding to the ROI is registered with the contrast image and the difference image is formed and displayed. (See Fig. 1.) The automatic step is executed iteratively. Each time an improved registration is discovered (according to the evaluation function), a new difference image is formed and displayed. The iterative improvement will continue for a preset time limit, or will be interrupted before the limit, if a human observer decides that a suitable registration has been achieved. Other ROI's may be selected from the same image pair and the same sequence repeated. When all the registrations are complete, a final composite difference image is formed consisting of the registered ROI's displayed together with the rest of the unregistered difference image to provide a context for diagnosis. (See, for example, Fig. 7 below). Our system consists of the software to facilitate operator selection of the images and the ROI's, to perform the iterative registration, to display the improved registrations as they are discovered, and to produce the final composite image.

## The Transformations

Our transformations employ the Jacobian factor as prescribed above in Section 2. In that section we describe an ideal image transformation as being based on a one-to-one, continuous, differentiable, computationally simple image mapping. A class of differentiable mappings which are computationally simple are the polynomial warping functions (Wong, 1977; Hall, 1979). In these mappings the coordinates, $x_1, y_1$, are polynomials in the coordinates, $x_2, y_2$. Unfortunately, without additional restrictions, polynomial mappings may not be one-to-one. However, a restricted class of polynomial mappings has been recently described by Fitzpatrick and Leuze (Fitzpatrick and Leuze, 1987) which is guaranteed to be one-to-one, and it is this class which we use in this work.

The mapping is based on a bilinear interpolation of the motion at the four corners of a rectangular ROI. The motion at the four corners is specified as shown in Fig. 2 by four motion vectors, $d_1$ through $d_4$, each of which is broken into its $x$ and $y$ components. These eight components are the parameters which specify the two dimensional image transformation. To show the algebraic formulation for the mapping, $x_1(x_2)$, it is convenient to set the origin at the center of the ROI and to define $x_0$ to be half the width and $y_0$ to be half the height of the ROI. The mapping is then calculated as a bilinear form:

$$x_1 = x_2 + [d_{1x}(x_0-x_2)(y_0-y_2) + d_{2x}(x_0+x_2)(y_0-y_2) \qquad (2)$$
$$+ d_{3x}(x_0-x_2)(y_0+y_2) + d_{4x}(x_0+x_2)(y_0+y_2)]/4x_0 y_0,$$

This mapping is a polynomial which includes terms of the form $a_{ij}x^i y^j$ for $i=0,1$ and $j=0,1$. It can be shown that the bilinear mapping is one-to-one as long as the following conditions are maintained:

$$|d_{ix}| < x_0/2; \quad |d_{iy}| < y_0/2$$

for $i = 1$ to 4. Arbitrarily complex one-to-one mappings can be formed by composing bilinear forms with different sets of d's obeying somewhat different sets of conditions (Fitzpatick and Leuze, 1987), but for the work described here we have used only the simple, eight parameter transformation as shown above. The Jacobian of the bilinear mapping reduces to a linear function and thus can be calculated quickly.

## The Evaluation Function

Our choice of function for the evaluation of the success of an image registration within an ROI is the mean of the absolute values of the pixels in the difference image. This function is large when the images are different and small when they are similar. Thus it measures, in some sense, the image difference as opposed to image similarity, as does, for example, the cross correlation. This function is simple to calculate and provides a large dynamic range. We have performed some simple experiments to determine whether this function exhibits agreement with the human visual system, as described above in Section 2. While we have not yet carried out a systematic study of the correlation, we have found that for our phantom at least, difference images with smaller mean values of absolute pixel difference are consistently judged to be superior by human observers with regard to the absence of motion artifacts. Fig. 5 in Section 5 illustrates this effect. These images are difference images for various transformations of the mask image, ranging from large mean values to small mean values of absolute pixel difference. It is clear that as the mean value gets smaller, the motion artifacts become less severe.

The difference function is, as discussed above in Section 2, sensitive to the inherent differences in the mask and contrast images arising from the influx of dye. Whether these differences are large enough to effect significantly the evaluation of the registration depends on the dye

420

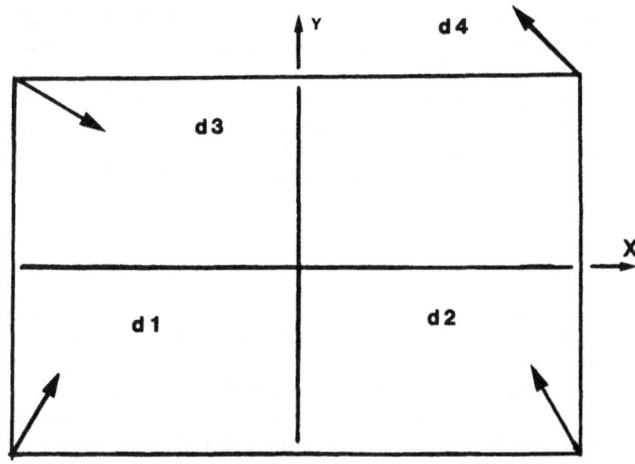

Fig. 2.    Schematic diagram of the motion at the corners of the ROI.
The motion at other points within the ROI is gotten by
bilinear interpolation.  Constraints on the d's insure that
the mapping is one-to-one.

concentration and the area of the image occupied by the arteries.  With our choice of the mean
of the absolute pixel difference we are tacitly assuming that the concentrations and the areas are
small enough such that the effect on the registration is negligible.  The assumption is reasonable
since the need for registration is present only for images of small arteries with low dye concentrations.  However, during the registration procedure, as the registration improves and the image
difference due to motion artifacts decreases, there will come a point at which the inherent difference is of the same magnitude as the difference due to motion artifacts.  The registration cannot
be expected to proceed consistently beyond this point (without some alteration of the evaluation
function).  At this point, the relative sizes of the area occupied by the arteries and that occupied
by the motion artifacts become important.  If the artery area is relatively small in comparison to
the area of the motion artifacts, then the signal due to the artery will be concentrated within a
small area and the image of the arteries will be distinct.  Otherwise, the arterial image may be
obscured by the artifacts and the registration may be unsuccessful.

The evaluation function must be calculated many times as different registrations are tried
by the optimization algorithm.  The evaluation must be based on the pixels of the difference
image, which in turn means that the image transformation must be applied to the mask image as
part of the evaluation procedure, a process involving many arithmetic operations. Even a simple
bilinear transformation requires, for each pixel, twenty-four arithmetic operations to produce the
mapping, four more to calculate and multiply by the Jacobian, and, because of fractional pixel
motion, still more to provide for some sort of interpolation among pixel values.  Our choice, bilinear interpolation, for example, requires twelve operations.  There are ancillary arithmetic operations required in order to calculate addresses of pixel values stored in the computer memory.
Because of the expensive nature of arithmetic operations and because of the large number of
such operations required to construct the complete difference image, the calculation of the
evaluation function becomes the major part of the calculations performed during the entire registration process.  In order to speed up the process of calculating the evaluation function, we use a
Monte Carlo approach which permits us to reduce drastically (by factors of 100 or so) the
number of pixels evaluated for a given set of parameters.  The idea is an outgrowth of the work
of Barnea and Silverman on stochastic similarity estimation (Barnea and Silverman, 1972) and is
related to the estimation technique employed by Potel and Gustafson (Potel and Gustafson,
1983).  Rather than evaluating the average absolute pixel difference exactly by inspecting every
point within the ROI, we estimate the average absolute pixel difference by sampling a randomly
selected set of points within that ROI.  The result is an inexact evaluation, but we have found
that the speedup in the evaluation more than compensates for the evaluation error when the
genetic search technique (described below) is employed (Grefenstette and Fitzpatrick, 1985).

The precision of the evaluation is related to the variance of the histogram of the difference image. The precision can be increased if detailed knowledge of the image is available, but even without that knowledge, it is possible to improve the precision in most cases with no danger of decreasing the precision by means of stratified sampling (James, 1980). We apply this technique in our sampling procedure. The technique involves partitioning the ROI into non-overlapping subregions (arranged in our case in a simple grid) and taking an equal number of samples from each subregion. The improvement comes about when there are significant differences among the variances of the histograms of the subregions.

## The Optimization Procedure

As pointed out above in Section 2, the success of the registration depends on the use of a robust optimization procedure. Because of their success in finding nearly global optima of non-linear multimodal functions in large search spaces, we have chosen to use genetic search algorithms. Genetic algorithms are adaptive generate-and-test procedures derived from principles of natural population genetics. This section presents a high level description of genetic algorithms. The reader is referred to (De Jong, 1980) for a more detailed account. A genetic algorithm maintains a fixed-size set, called a "population", of "structures", which are candidate solutions to the given problem. Each structure is evaluated by a problem-dependent evaluation procedure which assigns the structure a measure of its fitness as a solution to the problem at hand. For the image registration problem, each structure represents a vector of parameters which characterize an image transformation, and fitness is measured by the success of the transformation in producing a registration. When each structure in the population has been evaluated, a new population of structures is formed in two steps. First, structures in the current population are selected to be reproduced on the basis of their relative fitness. That is, high performing structures may be chosen several times for replication and poorly performing structures may not be chosen at all. Next, the selected structures are recombined using idealized genetic operators to form a new set of structures for evaluation. One of the most important genetic operators is the "crossover" operator, which combines the features of two "parent" structures to form two similar "offspring". Crossover operates by swapping corresponding segments of a binary representation of the parents. For example, if we use the structures

$$s_1 = 100|01010 \quad \text{and}$$

$$s_2 = 010|10100$$

as two selected parents and suppose that the crossover point has been chosen as indicated by the vertical bar, the resulting offspring structures would be

$$s_3 = 100|10100 \quad \text{and}$$

$$s_4 = 010|01010.$$

This simple operator has some important properties. First, the offspring share many of the combinations of features exhibited by the parents. In the preceding example, the combination $100\#\#\#\#0$ appears in both $s_1$ and in $s_3$. (The "$\#$" indicates that the value in this position is irrelevant.) This common trait implies that the offspring should share many of the performance characteristics of the parents. Second, crossover introduces new combinations of features into the population. In the above example, $s_4$ contains the combination $\#1001\#\#\#$, which does not occur in either parent. If $s_4$ exhibits high performance, then this new combination of features will tend to propagate through the population.

The theoretical properties of genetic algorithms have been extensively analyzed. Holland (Holland, 1975) shows that genetic algorithms perform a sophisticated search through the space of all feature combinations, quickly identifying and exploiting combinations which are associated with high performance. Genetic algorithms have been applied successfully in a variety of domains, including combinatorial optimization (Grefenstette et al., 1985), gas pipeline control systems (Goldberg, 1983), very large scale integrated (VLSI) circuit layout (Fourman, 1985), and machine learning (Smith, 1983; Schaffer and Grefenstette, 1985; Holland, 1986).

Our implementation of the registration system incorporates the GENESIS software system, developed by Grefenstette (Grefenstette, 1984), which facilitates the use of genetic optimization algorithms in specific applications. We provide an evaluation procedure which, when called by the GENESIS program, performs the Monte Carlo evaluation of a geometric transformation. The transformation to be evaluated is specified by a single argument passed to the procedure by GENESIS. The argument is a 64 bit structure which is partitioned by the evaluation procedure into eight substrings of eight bits each. Each eight-bit substring is decoded into one of 256 evenly spaced numbers in a specified range which falls within $[-x_0/2, x_0/2]$ or $[-y_0/2, y_0/2]$, representing an $x$ or $y$ component, respectively, of one of the $d$ vectors. These limits insure that the $d$'s satisfy the inequalities which follow Equation (2), and hence that the mapping is one-to-one. These components are then used in Equation (2) to calculate $x_1$ and the associated Jacobian for each sample point, $x_2$, within the ROI. The absolute difference, $|p(x_2, t_2) - p_c(x_2)|$, where $p(x_2, t_2)$ is the transformed mask image value, as in Equation (1), and $p_c(x_2)$ is the contrast image value, is determined for each randomly selected point, and the mean is calculated and returned to GENESIS. The GENESIS program chooses the structures with no knowledge of the algorithm used by the evaluation procedure to decode a structure into the eight $d$ components. In its first iteration of the search, GENESIS uses randomly selected structures. Thereafter, it bases its choice of structures upon a selection and crossover algorithm as described above. At the conclusion of each generation, GENESIS produces as output the structure with the best approximate evaluation. This structure is used as input by a second, independent procedure which produces a complete, warped mask image within the ROI, forms the difference image for the ROI, and displays it. As these procedures run, a series of progressively improving difference images appears before the user on the display screen. The program runs for a predetermined number of generations, or until the user determines that it has produced a satisfactory registration.

The program which implements the optimal registration algorithm is written in the computer language, "C", and is run under the BSD 4.2 Unix operating system on a Sun Microsystems, Inc., Sun-3/260 Deskside Workstation with floating point accelerator board, 8 MBytes of electronic memory, and a color display with 8 bits per pixel and 1152 by 900 resolution. The program is designed to permit parallel execution of the genetic search and image display. The genetic search is executed by one workstation, while a second workstation displays the difference images. The two workstations communicate by means of Sun's Network File System over an Ethernet connection. The image access routines employ the image handling utilities licensed by the University of North Carolina under the name "/usr/image". The images presented in this paper were displayed using displaytool (Chang, 1987), a program which provides interactive contrast and brightness adjustment and runs within Sun's "Suntool" windowing system.

## 4. EXPERIMENTS

### Phantom Images

A phantom has been constructed to be used in testing the optimal registration algorithm. It is designed to simulate structures which would normally contribute to a clinical image. These structures include rib bones, soft tissue, vessels, and the left ventricle of the heart. The phantom is shown in the diagram in Fig. 3. The flat acrylic plastic plates have a total thickness 4.1 cm. On the base plate rests a container which holds the plastic tubing that simulates arteries. These tubes are arranged in sequential order by increasing size. They are 0.58 mm, 0.76 mm, 1.14 mm, 1.57 mm, and 1.67 mm inside diameter to cover the spectrum of sizes from just below the resolving capabilities of the imaging system to the size of small coronary arteries. The tubes can be filled with dilute contrast solution or water during an imaging experiment and rest in a pan of water so that the tubes are just covered. This arrangement causes the tubes to be mostly invisible until the contrast solution is injected into them. Above the water bath is a support plate of acrylic plastic which is mounted so that its angle with respect to the base can be varied by adjusting the clamps on the aluminum supports. On this plate rests another plate on which several rib bones from a cadaver are placed. The two plates are not fixed together, so the plate with the rib bones can be positioned as necessary along the support plate. Above the bones is another support plate on which an inflatable bladder is attached. The bladder, from a blood pressure cuff, is connected to a reservoir which contains a dilute solution of contrast and water. The bladder can be inflated with fluid from the reservoir so that it appears to be a static left ventricle filled with a dilute contrast agent and blood. Furthermore, the bladder's inflation level can be varied between acquisition of a mask and acquisition of a contrast image, simulating the large motion that would be expected when imaging the heart without cardiac gating.

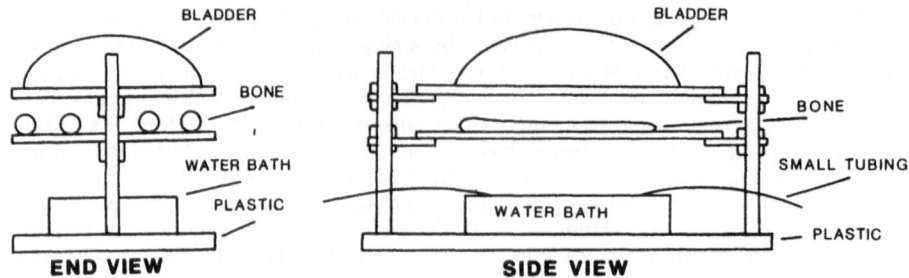

END VIEW          SIDE VIEW

Fig. 3.    Diagram of three dimensional motion phantom. The base plate of acylic plastic holds the water bath and tubing which simulates arteries. The second plate can be positioned at different angles and holds the rib bones. The third plate, also positionable, holds the bladder which can be filled with dilute contrast. A reservoir of contrast and the inflation pump are adjacent to the rest of the phantom. Aluminum supports hold the parts together.

An experiment was performed using the phantom to simulate three dimensional motion. Images were acquired on a commercial DSA system, a Technicare DR-960, coupled to a GE Fluorocon 300 X-ray imaging system. Digital images were acquired in 512 by 512 by 8 bit resolution with the image intensifier in the 6 inch mode. The X-ray technique used was 300 ma, 0.02 sec, at 80 kVp, log amplifier on. All image data were written to magnetic tape and transported to the Sun 3/260 systems for processing.

The first image acquired was a calibration image which is used in the optimal registration procedure to convert all of the images to approximations of projected density images (see Appendix), which we refer to as "calibrated images". The calibration image was obtained at the above specified radiographic technique by imaging the 2.4 cm thick base of the phantom. Each of the experimental images is subtracted from the calibration image to produce a calibrated image prior to further processing. A mask image, the image which is to be warped, was acquired next, with the support plates positioned parallel to the base plate. The tubing was immersed in 3 cm of water and the tubes were individually filled with water. The bladder was filled with a weak contrast solution so that it measured 3 cm thick at the center. The contrast image is quite similar to the mask image except that a small amount of three dimensional motion was present and dilute contrast agent was injected into the simulated arteries. The dilute solution contained about 72 mg/ml of iothalamate meglumine. Motion of the rib bones was achieved by moving the rib plate 1/4 cm along the support plate. Three dimensional motion was achieved by tipping the plate supporting the rib bones by about 4 degrees (motion at the edge of the plate of 1/4 cm). An ROI was selected to demonstrate the capabilities of the optimal registration algorithm.

Clinical Images

Several images obtained from routine clinical studies with the Technicare-GE DSA system have also been used to test the registration algorithm. These images are vascular studies of the humerus and of the elbow in one patient. Acquisitions were made at 512 by 512 by 8 bits with logarithmic amplification at normal radiographic levels. In both cases the patient moved during the imaging series, producing a motion artifact due to mispositioning of the bone. No information about the type of motion is known except for the artifacts in the subtraction images. Calibrated mask and contrast images were formed by subtracting from the calibration image as described above for the phantom images. ROI's were selected in areas where an obvious motion artifact obscured details of the arterial system, especially the secondary arterial branches.

In all of the results which follow, an eight parameter polynomial warp was used. The sample size used for the statistical estimate of the average absolute pixel difference in a ROI was 20 for the phantom images and 100 for the clinical images. Stratified stampling was employed as

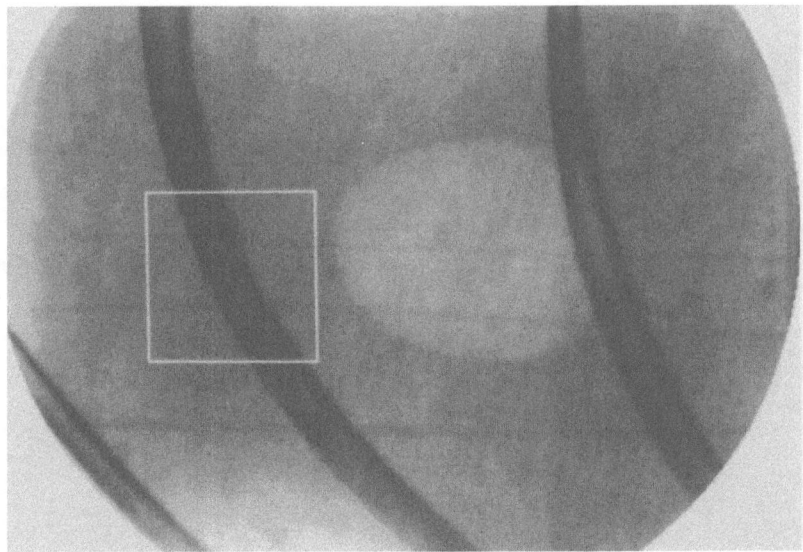

Fig. 4.  Digital radiograph of the three dimensional motion phantom. This image shows the region of interest selected for optimal registration. An air bubble is clearly visible in the center of the image, as well as several rib bones and contrast-filled tubes. The ROI is selected on the contrast image, but the geometric transformation is applied to the corresponding region on the mask image.

described above in Section 2 with four subregions at five sample points per subregion for the phantom images. The phantom registration was repeated with one point per subregion with essentially the same results (not shown) but shorter registration times. All clinical image registrations used one point per subregion. The optimal registration algorithm was permitted to run until the images showed the best removal of motion artifacts when compared by the human operator to the unprocessed subtraction image. At this point the registration procedure was halted.

## 5. RESULTS

Fig. 4 shows a digital image (before calibration) of the phantom with a 100x100 pixel ROI that includes portions of the 1.14 mm and 1.57 mm tubes. The rib bone can be seen clearly in the image, as well as the three larger tubes filled with contrast. A fourth tube is barely visible. In the center of the image is an air bubble in the bladder. The background is largely due to the dilute contrast solution in the bladder with some contribution from the acrylic plastic and water comprising the rest of the phantom. The mask image is similar in appearance except for the simulated motion and the absence of contrast in the tubing.

Fig. 5 has six images which show the action of the optimal registration algorithm as it processes the selected ROI on the mask image and performs the subtraction from the companion ROI on the contrast image. Fig. 5A is the subtraction of the mask from the contrast with no registration. The characteristic misregistration artifacts can be seen at those points for which the bone does not match in position at subtraction, obliterating part of the contrast-filled tubing in the image. Fig. 5B through Fig. 5E Show the progression of the optimal registration algorithm as it automatically seeks the best registration of the mask and contrast images by warping the mask image. Fig. 5F represents the optimal registration of this ROI for this image pair. The magnitudes of the d components for this registration ranged from 1.69 to 6.89 pixels. Of primary interest is the substantial reduction in the bone artifact when compared to Fig. 5A. A reduction

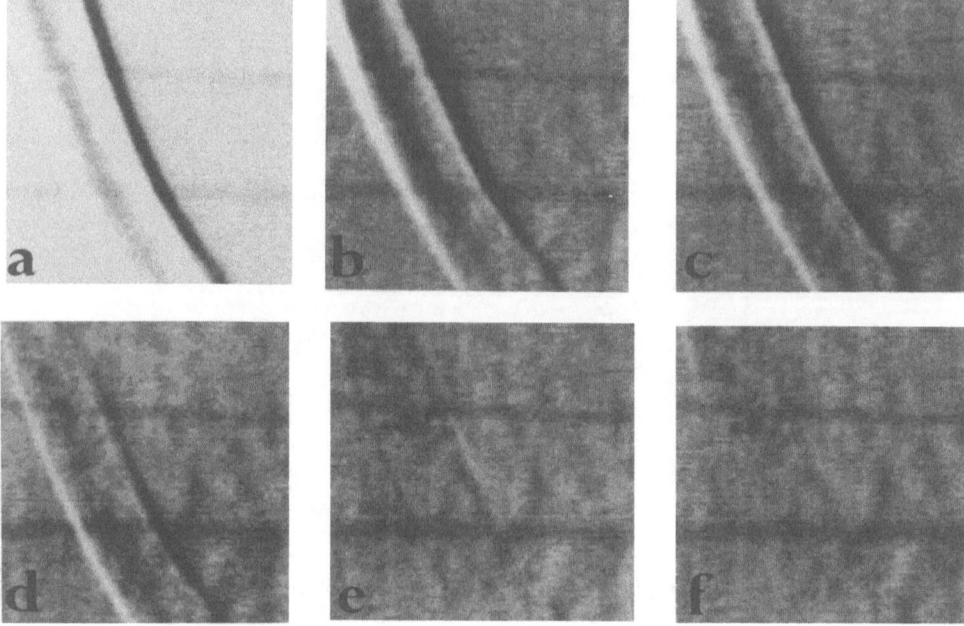

Fig. 5.    Subtraction images of the three dimensional motion phantom. These subtraction images show the successive stages in the optimal registration process from no registration in Fig. 5a through successive iterations by the optimal registration algorithm (Fig. 5b through 5e). Fig. 5f shows the final result of optimal registration where the bone artifacts present in Fig. 5a have been nearly completely removed.

in the background signal is also noticeable. The genetic search algorithm has found a mapping which, in conjunction with the Jacobian factor, registers both the bladder and the independently moving bone simultaneously. The residual background variation is caused by noise in the acquisition system. For this ROI, 6,102 calls to the evaluation procedure occurred with 20 samples per evaluation. The time required to register the ROI was 40 seconds.

The next image, Fig. 6, is a subtraction image of the upper arm of a patient who was undergoing a DSA study for evaluation of vascular disease. The brachial artery and its branches can be seen. Considerable motion artifact is present at the edge of the bone and can be seen distorting the arterial image in several places. Four ROI's were selected to cover the artery as it crosses the bone. The dimensions of the ROI's are, from left to right, 100x80, 100x80, 100x100, and 80x80. Each ROI was processed independently of the others. With 100 samples per evaluation, the optimal registration algorithm executed 33,545 evaluations for a combined time of 714 seconds for all ROI's. Fig. 7 shows the results of optimal registration of all four ROI's. The magnitudes of the d components ranged from 0.16 to 3.98 pixels. Within the ROI, the artifacts due to the bone misregistration are significantly reduced or eliminated. This largely removes the distortion of the brachial artery as it crosses the edge of the humerus (arrow A). Furthermore, after registration it is possible to follow a branch of the brachial artery (arrow B) much farther than was possible in the unregistered subtraction image. Some increase in the noise of the background is also seen in the optimally registered ROI's.

Fig. 7 reveals a difficulty with the technique. While the restrictions stated in Section 2 concerning suitable mappings are obeyed within a given ROI, they are not obeyed over the composite image. The problem is that the ROI's are independently registered, and since there is no provision for reconciling the motion of adjacent ROI's, there is the possibility of discontinuities in the transformations at the borders. Such a discontinuity is visible at the border between the two leftmost ROI's in Fig. 7. To highlight the problem we have in the inset of Fig. 8 magnified a

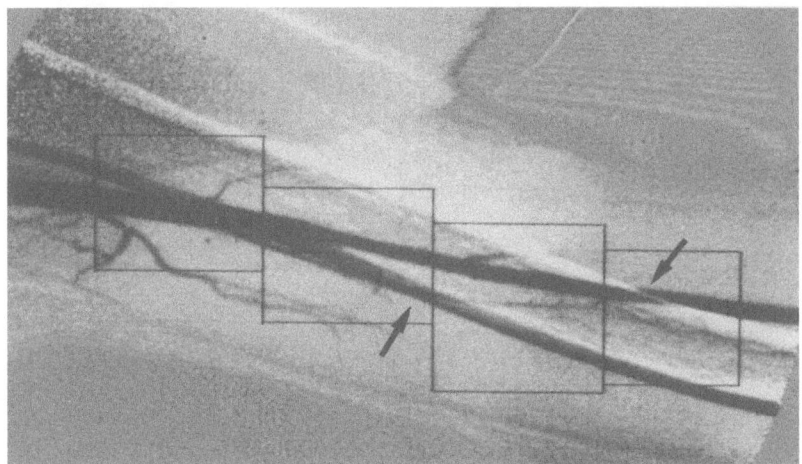

Fig. 6. DSA image of the upper arm. A patient undergoing evaluation for vascular disease moved between acquisition of the mask and contrast images. The motion is seen in the subtraction image by the white-black artifacts at the edges of the humerus (arrows). These artifacts affect visualization of those places where the artery crosses the bone. Four regions of interest are shown which define the mask subimages processed by the optimal registration algorithm.

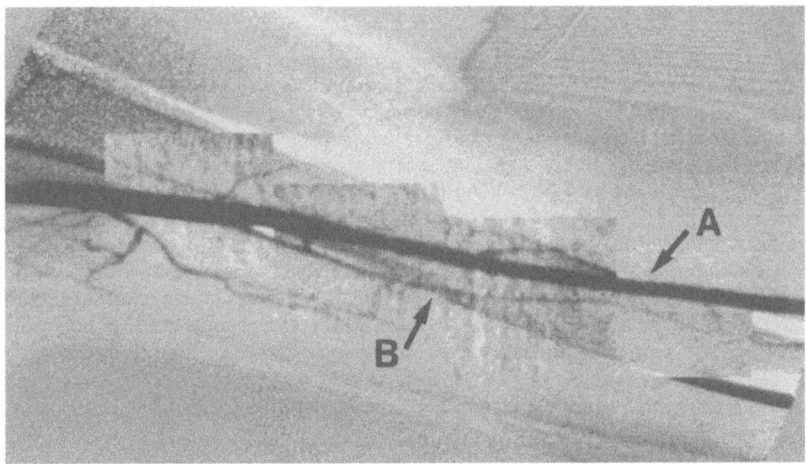

Fig. 7. DSA image of the upper arm processed by optimal registration. Each of the mask subregions shown in Fig. 6 were transformed independently and subtracted from the corresponding contrast subregion to form the processed image. Arrow A shows the brachial artery where a major artifact was removed. Arrow B indicates a branch of the brachial artery which is visible for a much greater distance along the bone after processing.

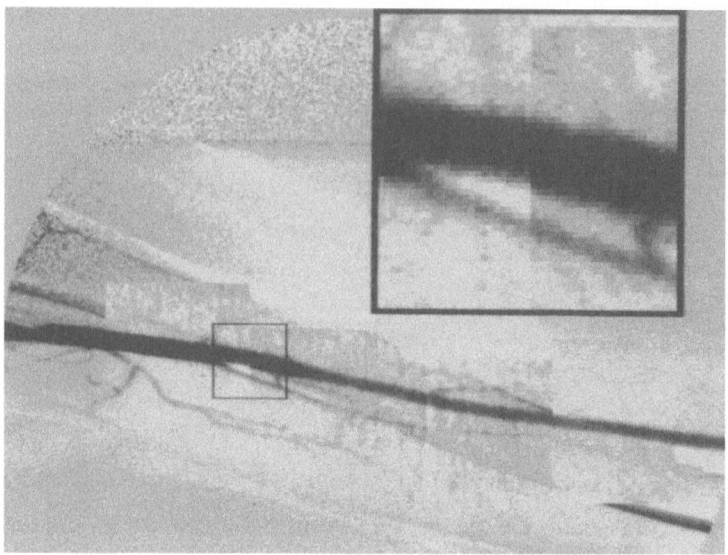

Fig. 8.  Boundary effect of adjacent ROI's in optimally registered images. The ROI in the inset has been enlarged by 4 times to show that there is no offset along the arteries, since only the mask is warped. Density differences between subregions are apparent, however. In this image no attempt has been made to join the regions smoothly.

region surrounding the discontinuity. (The magnification is accomplished by means of 4x4 pixel replication.) The principal effect seems to be a discontinuity of gray levels at the interface. There is no misregistration of the contrast-filled vessels since only the mask, in which the vessels are not visible, is warped.

A third image set illustrates the capabilities of the optimal registration algorithm to remove the motion artifacts in a relatively complex area surrounding the elbow. Fig. 9 shows a DSA image in the region of the elbow of the same patient. Motion artifacts from the humerus, radius, ulna, and the joint, as well as the brachial artery branching into the radial and ulnar arteries are visible. The smaller branches of the brachial artery around the joint are not readily seen and a significant misregistration artifact (arrow A) falls across the ulnar artery. The ROI's were selected to improve the visibility of the arterial segments in areas where the artifacts appear to be most significant. Four 70x70 pixels ROI's were used, and each ROI was processed independently. With 100 samples per evaluation, 51,920 evaluations were executed for a combined time of 1117 seconds for all ROI's. The magnitudes of the d components varied from 0.00 to 3.19. After processing, as is shown in Fig. 10, the motion at the elbow joint itself is noticeably reduced in severity in the ROI's when compared to the unregistered image. Especially apparent is the improved visualization of branches of the brachial artery which run into the joint capsule (arrow A). Similarly, a significant reduction in motion artifact overlying the ulnar artery can be seen as indicated by arrow B.

## 6. DISCUSSION

The phantom images provide the optimal registration algorithm with a controlled test which includes the essential features of a clinical imaging situation. Both bone and soft tissue in the presence of scatter and three dimensional motion are present. The images which result from the registration procedure clearly indicate that three dimensional motion can be corrected by the eight parameter polynomial warp function which was applied during this work. The registration of the bone is very good by any standards when compared to the unprocessed subtraction image. It is interesting, however, to compare the signal in Fig. 5f arising from the the inherent

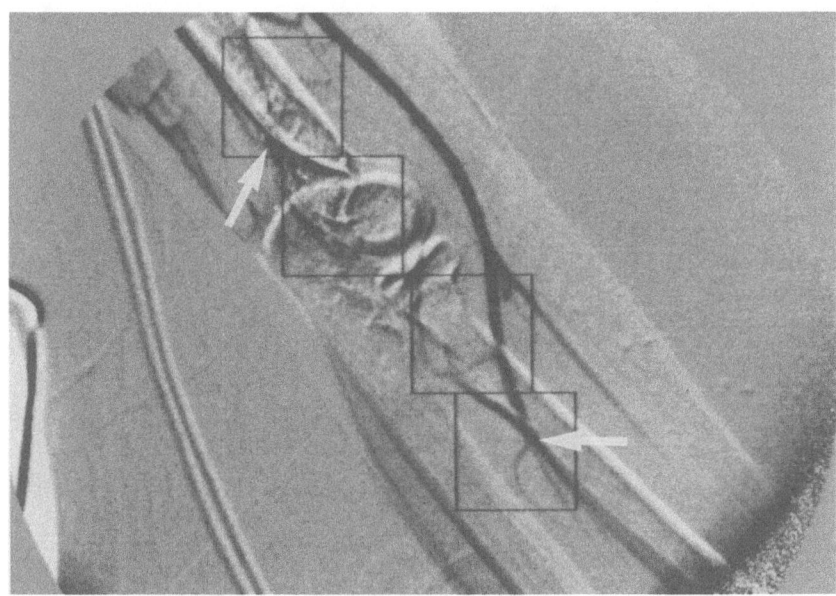

Fig. 9.    DSA of the elbow. Motion between the mask and contrast images
yielded the subtraction image shown which exhibits artifacts along the
bone and around the joint. Four ROI's were selected for processing
based the locations of branches of the brachial and ulnar arteries.
Misregistration artifacts, indicated by arrows, falls across the artery.

differences between the mask and contrast images due to the influx of dye, to that arising from
the motion artifacts. As discussed above in Section 3, the registration cannot be expected to
proceed consistently beyond the point at which the signal from the motion artifacts has been
reduced to the level of the inherent difference signal. At this point the relative areas of these
two components become important. In Fig. 5e it can be seen that these areas are approximately
equal, and, as expected for such a case, the arteries are barely visible in the vicinity of the
artifacts. Fig. 5f shows the small improvement achieved beyond this point.

A secondary effect in the phantom images is the change in background signal which is seen
in the optimally registered images. As stated above in Section 5, the change is achieved by finding a transformation of the form of Eq. (1) which registers both the bladder and the bone. In
the phantom image, the resulting decrease in signal in the background may be more pronounced
than would ordinarily be expected in clinical images, but no specific investigation of this effect
has been completed. The soft tissue signal seems in fact to be increased in most of the processed
ROI's on clinical images, but the overall effect of the processing is to increase the visualization of
the vascular structures by removing bone artifacts. Further study of the problem of reducing
both bone and soft tissue signal is proceeding.

There are a number of questions concerning optimal registration which remain to be
resolved. (a) As pointed out in Section 2, the success of automatic registration depends on there
being a correlation between the evaluation function used by the registration algorithm and the
evaluation made by a human observer. A systematic study of human evaluation of difference
images may provide guidance in the formulation of improved evaluation functions. (b) The statistical evaluation technique has proven to be essential in the development of algorithms which
register images quickly. Grefenstette and Fitzpatrick investigated the effect of changing the sample size (Grefenstette and Fitzpatrick, 1985), but no method for choosing an optimal size based
on characteristics of the image pair has been developed. Furthermore, in addition to the method
of stratified sampling, other methods for improving the precision of the statistical estimate, such
as the method of "control variates" (James, 1980) should be tried. (c) The search space is large

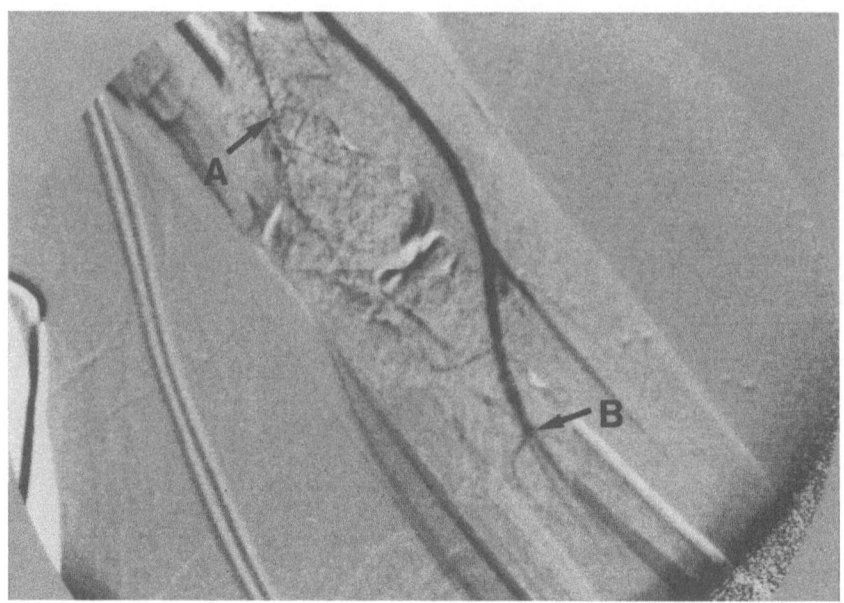

Fig. 10.    DSA of the elbow processed by optimal registration. Each of the subregions shown in Fig. 9 was transformed independently by the optimal registration algorithm and subtracted from the corresponding contrast subregion to form the processed image. A branch of the brachial artery running into the joint capsule area (arrow A) is much more clearly visible after processing. Arrow B shows that the bone artifact which affected the ulnar artery has been removed, greatly improving visualization of the artery.

for these problems and is somewhat coarse, since the continuous **d** vectors are varied by discrete increments. The size of these increments can be reduced by increasing the number of bits in the structures used to specify the **d**'s, a change which also increases the size of the search space, or by decreasing the range of values for their components (See Section 3.). The minimum number of bits required depends on the fractional pixel motion required to achieve a registration, and the component range depends on the distance which must be moved to achieve a registration. Methods for estimating the minimum number of bits and minimum range for a successful registration need to be developed. (d) Finally, the problem of boundary discontinuities, as illustrated by Fig. 8, must be solved. One approach is to use a grid of contiguous ROI's which share **d** vectors with their neighbors. A structure which encodes all **d**'s for all ROI's could be used in the registration algorithm. The problem with such an approach is that the search space becomes much larger, and the time for a registration is likely to become unacceptably long. Some method should be devised to allow separate registrations for each such ROI, with an integration of the separate intra-ROI transformations into one inter-ROI transformation.

An important feature of the algorithm described here is that it is used in an interactive mode rather than a totally automatic mode. After manual selection of the ROI from which the mask image will be processed, the algorithm continuously tries new sets of parameters. The algorithm can be allowed to function until a best match is determined by the minimization of the mean of the absolute value of the difference image, but it has been found that the process creates acceptable warpings on its way towards the minimum value of the difference function. If the operator is permitted to halt the warping function evaluation when a satisfactory trial is completed, the process of producing acceptable results is in some cases much quicker. A disadvantage to this approach is that it requires the operator to be much more knowledgeable about the images that he is viewing in order to make an appropriate decision about stopping the warping process. Further investigation into the need for operator interaction versus more automated stopping criteria is warranted.

Scatter and beam hardening are effects which exist in all clinical images. Time-varying scatter can produce image noise which might affect the optimal registration algorithm. However, in clinical images, the scatter between mask and contrast images will tend to be similar. In our studies to date, scatter has not seemed to confuse the registration algorithm. Likewise, beam hardening, which causes the assumption of proportionality between line integral of attenuation and the logarithmically transformed beam intensity to be invalid (see the Appendix), does not appear to present significant problems for the optimal registration algorithm. Since the method is not sensitive to the absolute measure of the line-integral of attenuation, but only to is temporal and spatial variation, little effect is expected in clinical images because of the overall similarity between the composition and thickness of the tissues in the mask and contrast images.

It is not expected that such algorithms can ever be developed to the extent that they remove all motion artifacts in DSA. Furthermore, more complex motion may very well cause the algorithm to increase greatly the time required to obtain a satisfactory subtraction. However, the results shown indicate that there is likely to be a considerable improvement in the appearance of some DSA images of small vessels after optimal registration.

## 7. ACKNOWLEDGEMENTS

The authors wish to express their gratitude to Hsuan Chang and Venkateswara R. Mandava for their help with the system development, the experiments, and photography.

This work has been supported by grants from the National Institutes of Health (HL34703), the National Science Foundation (ECS-8608588), and the Whitaker Foundation.

## 8. APPENDIX

Our proof of the existence of a two dimensional geometrical image transformation which duplicates the effects of the three dimensional motion of the objects being imaged depends upon the assumption that the image formation procedure produces a "projected density" image. We define a projected density image to be such that the image value at each point in the image is proportional to the line-integral of the density of some conserved quantity, where a conserved quantity is one whose value for a given region can change only as the result of flux across the boundaries of that region. We can state the definition as follows:

$$p(x,y,t) \equiv a \int_{z_1}^{z_2} \mu(x,y,z,t)\,dz, \tag{3}$$

where $p$ is the image, $\mu$ is the density, and $a$ is some constant of proportionality. In our case $p$ represents a calibrated X-ray projection image (see below), and $\mu$ represents the linear X-ray attenuation coefficient. It can be seen that $\mu$ is the density of a conserved quantity by noting that it is equal to mass per unit volume multiplied by the mass attenuation coefficient (Macovski, p. 27, 1983). Since both the mass and the mass attenuation coefficient of a given particle are independent of time and position, a change, for any region, in the quantity represented by their product must be the result of particle flux across the boundaries of the region. (An alternative argument may be based on the physical interpretation of $\mu$ as representing cross-sectional area per unit volume.)

The production of an approximate projected density image is possible with a conventional X-ray system by means of logarithmic amplification during image acquisition, followed by subtraction from a "calibration image". The approximation, which ignores the finite energy spread of the X-ray spectrum, is based on the assumption made in early computed tomography (CT) (Stonestrom et al., 1981) that the image, $i(x,y,t)$, is an exponential function of the line integral of the attenuation coefficient,

$$i(x,y,t) = i_0(x,y) \exp\left( - \int_{z_1}^{z_2} \mu(x,y,z,t)\,dz \right),$$

where $i_0(x,y)$ is the image which is obtained without the imaged object present. The spatial variation in $i_0$ results from variations in both the X-ray flux and the gain of the image intensifier. Taking the logarithms of both sides of this equation, we obtain

$$\log i(x,y,t) \; = \; \log i_0(x,y) \; - \; \int_{z_1}^{z_2} \mu(x,y,z,t)\,dz.$$

If the logarithmically amplified image is subtracted from a calibration image, obtained without the imaged object present, the result with the use of Equation (3), is a calibrated projection image,

$$p(x,y,t) \; = \; \log i_0(x,y) \; - \; \log i(x,y,t).$$

This calibration step accomplishes two things: it compensates for the $i_0$ offset, so that when the line integral of attenuation changes, $p(x,y,t)$ changes proportionally, rather than just linearly; and it removes the spurious spatial variation arising from variations in X-ray flux and intensifier gain. The resulting image is only an approximation of a projected density image. If the errors in this approximation are ultimately shown to cause serious problems in image registration, it may be helpful to apply the corrections for "beam hardening" developed for CT (Stonestrom et al., 1981).

Because it is the density of a conserved quantity, $\mu$ obeys the continuity equation of continuum mechanics and fluid dynamics,

$$\frac{\partial \mu}{\partial t} + \nabla \cdot (\mu \mathbf{u}_f) \; = \; 0, \tag{4}$$

where $\mathbf{u}_f = \mathbf{u}_f(x,y,z,t)$ is the fluid velocity and $\nabla$ is the three dimensional divergence operator. If we integrate Equation (4) over $z$ from $z_1$ to $z_2$, multiply both sides by $a$, and define the two dimensional mean velocity,

$$\mathbf{u}(x,y,t) \; = \; = \; \int_{z_1}^{z_2} \mu \mathbf{u}_p \, dz \, / \, p(x,y,t),$$

where $\mathbf{u}_p$ is the component of $\mathbf{u}_f$ in the image plane, we obtain a two dimensional continuity equation for $p$,

$$\frac{\partial p}{\partial t} + \nabla \cdot (p\mathbf{u}) \; = \; 0, \tag{5}$$

where $\nabla$ now represents the two dimensional divergence operator. The time-dependent, two dimensional image produced by the three dimensional motion is a solution to Equation (5).

Letting the vector $\mathbf{x}$ represent the the coordinates, $x, y$, we next consider the path produced by starting at some point $\mathbf{x}_1, t_1$, and moving continuously at the current image plane velocity, $\mathbf{u}$, to the point $\mathbf{x}_2, t_2$. For continuous, differentiable functions, $\mu$ and $\mathbf{u}$, it can be shown (Fitzpatrick, 1986) that the resulting transformation from $\mathbf{x}_1$ to $\mathbf{x}_2$ is one-to-one, continuous, and differentiable. Thus, for a given pair, $t_1$ and $t_2$, both of the functions, $\mathbf{x}_1(\mathbf{x}_2)$ and $\mathbf{x}_2(\mathbf{x}_1)$, exist and are continuous and differentiable.

We now note that the rate of change with time of any continuous, differentiable function $f(\mathbf{x},t)$, measured along the path produced by moving at $\mathbf{u}(\mathbf{x},t)$ can be expressed in terms of partial derivatives as follows,

$$\frac{df}{dt} \; = \; \frac{\partial f}{\partial t} + \mathbf{u} \cdot \nabla f.$$

We then consider the special case, $f = pJ$, the image intensity multiplied by the Jacobian. For this case we have

$$\frac{d}{dt}(pJ) \; = \; p\left(\frac{dJ}{dt}\right) + J\left(\frac{\partial p}{\partial t} + \mathbf{u} \cdot \nabla p\right). \tag{6}$$

We note by expanding the second term in Equation (5) that

$$\frac{\partial p}{\partial t} + \mathbf{u} \cdot \nabla p \; = \; -p\nabla \cdot \mathbf{u}, \tag{7}$$

and we make use of Euler's formula for the rate of change of the Jacobian (Serrin, 1959),

$$\frac{dJ}{dt} \; = \; J\,\nabla \cdot \mathbf{u}. \tag{8}$$

By using Equations (7) and (8) in Equation (6) we find that

$$\frac{d}{dt}(pJ) \ = \ 0.$$

Thus, $pJ$ is a constant of the motion. Noting that $J(\mathbf{x}_1(\mathbf{x}_1)) = 1$, we have for two specific points in space-time, $\mathbf{x}_1, t_1$ and $\mathbf{x}_2, t_2$,

$$p(\mathbf{x}_1, t_1) \ = \ J(\mathbf{x}_2(\mathbf{x}_1)) \ p(\mathbf{x}_2(\mathbf{x}_1), t_2). \tag{9}$$

Furthermore, since the transformation is continuous and one-to-one, J is nonzero and finite and obeys the inverse relationship,

$$J(\mathbf{x}_1(\mathbf{x}_2)) \ = \ 1 \ / \ J(\mathbf{x}_2(\mathbf{x}_1)).$$

Therefore, we have the inverse of Equation (9) as well,

$$p(\mathbf{x}_2, t_2) \ = \ J(\mathbf{x}_1(\mathbf{x}_2)) \ p(\mathbf{x}_1(\mathbf{x}_2), t_1),$$

which is identical to Equation (1). The derivation of Equation (1) constitutes the proof of the existence of the desired two dimensional geometrical transformation. The proof depends on the aptness of Equation (4), which requires that $\mu$ and $\mathbf{u}$ be continuous and differentiable. The proofs can be extended to the case of discontinuous and non-differentiable images, provided that the point-spread function of the imaging system is itself continuous and differentiable or that post-processing is performed by convolution with a continuous, differentiable kernel (Fitzpatrick, 1986).

## 9. REFERENCES

Akisada, A., Ando, M., Hyodo, K., Hasegawa, S., Konishi, K., Nishimura, K., Maruhashi, A., Toyofuku, F., Suwa, A., and Kohra, K. (1986). An attempt at coronary angiography with a large size monochromatic SR beam, Nucl. Instruments and Methods Phys. Res., A246, 713-718.

Barnea, D. I. and Silverman, H. F. (1972). A class of algorithms for fast digital image registration, IEEE Trans. Comp., 21, 179-186.

Brody, W. R. (1984), Digital Radiography, Raven Press, New York.

Chang, H. (1987). Displaytool: A Window-Based Image Display Tool for Sun Workstations, Technical Report, Dept. Comp. Sci, Vanderbilt University.

DeJong, K. A. (1980). Adaptive system design: a genetic approach, IEEE Trans. Syst., Man, and Cyber., SMC-10, 566-574.

De Vries, N., Miller, F. J., Wojtowycz, M. M., Brown, P. R., Yandow, D. R., Nelson, J. A., and Kruger, R. A. (1985). Tomographic digital subtraction angiography: initial clinical studies using tomosynthesis, Radiology, 157, 239-241.

Fitzpatrick, J. M., Grefenstette, J. J., and Van-Gucht, D. (1984). Image registration by genetic search, Proceedings of Southeastcon '84, R. T. Coomes, ed., IEEE Publishing Services, NY, 460-646.

Fitzpatrick, J. M. (1986). The existence of geometrical density-image transformations corresponding to object motion, manuscript under review by Computer Vision, Graphics, and Image Processing.

Fitzpatrick, J. M. and Leuze, M. R. (1987). A class of one-to-one two dimensional transformations, Computer Vision, Graphics, and Image Processing, to appear September, 1987.

Frei, W., Shibata, T., and Chen, C. C. (1980). Fast matching of non-stationary images with false fix protection, Proc. 5th Intl. Conf. Patt. Recog., vol. 1, T. Pavlidis, ed., IEEE Publishing Services, NY, 208-12.

Fourman, M. P. (1985). Compaction of symbolic layout using genetic algorithms, Proc. Intl. Conf. on Genetic Algorithms and Applicat., John J. Grefenstette, ed., Carnegie-Mellon Univ., Pittsburgh, PA, 141-153.

Grefenstette, J. J. (1984). A user's guide to GENESIS, Tech. Report CS-84-11, Dept. Comput. Sci., Vanderbilt University, Nashville, TN.

Grefenstette, J. J. and Fitzpatrick, J. M. (1985). Genetic search with approximate function evaluations, Proc. Intl. Conf. on Genetic Algorithms and Applicat., John J. Grefenstette, ed., Carnegie-Mellon Univ., Pittsburgh, PA, 112-118.

Grefenstette, J. J., Gopal, R., Rosmaita, B. J., Van Gucht, D. (1985). Genetic algorithms for the traveling salesman problem, Proc. Intl. Conf. on Genetic Algorithms and Applicat., John J. Grefenstette, ed., Carnegie-Mellon Univ., Pittsburgh, PA, 160-168.

Goldberg, D. (1983), Computer aided gas pipeline operation using genetic algorithms and rule learning, Ph. D. Thesis, Dept. Civil Eng., Univ. of Michigan.

Hall, E. L. (1979), Computer Image Processing and Recognition, Academic Press, New York.

Holland, J. H. (1975), Adaptation in Natural and Artificial Systems, Univ. Michigan Press, Ann Arbor.

Holland, J. H. (1986), Escaping brittleness in: Machine Learning, Vol. 2, R.S. Michalski, J. G. Carbonell, and T. M. Mitchell, eds., Morgan Kaufman, 593-623.

Horn, B. K. P. and Bachman, B. L. (1979). Registering real images using synthetic images, in: Artificial Intelligence: An MIT Perspective, vol 2, P. H. Winston and R. H. Brown, eds., MIT Press, Cambridge.

Hughes, E. B., Rubenstein, E., Zeman, H. D., Brown, G. S., Buchbinder, M., Harrison, D. C., Hofstadter, R., Kernoff, R. S., Otis, J. N., Sommer, H. A., Thompson, A. C., and Walton, J. T. (1985). Prospects for non-invasive antiogarphy with tunable X-rays, Nucl. Instruments and Methods Phys. Res., B10/11, 323-328.

James, F. (1980). Monte Carlo theory and practice, Rep. Prog. Phys., 43, 73-1189.

Kinsey, J. H. and Vannellii, B. D. (1975). Application of digital image change detection to diagnosis and follow-up of cancer involving the lungs. Proc. Soc. Photo-optical Instrum. Eng., 70, 99-112.

Kruger, R. A. (1981). A method for time domain filtering using computerized fluoroscopy, Med. Phys., 8, 466-470.

Kruger, R. A., Sedaghati, M., Roy, D. G., Liu, P., Nelson, J. A., Kubal, W., and Del Rio, P. (1984). Tomosynthesis applied to digital subtraction angiography, Radiology, 152, 805-808.

Kruger, R. A. and Riederer, S. J. (1984), Basic Concepts of Digital Subtraction Angiography, G. K. Hall Medical Publishers, Boston.

Levin, D. C., Schapiro, R. M., Boxt, L. M., Dunham, L., Harrington, D. P., and Ergun, D. L. (1984). Review--digital subtraction angiography: principles and pitfalls of image improvement techniques, Am. J. Roent, 135, 1153-1160.

Macovski, A. (1983), Medical Imaging Systems, Prentice-Hall, Inc., Englewood Cliffs, NJ.

Miller, J. W. V., Windham, J. P., and Kwatra, S. C. (1984). Optimal filtering of radiographic image sequences using simultaneous diagonalization, IEEE Trans. Med. Imaging, MI-3, 116-123.

Oung, H. and Smith A. M. (1984). Real time motion detection in digital subtractive angiography, Proc. ISMII, A. Duerinckx, M. H. Loew, J. M. S. Prewitt, eds., IEEE Publishing Services, NY, 336-339.

Pfeiler, M., Marhoff, P., and Schipper, P. (1984). The digital imaging technique in conventional radiography: present and future possiblilties, Electromedica, 52, 2-12.

Potel, M. J. and Gustafson, D. E. (1983). Motion correction for digital subtraction angiography, Proc. IEEE Frontiers Eng. and Computing in Health Care, 166-169.

Price, R. R., Lindstrom, D. P., Hillis, S., Friesinger, G. C., and Brill, A. B. (1975). Analytical techniques for image superposition, Proc. 5th Symp. on sharing of Comp. Programs and Tech. in Nuc. Med., 241-250.

Riederer, S. J., Enzmann, D. R., Hall, A. L., Pelc, N. J., and Djang, W. T. (1983). The application of matched filtering to X-ray exposure reduction in digital subtraction angiography: clinical results, Radiology, 146, 349-354.

Riederer, S. J. and Kruger, R. A. (1983). Intravenous digital subtraction: a summary of recent developments, Radiology, 147, 633-638.

Rosenfeld, A. and Kak, A. (1982), Digital Picture Processing, 2nd ed., Academic Press, New York.

Schaffer, J. D. and Grefenstette, J. J. (1985). Multi-objective learning via genetic algorithms, Proc. 9th Intl. J. Conf. Artif. Intel., 593-595.

Serrin, J. (1959). Mathematical principles of classical fluid mechanics in: Encyclopedia of Physics, vol 8, Flugge, S., ed., Springer-Verlag, Berlin, 126ff.

Smith, S. F. (1983). Flexible learning of problem solving heuristics through adaptive search, Proc. 8th Intl. J. Conf. Artif. Intel.

Stonestrom, J. P., Alvarez, R. E., and Macovski, A. (1981). A framework for spectral artifact corrections in X-ray CT, IEEE Trans. Biomed. Eng., BME-28, 128-141.

Svedlow, M., McGillem, C. D., and Anuta, P. E. (1977). Image registration: similarity measure and preprocessing method comparisons. IEEE Trans. Aerospace Electronic Syst., AES-14, 141-150.

Tobis, J. M., Henry, W. L., and Nalcioglu, O. (1983). Cardiac applications of digital subtraction angiography, Appl. Radiology, 61-67.

Van-Lysel, M. S., Dobbins, J. T., III, Peppler, W. W., Hasegawa, B. H., Lee, C, Mistretta, C. A., Zarnstroff, W. C., Crummy, A. B., Kubal, W., Bergsjordet, B., Strother, C. M., and Sackett, J. F. (1983). Work in progress: hybrid temporal-energy subtraction in digital fluoroscopy, Radiology, 147, 869-874.

Venot, A. and Leclerc, V. (1984). Automated correction of patient motion and gray values prior to subtraction in digitized angiography, IEEE Trans. Med. Imaging MI-3(4), 179-186.

Venot, A., Liehn, J C., Lebruchec, J. F., and Roucayrol, J. C. (1986a). Automated comparison of scintigraphic images, J. Nucl. Med., 27, 1337-1342.

Venot, A., Pronzato, L., Walter, E., and Lebruchec, J. F. (1986b). A distribution-free criterion for robust identification, with applications in system modelling and image processing, Automatica, 22, 105-109.

Yanagisawa, M., Shigemitsu, S., and Akatsuka, T. (1984). Registration of locally distorted images by multiwindow pattern matching and displacement interpolation: the proposal of an algorithm and its application to digital subtraction angiography, Seventh Intl. Conf. Pattern Recog., M. D. Levine, ed., IEEE Publishing Services, NY, 1288-1291.

Wong, R. Y. (1977). Image sensor transformations, IEEE Trans. Syst. Man Cyber. SMC-7 (12), 836-841.

# ON THE INFORMATION CONTENT OF DIAGNOSTIC ULTRASOUND

M.F. Insana, R.F. Wagner, D.G. Brown, and B.S. Garra[*]

Office of Science and Technology, Center for Devices and
Radiological Health, FDA, Rockville, MD 20857 USA

[*]Dept. of Diagnostic Radiology, National Institutes of Health,
Bethesda, MD 20892 USA

## INTRODUCTION

Echo signals in medical ultrasound are rich in information about
tissue composition and structure. But not all of this information is
readily apparent from the image. For example, the average size, density
and organization of microscopic tissue structures which may be obtained
from the first- and second-order statistical properties of the data are
difficult to visualize directly from the image. Yet these acoustic
parameters have been shown to be sensitive indicators of changes brought on
by disease processes in the liver and spleen (Fellingham and Sommer 1984,
Insana et al. 1987), and therefore make good classifiying features for
tissue characterization. Realizing the full potential of these features
requires the use of pattern recognition techniques in order to minimize
classification errors due to measurement uncertainty and patient
variability.

It is our purpose in this paper to describe a computer assisted
approach for the detection and classification of disease using
backscattered ultrasound. We will demonstrate the utility of these
techniques by comparing their accuracy with that of human observers for
detection tasks using both computer simulation and actual clinical data.

## THE INVERSE PROBLEM: TISSUE PROPERTIES FROM IMAGE SPECKLE

Characteristic of diagnostic ultrasound images is the textured
appearance of the tissues. This image property is known as speckle and is
generated by a coherent summation (or interference), at the detector
surface, of acoustic echoes arising from a distributed source of scatterers. Speckle properties are determined in a complex way by the composition
and distribution of tissue components and by properties of the imaging
system, e.g., aperture and bandwidth. Although speckle reduces the visual
detectability of target signals in the image, it is a rich source of
information about the tissue type and condition. Unfortunately much of
that information is found in the second-order statistics of the image
speckle, which is of limited accessibility to the human visual system
(Julesz 1981).

One way to recover some of this information for use in diagnosis is to search for a consistent set of data features that quantitatively describe physical properties of the tissues and are sensitive to disease processes. Work in this area has progressed along two paths. The first approach uses the established theory of the interaction between sound and inhomogeneous media, such as the body, to propose rigorously-defined <u>physically-based</u> quantitative features for classification. However, precise measurements of such physical features as scattering, attenuation, and the speed of sound propagation in tissues are quite difficult because of the coherent nature of the detector and the complexity of the body. Alternatively, a heuristic approach has been used in which a large number of <u>statistical</u> features (as many as 100 or more) are extracted from the acoustic signal, often without prior knowledge of discrimination relevancy, and tested for their ability to distinguish among different tissues and disease conditions. This approach uses statistical learning concepts to find the smallest number of features which offer the greatest discriminability. The first approach provides a sound physical basis for the choice of discriminating features and the second approach allows the development of a system capable of adapting to a diverse clinical environment.

We have combined the two approaches and developed a multiparameter technique that uses physically-based features derived from the first- and second-order statistics of the echo signal to describe clinically relevant aspects of the tissue macro- and microstructure and tissue composition. The methods of statistical pattern recognition and decision theory are then applied to select the most discriminating features, establish optimal decision boundaries within the feature space, and evaluate the diagnostic performance for comparison with established diagnostic methods. This method requires a thorough understanding of the statistical properties of acoustic signals in terms of the scattering physics. Recently, such an analysis has become available (Wagner et al. 1987a), and is based on the principles of coherent imaging as established from the literature on laser speckle and radar imaging (e.g., Goodman 1985, Middleton 1960). Wagner et al. (1987a) have derived the statistical properties of the radiofrequency (rf) echo signal, its envelope (B-scan or magnitude signal), and the squared envelope (intensity signal) for the scatter signals arising from simple and complex media. From the intensity and rf spectra, a total of six features have emerged as a basis set for characterizing soft tissues.

Tissue Features From the Intensity Signal

For most ultrasonic imaging systems, it is the envelope of the echo signal that is displayed. However, the relationship between image statistics and scattering physics is much simpler when the analysis is performed using the squared envelope or intensity data. From the intensity data, soft tissue macrostructure (on the order of 1 mm) may be described with four scattering features. The exact method for calculating three of these features using data from a clinical sector scanner is described by Insana et al. (1986a). These features describe the scale and strength of tissue scatterers and are summarized in Table 1.

The analysis assumes that soft tissues may be represented as an acoustically uniform medium populated by three distinct classes of discrete scatterers. These are shown schematically in Fig 1.

Class I consists of small randomly positioned (diffuse) scatterers of sufficient concentration to give an echo signal with circular Gaussian statistics, i.e., the rf echo signal is a complex, zero-mean Gaussian random variable in which the real and imaginary parts have equal variance,

$\sigma^2$. Approximately seven to ten scatterers per resolution cell are sufficient to assume Gaussian statistics to second order. A histogram of the intensity values will follow an exponential probability density function (pdf)

$$p(I) = \frac{1}{2\sigma^2} \exp\left(-\frac{I^2}{2\sigma^2}\right) \qquad I \geq 0 \qquad (1)$$

and the square of the point signal-to-noise ratio is

$$SNR_o^2 = \frac{\langle I \rangle^2}{(\langle I^2 \rangle - \langle I \rangle^2)} = 1.0 \qquad . \qquad (2)$$

The medium is entirely characterized by one first-order quantity; the average incoherent (or diffuse) backscattered intensity, $I_d = 2\sigma^2$. $I_d$ has been accurately quantified by such measures as the backscatter coefficient (Madsen et al. 1984).

Table 1. Intensity Tissue Structure Signature[*]

| Distribution Function | 1st-Order Signature ($SNR_o^2$) | 1st- and 2nd-Order Structure Analysis | Classification Features |
|---|---|---|---|
| Sub-Rayleigh | $\bar{N}/(\bar{N}+1) < 1$ | Non-Gaussian / few diffuse scatterers | $\bar{N}$ |
| Rayleigh | 1 | Gaussian / many diffuse scatterers | $I_d$ |
| Rician | $\dfrac{(1+r)^2}{1+2r} \geq 1$ | Unresolved coherent component (spacing < pulse width) | $I_d, I_s$ |
| Generalized Rician | ambiguous | Resolved coherent component (spacing > pulse width) | $I_d, I_s, \sigma_s^2, \bar{d}$ |

[*]Trends and inhomogeneities (e.g., large vessels) must be removed.

Class II scatterers consist of small but nonrandomly distributed tissue scatterers with regular, quasi-periodic and long-range order. This class of scatterer contributes a coherent scattering or specular component to the echo signal that is spatially varying with mean $I_s$ and variance $\sigma_s^2$. If both class I and II scatterers are present, and if the scale of the regular stucture is well below the resolution of the imaging system, then $\sigma_s 2$ is negligible and the intensity $SNR_o$ is larger than one. $SNR_o$ is unity when only class I scatterers are present. Defining the value $r = I_s/I_d$, the $SNR_o^2$ is given by

$$SNR_o^2 = \frac{(1+r)^2}{1+2r} \geq 1 \qquad . \qquad (3)$$

We refer to this case as distributed specular scattering, and now the nature of the image texture becomes dependent on several properties of the scattering medium. This medium is characterized by two first-order statistical quantities, the average backscatter intensities $I_d$ and $I_s$. The

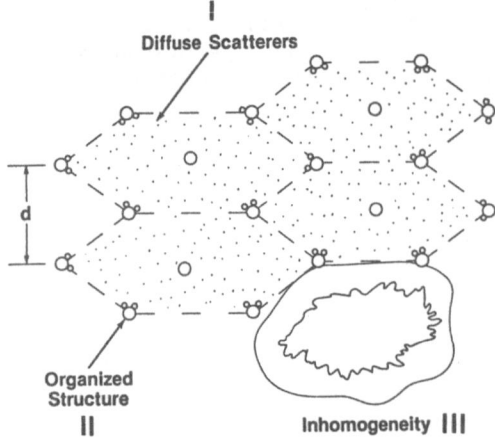

Fig. 1. A schematic diagram of human liver parenchyma showing three types of scatterers.

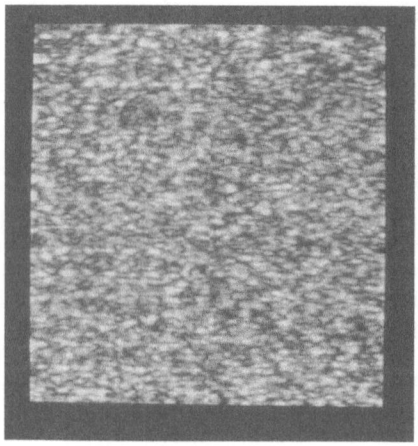

Fig. 2. Two computer simulated speckle fields. The left half was simulated using both class I (diffuse) scatterers and class II (organized) scatterers. The right half is a simulation of a non-Gaussian field in which there are an average of two scatterers per resolution cell.

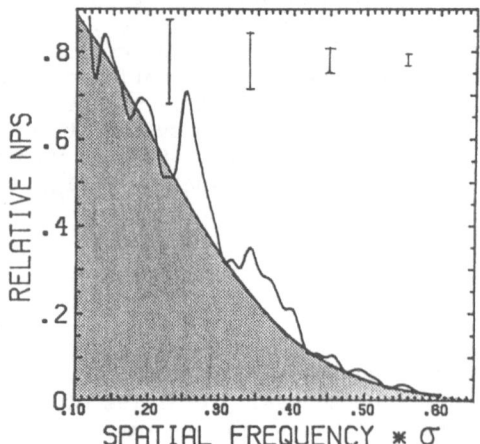

Fig. 3. The average power spectrum of the intensity data for normal human liver, in vivo. The shaded area is the Rician variance while the unshaded area represents variance due to the organized structure. The average scatterer spacing, d, is found from spectral peaks with height greater than 2 standard deviations (see error bars).

statistics of the speckle follow a Rician pdf,

$$p(I) = \frac{1}{I_d} \exp\left(-\frac{I+I_s}{I_d}\right) I_o\left(2\frac{\sqrt{II_s}}{I_d}\right) \qquad I \geq 0 , \qquad (4)$$

where $I_o$ is a modified Bessel function of the first kind, zero order.

If the quasi-periodic class II scatterers are resolved by the system, $\sigma_s^2$ is greater than zero and an average scatterer spacing $\bar{d}$ can be estimated. A modified Rician pdf generalized to include a spatially structured specular signal describes the statistics of this speckle. Its properties have been derived by Wagner et al. (1987a). Examples in tissues of specular scatterers with organization or long-range order are the portal triads in liver parenchyma and the collagenous sheaths that surround muscle fascicles. Not one, but many levels of organization are present in most tissues. The spatial frequency "window" for observing the different levels of tissue structure is determined by the center frequency and bandwidth of the interrogating acoustic pulse.

The parameters $\bar{d}$ and $\sigma_s^2$ are calculated from the second-order statistics of the intensity data and, when resolvable periodicities are present, are necessary to uniquely identify the medium. If one were to work only with the first-order statistics of the intensity signal to estimate the parameter r without accounting for the variance in $I_s$, the results would suggest that there were too few scatterers to give Gaussian statistics, i.e., the intensity $SNR_o$ would be less than one. For example, the right half of the image in Fig. 2 was generated using approximately 2 scatterers per resolution cell -- clearly a simulation of a non-Gaussian medium. The left side is an image with modified Rician statistics, simulating a medium with class I (diffuse) scatterers and resolvable class II (organized) scatterers. The intensity $SNR_o$ for both halves is 0.88, and the speckle patterns are visually quite similar. Only by analyzing the second-order statistics can the two patterns be differentiated and an unambiguous signature be obtained. In clinical data, we often find that the intensity $SNR_o$ is less than one. For normal human liver measured in vivo, the values range between 0.6 and 1.1. Because we measure a periodicity of approximately 1.1 mm, we know that we must separate the variance due to the structured scattering, $\sigma_s^2$, from the rest of the power spectrum if we are to unambiguously sense the structure of the organ.

Class III scatterers are nonrandom and specular, but with short-range order, such as organ surfaces and blood vessels. They represent inhomogeneities which violate the assumption of a homogeneous medium needed for tissue characterization, and therefore are eliminated from the data in a preprocessing procedure. A simple matched filter technique to automatically identify suspected blood vessels has been reported by Insana et al. (1986a).

The above information is summarized by three tissue characterization features which are measured from the power spectrum of the intensity signal. For example see Fig. 3. The features are $\bar{d}$, the average spacing of quasi-periodic scatterers, $r = I_s/I_d$ and $\sigma_s' = \sigma_s/I_d$. The ratio r is a measure of the relative strength of class II and class I scatterers; it is a first-order statistical measure. The parameters $\bar{d}$ and $\sigma_s'$, on the other hand, are principally second-order tissue features. They describe the macroscopic scattering structure (macroscopic because the structure probed is resolvable and on the order of 1 mm), in particular the characteristic scale of the structure and the relative variability in the structured scattering strength.

For tissues where the image speckle is the result of a small number of scatterers per resolution cell, non-Gaussian conditions apply. In this case, a fourth feature, the average scatterer density $\bar{N}$, may then be estimated from the speckle statistics (Wagner et al. 1987b) by making use of the statistical models of Jakeman (1984). If we assume that the number density has a Poisson distribution with parameter $\bar{N}$ and that all scatterers contribute equally, the intensity $SNR_o^2$ is given by

$$SNR_o^2 \sim \bar{N}/\bar{N}+1 \quad .$$

The Gaussian limit is reached asymptotically as $\bar{N} \to \infty$. The applicability of this feature in the characterization of tissues is still unknown, but will become apparent as the sources of tissue scattering are more clearly understood.

## Tissue Features From the rf Echo Signal

The Attenuation Coefficient. Ultrasonic attenuation coefficients, $\alpha_o$, measure the lineal loss in energy of an acoustic pulse as it travels through tissue. It is a function of frequency and has the units $[dB\ cm^{-1}\ MHz^{-1}]$. Attenuation is often a sensitive indicator of material composition; in particular, $\alpha_o$ is sensitive to the fat content of tissues (Taylor et al. 1986, Garra et al. 1987a). We used a new broadband amplitude method developed by Garra et al. (1987a) for measuring ultrasonic attenuation coefficients in vivo. This method requires that a number of assumptions be made about the imaging system and the tissues. With regard to the system, it assumes that the transducer is weakly focused and that the transmitted acoustic pulses have a Gaussian-shaped spectrum. With regard to the tissues, the method assumes that the backscatter coefficient for the medium is constant over the region of interest and has a known frequency dependence. It also assumes that the attenuation coefficient is a linear function of frequency.

The attenuation coefficient was estimated from the root mean square (rms) amplitudes of the rf echo signal. The echo signal was segmented into relatively short depth intervals so that the signal was approximately stationary over the interval. The nonstationary effects of focusing, diffraction and variable gain were accounted for by phantom calibrations. The best estimate of attenuation was then found by iteratively searching for the attenuation coefficient that gave an rms amplitude that was constant with depth. Estimates based on this method were found to be as accurate as other attenuation measurement techniques, such as the spectral difference method, in spite of the many assumptions made, and yet show less within-group patient variability and less day-to-day variability for a given patient.

Average Scatterer Size. With the features described above, we have concentrated on estimating properties of large-scale structure or bulk attenuation properties. As seen in the next section, these features are quite sensitive to disease processes, but require regions of interest (ROIs) in excess than 1 $cm^2$ to obtain reasonable accuracy.

To obtain information about microscopic tissue changes we use a method based on the rf spectrum to estimate the average size of tissue scatterers in the 25 to 250 micron range. Such a tool could aid investigators in the basic research of identifying, in vivo, the sources of soft tissue scattering, improve the detection of early changes that often accompany the presence of disease, and provide a probe to study disease mechanisms.

The analysis uses a well-known theoretical model for power spectra of incoherent backscatter signals. (See Morse and Ingard 1968, Lizzi et al. 1987, Wagner et al. 1987a.) The interaction between acoustic pulses and tissues may be considered, to first order, as a linear system, and therefore the rf power spectrum $W(k)$ is separable and may be written as the product of the differential backscattering cross section $d\sigma$, the imaging system response $|H(k)|^2$, and an exponential attenuation factor,

$$W(k) = d\sigma \ |H(k)|^2 \ \exp(-4\alpha_o \underline{fx}), \tag{5}$$

The wave vector $\underline{k}$ is the frequency space variable conjugate to the vector position variable $\underline{x}$, and the wave number $k = |\underline{k}| = \omega/c$.

In the focal region of the tranducer, the point spread function can be separated into a transverse component due to diffraction and a range component due to the pulse:

$$h(\underline{x},k_o) = h_t(x,y,k_o) \ h_r(z,k_o). \tag{6}$$

Lizzi et al. (1983) have shown that for typical pulse-echo geometries, the autocorrelation of the tissue scatterer decorrelates at much smaller distances than that of the transverse component of h. Therefore, for this non-imaging application of estimating target sizes, i.e., for the purposes of Eq.(5), the system response in k-space may be approximated by the range component:

$$|H(k)|^2 \ \sim \ |H_r(k)|^2 \ , \tag{7}$$

where $H_r(k)$ and $h_r(z,k_o)$ are Fourier transform pairs. The system response may be estimated, for example, from the echo signal off a planar interface.

The differential backscattering cross section for the weak-scattering condition (Born approximation) may be written as the product of two factors

$$d\sigma = d\sigma_o \ \Gamma_o^2(2k) \ . \tag{8}$$

The first quantity represents the scattering strength assuming point targets, and the second quantity describes the size and shape of the scattering targets. Assuming spherical targets, the familiar Rayleigh scattering expression in the long-wavelength limit is (Morse and Ingard 1968)

$$d\sigma_o = \frac{1}{9} \ k^4 \ a_o^6 \ \bar{\gamma}_\kappa^2 \ . \tag{9}$$

The radius of the scatterer is $a_o$ and $\bar{\gamma}_\kappa$ is the average fractional change in compressibility of the scatterer relative to its surrounding material. (We have assumed that density changes make a negligible contribution to the scattering.)

The quantity $\Gamma_o(2k)$ in Eq.(8) is referred to, in various scattering experiments (e.g., see Kittel 1966), as a normalized scattering form factor. It is the ratio of the scattering amplitude of a finite-dimensional source to that scattered by a point source, and is therefore a function of the size and shape of the individual scattering targets.

$\Gamma_o^2(2k)$ is expressed mathematically as the spatial Fourier transform of the autocorrelation of the scattering process $\gamma_\kappa(\underline{x})$, or

$$\Gamma_o^2(2k) = \frac{k^4}{16\pi^2 d\sigma_o} \int d\underline{x}_1 \int d\underline{x}_2 \, \langle\gamma_\kappa(\underline{x}_1) \, \gamma_\kappa(\underline{x}_2)\rangle \, \exp(-2i\underline{k}\cdot\Delta\underline{x}) \qquad (10)$$

where $\Delta x = x_2 - x_1$. Wagner et al. (1987a) showed that for Rayleigh scattering ($ka_o \ll 1$, see Fig. 4), only the target size and not the details of the shape are important. Unfortunately, in the Rayleigh region, we expect the form factor to be relatively insensitive to changes in scattering size because, for small $ka_o$, $\Gamma_o(2k)$ is only weakly dependent on $a_o$. At the other end of the frequency spectrum, in the Mie scattering region where $ka_o > 1$, the form factor is very sensitive to changes in $a_o$, but requires precise knowledge of the scattering target shape as described by the target autocorrelation $\langle\gamma_\kappa(\underline{x}_1) \, \gamma_\kappa(\underline{x}_2)\rangle$. (Furthermore, if the scatterers are non-rigid, strong resonance peaks and minima occur in the scattering intensity as a function of $ka_o$ due to sound waves penetrating the target. The minima in Fig. 4 are not the result of resonance, but are the consequence of scattering from rigid spheres.)

To compromise between trade-offs in sensitivity to target size and the need for prior knowledge of target shape, we estimate $a_o$ in the transition zone between the Rayleigh and Mie scattering regions, i.e., where the size of the target is comparable to the wavelength of sound ($ka_o \sim 1$). This means that, for the the range of diagnostic ultrasound frequencies (1 to 10 MHz), target sizes between 25 and 250 microns may be determined in this straight-forward manner. (See Table 2.)

The first test of the theory involved four scattering phantoms with well-defined properties. The samples contained glass spheres that were randomly positioned in agar, each sample having spheres with a different average diameter. The distribution of sphere diameters was strongly peaked about the mean (Insana et al. 1986b).

The diameter of the spheres was estimated from echo signals by combining Eqs.(5) and (8), and solving for $\Gamma_o^2(2k)$, i.e.,

$$\Gamma_{meas}^2 = \frac{A \, W(k) \, e^{4\alpha_o fz}}{k^4 \, |H(k)|^2} \qquad (11)$$

where A is a normalization constant. Eq.(11) was compared with a squared

Table 2. Radiofrequency Tissue Signature

| Scattering Regime | Scatterer Size | Particle size Signature |
|---|---|---|
| Rayleigh | $ka_o \ll 1$ (small)<br>$ka_o \sim 1$ (intermediate) | None/weak<br>Form factor: size only |
| Mie | $ka_o > 1$ (large) | Form factor: size and shape |

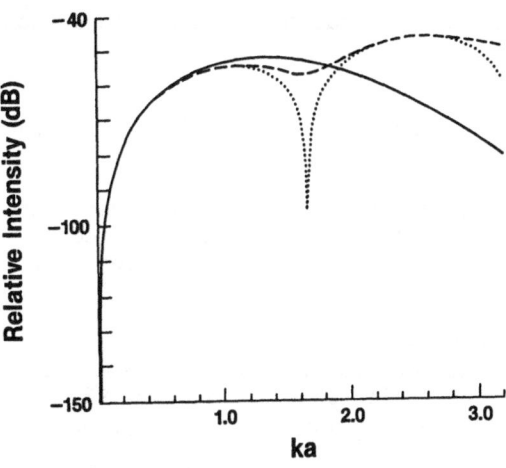

Fig. 4. Acoustic scattering functions for three theoretical models. Solid curve, $f^4$ weighted by a squared Gaussian form factor; dotted curve, $f^4$ weighted by a squared spherical form factor; and dashed curve, calculation using the exact theory of Faran (1951) for glass spheres in gelatin.

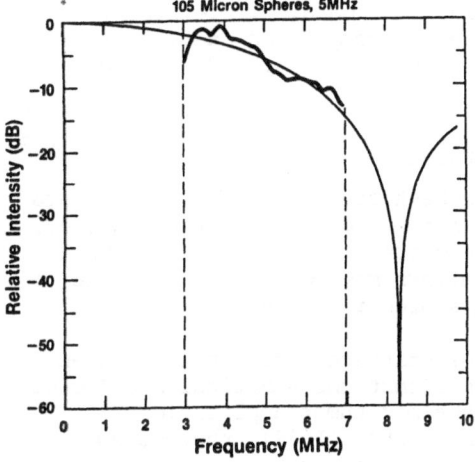

Fig. 5. Illustration of particle sizing technique using acoustic form factors. The MMSE was found between the data for 105 micron glass spheres Eq.(11) (bold line) and the spherical model Eq.(12) assuming a sphere diameter of 93 microns. A 5.0 MHz/13 mm transducer with an 8 cm focus and a −12 dB bandwidth of 4 MHz was used.

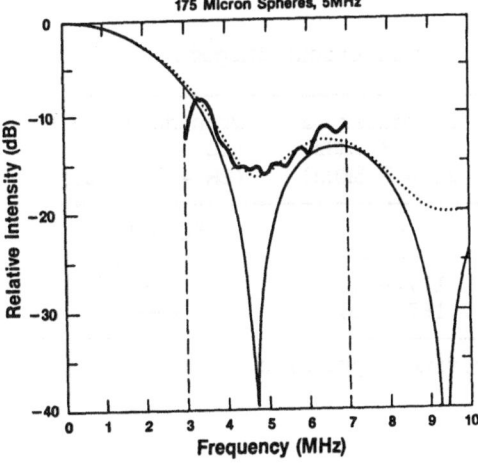

Fig. 6. Illustration of the particle sizing technique in the shorter wavelength limit ($ka_o \sim 2$). In the 3 to 7 MHz frequency range, the simple spherical model (solid line) is insufficient to represent the data (bold line) for 175 micron spheres. However, using an exact scattering expression and Eq.(13) (dotted line), we find the MMSE when we assume a sphere diameter of 165 microns. If details of the target shape and composition are known, the size may be estimated even for $ka_o > 1$.

form factor that was calculated assuming a spherical model with interaction only at the surface (rigid sphere):

$$\Gamma^2_{calc} = \left(\frac{\sin 2ka_o}{2ka_o}\right)^2 = j_o^2(2ka_o) \; , \tag{12}$$

where $j_o$ is a spherical Bessel function of the first kind, zero order. The sphere diameter, $2a_o$, was estimated by fitting Eq.(12) to the measured data, Eq.(11), for various values of $2a_o$ to find the sphere diameter that gave the minimum mean-square error (MMSE).

An example is given in Fig. 5. A sample containing 105 micron diameter spheres was scanned using a 5 MHz focused transducer with a -12dB bandwidth of 4 MHz. From the analysis, we estimated a diameter of 93 microns using a 4 cm$^2$ ROI. For the appropriate choice of frequency, estimates were generally within 15 percent of the known value. A summary of the results using three transducers and four samples is given in Table 3.

Of particular interest is the measurement of the 175 micron sample at 5 MHz, where $ka_o \sim 2$. See Fig. 6. We found that the simple spherical form factor of Eq.(12) was inadequate to explain the data. Therefore, the scattering theory of Faran (1951) was used to compute an exact differential scattering cross section for the spherical target to provide a more representative form factor, i.e.,

$$\Gamma^2_{calc} = B\,k^{-4}\,d\sigma_{Faran} \; , \tag{13}$$

where B is a normalization constant. The best fit of Eq.(13) to the data was achieved using a target diameter of 165 microns. A plot of Eq.(13), using $2a_o$ = 165 microns, is shown by the dotted curve in Fig. 6. This result demonstrates that scattering diameters may be estimated for $ka_o > 1$ if detailed knowledge of the scattering source is known.

Although the form factors for tissue scatterers have not yet been determined, Lizzi et al. (1987) have found that the spherical and Gaussian models produce consistent results in opthalmic tumor applications. However, as mentioned earlier and also by Bamber (1979), these simple models may not provide a realistic description of scattering structure in multi-structured media such as the human liver.

Table 3.  Size Measurements for Spherical Targets

| Nominal Sphere Diameter (microns) | Transducer 1 (fo = 5.0MHz) (BW = 4.0MHz) | Transducer 2 (fo = 3.1MHz) (BW = 3.5MHz) | Transducer 3 (fo = 4.1MHz) (BW = 3.4MHz) |
|---|---|---|---|
| 39 ± 2   | 34 ± 11  | ——       | 56 ± 14 |
| 75 ± 3   | 71 ± 6   | ——       | 75 ± 11 |
| 105 ± 4  | 93 ± 9   | 117 ± 12 | ——      |
| 175 ± 6  | 165*     | 167 ± 26 | ——      |

*From form factor using exact scattering expression.

446

Fig. 7 is an outline of the procedure for choosing the most discriminating features for classification, and developing decision rules that optimize the diagnostic performance of a multivariate tissue classifier. The clinical application described is the discrimination among data for normal liver tissue (36 volunteers) and two diffuse liver diseases -- chronic hepatitis (109 cases) and Gaucher's disease (68 cases) -- using four of the features described above. (Measurements of the average scatterer size and density are not included in this study.) The normal group consisted of volunteers with no evidence of disease and the condition of all patients was confirmed by biopsy. Further details on the patient histories are given by Garra et al. (1987b).

Feature Selection

Once the features are extracted from the data, the next step is to reduce the total number to include only the least correlated features with the largest object-class separability. For this we need a training set -- a set of measurements from patients with known class membership -- consisting of N-dimensional feature vectors, M total number of patient observations, and L classes, e.g., normal, disease 1 and disease 2. Each feature vector is a point on a scatter diagram as shown for 3 features, 2 classes, and 73 observations in Fig. 8. From the mean feature vector and the covariance matrix of each class, two N x N scatter matrices, $[S_w]$ and $[S_b]$ are calculated. The within-class scatter matix $[S_w]$ is the sum of all the covariance matrices weighted by the class prevalence. $[S_w]$ describes the average variation of feature vectors about the mean. $[S_b]$ is the between-class scatter matrix which describes the separation between class means.

A useful summary measure of class separability is the Hotelling trace (Gu and Lee 1984, Barrett et al. 1986), defined as

$$J = tr \left\{ [S_w]^{-1} [S_b] \right\} , \qquad (14)$$

where tr{ } is the trace of the matrix. This quantity is large when the classes are distinct and is small when the classes are similar. Features were selected to maximize the quantity J, while taking into consideration the cost of measurement and their degree of correlation.

The Hotelling trace was calculated for feature vectors consisting of permutations of the four acoustic parameters, $\bar{d}$, $r$, $\sigma'_s$ and $\alpha_o$. The results are displayed in Fig. 9. There were three clinical tasks: discrimination between (o) normal liver and livers with chronic hepatitis, (Δ) normals and Gaucher's disease, and (▼) chronic hepatitis and Gaucher's disease.

Four points are immediately apparent from Fig. 9. The first is, of the three tasks, this feature space is most sensitive to differences between normals and Gaucher's disease. Second, the importance of each feature for discrimination depends on the task. Third, the use of all four features gives the largest class separability for all three tasks. And fourth, the quantitative measurements of class separability permit a rational trade off between system performance and the cost of making additional measurements.

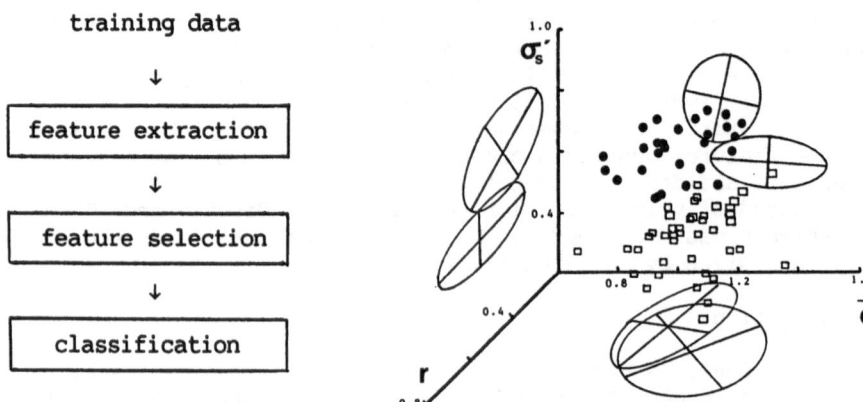

training data

↓

feature extraction

↓

feature selection

↓

classification

Fig. 7. Supervised classifier design.

Fig. 8. Scatter diagram of normal (●) and Gaucher's disease (□) liver data in three dimensions. The ellipses are projections of the data onto the measurement planes, and the major and minor axes are the first two principal components.

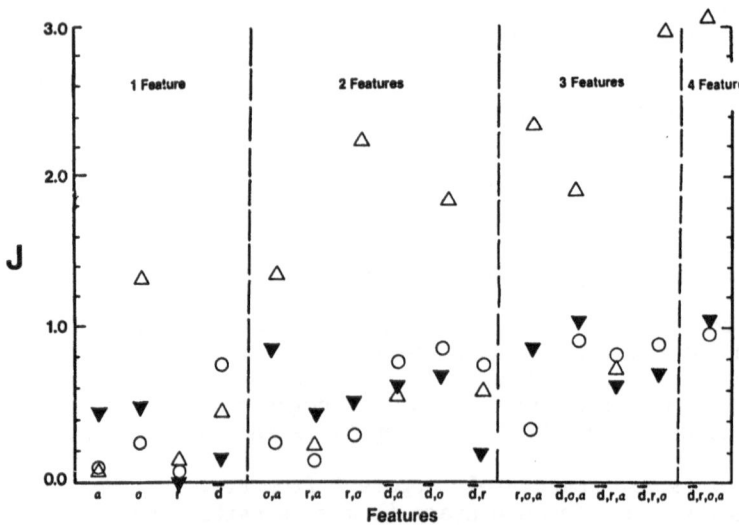

Fig. 9. Comparison of the Hotelling trace for combinations of four measurement features. Three discrimination tasks are considered: (o) normal vs chronic hepatitis, (△) normal vs Gaucher's disease, and (▼) chronic hepatitis vs Gaucher's disease. Note that $a \equiv \alpha_o$ and $\sigma \equiv \sigma'_s$.

## Linear Classifiers

A data classifier establishes decision boundaries to divide data into classes by the use of discriminant functions. The form of the discriminant function depends on the distribution of data. An example of a linear decision function is given in Fig. 10a.

Let $\underline{x}$ be a feature vector for a patient and suppose there are only two classes possible, $\omega_1$ and $\omega_2$. The Bayes classifier, which is based on the likelihood ratio test, has been shown to be the optimal decision rule, in the sense that it minimizes the expected cost or probability of error (Fukunaga, 1972). In general the Bayes classifier is quadratic, but when the covariance matices for each class are similar, the simpler linear classifier may be used. If the mean feature vector and covariance matrix of the ith class are $\overline{x}_i$ and $[S_i]$, respectively, and if $P(\omega_i)$ is the a priori probability of observing $\omega_i$, then the linear discriminant function is given by

$$\underline{m}^T \underline{x} - 0.5 \, \underline{m}^T (\overline{x}_1 + \overline{x}_2) \leq \iota' \, , \tag{15}$$

where
$$\underline{m}^T = (\overline{x}_1 - \overline{x}_2)^T [S]^{-1} \, ,$$

$$[S] = P(\omega_1) [S_1] + P(\omega_2) [S_2]$$

and
$$\iota' = \ln \{P(\omega_1)/P(\omega_2)\} \, .$$

Eq.(15) may be interpreted as follows: Use the pre-whitening matched filter $\underline{m}^T$ to weight the data $\underline{x}$ so that features with large differences in class means and small inter-class variances are emphasized. Then compare the weighted data $\underline{m}^T \underline{x}$ with the weighted balance point $0.5 \, \underline{m}^T (\overline{x}_1 + \overline{x}_2)$ and decide $\omega_1$ if the result is less than or equal to the threshold $\iota'$, otherwise decide $\omega_2$. A classifier makes a decision by detecting the sign of the discriminant function. This concept can be easily extended to more than two classes (see Fig. 10b, from Insana et al. 1987).

## Classifier Evaluation

The quality of the diagnostic decisions made using the linear classifier described above was evaluated using ROC (Receiver Operating Characteristic) analysis (Metz 1986). With ROC analysis, the performance of alternative diagnostic methods can be compared directly, including comparisons with human observers.

The ROC curves in Fig. 11 show that our quantitative methods provide excellent discrimination for the three clinical tasks studied. The true positive fraction (TPF) and false positive fraction (FPF) pairs were calculated for a range of discriminant function thresholds by varying the right side of Eq.(15). The curves are plotted on normal probability scales and the error bars indicate one standard deviation. The area under the ROC curve, as measured on a linear scale, is $A_z^*$, which can be related to the Hotelling trace criterion (Fiete et al. 1987, Insana et al. 1986). The range of this commonly used summary measure of performance is 0.5 (no discrimination) to 1.0 (perfect discrimination). (To orient the reader

---

[*] $A_z$ values and error bars for the ROC curves were calculated using the programs ROCFIT and INDROC written by Charles E. Metz and colleagues at the University of Chicago (Metz and Kronman 1980).

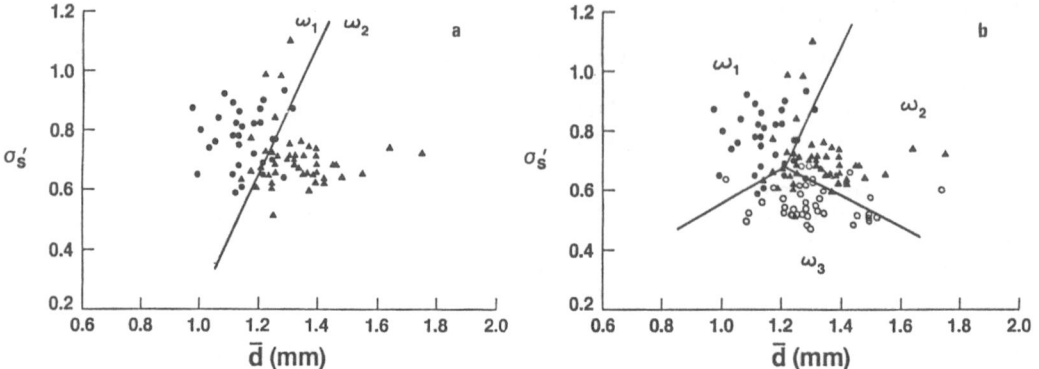

Fig. 10. Linear (a) and piecewise linear (b) discriminant functions for separating normal liver data (●) from chronic hepatitis (▲) and Gaucher's disease (o). The thresholds have been set equal to $\iota' = 0$.

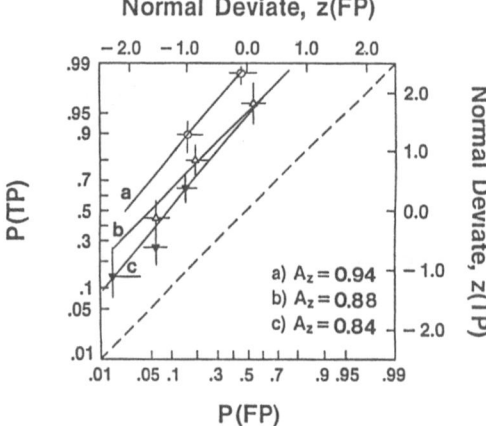

Fig. 11. ROC curves for the task of discriminating normals from Gaucher's disease (a), normals from hepatitis (b), and hepatitis from Gaucher's disease (c). Four features were used and the error bars denote one standard deviation.

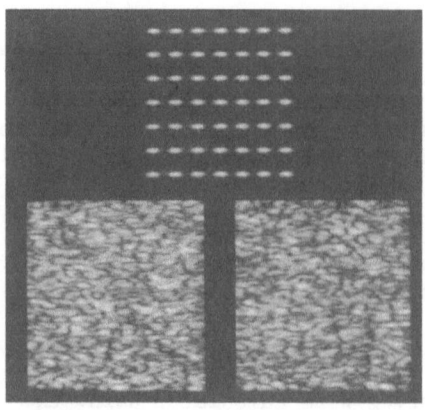

Fig. 12. The two speckle fields are an example of image pairs used in a 2AFC experiment. The goal of the experiment was to measure the efficiency of human observers at detecting a lattice structure. The lower right image is an example of Rayleigh statistics (no structure) while the lower left image is an example of modified Rician statistics; i.e., it contains a low-contrast copy of the lattice in the upper image.

unfamiliar with ROC analysis, the following examples from the literature are given for comparison. Swets et al. (1979) reported average $A_z$ values for detection of brain lesions using CT and radionuclide imaging as 0.97 and 0.87, respectively. Bacus et al. (1984) reported an average $A_z$ value of 0.87 for the detection of cervical carcinoma using the PAP smear.)

## HUMAN OBSERVER EFFICIENCIES

We studied the relative efficiency of human observers at the task of detecting the subtle changes in speckled images often found in clinical practice. Depending on the detection efficiency of human observers, signal processing methods may offer new opportunities for diagnostic information.

Burgess et al. (1981) found that the human eye-brain system is very efficient at extracting first-order information for well-specified tasks. Given the task of detecting sinusoids in additive Gaussian white noise fields, they measured statistical efficiencies as high as $0.83 \pm 0.15$.

In ultrasonic imaging, the noise (speckle) is multiplicative, Rician, and correlated. Smith et al. (1983) have derived the detectability of low contrast lesions in speckled fields, and have shown (Wagner et al. 1987b), along with Trahey (1985), the utility of spatial and frequency compounding techniques for increasing detectability. In compounding, independent images are incoherently summed to produce an increase in the area-wise SNR, and hence detectability, for first-order tasks. However, as discussed above, ultrasonic speckle often carries diagnostic information at the level of second-order statistics. Therefore it is of interest to determine the human observer's efficiency for extracting this information relative to the ability of the signal processing algorithm to extract the same information.

## Detecting Regular Structures in Speckled Images: Simulation

The first example involves estimating the efficiency of human observers for detecting a two-dimensional lattice structure embedded in a computer-generated speckle field -- a task similar to reading liver and spleen scans. In a two-alternative forced-choice (2AFC) experiment, observers were presented with a pair of images and asked to choose the field that contained the lattice. Hundreds of image pairs such as those in Fig. 12 were presented. For the same images, we also calculated the second-order feature $\sigma_s^2$, described above. This quantity was chosen as the decision function for the machine because it is the most discriminating, giving the larger value for the field containing the lattice. Care was taken to ensure that no reliable first-order differences between the two alternatives were provided to the human observers.

The percent correct for the human and machine observers was converted into detectability d' (Elliot 1964), and the efficiency of visual detection relative to the machine was calculated using

$$\eta = (d'_{human}/d'_{machine})^2 . \tag{16}$$

The efficiencies of five observers are given in Table 4, for the observation time of 2 seconds, and for one observer $\eta$ is plotted as a function of observation time in Fig. 13.

Table 4.
Observer efficiencies
(2 sec observation time)

| Observer | η |
|----------|------|
| 1 | 0.56 |
| 2 | 0.24 |
| 3 | 0.15 |
| 4 | 0.12 |
| 5 | 0.07 |

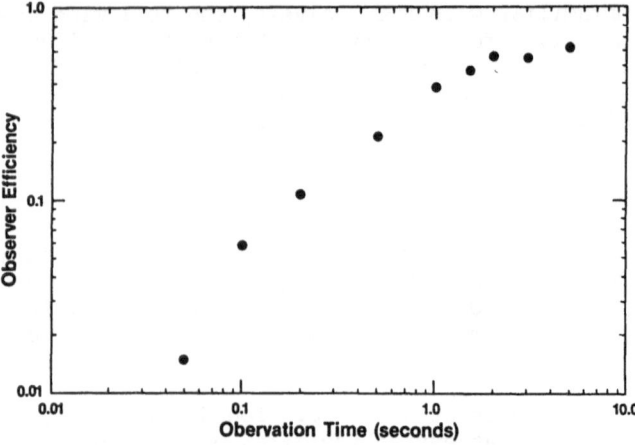

Fig. 13. The efficiency of observer 1 for detecting a regular lattice structure in a speckle field vs the time of observation.

For regular lattice structure, the efficiency of detection was found to increase with observation time up to approximately 2 seconds, where for that one observer the greatest value was approximately 0.6. However, performance strongly depended on the observer as seen in Table 4, and, we expect, will decrease with increasing perturbations in the lattice structure. In addition clinical observers, in our experience, tend to be conservative in their reading, being more likely to call a difficult case negative then positive. This tendency could have the effect of further reducing observer efficiency in clinical situations. We conclude therefore that, although performance varies with the conditions and the observer, humans have demonstrated significantly poorer performance than the signal processing algorithms for this second-order detection task.

### Tissue Differentiation from Image Texture: Clinical Results

One clinical imaging example of a second-order detection task is the grading of subtle changes in image texture needed to detect isoechoic focal lesions. A second example, which we have focused on, is the detection of a diffuse disease process. We asked four trained clinical observers to detect diffuse liver disease by reading, from film, 30 liver/spleen exams from each of the three groups: normals, chronic hepatitis, and Gaucher's patients. Presented two groups at a time (60 exams), the observer was asked to decide, on a 5-point rating or confidence scale, if the patient belonged to group 1 or group 2. The exams were viewed in two ways. In one study, the entire set of films were presented (typically 6 films including kidney and spleen images). A second study limited the presentation to three liver images displaying essentially second-order textural information (Garra et al. 1987b). The exams were taken from the same volunteer and patient populations described above.

ROC curves for the human observers were averaged and compared with the machine "observer" in Fig. 14 for the task of discriminating between normals and chronic hepatitis. The indices $A_z$ for all the tasks considered are summarized in Table 5 along with the corresponding efficiencies.

Efficiencies were calculated using Eq.(16), assuming d' ~ $\sqrt{2}$ z(A).
The quantity z(A) is the perpendicular distance from the origin (z(TPF) =
z(FPF) = 0) to the ROC curve when it is plotted on normal-deviate axes
(Swets and Pickett 1982). The above relationship between d' and z(A) is
exact when the ROC curves have unit slope.

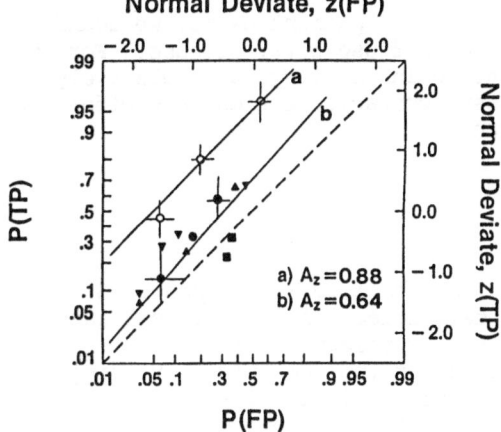

Fig. 14. ROC curves for the
detection of chronic hepatitis
using ultrasound. Curve (a)
summarizes the machine performance
for four features using linear
discriminant analysis. Curve (b)
is the average performance of
four trained clinicians.

When limited to textural information, the efficiency of clinical
observers relative to the tissue characterization algorithms was very low.
Given the entire exam, the efficiencies were also low for detecting
hepatitis, but increased to order 1 for detecting Gaucher's disease. This
high detection efficiency is probably due to the obvious cue of increased
liver size for Gaucher's patients. Overall liver size is a reliable visual
cue that was not a part of the feature space.

Table 5. Performance Comparison for Machine and Human "Observers"

| Task | Binormal ROC Area, $A_z$ | | | Detection Efficiency, $\eta$ | |
| | Machine | Humans | | Human/Machine | |
| | 4 Classification Features | All Images | Texture Only | All Images | Texture Only |
|---|---|---|---|---|---|
| Normal vs. Chronic Hepatitis | 0.88+0.03 | 0.64+0.08 | 0.53+0.08 | 0.09 | 0.01 |
| Normal vs. Gaucher's Disease | 0.94+0.03 | 0.92+0.04 | 0.67+0.08 | 0.77 | 0.10 |
| Gaucher's vs. Chronic Hepatitis | 0.84+0.04 | 0.87+0.05 | 0.71+0.07 | 1.19 | 0.32 |

# CONCLUSIONS

Acoustic signals contain a considerable amount of diagnostic tissue information that is not always visually apparent from the B—scan image. A description of the macroscopic tissue structure is most easily obtained from signal processing using the intensity spectrum, while information about the composition and microscopic structure may be obtained from the rf spectrum. In all, six physically—based features form our basis set for tissue classification.

Using just four features and more than 200 patient exams, we found excellent performance for the detection of diffuse liver disease. For the same detection tasks, we also found that human observers are relatively inefficient. Therefore, ultrasonic tissue characterization does offer new opportunities for diagnostic information.

# REFERENCES

Bacus, J.W., Wiley, E.L., Galbraith, W., Marshall, P.N., Wilbanks, G.D. and Weinstein, R.S. (1984). Malignant cell detection and cervical cancer screening, Analytical and Quantitative Cytology, 6, 125.

Bamber, J.C. (1979). Theoretical modelling of the acoustic scattering structure of human liver, Acoustic Letters, 3, 114–119.

Barrett, H.H., Myers, K.J. and Wagner, R.F. (1986). Beyond signal-detection theory, in: Proc. of the SPIE, R.H. Schneider and S.J. Dwyer III, eds., 626, 231–239.

Elliott, P.B. (1964). Tables of d', in: Signal Detection and Recognition by Human Observers, John A. Swets, ed., John Wiley and Sons, New York.

Faran, J.J. (1951). Sound scattering by solid cylinders and spheres, J. Acoust. Soc. Am., 23, 405–418.

Fellingham, L.L. and Sommer, F.G. (1984). Ultrasonic characterization of tissue structure in the in vivo human liver and spleen, IEEE Trans. Sonics Ultrason., SU–31, 418–428.

Fiete, R.D., Barrett, H.H., Smith W.E., and Myers, K.J. (1987). Hotelling trace criterion and its correlation with human—observer performance, J. Opt. Soc. Am. A, 4, 945–953.

Fukunaga, K. (1972). Introduction to Statistical Pattern Recognition, Academic Press, New York.

Garra, B.S., Insana, M.F., Shawker, T.H., and Russell, M.A. (1987a). Quantitative estimation of liver attenuation and echogenicity: Normal state versus diffuse disease, Radiology, 162, 61–67.

Garra, B.S., Insana, M.F., Shawker, T.A., Wagner, R.F., Bradford, M., Russell, M.A. (1987b). Quantitative US detection and classification of liver and spleen disease: Comparison with human observer performance, Radiology (submitted).

Goodman, J.W. (1985). Statistical Optics, John Wiley and Sons, New York.

Gu, Z.H. and Lee, S.H. (1984). Optical implementation of the Hotelling trace criterion for image classification, Opt. Eng., 23, 727–731.

Insana, M.F., Wagner, R.F., Garra, B.S., Brown, D.G., and Shawker, T.H. (1986a). Analysis of ultrasound image texture via generalized Rician statistics, Opt. Eng., 25, 743–748.

Insana, M.F., Madsen, E.L., Hall, T.J., and Zagzebski, J.A. (1986b). Tests of the accuracy of a data reduction method for determination of acoustic backscatter coefficients, J. Acoust. Soc. Am., 79, 1230–1236.

Insana, M.F., Wagner, R.F., Garra, B.S., Momenan, R., and Shawker, T.H. (1986c). Pattern recognition methods for optimizing multivariate tissue signatures in diagnostic ultrasound, Ultrasonic Imaging, 8, 165–180.

Insana, M.F., Wagner, R.F., Garra, B.S., Momenan, R., and Shawker, T.H. (1987). Supervised pattern recognition techniques in quantitative diagnostic ultrasound, in: Proc. of the SPIE, R.H. Schneider and S. J. Dwyer III, eds., 768, (in press).

Jakeman, E. (1984). Speckle statistics with a small number of scatterers, Opt. Eng., 23, 453–461.

Julesz, B. (1981). Textons, the elements of texture perception, and their interactions, Nature, 290, 91–97.

Kittel, C. (1966). Introduction to Solid State Physics, John Wiley and Sons, New York.

Lizzi, F.L., Greenebaum, M., Feleppa, E.J., and Elbaum, M. (1983). Theoretical framework for spectrum analysis in ultrasonic tissue characterization, J. Acoust. Soc. Am., 73, 1366–1373.

Lizzi, F.L., Ostromogilsky, M., Feleppa, E.J., Rorke, M.C. and Yaremko M.M. (1987). Relationship of ultrasonic spectral parameters to features of tissue microstructure, IEEE Trans. Ultrason. Ferro. Freq. Control, UFFC-33, 319–329.

Madsen, E.L., Insana, M.F., and Zagzebski, J.A. (1984). Method of data reduction for accurate determination of acoustic backscatter coefficients, J. Acoust. Soc. Am., 76, 913–923.

Metz, C.E. and Kronman, H.B. (1980). A test for the statistical significance of differences between ROC curves, in: Information Processing in Medical Imaging, R. DiPaola and E. Kahn, eds., Paris.

Metz, C.E. (1986). ROC methodology in radiological imaging, Invest. Radiol., 21, 720–733.

Middleton, D. (1960). An Introduction to Statistical Communication Theory, McGraw-Hill, New York.

Morse, P.M. and Ingard, K.U. (1968). Theoretical Acoustics, McGraw-Hill, New York.

Schlaps, D., Raeth, U., Volk, J.F., Zuna, I., Lorenz, A., Lehmann, K., Lorenz, D., Van Kaick, G., and Lorenz, W.J. (1986). Ultrasonic tissue characterization using a diagnostic expert system, in: Information Processing in Medical Imaging, S.L. Bacharach, ed., Martinus Nijhoff Publ., Dordrecht.

Smith, S.W., Wagner, R.F., Sandrik, J.M. and Lopez, H. (1983). Low contrast detectability and contrast/detail analysis in medical ultrasound, IEEE Trans. Sonics Ultrason., SU-30, 164–173.

Swets, J.A. (1979). ROC analysis applied to the evaluation of medical imaging techniques, Invest. Radiol., 14, 109–121.

Swets, J.A. and Pickett, R.M. (1982). Evaluation of Diagnostic Systems: Methods from Signal Detection Theory, Academic Press, New York.

Taylor, K.J.W., Riely, C.A., Hammers, L., Flax, S., Weltin, G., Garcia-Tsao, G., Conn, H.O., Kuc, R. and Barwick, K.W. (1986). Quantitative US attenuation in normal liver and in patients with diffuse liver disease: Importance of fat, Radiology, 160, 65–71.

Trahey, G.E. (1985). Speckle reduction in ultrasonic B-mode images via spatial compounding, Ph.D. Thesis, Duke University, Durham, NC.

Wagner, R.F., Insana, M.F. and Brown, D.G. (1986). Unified approach to the detection and classification of speckle texture in diagnostic ultrasound, Opt. Eng., 25, 738–742.

Wagner, R.F., Insana, M.F. and Brown, D.G. (1987a). Statistical properties of the radiofrequency and envelope-detected signals with applications to medical ultrasound, J. Opt. Soc. Am. A, 4, 910–922.

Wagner, R.F., Insana, M.F. and Smith, S.W. (1987b). Fundamental correlation lengths of coherent speckle in medical ultrasonic images, IEEE Trans. Ultrason. Ferro. Freq. Control, (in press).

# LEFT VENTRICULAR MOTION AND SHAPE ANALYSIS

# USING MULTIPLE IMAGING MODALITIES

James S. Duncan[†,*] and Lawrence H. Staib[*]

Departments of [†]Diagnostic Radiology and [*]Electrical Engineering
Division of Imaging Science
Yale University, New Haven, CT 06510

## ABSTRACT

An image understanding system is discussed that will analyze cardiac dysfunction found by combining information from multiple, noninvasive imaging modality studies. The system is a model for intelligent multimodality image understanding in general, but is applied to a very specific problem: detection and rating of left ventricular (LV) aneurysms. Key features of the system are: 1) its ability to handle and quantify uncertain or partial image-derived information in a concise way using probabilistic evidential reasoning, 2) its ability to fuse pertinent relative information from independent diagnostic images of the same patient to achieve an algorithm-assembled, consensus, quantitative opinion of cardiac shape and motion, and finally 3) to arrive at a decision level set of numbers that quantify and localize left ventricular aneurysm formation for each patient. The availability of data such as described in 3) will enable more precise prognostic or diagnostic risk classification for patients, making therapy alternatives more rational. Because of the subjective probabilistic reasoning strategy (based on the principle of maximum entropy) the final quantitative results will carry not only the system's assessment of a particular patient's heart, but also the degree of confidence that the automated analysis system has in the result it presents. This confidence is increased when similar LV motion and shape is perceived by the multiple imaging modalities.

## INTRODUCTION

Widespread use of equilibrium radionuclide angiography (RNA) and two-dimensional echocardiography (2DE) for evaluating cardiac problems has centered primarily on the qualitative (i.e. a cardiologist's or a radiologist's visual impression) or semi-quantitative gross analysis of global and regional motion and shape events. Each modality has its own advantages and disadvantages in this regard, as is true in all areas of diagnostic imaging. RNA yields a sequence of volumetric projection images, which are very good for computing volumetric parameters such as global and regional left ventricular (LV) ejection fraction. However, the images are of very low spatial resolution making it difficult to outline certain anatomical regions in views needed to compute these parameters. In addition, the projection image obscures certain structures from being fully viewed (e.g. the anterior wall of the left ventricle in the left lateral view). 2DE is a tomographic rather than a projection image, which is poor for volumetric computations, but gives a clearer picture of the endocardial boundary in a particular image plane. Also, whereas RNA defines only the extent of the radiolabeled blood pool within a chamber, 2DE can look at the inner and outer walls of a chamber, enabling measurement of wall thickness (e.g. LV hypertrophy) or combine the measurement of the epicardial and endocardial outlines into a single wall thickening measure. The 2DE image frames are higher in spatial resolution than the RNA frames, but often don't give as complete an impression of the heart, or in particular, the left ventricle, due to the signal dropout in certain regions (especially the apex) and/or the fact that certain anatomical structures cannot be specifically defined (e.g. papillary muscle merging with the inferior LV wall). Also, many adult patients cannot be fully examined by 2DE due to air in the lung that obscures the acoustic window to the heart.

In an effort to maximize information derivable from these noninvasive imaging techniques, it is tempting to try to take the most useful information from each technique and combine it in some optimum way for analysis. Recently, a whole subfield (Marion, 1983), termed PACS, for Picture Archiving and Communication Systems, has developed within diagnostic imaging, aimed at providing the computer networking technology to allow multimodal imaging studies to be moved to single viewing stations. However, without a quantitative approach to some integrated form of analysis, it is not clear how optimally this information will be used. The ability of a human observer to effectively integrate information from two images is limited. The observer tends to study a single modality's image at a time, rather than perform any true simultaneous analysis. This is further limited in cardiac diagnosis by the observer's severe difficulty with tracking two moving regions simultaneously, a near-impossible human perceptual task.

## OVERVIEW

### Multisensor Quantitative Image Analysis

The work discussed here is aimed at more fully integrating multimodal image information using mathematical image understanding and analysis techniques. The automated approach will merge relevant quantitative parameters gathered from two modalities in a way that will yield a higher level consensus result. The objective reasoning strategy proposed here embodies several advantages over qualitative or semi-quantitative human image analysis. Primarily, more factors or types of information, i.e. the multiple modalities, can be considered simultaneously, and the weighting of these can be controlled in a quantifiable and reproducible manner.

The integration of meaningful information from multisensor data is a rather difficult problem which is of current interest not only in medicine, but in other fields as well, including robotics and aerospace. Several approaches have been proposed, ranging from integrated approaches to region segmentation at the conceptually lower levels of image understanding to the use of scene descriptions formed by separately processing each sensor's images to generate high level hypotheses about simple geometric shapes (Belknap et al., 1986). The data fusion work that will be discussed here will separately process low level information from two modalities, compare combined forms of this information at higher levels of processing, and iteratively modify the system's probabilistic confidence in the low level information in order to seek a consensus opinion about the underlying scene.

### Application to Cardiac Problems

Although the proposed system will be a general approach and model for multimodality cardiac image analysis, this paper will address a very specific cardiac problem as an initial testbed, namely left ventricular aneurysm formation. It was important that this initial application of the system be such that multimodality-derived information is both obtainable and is qualitatively determined a priori to be advantageous as compared to similar information derived from any one of the individual modalities. The derivation of information necessary to rate LV aneurysm formation from RNA and 2DE image sequences meets these requirements. RNA and 2DE scans are both often routinely performed on many cardiac patients, providing a readily available test data base. In addition, some qualitative/semi-quantitative work which has previously been published points to improved LV aneurysm detection when combining independent RNA and 2DE assessments (Sorenson et al., 1982).

However, the anatomical and physiological characteristics of left ventricular aneurysms are not well enough defined by noninvasive techniques to warrant accurate qualitative analysis. Historically, the commonly accepted cardinal manifestation of aneurysm, i.e. regional motion dysfunction as analyzed by using RNA or 2DE, cannot alone discriminate the severity of an aneurysm using qualitative visual analysis. Meizlish et al.(1984) showed that qualitative evaluation of end diastolic shape may help in this regard, but it is difficult to separate patients into more than a few categories using this technique (and even this may be difficult for certain patients). Recent work done comparing regional qualitative analysis of postmortem hearts with regional qualitative RNA wall motion analysis showed excellent correlation in regions of normal tissue and in regions with severe (transmural) infarcts. However, poorer agreement was seen in areas that were less clearly defined, i.e. focal infarcts as defined by pathological measurements and hypokinetic motion as read by RNA (Cabin et al., 1984). It is in these areas that quantitative techniques can potentially provide more reliable stratification of the diagnostic and prognostic status of a specific patient.

Thus, the analysis system described in this paper is aimed at deriving quantitative low level information from RNA and 2DE image sequences from a single patient, and combining the information in a profitable manner to form a consensus opinion of left ventricular regional wall motion and end diastolic shape (end systolic shape is not used since it is perceived to be directly dependent on end diastolic shape and wall motion). This consensus quantitative information is intended for use in stratifying patients with regard to degree of aneurysm formation.

The common reference from which intermodality information will be compared and combined is through geometric information derived from comparable views of the heart in each modality. The end diastolic to end systolic regional wall motion and the regional end diastolic shape of the left ventricular (LV) silhouette in the optimal lateral RNA view and the apical long axis 2DE view are the geometrically-derived properties chosen for comparison in the proposed system.

## Consideration of Uncertainty

The probabilistic reasoning methodology is included in order to allow the system to consider the inherent uncertainty associated with comparing medical images. For instance, at the lowest level, image-derived quantitative evidence of anatomical and physiological events that are often only either partial or obscured can only be known to some degree of confidence. For the multimodality problem at hand, a priori perceived angulation differences (which may initially have to be inserted manually) may be indicated by lower prior probabilistic confidence. In either case, this uncertainty is propagated to the high levels of the system and included in the system's own confidence rating of it's combined output. A multi-modality consensus motion and shape analysis with less than maximum confidence may still be better than results stemming from a single modality's result in certain LV border regions or no result at all (due to obscured segments, for instance).

Recent developments in the research areas of Artificial Intelligence and Image Understanding address the difficult problem of handling uncertainty using various techniques, many of which appear quite mathematically informal. Examples of these are the confidence factors used in MYCIN (an "expert" system for medical diagnosis), fuzzy set theory (which has been previously applied to cardiac analysis by Niemann et al. (1985) ) and the Dempster-Shafer theory (see Cheeseman (1985) for these references). The use of non-rigorous techniques precludes the use of years of mathematical knowledge dealing with problems that arise while trying to appropriately consider uncertainty. A specific example of this is the treatment of dependent evi-

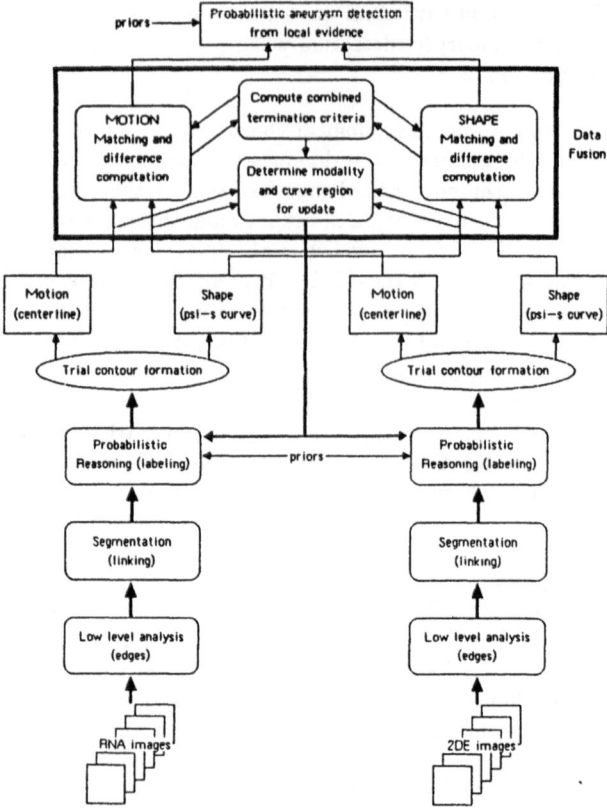

Figure 1: System Block Diagram

dence in decision-making. The work proposed here will incorporate an approach to dealing with uncertainty based on the mathematics and statistics principle of maximum entropy or least commitment. This technique is firmly based in formal statistics concepts, stemming from Bayesian statistical theory, and was first applied to information theory by Jaynes (1957). It yields the most unbiased subjective probability estimate given the available constraining evidence. The use of a modified version of this approach here is attractive for considering uncertainty at two levels, first making initial anatomical assignments to grouped low level information (i.e. edge segments) and secondly combining information from various segments to provide a consistent contextual result for a group of segments.

## SYSTEM DESCRIPTION

The system block diagram is shown in figure 1. This represents a complete strategy for integrated, geometrically-based multimodality left ventricular image analysis. Note that at the low and intermediate levels of the system, identical processing operations are performed on each modalities' images. As can be seen, an important feature of this system is the presence of a feedback loop between the upper and lower levels of the system. This feedback is intended to drive the analysis toward obtaining a consensus interpretation of LV motion and shape from multiple modalities. Each of the system modules is described in more detail below, with emphasis placed on the approach to reasoning from uncertainty. This part of the system has received the bulk of the attention in the initial development, since much of the remainder of the processing depends on how partial and uncertain information is handled.

## Low Level Analysis: Edge Finding

At the lowest level of the system, image feature information will be extracted from RNA and 2DE images using local neighborhood gradient convolution operators to find magnitudes and directions of gray level gradients in the image. The decision to use this type of operator was made in conjunction with the overall planned approach to boundary finding (discussed below) and after considering several alternatives (e.g. Gerbrands et al., 1982, Geiser and Oliver, 1984). The details of this approach are described in Duncan (1984). Briefly, the strength of discontinuities are found in two orthogonal directions and from this information, the magnitude and direction of each edge vector is easily computed. Depending on the size of the convolution operators (typically 3x3 or 5x5), several edge vectors may be produced across a given edge region. In the context of this system it is worthwhile to "thin" the vectors in a region down to a single maximum edge vector for the eventual purpose of boundary tracking. This thinning process is the same that is used in Duncan (1984). The results of running the edge finding and thinning operations on an example left lateral view RNA study is shown in the upper 2 images of figure 3.

## Segmentation: Grouping Into Partial Boundary Segments

Second level algorithms are aimed at grouping or linking homogenous lower level information so that these groupings may be symbolically and quantitatively described in preparation for the higher level reasoning strategies. An edge linking approach used in earlier work (Duncan, 1984) was modified and used here to obtain and describe the curve segments. The algorithm's basic operation relies on a stack data structure, which pushes candidate edge vectors onto the stack until either an end point (no linkable surrounding vectors) or a branch point occurs. The edge vector linking criteria include the following: similar orientation, closeness of spatial location, and closeness of surrounding gray level values. Segments are marked as "fathers" or "sons" of other segments in an indexed hierarchy, and branching can go on indefinitely. Somewhat relaxing a strict spatial adjacency criteria allows for possible branches to also be included in the final tree. The output list data structure was tailored specifically to provide the appropriate information for the reasoning system described in the next section. The primary information passed from the intermediate level to higher level logic and analysis, consists of lists of linked edge segments with associated attributes (such as: location, adjacent segments, number of branches, directions and positions of vectors that form segment).

The linked lists of edge points are thus assumed to contain all of the evidence regarding the presence or absence of an endocardial left ventricular boundary that can be found from the particular image frame from a particular modality. Thus any higher level decisions about left ventricular motion or shape will be made primarily considering this partial boundary evidence.

## Probabilistic Reasoning Using A Maximum Entropy Approach

The degree of confidence in the partial and uncertain image-derived information is tracked with subjective probabilities using the principle of maximum entropy. Maximum entropy has been considered as a means of tracking probabilistic evidence by Cheeseman (1983). It has the advantage of not requiring the assumption of independent evidence, as does traditional Bayesian updating and Dempster-Shafer theory (Cheeseman, 1985). The maximum entropy method calculates the most conservative estimate of the probabilities given constraints on the probability space, or event group, taken from the model and the data. Here, we will use it to solve the problem of labeling the edge segments according to our model for the left ventricle ("Probabilistic Reasoning" in figure 1).

For each modality, each piece of segmental evidence is considered first separately and then together with other segments to determine the likelihood of it being labeled as a part of the left ventricular boundary, according to an initial model of what the regions of a left

461

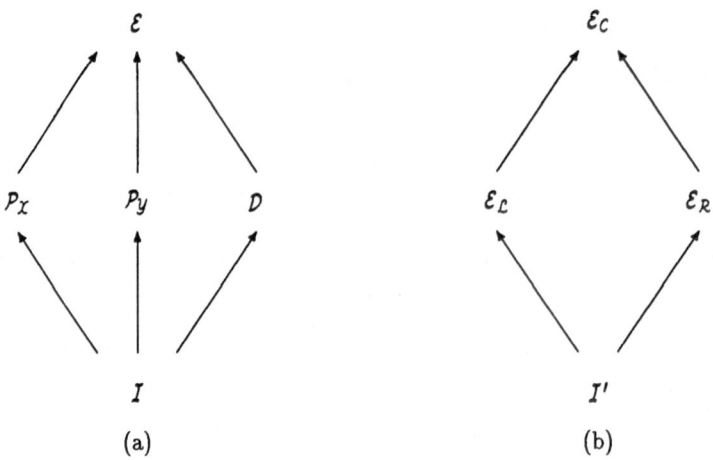

Figure 2: Local event groups for labeling

ventricular boundary should look like. Because of the range of shapes and sizes in both normal and abnormal hearts, the creation of this model is a difficult task. The constraints derived from this model constitute the system's prior bias on the analysis. The desirable neutral prior of an ideal "normal" heart is chosen, and is created by incorporating the statistical distributions of a range of ideal normal patient's left ventricular boundary data into discrete mathematical constraints with regards to the direction and relative position of anatomical regions that make up the heart. In addition to relative direction and position, priors will be built into the system which contain biases regarding known angulation differences between views.

The distribution of probabilistic confidence to the different labeling possibilities for each edge segment is done in two stages. This separation of stages is done in order to limit the size of the event groups and thus the corresponding computational burden. In order to update the labeling probabilities of an edge segment based on new information, the principle of maximum entropy is applied, in conjunction with the constraints arising from the data and the model, to the event group corresponding to the edge under consideration. At the first stage, shown in figure 2(a), the event group consists of the following events: $\mathcal{E}$ is the edge segment to be updated, $P_x$ is the x-position of the segment, $P_y$ is the y-position of the segment, $D$ is the direction of the segment, $I$ is the node representing the presence of the image derived information $P_x$, $P_y$ and $D$. This event group forms an initial estimate of the probabilities based only on the low level information.

The second stage, shown in figure 2(b), is formed to incorporate contextual information into the label probabilities for each edge segment by including the edge segments nearest to the edge in question. Thus, the events in the group are: $\mathcal{E}_C$ is the edge segment to be updated, $\mathcal{E}_L, \mathcal{E}_R$ are neighboring segments, $I'$ is the node representing the presence of the image derived information used for $\mathcal{E}_L$ and $\mathcal{E}_R$.

We will now follow the mathematics for the second stage in detail. The first stage is solved in a corresponding way using the same methodology. $\mathcal{E}_C, \mathcal{E}_L$ and $\mathcal{E}_R$ have possible values ranging over the number of segments in the object model (i.e. $O_1 =$ apex, $O_2 =$ posterior, ...). We also include a noise segment in the object model to account for segments which do not belong to the actual LV boundary. $I'$ is either true or false (i.e. 1 or 0). This defines the events in our probability space, designated $P_{i,j,k,l}$. We now constrain certain marginal and conditional probabilities defined on the space, all of which are expressable as partial sums. First, the probability space must be normalized by making the probability of the certain event equal to 1:

$$P(\mathcal{S}) = 1 \qquad \text{or} \qquad \sum_{i,j,k,l} P_{i,j,k,l} = 1$$

The labeling probabilities for edge segment $\mathcal{E}_C$ derived from low level information are known from the first stage, and thus impose a constraint on the space:

$$P(\mathcal{E}_C = O_i) = A_i \qquad \text{or} \qquad \sum_{j,k,l} P_{i,j,k,l} = A_i$$

The labeling probabilities for edge segments $\mathcal{E}_L$ and $\mathcal{E}_R$ derived from low level information are also known from the first stage. These are conditioned off $I'$ to allow for the updating of $\mathcal{E}_C$ based on this information.

$$P(\mathcal{E}_L = O_j | I' = 1) = B_j \qquad \text{or} \qquad \frac{\sum_{i,k} P_{i,j,k,1}}{\sum_{i,j,k} P_{i,j,k,1}} = B_j$$

$$P(\mathcal{E}_R = O_k | I' = 1) = C_k \qquad \text{or} \qquad \frac{\sum_{i,j} P_{i,j,k,1}}{\sum_{i,j,k} P_{i,j,k,1}} = C_k$$

The likelihood of particular adjacencies of segments as imposed by the model further constrains the space.

$$P(\mathcal{E}_C = O_i | \mathcal{E}_L = O_j) = D_{i,j} \qquad \text{or} \qquad \frac{\sum_{k,l} P_{i,j,k,l}}{\sum_{i,k,l} P_{i,j,k,l}} = D_{i,j}$$

$$P(\mathcal{E}_C = O_i | \mathcal{E}_R = O_k) = E_{i,k} \qquad \text{or} \qquad \frac{\sum_{j,l} P_{i,j,k,l}}{\sum_{i,j,l} P_{i,j,k,l}} = E_{i,k}$$

In order to determine the most conservative values for the probability space consistent with the constraints, we must maximize the entropy, $H$, over the possible $P_{i,j,k,l}$ values where:

$$H = - \sum_{i,j,k,l} P_{i,j,k,l} \log P_{i,j,k,l}$$

This constrained optimization can be solved using Lagrange multipliers by first forming the function $H'$ that incorporates the constraints as follows:

$$H' = H + \sum_{i=1}^{m} \lambda_i \phi_i$$

where the $\phi$'s are the constraints written to equal zero and the $\lambda$'s are constants to be determined, along with the values of $P_{i,j,k,l}$ at the extreme point. The derivative of $H'$ with respect to each $P_{i,j,k,l}$ is set to zero. This set of equations, along with the original constraints, is solved, thus determining the probability space. In our case, $H'$ will have the form (showing only the first few terms):

$$H' = -\sum_{i,j,k,l} P_{i,j,k,l} \log P_{i,j,k,l} + \lambda \left(1 - \sum_{i,j,k,l} P_{i,j,k,l}\right) +$$

$$\lambda_{a2} \left(\sum_{j,k,l} P_{i,j,k,l} - A_2\right) + \lambda_{b4} \left(B_4 \sum_{i,j,k} P_{i,j,k,1} - \sum_{i,k} P_{i,4,k,1}\right) + \cdots$$

The derivative equations will have different terms, depending on the index of $P$, as shown.

$$0 = \frac{\partial H'}{\partial P_{w,x,y,z}} = -\log P_{w,x,y,z} - 1 - \lambda + \underbrace{\lambda_{a2}}_{\text{if } w=2} + \underbrace{\lambda_{b4} B_4}_{\text{if } z=1} - \underbrace{\lambda_{b4}}_{\text{if } z=1 \text{ and } x=4} + \cdots$$

This gives:

$$P_{w,x,y,z} = \exp\left(1 + \lambda - \underbrace{\lambda_{a2}}_{\text{if } w=2} - \underbrace{\lambda_{b4} B_4}_{\text{if } z=1} + \underbrace{\lambda_{b4}}_{\text{if } z=1 \text{ and } x=4} + \cdots \right)$$

Using the substitutions $e^{-(\lambda+1)} = \alpha_0$, $e^{\lambda_{a2}} = \alpha_{a2}$, and $e^{\lambda_{b4}} = \alpha_{b4}$ we get:

$$P_{w,x,y,z} = \alpha_0 \underbrace{\alpha_{a2}}_{\text{if } w=2} \underbrace{\alpha_{b4}^{B_4}}_{\text{if } z=1} \underbrace{\alpha_{b4}^{-1}}_{\text{if } z=1 \text{ and } x=4} \cdots$$

Since we can now express $P_{i,j,k,l}$, and thus the original constraints, in terms of the $\alpha$'s, we have an equation for each $\alpha$. This set of simultaneous equations is then solved using standard techniques. Since the original entropy function is strictly concave upwards and the constraints are linear, the extremum is unique and global. The updated label probabilities for segment $\mathcal{E}_C$ is then determined by calculating $P(\mathcal{E}_C = O_i \mid I' = 1)$ from the newly derived expression for $P_{i,j,k,l}$ in terms of the $\alpha$'s. The low-level stage, along with parts of the high level stage, have been run on simulated edge segment data.

## Forming Trial Contours

Once probabilistic labeling on all candidate segments is complete, the segments are now combined into a trial LV contour. This operation is performed separately on each frame within each modality. The algorithm to perform this linking is currently only partially implemented. The approach is centered around treating the problem as a graph search, where the linked edge segments are the nodes of the graph and metrics such as spatial adjacency and low curvature determine the whether arcs between the nodes exist and to what degree. The search for a complete LV contour in each RNA lateral view or 2DE apical long axis view frame proceeds by beginning with segments labeled as very likely to be part of the anterobasal wall, and ends with segments very likely to be part of the posterobasal wall. By allowing only local neighbors to interact in the tracking process, yet still searching for a global optimal boundary, dynamic programming is invoked as the search method of choice. The search is carried out on the basis that the final LV contour in each frame should have a logical progression of regional anatomical labelings and be smooth in terms of local curvature variations. Gap filling will be initially performed by connecting the end points of high probability segments accepted by the dynamic programming search procedure. Boundary regions created by this filling process will be assigned low probability labels for further processing. Some curve smoothing may be required to create usable contours, and probabilities will be reduced as they deviate from original values. The entire border with associated regional labels and label probabilities is stored in a list data structure. Note that this approach differs from methods typically used in more standard RNA (e.g. Gerbrands et al., 1982) and 2DE (e.g. Geiser and Oliver, 1984) contour analysis. Many of these approaches focus on studies that have some approximate circular symmetry (e.g. transaxial 2DE views or LAO RNA views) and employ radial search techniques for finding boundary points. The more ellipse-like shape of the views used here require an alternate approach, such as what is presented here.

## Motion and Shape Analysis

The two trial contours (at end diastole and end systole) from each of the two modalities may now be used to decipher local motion and local shape. The contours are continuous curves and may be treated as such for further analysis. The probabilistic confidence for the regions of the curves as discussed in the last section is maintained, however, and will in fact be used in the inter-modality data fusing.

The centerline algorithm, developed initially for use with contrast angiograms by Bolson et al. (1980), will be used for motion quantification. This approach has been adapted for use with both RNA left lateral and 2DE apical long axis view studies. Results for RNA studies are shown in Duncan (1984). A final plot of chord motion is used for intermodality comparison (described below). In this plot, the horizontal axis represents a chord numbering starting at one end and wrapping around to the other end of the ED ventricular contour (nominally 100 equally spaced chords are used), and the vertical axis is the degree of motion, i.e. the length of each chord (normalized to the end-diastolic perimeter). Normal ranges of motion are recorded to help delineate abnormalities. It is important to realize that although only the ED and ES curves are used for the centerline motion analysis, that boundary segments are found at each intermediate frame between ED and ES and are used to temporally track the segments that are most likely part of the LV boundary. This attempt at maintaining temporal continuity between the ED and ES boundaries is incorporated via the constraints in the probabilistic reasoning system, operating on the segments in each frame.

The measurement of shape, although a much addressed problem in computer vision and image understanding in general (Ballard and Brown, 1982), has its own unique problems in this context. It is desired to use a local measure that necessarily carries sufficient surrounding point information to be meaningful. The desired ED shape information must relate smoothness within a neighborhood as well as a degree of curvature from some starting axis. These ideas are manifested in the $\psi - s$ curve as discussed in Ballard and Brown (1982). In this representation, and for the purposes of measuring shape of the trial ventricular contours, $\psi$ is the angle made between a fixed line, which will be the line formed by the tangent to the anterobasal wall of the heart at the point it intersects the valve plane in the optimal lateral (RNA), and apical long axis (2DE) views, and a tangent to each point along the boundary of the ventricular border. This is then plotted against $s$, which is the arc length of the amount of the total trial left ventricular border that has been traversed. Note that horizontal lines in the $\psi - s$ curve correspond to straight lines (no change in $\psi$) on the left ventricular contour, and any vertically sloping $\psi - s$ lines correspond to a degree of curvature. Because $s$ is a relative measure of spatial distance, it can be exactly compared with the distance of each of the motion chords from the same starting point (i.e. the intersection of the anterobasal wall with the valve plane). This algorithm has been tested on clinical data and described by Duncan et al. (1986), where the use of the $\psi - s$ and $\psi' - s$ derivative curves to identify location, extent and severity of shape abnormalities is delineated.

Thus, spatially localized relative measures of motion and end diastolic shape have now been realized. For each point on the centerline and $\psi - s$ curve a probability value is stored. These values are computed during the probabilistic reasoning process.

Examples of quantitative motion analysis by the centerline method and quantitative shape analysis using $\psi - s$ plots are shown in figures 3, 4, 5 and 6 for the multimodality-based study of a single patient's heart. In the images shown in the upper portion of figure 3, complete LV contours at end diastole (left upper and lower gray scale images) and end systole (right upper and lower gray scale images) for a left lateral view RNA study were manually traced using the thinned edges (shown in black) as a guide in order to simulate trial contour formation. The final contours are shown in white and their centerline chord motion plot is shown on the right side of figure 3. The plots on the bottom of figure 3 represent the quantification of the centerline motion information. Manually traced (without using thinned edges as a guide) end diastolic and end systolic contours from the 2DE apical long axis view taken from the same patient whose RNA images are presented in figure 3 are shown overlayed on the 2DE end systolic image in figure 4. The centerline plots of this 2DE-based motion information are shown in figure 5. Note

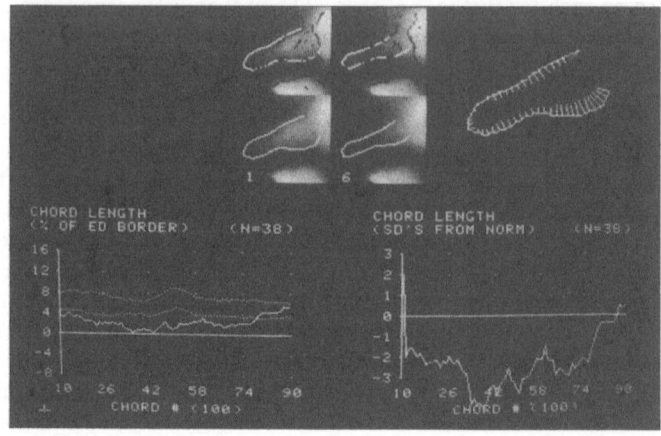

Figure 3: Simulated RNA trial contours with regional wall motion analysis. Gray scale images: left lateral view ED (two leftmost images) and ES (two rightmost images) frames shown with manually traced contours overlayed on the thinned edge results (two uppermost images) and smoothed original data (two lowermost images). Chord plot (upper right): centerline motion plot using ED and ES trial contours shown. Quantified wall motion: chord position (no. 1 = top right, no. 100 = lower right chords in chord plot) vs. normalized chord length (motion) (left lower graph) and vs. deviation of length from normal mean motion (lower right graph). The dotted lines in the lower left graph represent ±1 standard deviation from the normal mean of 35 patients.

the similarity of the final quantitative motion plots in each of the two modalities (bottom left of figure 3 and right side of figure 5), especially in the akinetic anteroapical wall region. Finally, $\psi - s$ and $\psi' - s$ shape plots of the end diastolic left lateral view RNA contour are shown in figure 6.

Fusing Shape and Motion Information: Coming to a Multimodality, Consensus Opinion

Once both motion and shape measures have been developed, it is desired to compare the results and, if necessary, iteratively check to see if alternate choices at the low level of analysis were possible in either modality to form a system consensus opinion about the shape and motion of the particular patients' left ventricle. As was evident from the earlier discussion, the trial contours passed from the lower and intermediate levels of processing were only the best estimates of a left ventricular contour given the available information from one modality. It is possible that a different trial contour could have been formed using a slightly different combination of edge segment groupings, had additional information been provided (i.e. bias from a second modality). Thus the proposed system will iteratively feed back such additional information about regions of the left ventricular endocardial border after looking at two modalities opinions of motion and shape, possibly causing a different trial contour on the next iteration. An important observation is that consensus is sought at the reasonably higher cognitive levels of the system's analysis, namely shape and motion (and eventually thickening), rather than trying to force the gray level edge segments to precisely match pixel-by-pixel. This allows the lower level analysis to proceed optimally for each modality. The angulation of the heart (to some extent) and the different scale of the heart for each modality are effectively normalized out of the problem. In addition, the most

466

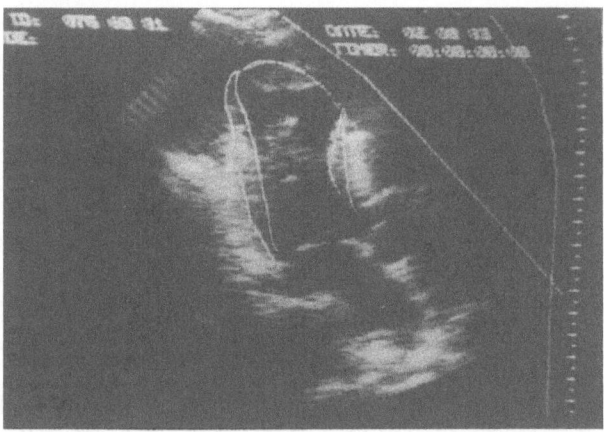

Figure 4: Simulated 2DE trial contours. Manually traced LV trial contours from the ED and ES frames of an apical long axis view study overlayed on the ES frame. This study was performed on the same patient whose RNA study is described in figure 3.

prominent gray level edges in each modality determine that modality's evidential contribution to the analysis, as is appropriate.

The approach to this problem is as follows. First, the $\psi - s$ shape(ED) and centerline motion (ED to ES) curves will both be run through a matching algorithm to look for gross curvature and motion variations that best line up (i.e. the assumption is made that the two curves must roughly agree initially). The matching process shifts one modality's motion and shape curves until they best agree according to a weighted cross correlation with the second modality's curves. Matching of these plots helps account for acquisition angulation differences between RNA and 2DE studies. The goal of the matching process is to line up the discrete spatial positions on the motion and shape maps in the planes of the contours, so that probabilistic statements can be made about motion and shape as derived from the original (gray-level gradient) evidence.

Now that the curves have been lined up in an optimal way, it is desired to compute the agreement or disagreement between the modalities separately for shape and motion. This is done by simply computing the least squares error on a point by point basis and plotting an error curve, one each for shape and motion (although the use of a combined correlation curve is also being considered). In this way, full agreement is represented as zero error and disagreement is a large number. These curves are now weighted by the multiplicatively combined probabilities, propagated from the lower levels of analysis. Now, regions of low agreement with regard to motion and/or shape are isolated by simply comparing the areas under the least squares error plot. The largest area is considered first, and then smaller and smaller regions within a predetermined bound. As an isolated region is considered, several things occur: first, the propagated motion and shape confidence is considered, if one modality was considerably less confident in its analysis, that is the one considered for new trial contour formulation. If just shape is less confident or just motion is less confident, still the weaker modality is chosen. If there is a conflict, the parameter with the most disagreement is used as the deciding factor. The isolated region of points in the chosen modality is now considered at the TRIAL CONTOUR FORMATION level (see Figure 1). A search window around the region of concern is created for both the diastolic and systolic frames in that modality. Diastole is considered first: depending on whether the mismatch of motion was due to more or less perceived motion and/or the mismatch

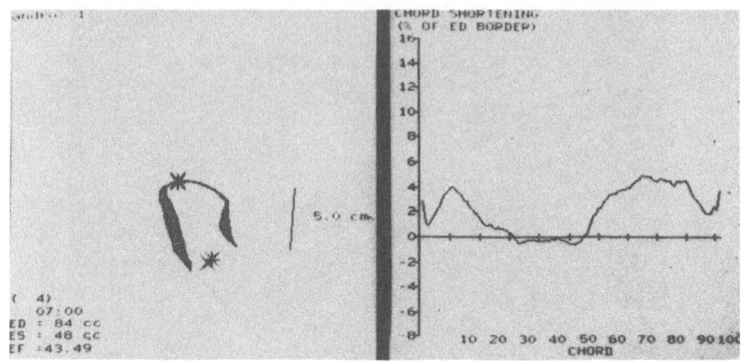

Figure 5: 2DE regional wall motion analysis. Left: centerline motion plot using ED and ES contours shown in figure 4. Right: quantified wall motion graph of chord position (no. 1 = lower right, no. 100 = lower left) vs. normalized chord length (motion).

of shape is due to more or less curvature, the local probabilistic models for label direction and relative position are modified accordingly. Disagreement of intermodality motion and ED shape information causes the reconstraining of the low level maximum entropy probabilistic labeling problems and new labelings are generated. For example, a perceived high curvature region by the second modality would spread out the direction probability distribution in a usually low curvature corresponding region in the first modality. Disagreement in regional motion according to the centerline plot matching causes a change in the probabilistic low level models for both the end diastolic and end systolic frames. Once these probabilistic models have been modified by this feedback process, a new trial contour is formed and its linked list with stored probabilistic confidence is sent to the upper level shape and motion algorithms. The entire process is repeated (iterated) until either no further modifications can be made or the system converges to full agreement (within an $\epsilon$-error bound).

For the initial practical consideration of building a simplified stable working system, as soon as the inter-modality correlation gets worse in any way, no further reasoning is allowed for that region and a new region is considered or the feedback process stopped and in both cases the last best result is maintained. Obviously this monotonic approach will not be able to reason out of local valleys and a more sophisticated overall optimization scheme is eventually be considered. The computational speed of the algorithm is also of concern. However, the maximum amount of grossly uncorrelated regions is expected to be on the order of only 10–20 according to initial trials.

Final Assessment of Presence and Degree of Aneurysm Formation

The consensus opinion curves of shape and motion weighted by multiplicatively combined probabilities must now be combined to assess aneurysm formation likelihood. Before discussing this, an important point about the probabilistic evidence should be made: although the combined probabilities for local shape and motion of the multimodality system are available, the individual modality motion and shape curves and regional subjective probabilities (confidence) are retained as well. Thus, the system may be probed as to where and how it came to the decision it did. In other words, the system can alter its opinion based on a user bias, and pass this result through the iterative scheme.

The logic used to finally assess LV aneurysm formation follows that proposed by Meizlich (1984). Each of the 100 defined points on the consensus motion and shape curves (which are

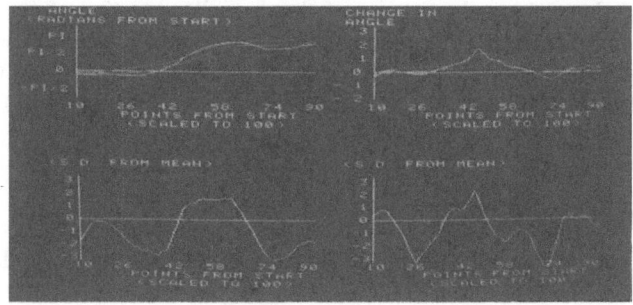

Figure 6: RNA regional shape analysis. $\psi - s$ (2 leftmost graphs) and $\psi' - s$ (two rightmost graphs) plots for the end diastolic perimeter shown in figure 3. The two upper plots' vertical axes are actual angles in radians and the dotted lines represent $\pm 1$ standard deviation from the normal mean. The two lower plots are in units of standard deviation from the normal mean.

exactly registered and are the average of the final values found for each modality) are investigated for the three properties and thus a final plot is generated. These three properties are 1) Is the point part of a motion minimum?, i.e. is it dyskinetic or akinetic and surrounded by at least two other minima; 2) are there surrounding groups of normal points?, i.e. does the local motion return to plateaus of normal motion on either side; and 3) is the ED shape in that region part of a bulging region?, i.e. is the point on the derivative of the $\psi - s$ curve surrounded by maxima? Each of these factors, weighted by the probabilistic confidence that each is evident, is combined to form a likelihood of that point being part of an aneurysm.

## SUMMARY

In summary, an approach to multimodality cardiac image analysis has been presented that has the following characteristics:

1) First, a complete and detailed logical strategy has been developed for the overall system. This approach considers low level uncertainties via a probabilistic reasoning algorithm, groups locally smooth low level information (edge segments), creates complete trial left ventricular end diastolic and end systolic contours using an interpolation procedure and includes feedback from the high to the low levels in order to seek an intermodality consensus opinion of left ventricular ED shape and motion.

2) Edge finding, thinning and linking algorithms have been adapted from previous work for use here and have been tested on clinical RNA and 2DE data.

3) A maximum entropy (least information) probabilistic reasoning approach to assigning and updating labelings on low level information has been developed and initial testing on simulated edge segment data performed. This approach allows the full consideration of dependent probabilistic information within local event groups.

4) The quantitative analysis of left ventricular aneurysms has been identified as a useful clinical problem to which the multimodality analysis developed in this work can be initially applied. The measurement of regional wall motion and regional ED shape are exactly the features that are relevant to this difficult clinical problem. Approaches to the quantification of these measurements have been presented and initial testing on semi-automatically derived data has been performed.

Integration of the various algorithm modules as well as testing of the entire system on simulated and real data are planned as the next steps in the development process. In addition, it is planned to test the usefulness of this approach in obtaining a multimodality consensus opinion regarding other cardiac parameters and other modalities (e.g. wall thickening as perceived by 2DE and gated Magnetic Resonance Imaging).

ACKNOWLEDGEMENTS

The authors gratefully acknowledge the support of the Whitaker Foundation.

REFERENCES

Ballard, D. H. and Brown, C. M. (1982). Computer Vision, Prentice Hall, Englewood Cliffs.

Belknap, R., Riseman, E. M. and Hanson, A. R. (1986). The information fusion problem and rule-based hypotheses applied to computer aggregations of image events, in: Proc. IEEE Conf. on Computer Vision and Pattern Recognition, IEEE Computer Society Press, Washington, D.C., 227–237.

Bolson, E. L., Kliman, S., Sheehan, F. and Dodge, H. T. (1980). Left ventricular segmental wall motion – A new method using local direction information, in: Proc. Computers in Cardiology, IEEE Computer Society Press, Washington, D.C.

Cabin, H., Vita, N., Clubb, K. and Zaret, B. L. (1984). Regional wall motion post-myocardial infarct: A predictor of the site and severity of necrosis and scar at necropsy, in the 57th American Heart Association Scientific Sessions, Washington, D.C. (abstract).

Cheeseman, P. C. (1983). A method of computing generalized bayesian probability values for expert systems, in: Proc. Intl. Joint Conf. on Artificial Intelligence, Morgan Kaufmann, Los Altos, CA, 198–202.

Cheeseman, P. C. (1985). In defense of probability, in: Proc. Intl. Joint Conf. on Artificial Intelligence, Morgan Kaufmann, Los Altos, CA, 1002–1009.

Duncan, J. S., Koster, K., Zaret, E., Wackers, F. and Zaret, B. (1987). Quantitative analysis of diastolic shape deformity from equilibrium radionuclide angiography, in: Society of Nuclear Medicine 34th Annual Meeting, Toronto, Canada. (Abstract).

Duncan, J. S. (1984). Intelligent determination of left ventricular wall motion from multiple view, nuclear medicine image sequences, in: Proc. Joint Intl. Symposium on Medical Images and Icons, Arlington, VA, 265–269.

Geiser, E. and Oliver, L. (1984). Echocardiography: Image processing in two-dimensional echocardiographic images, Automedica, 5, 171.

Gerbrands, J., Hoek, C., Reiber, J., Lie, S. and Simoons, M. (1980). Minimum cost contour detection in technetium-99m gated cardiac blood pool scintigrams, in: Proc. Computers in Cardiology, IEEE Computer Society Press, Washington, D.C., 281–284.

Jaynes, E. T. (1957). Information theory and statistical mechanics, Phys. Rev., 106, 620–630.

Marion, J.L. (1983). Analysis of justification for modality integration, in: Proc. 2nd Intl. Conf. and Workshop on Picture Archiving and Communication Systems for Medical Applications, 17–23.

Meizlish, J. L., Berger, H., Plankey, M., Errico, D., Levy, W. and Zaret, B. L. (1984). Functional left ventricular aneurysm formation after acute transmural myocardial infarction, The New England Journal of Medicine, 311, 1001–1006.

Niemann, H., Bunke, H., Hofmann, I., Sagerer, G., Wolf, F. and Feistel, H. (1985). A knowledge-based system for analysis of gated blood pool studies, IEEE Trans. on Pattern Analysis and Machine Intelligence, 7, 246–259.

Sorenson, S. G., Crawford, M., Richards, K. L., Thaudhuri, F. and O'Rourke, R. (1982). Noninvasive detection of ventricular aneurysm by combined two-dimensional echocardiography and equilibrium radionuclide angiography, American Heart Journal, July, 145–152.

# A SYSTEM FOR THE DIAGNOSTIC USE OF TISSUE CHARACTERIZING

# PARAMETERS IN  N M R - TOMOGRAPHY

M. Jungke, W. von Seelen, G. Bielke,
S. Meindl, M. Grigat, and P. Pfannenstiel

Deutsche Klinik f. Diagnostik, Abt. NMR
Aukammallee 33, D-6200 Wiesbaden, FRG

## INTRODUCTION

In the last years Nuclear Magnetic Resonance (NMR) tomography of hydrogen nuclei has become a well-established technique of non-invasive diagnostics. Both the kind of tissue specific information being distributed to several series of images and the importance of the physician as a user with final competence and responsibility make the task of tissue characterization and differentiation special in applied classification methodology. The following chapters will outline progress and results of developmental work of several components of an image analysis and classification system, which is superimposed by a system of control and information management. Additionally the design of tools to include the user in the decision process will be discussed.

## DATA PREPROCESSING

The separation of different tissues in NMR-tomography may be achieved by the spin lattice relaxation time T1, the spin spin relaxation time  T2 and the relative spin density of hydrogen nuclei RHO. Provided the NMR-image data result from a CPMG - sequence, the intensity of an image point S(x,y) with the coordinates x,y can be described by the simplified solution of the Bloch equations, Bielke et al.(1984), Crooks (1986).

$$S(x,y) = Rho(x,y)*[1-exp[-TR/T1(x,y)]]*exp[-TE/T2(x,y)]$$

(1)

The terms TR and TE indicate 'recovery time' and 'echo delay time'.

Studies concerning the distribution of the parameters mentioned above  belonging to homogenous phantom media showed some variations due to measurement noise, which had been propagated

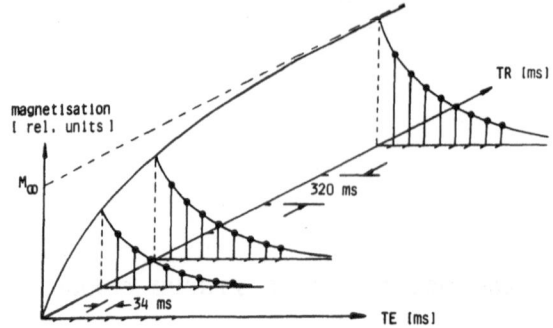

Fig. 1    Response to excitation
          sequence (ideal case)

into the parameter estimation. Improvements on this early level
of data transformation turned out to be of fundamental necessity
to further steps of processing. The following chapters will show
the way we succeeded in reducing the sensitivity of the estimation algorithms to signal noise.

MEASUREMENT CONDITIONS

        Subject of our research is brain tissue. Data acquisition
was done on a  0.28 T iron shielded resistive system. The measurement sequence was modified to a combination of three CPMG-
spin-echo-trains of eight echoes each, with different recovery
times interlaced for each projection. The time between two
echoes is 34 ms, the three TR values are 320 ms, 640 ms and
1920 ms. Fig. 1 shows the principle method of decoupling the
three parameters by extrapolating the responses to the CPMG-
excitation to TE = 0. However, the problem of noise propagation
is obvious.

ESTIMATION OF SPIN SPIN RELAXATION TIME BY DIFFERENCE EQUA-
TION MODELLING COMBINED WITH DIGITAL FILTERING

        A normal way of preprocessing is filter application. We
made a digital filter algorithm part of the T2 estimation procedure. Considering the fact of starting data sampling at 34 ms,
we assume data to belong to a monoexponential decay curve and
estimate T2 by an approach based on the theory of time discrete
system modelling.

        The T2 decay curve is considered to be the discrete output
signal $y(k)$ of a black box model (fig. 2) with the input signal
$u(k)$, which in this special case will turn out to be of a hypothetic form.  The letter 'k' scales the time axis equidistantly,
$T_0$ is the time interval between two echoes. Concerning our type
of monoexponential function, the general difference equation

$$y(k) - a_1 y(k-1) - \ldots - a_m y(k-m) =$$

$$b_0 u(k) + b_1 u(k-1) + \ldots + b_m u(k-m) \qquad (2)$$

reduces to the expression :

$$u(k) = \begin{cases} 1 & k=0 \\ 0 & k\neq0 \end{cases} \qquad y(k) = \begin{cases} 0 & k<0 \\ a_1\,y(k-1) + b_0\,u(k) & k\geq0 \end{cases}$$

The notation 'k-1' describes a time shift operation to the sample point before 'k'. Parameter $a_1$ substitutes the exponential expression

$$a_1 = \exp(-T_0/T2) \tag{3}$$

while parameter $b_0$ represents the magnitude of the first output signal. Now we apply a digital smoothing filter to the whole set of data, which in the black box model means that real output data and hypothetic input data will pass the same type of filter. The scheme of the filtered T2 estimation is demonstrated in fig. 2 showing y(k) superimposed by an additive zero mean noise signal n(k), which, however, can't be measured explicitly.

An example for a filter algorithm, an ideal low pass filter is given by

$$r(k) \longrightarrow \boxed{\begin{array}{c}\text{ideal}\\\text{low pass}\end{array}} \longrightarrow w(k) \qquad w(k) = \begin{cases} 0 & k<0 \\ w(k-1) + r(k) & k\geq0 \end{cases}$$

The filtered output data (marked with '*') are written as a vector and, together with the input data, they fill a measurement matrix $\Phi$.

$$\begin{bmatrix} y^*(0) \\ y^*(1) \\ \vdots \\ y^*(N) \end{bmatrix} = \begin{bmatrix} 0 & u^*(0) \\ y^*(0) & u^*(1) \\ \vdots & \vdots \\ y^*(N-1) & u^*(N) \end{bmatrix} \cdot \begin{bmatrix} a_1 \\ b_0 \end{bmatrix} \tag{4}$$

This is equivalent to

$$\underline{y} = \underline{\Phi} * \underline{\Theta} . \tag{5}$$

The final solution of the overestimated system of equations is

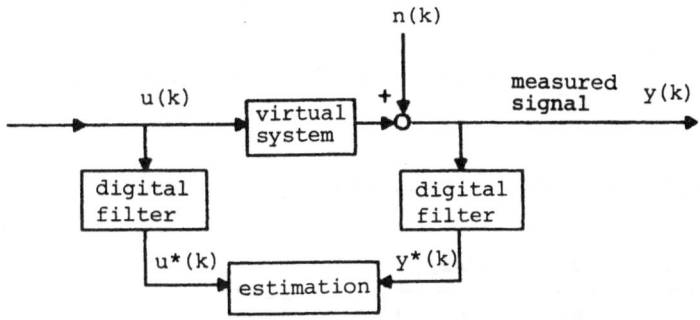

Fig.2 Black box model of a system with time discrete input and output, digital filters added for parameter estimation

achieved by a least squares fit, leading to the covariance matrix $\underline{\Phi}^T\underline{\Phi}$ of rank two which allows the calculation of $a_1$ and $b_0$, the components of vector $\underline{\Theta}$.

$$\underline{\Phi}^T\underline{\Phi} \cdot \underline{\Theta} = \underline{\Phi}^T\underline{y} \qquad (6)$$

In this context it should be remembered that there is no need for logarithmic operations to the original input data up to this point of calculation. By avoiding the unfavourable noise increassing effect of the input data being logarithmed before applying a linear least squares fit, the variation of parameter T2 decreased rapidly. As a consequence of estimating $a_1$ one component of the feature vector and, according to it, one axis of the feature space may be replaced by this parameter instead of using T2.

ESTIMATION OF SPIN-LATTICE RELAXATION TIME AND RELATIVE DENSITY OF HYDROGEN NUCLEI

As to T1 and RHO we use the three values extrapolated to TE = 0 at TR1 = 320 ms, TR2 = 640 ms and TR3 = 1920 ms for estimation (fig. 1). The algorithm bases on splitting the factor RHO of the simplified image equation into two constants $\alpha$ and $\beta$,

$$S(TR) = \alpha + \beta*\exp(-TR/T1) \qquad (7)$$

which are connected by the additional equation

$$\alpha = -\beta \qquad (8)$$

Applying a linear least squares fit, with the loss function

$$\Gamma^2 = \sum_{n=1}^{3} [ S(TRn) - \alpha - \beta*\exp(-TRn/T1) ]^2$$
$$\rightarrow \alpha_{opt}(1/T1), \beta_{opt}(1/T1) \qquad (9)$$

we obtain an optimal $\alpha$ and $\beta$, both being functions of T1. The next step forces $\alpha_{opt}$ and $\beta_{opt}$ to fulfill eq.(7) by variation of (1/T1). The task of detecting but one zero crossing is done iteratively by a Newton-Raphson algorithm, Garnir and Garnir - Monjoie (1981).

$$\frac{1}{T1_{(j+1)}} = \frac{1.1}{T1_j} + \frac{0.1}{T1_j} * f(1.1/T1_j)/[f(1/T1_j)-f(1.1/T1_j)] \qquad (10)$$

The condition of stopping iterations

$$\frac{|\alpha_{opt}(1/T1_j) + \beta_{opt}(1/T1_j)|}{|\alpha_{opt}(1/T1_j) - \beta_{opt}(1/T1_j)|} < 10^{-5} \qquad (11)$$

is achieved within a few steps. The method showed to be quite insensitive to the starting value of T1. Optimal RHO is considered to be the mean of last $\alpha_{opt}$ and $\beta_{opt}$ optimizing T1.

$$RHO = \frac{\alpha_{opt}(1/T1_j) - \beta_{opt}(1/T1_j)}{2} \qquad (12)$$

Parameter images obtained by the methods described before are shown in fig. 3. (Please refer to the results of the next chapter.)


## INITIALIZATION OF THE FEATURE SPACE BASED ON SIMULTANEOUS REFERENCE MEASUREMENTS

The absolute parameter values are intraindividually suitable for the identification of the tissues which are detectable as 'cluster' in the feature space. However the evaluation of these data for the interindividual classification of the findings raises problems due to partly considerable differences in the parameter values for histologically comparable tissues of different patients. Moreover, the parameter RHO escapes from any interindividual comparability on account of its being dependent on the adjustment of the magnet system as relative measurement value.

The reliability of the calculated parameters describing the tissue is subject to various changing noise influences; effects on the 'real' parameters may be reduced provided a sufficient number of measurement values are realized. It is just this restriction which as a rule is neglected during routinely performed examinations for reasons of a limited measuring time. However, the parameter failures which are unable to be avoided in the case of a small number of measurement values can be estimated by means of a reference phantom simultaneously measured to the patient's examination in order to limit their effects on tissue classification.

On account of the parameter values of both the relaxation time constants and the relative spin density of hydrogen nuclei being highly similar to those of white brain matter, a linear polymere dimethylsiloxane with a viscosity of 12500 cSt serves as reference quantity for brain tissue characterisation. Transverse and longitudinal relaxation of this silicone can be well described by means of a monoexponential model formulation at a field of 0.28 T and 0.47 T. The measured signal mainly is determined by the behaviour of the methyl groups in the magnetic field, long time stability of relaxation times and spin density were checked by reproducing the parameters at room temperature within a period of ten months, showing recurrently identical values within the degree of measurement exactness.

Based on the observation that adjacent points in the feature space are highly correlated with functional neighbourhood in the image domain, the position of the cluster of the reference substance in the feature space serves as reference point for parameter standardization. The detection and classification of this cluster is achieved by marking the reference substance by means

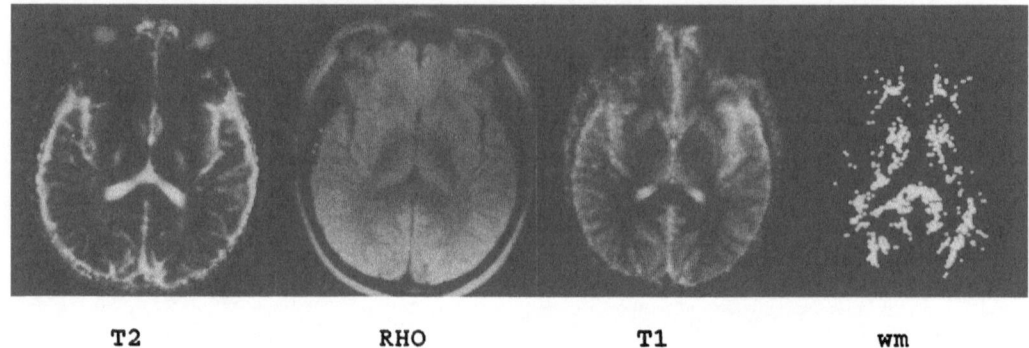

T2         RHO        T1        wm

Fig. 3  Detecting a volunteer's white matter (wm) based on a reference medium

of a freely movable standardized cursor matrix within the original image domain. Following the determination of the coordinates of the actual reference vectors, the parameters with scaling and rotation operations are standardized by applying them to the vectors of the feature space. As illustrated in fig. 3 where the classification of white brain matter is exemplified, we succeeded – additionally to T1 and T2 – in considering the parameter RHO for the interindividual comparison of the tissue-characterising values.

## CONFIGURATION OF THE CLASSIFIER

Based on measurement values being available in form of a feature vector $\underline{v}$, the recognition system has to come to a decision as reliable as possible with respect to a tissue voxel actually belonging to a tissue group. In case the feature vectors of all patients are part of global entities, an optimal statistical classifier may be derived. The classification algorithm self-adaptively adjusts the decision boundaries by means of the aposteriori statistic of prior classifications. The result of a classification is an image with the pixels being displayed in tissue specific colours, demonstrating type and extension of the tissue.

## MAXIMUM LIKELIHOOD CLASSIFIER

Due to the structure of the problem, we will discuss the application of a maximum likelihood classifier, which is the solution to the decision theoretical approach. Fundamental to the design of the decision system is the knowledge of the type of distribution function to describe the real statistical distribution of the feature vectors in a reasonable way. In the following the statistical process will be assumed to consist of independent subprocesses $\{\underline{v}|k\}$

$$p(\underline{v},k) = p(\underline{v}|k)*p(k) \tag{13}$$

each of them generated by tissue of one of the classes k. A sub-process is supposed to belong to the type of conditional distribution function ( $N$: number of components of $\underline{v}$ )

$$p(\underline{v}|k) = \frac{1}{\sqrt{(2\pi)^N \det \underline{K_k}}} * \exp[ -0.5*(\underline{v} - \mu_k)^T \underline{K_k}^{-1} (\underline{v} - \mu_k)]$$

(14)

with mean

$$\mu_k = E\{\underline{v}(k)\}$$

(15)

and class specific covariance matrix

$$\underline{K_k} = E\{(\underline{v} - \mu_k)(\underline{v} - \mu_k)^T|k\}$$

(16)

Computation may be done recursively as demonstrated for class k,

$$\underline{\hat{K}_I^k} = \frac{I-1}{I} [ \underline{\hat{K}_{I-1}^k} + \frac{1}{I} ( \underline{v_I} - \mu_{I-1})( \underline{v_I} - \mu_{I-1})^T]$$

(17)

$$\underline{\hat{\mu}_I^k} = ( 1 - \frac{1}{I} ) \underline{\hat{\mu}_{I-1}^k} + \frac{1}{I} \underline{v_I} .$$

(18)

Choosing the elements of the cost matrix inversely proportional to the expected probability of occurence leads to the decision rule

$$D_k(\underline{v}) = \max \{p(\underline{v}|k)\} .$$

(19)

As the result of the comparison doesn't change with monotone transformation, $D_k$ may be replaced by

$$\tilde{D}_k(\underline{v}) = \ln(D_k(\underline{v}) \sqrt{[2\pi]^N}) .$$

(20)

Finally the maximum of

$$\tilde{D}_k(\underline{v}) = -0.5*\ln \det(\underline{K_k}) -0.5*[(\underline{v} - \mu_k)^T \underline{K_k}^{-1} (\underline{v} - \mu_k)]$$

(21)

has to be detected.The decision is rejected if $\tilde{D}_k(\underline{v})$ is below a minimum level.  The part underlined in eq.(21) is called Mahalanobis distance. It describes locations of constant density in the feature space , thus serving as a criteria to reject decisions due to an insufficent amount of probability.


SUPERVISION - AND INFORMATION SYSTEM

    Apart from developmental work done in the field of data preprocessing and  standardization, the aspect of including the user in the process of decision and classification increases in importance. As the physician is responsible for the diagnosis, he must be able to judge the internal course of the decision finding and the result of classification. He is supported by a

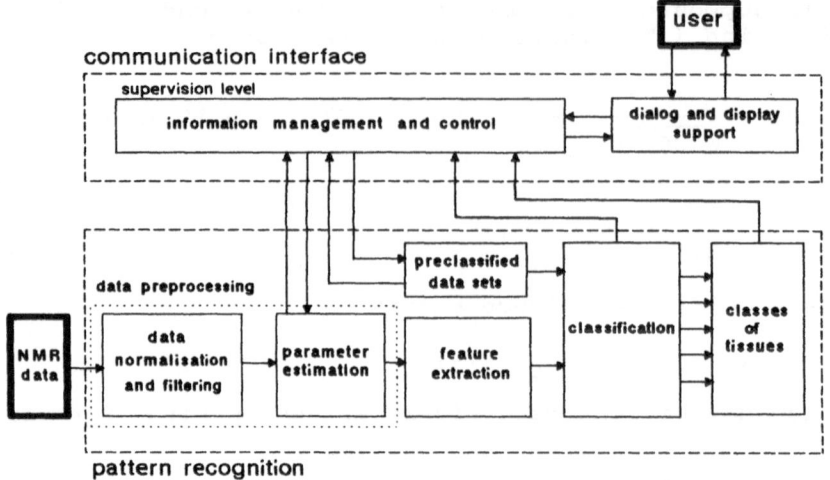

Fig. 4  System for the diagnostic use of tissue characterizing parameters in NMR – tomography

supervision level, which, including tools of observation and
information management, superimposes the feature extraction
process.

Connected by several input and output channels to each
partial step of the tissue characterizing  process (fig. 4),
functions of the supervision level check plausibility and consistency of partial and intermediate results by means of internal or externally defined quality criteria. The data structures
which vary according to the requirements of the different algorithms are converted to an image or graphic output on demand of
the supervisory level or at the request of the user. On the
other hand medical knowledge has to be inserted into different
steps of the processing. In the following some functions of the
supervision and information management level will be discussed
parallel to the feature extraction and classification steps respectively in order to illustrate the specific structures of
the system.

To start the classification algorithms, the system needs
a priori information, usually given as sets of preclassified
tissue-characteristic regions. The definition of these regions
by manually bordering  areas in the image domain with the help
of a cursor is a time consuming method, which requires training
in collecting a statistically sufficient amount of tissue-specific pixels due to problems of diminishing contrast in the
image domain.

The observation that adjacent points in the feature space
are closely correlated with functional neighbourhood within the
image domain is made use of as a tool of the information mana-
ging part of the supervision level. Following a standardized
path that links tissue-specific locations, (fig. 5), sectors of
the feature space are projected into the image domain, thus proposing tissue-characteristic regions to the user (fig. 6) which
he either accepts by pressing a key, rejects or marks as 'being
of special interest'. The beginning of the path through the fea-

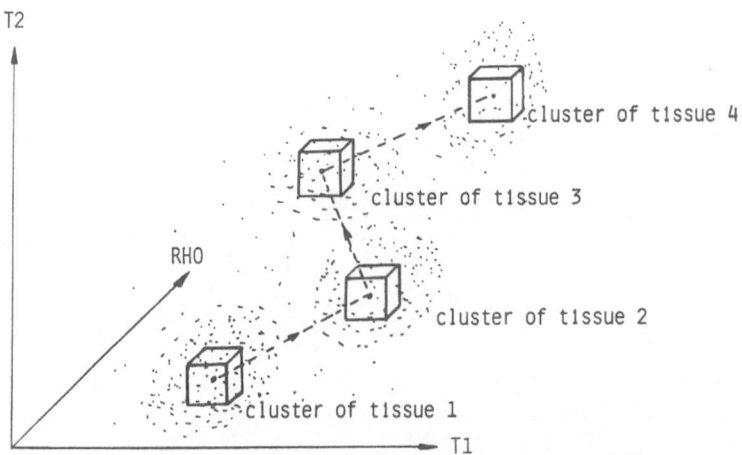

Fig. 5   Path in the feature space for semi-
automatical image segmentation

ture space is derived from the position of the reference medium,
which is close to the feature vectors of white matter.

As the user has to place every confidence in this system,
we support the system component of information management with
a decision board, displaying the values which are referred to
for the system-imminent decision-finding. For this purpose we
use the monitor as a combined image and graphic unit. Several
windows are simultaneously available requested on mouse or ascii

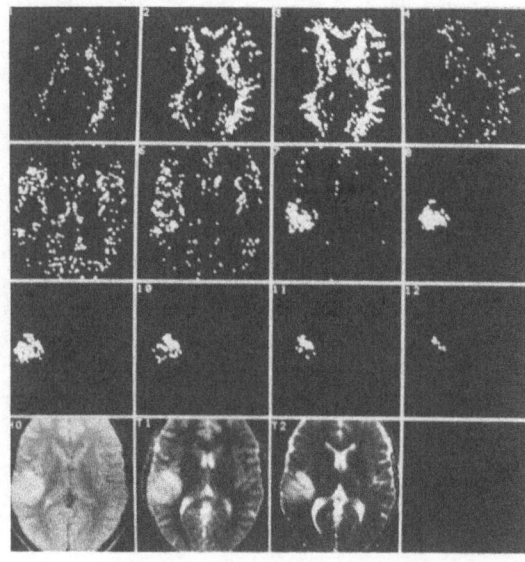

Fig. 6   Set of regions proposed
out of the feature space

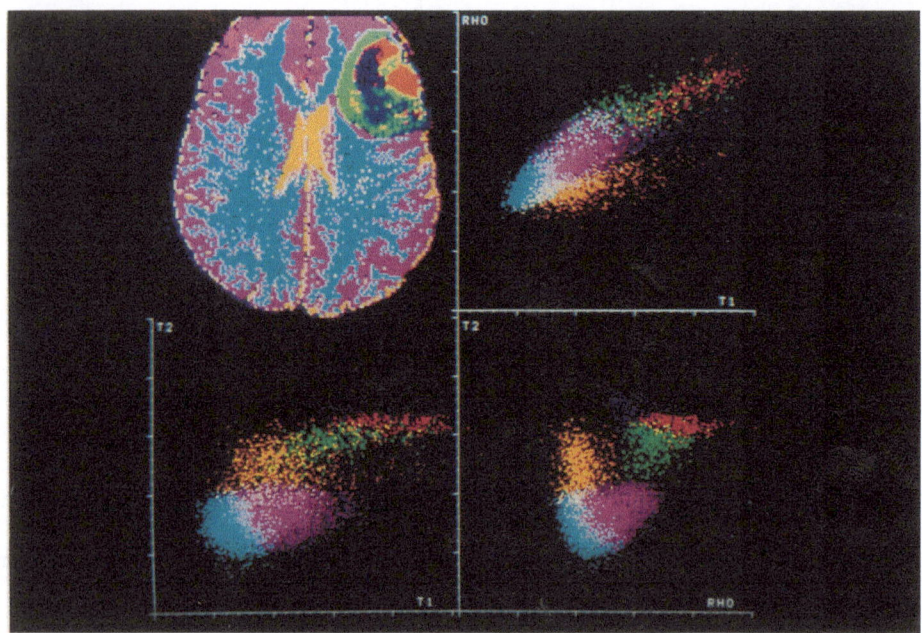

Fig. 7  Decision board: Distribution of feature
vectors (tissue-specific colour code)

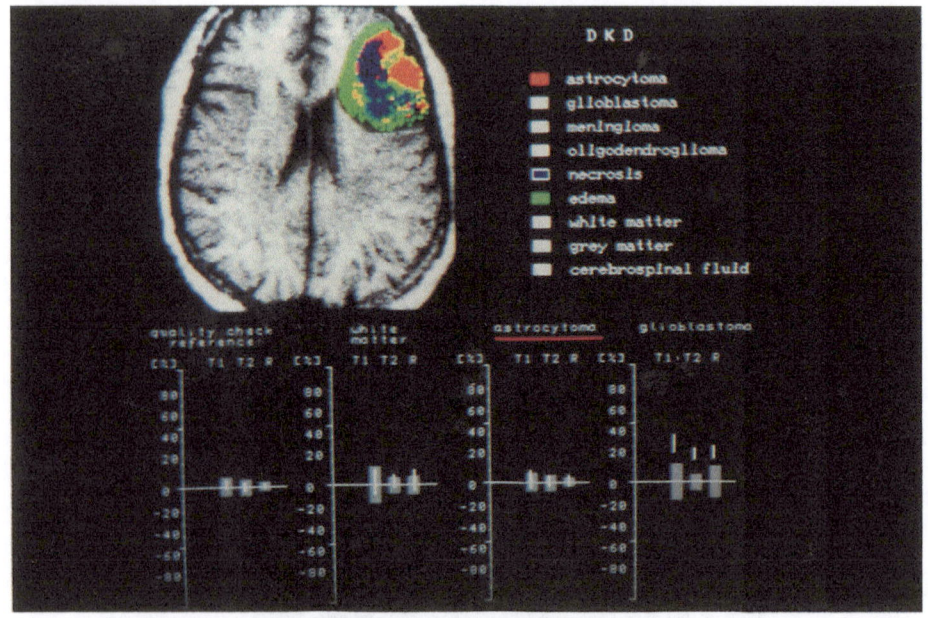

Fig. 8  Decision board: discussion of findings
(tissue-specific colour code)

input. An example of the version used commonly is shown in fig.7. This function of the supervision system allows views into regions of the feature space by projecting selected volumes on planes defined by the user. This approach enables the physician to judge the boundaries proposed by the classification process in comparison with the representation of tissue in the feature space

Another window to display NMR information consists of a synthetic grey value image, which is the result of resubstituting the three parameters T1, T2 and RHO of eq.(1), computed according to the constraint of optimal contrast versus grey and white matter. This image serves for morphologic orientation and is superimposed by coloured areas, which are, out of the classification algorithms view, of suspicious similarity to pathological findings. The colour code is simultaneously referred to in a list of pathological tissues (fig.8).

To simplify the judgement of the computer proposal, additional windows display actual statistics in comparison to inter-individual mean and standard deviation of tissue types which are of competitive similarity to the finding proposed as classification decision. One set of bar graphs serves for a visual a posteriori quality check of the examination itself, projecting the actual parameters of the reference medium together with the long time values.

ACKNOWLEDGEMENT

This work was supported by the Federal Ministry of Technology and Research.

REFERENCES

Bielke, G., Meves, M., Meindl, S., Brückner, A., von Seelen, W., Rinck, P., Pfannenstiel, P.,(1984). A systematic approach to optimization of pulse sequences in NMR-imaging by computer simulations, in: Technology of Nuclear Magnetic Resonance, P.D. Esser, R.E. Johnston, eds., The Society of Nucl. Med., New York, NY 10016

Crooks, L.E.(1986). Image contrast mechanisms in MRI, in: Medical Magnetic Resonance Imaging and Spectroscopy - A Primer, T.F. Budinger and A.R. Margulis, eds., Society of Magn. Res. in Med., Berkley, CA 94704

Garnir,H.P. and Garnir-Monjoie, F.S.(1981). Fit of the function y(x)=A(1-exp(-kx)) to data strongly embeded in noise, Nucl. Instr. and Meth. 190, 333-336.

# CONCERNING THE DERIVATION AND REPRESENTATION OF PARAMETER IMAGES

## IN NMR IMAGING

M. A. Moerland, C. J. G. Bakker, and C. N. de Graaf

University Hospital Utrecht
Catharijnesingel 101
3511 GV Utrecht, The Netherlands

## INTRODUCTION

In this work several aspects of the derivation and representation of parameter images in NMR imaging are taken into consideration. First we discuss the use of statistical parameter estimation techniques to determine the minimum variance bound (MVB) on the precision of any parameter determined from an NMR experiment and give some practical examples. Then we explore the effect of experiment design, i.e. the choice of sequence type and timings, on the precision of the estimated parameters achievable per unit experiment time. In the third section we compare some practical methods to extract $\rho$, $T_1$ and $T_2$ images from a set of partial saturation, saturation recovery or inversion recovery experiments which to a greater or less extent take into account the fact that a multiple echo/multiple repetition time experiment provides a set of largely independent $T_1$ and $T_2$ measurements. In the final section a provisional attempt is made to develop a non-linear gray scale for the display of $\rho$, $T_1$ and $T_2$ images which takes into account the estimated precision of the displayed parameter values.

## PARAMETER ESTIMATION

In an NMR experiment non-systematic errors in the observations can be modelled as zero-mean stochastic variables. A particular set of observations then constitutes a set of observations made on stochastic variables and the parameters to be estimated are parameters of the probability density function defining those stochastic variables. The measurement problem has thus taken the form of a statistical parameter estimation problem for the solution of which use can be made of the extensive collection of theories and methods available from mathematical statistics, econometrics and many other fields.

The statistical parameter estimation approach offers the possibility, if knowledge about the non-systematic errors in the observations is sufficiently detailed, to compute the lower bound on the variance of any unbiased estimator of a particular parameter for a given set of observations. This lower bound, the minimum variance bound, enables one to investigate the feasability of a set of observations for the parameter objectives concerned. Further, a statistical model of the observations may be used for minimizing the variance of an estimator through experiment design, i.e. through manipulating independent variables that can be freely chosen.

In the following the theory behind the application of statistical parameter estimation techniques to physical observations is briefly summarized (for a review the reader is referred to Van den Bos,1982) and illustrated by some examples from the NMR domain (see also Van der Lende,1985).

## The minimum variance bound

The minimum variance bound, also called Cramer-Rao lower bound, is a lower bound on the variance of any unbiased estimator. Since it is independent of any particular method of estimation it provides a bound on the precision that can be achieved given the observations. The MVB is a useful tool for investigating the feasability of the observations for the parameter estimation objectives concerned, the more so as a class of estimators exists, which, at least asymptotically, achieves this bound. These estimators are the so-called maximum likelihood estimators.

In the following underlined characters, e.g. $\underline{w}$, refer to stochastic variables, whereas vectors and matrices are denoted by a tilde, e.g. $\tilde{x}$. The minimum variance bound is derived as follows. Let $\underline{w}_1,.....,\underline{w}_N$ be the observations and let $\underline{\tilde{w}}$ be the column vector of these observations. Furthermore let the probability density function of $\underline{\tilde{w}}$ be $f(\underline{\tilde{w}};\tilde{\Theta})$, where the k elements of the vector $\tilde{\Theta}$ are the unknown parameters. If we now define the kxk information matrix $\tilde{M}$ by:

$$\tilde{M}=E[(\partial \ln \underline{L}/\partial \tilde{\Theta})^T(\partial \ln \underline{L}/\partial \tilde{\Theta})] \tag{1}$$

where $\underline{L} = f(\underline{\tilde{w}};\tilde{\Theta})$ and E is the expectation operator, then the Cramer-Rao inequality states (Van den Bos,1982) that

$$\text{cov}(\tilde{\Theta},\tilde{\Theta}) \geq \tilde{M}^{-1} \tag{2}$$

where $\text{cov}(\tilde{\Theta},\tilde{\Theta})$ is the kxk covariance matrix of $\tilde{\Theta}$. The Cramer-Rao inequality expresses that $\text{cov}(\tilde{\Theta},\tilde{\Theta})-\tilde{M}^{-1}$ is a positive semi-definite matrix. The right-hand term of the Cramer-Rao inequality defines the minimum variance bound (MVB) of any unbiased estimator.

Suppose we have the following model of observations:

$$\underline{w}_n=g(\tilde{x}_n;\tilde{\Theta})+\underline{v}_n \qquad n=1,....N \tag{3}$$

with $\underline{w}_n$ is an observation, $\tilde{x}_n$ are exactly known independent variables, $\tilde{\Theta}$ is the vector of unknown parameters, $\underline{v}_n$ are stochastic variables representing non-systematic errors and $g(\tilde{x}_n;\tilde{\Theta})$ is a function which describes the physical model. If the errors $\underline{v}_n$ are normally distributed with covariance $\tilde{V}=\text{cov}(\underline{\tilde{v}},\underline{\tilde{v}})$ then the joint probability density of $\underline{v}_1,......,\underline{v}_N$ is described by:

$$f_{\underline{\tilde{v}}}(\tilde{v})=(2\pi)^{-N/2}(\det\tilde{V})^{-1/2}\exp(-(1/2)\tilde{v}^T\tilde{V}^{-1}\tilde{v}) \tag{4}$$

Hence the probability density of $\underline{w}_1, \ldots, \underline{w}_N$ is:

$$f_{\underline{\tilde{w}}}(\tilde{w};\tilde{\Theta})=(2\pi)^{-N/2}(\det\tilde{V})^{-1/2}\det(\partial\tilde{v}/\partial\tilde{w})\exp(-(1/2)(\tilde{w}-\tilde{g})^T\tilde{V}^{-1}(\tilde{w}-\tilde{g})) \tag{5}$$

where: $\tilde{g}=(g(\tilde{x}_1;\tilde{\Theta}),.....,g(\tilde{x}_N;\tilde{\Theta}))^T$. Since $\underline{w}_n=g(\tilde{x}_n;\tilde{\Theta})+\underline{v}_n$ , $\partial\tilde{v}/\partial\tilde{w}=1$ and $\det(\partial\tilde{v}/\partial\tilde{w})=1$. Therefore

$$\ln\underline{L}=-(N/2)\ln(2\pi)-\ln(\det\tilde{V})^{-1/2}-(1/2)(\tilde{w}-\tilde{g})^T\tilde{V}(\tilde{w}-\tilde{g}) \tag{6}$$

Then from the definition of the information matrix $\tilde{M}$ and the Cramer-Rao inequality it follows that:

484

$$\text{cov}(\tilde{\Theta},\tilde{\Theta})\geq(E(\partial \underline{g}/\partial \tilde{\Theta})^T\tilde{V}^{-1}(\partial \underline{g}/\partial \tilde{\Theta}))^{-1} \qquad (7)$$

If the errors are independent and normally distributed with mean equal zero and standard deviation σ, then $\tilde{V}=\sigma^2 I$ and the Cramer-Rao inequality becomes:

$$\text{cov}(\tilde{\Theta},\tilde{\Theta})\geq\sigma^2(E(\partial \underline{g}/\partial \tilde{\Theta})^T(\partial \underline{g}/\partial \tilde{\Theta}))^{-1} \qquad (8)$$

In the next section this formula will be used to calculate the MVB on the covariance of any parameter estimated from an experiment.

Finally some remarks about estimators which achieve the minimum variance bound. A class of estimators which, at least asymptotically, achieves the MVB is the class of maximum likelihood (ML) estimators. These estimators maximize the function L. In practice ,however, ML estimators are not often used because they require a priori knowledge of the distribution function of the errors. Furthermore ML estimators are often very complicated and difficult to calculate. In practice, therefore, one usually resorts to non-linear least squares estimation techniques. According to equation 6, maximizing the function L with respect to Θ is equivalent to minimizing $(\underline{w}-\underline{g})^T\tilde{V}^{-1}(\underline{w}-\underline{g})$. Hence, if the errors are normally distributed with known covariance matrix, maximum likelihood estimation of the parameters is equivalent to weighted least squares estimation with the elements of the inverse covariance matrix as weights. The MVB, given in eq. 8, will thus be achieved asymptotically by a least squares estimator under the mentioned conditions on the errors ($\tilde{V}=\sigma^2 I$).

Some NMR experiments and the minimum variance bound

In NMR imaging ρ, $T_1$ and $T_2$ are usually calculated from a set of Partial Saturation Multiple Echo (PSME) or Inversion Recovery Multiple Echo (IRME) experiments. Besides, on many MRI machines a mixed sequence (MS), which is a combination of an IRME and a PSME experiment, is available for this purpose. The mentioned NMR experiments are schematically represented in table 1. The dependency of the signals on ρ, $T_1$ and $T_2$ is described by the formulae in table 1, which have been shown valid by Lee and Riederer (1986) on the assumption of ideal pulses, absence of flow and movement, uniexponential relaxation, zero transverse magnetization at the onset of each pulse cycle and negligible longitudinal magnetization at echo maxima.

In this section we elaborate the concept of the MVB for the parameters $T_1$ and $T_2$ derived from a PS experiment. A similar approach is valid for other NMR experiments. The parameter $T_1$ can be estimated from a Partial Saturation experiment with multiple waiting times $tw(i),i=1,....,nw$ and one particular echo time te. The physical model is decribed by:

$$g(tw(i);(\rho,T_1,T_2)^T)=\rho(1-\exp(-tw(i)/T_1))\exp(-te/T_2) \qquad i=1,....,nw \qquad (9)$$

In this experiment te has a fixed value, so $C=\rho.\exp(-te/T_2)$ is a constant and equation 9 becomes:

$$g(tw(i);(C,T_1)^T)=C(1-\exp(-tw(i)/T_1)) \qquad i=1,....,nw \qquad (10)$$

In a statistical model the errors are included:

$$\underline{w}_i=g(tw(i);(C,T_1)^T)+\underline{v}_i \qquad i=1,....,nw \qquad (11)$$

where $\underline{w}_i$ is an observation and $\underline{v}_i$ is a non-systematic error. The Cramer-Rao inequality states that $\text{cov}(\tilde{\Theta},\tilde{\Theta})\geq\tilde{M}^{-1}$ with in this case $\tilde{\Theta}=(C,T_1)^T$. We suppose that the errors are independent and normally distributed with mean equal zero and standard deviation σ. Then the information matrix $\tilde{M}$ is (see

Table 1: Schematic representation and signal formula of a partial saturation, an inversion recovery and a mixed sequence experiment with data collection by the spin echo technique.

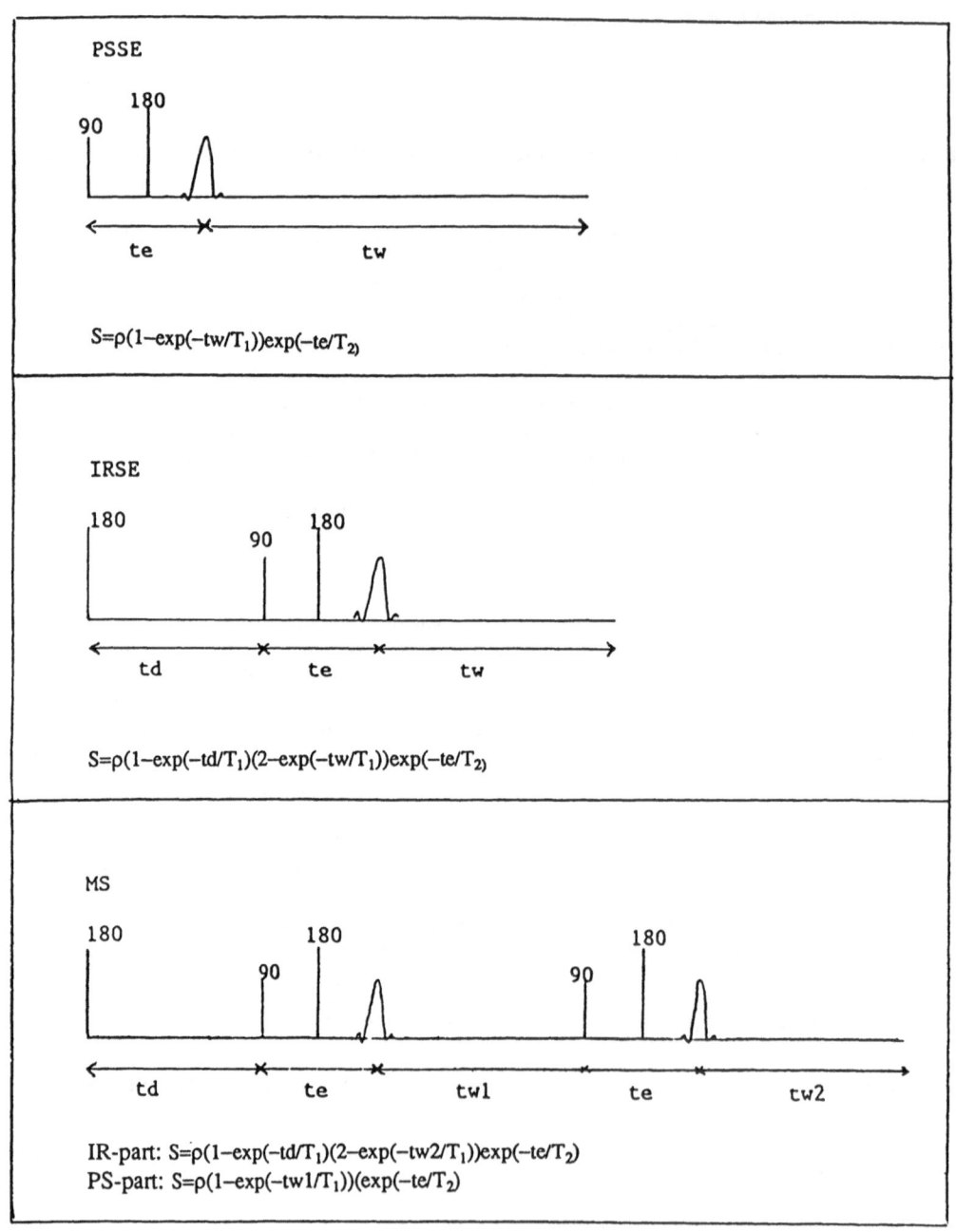

PSSE

$S=\rho(1-\exp(-tw/T_1))\exp(-te/T_2)$

IRSE

$S=\rho(1-\exp(-td/T_1))(2-\exp(-tw/T_1))\exp(-te/T_2)$

MS

IR-part: $S=\rho(1-\exp(-td/T_1))(2-\exp(-tw2/T_1))\exp(-te/T_2)$
PS-part: $S=\rho(1-\exp(-tw1/T_1))(\exp(-te/T_2))$

eq. 8):

$$\tilde{M}=\sigma^2(E(\partial\tilde{y}/\partial\tilde{\Theta})^T(\partial\tilde{y}/\partial\tilde{\Theta}))$$

(12)

The elements of the matrix $(\partial g/\partial \Theta)$ follow from eq. 10:

$$\partial g(tw(i))/\partial C = 1 - \exp(-tw(i)/T_1) \tag{13}$$

$$\partial g(tw(i))/\partial T_1 = -(C/T_1^2).tw(i).\exp(-tw(i)/T_1) \tag{14}$$

The information matrix becomes:

$$\bar{M} = \sigma^2 \begin{bmatrix} \sum_{i=1}^{nw}(\partial g_i/\partial C)^2 & \sum_{i=1}^{nw}(\partial g_i/\partial C)(\partial g_i/\partial T_1) \\ \sum_{i=1}^{nw}(\partial g_i/\partial C)(\partial g_i/\partial T_1) & \sum_{i=1}^{nw}(\partial g_i/\partial T_1)^2 \end{bmatrix} \tag{15}$$

where $g(tw(i))$ has been abbreviated to $g_i$. The diagonal elements of the inverse information matrix $\bar{M}^{-1}$ are the minimum variance bounds on the parameters C and $T_1$. Obviously, these variance bounds depend on the particular choice of the waiting times. This dependency is further examined in the next section.

The parameter $T_2$ can be estimated from a PS experiment with a particular waiting time tw and multiple echo times te(i),i=1,....,ne. The statistical model is described by :

$$\underline{w}_i = g(te(i);(C,T_2)^T) + \underline{v}_i \qquad i=1,...,ne \tag{16}$$

$$\text{where: } g(te(i);(C,T_2)^T) = C.\exp(-te(i)/T_2) \tag{17}$$

$$C = \rho(1 - \exp(-tw/T_1)) \tag{18}$$

The elements of the matrix $(\partial g/\partial \Theta)$ with $\Theta = (C,T_2)^T$ are:

$$\partial g(te(i))/\partial C = \exp(-te(i)/T_2) \tag{19}$$

$$\partial g(te(i))/\partial T_2 = (C/T_2^2).te(i).\exp(-te(i)/T_2) \tag{20}$$

The information matrix $\bar{M}$ becomes:

$$\bar{M} = \sigma^2 \begin{bmatrix} \sum_{i=1}^{ne}(\partial g_i/\partial C)^2 & \sum_{i=1}^{ne}(\partial g_i/\partial C)(\partial g_i/\partial T_2) \\ \sum_{i=1}^{ne}(\partial g_i/\partial C)(\partial g_i/\partial T_2) & \sum_{i=1}^{ne}(\partial g_i/\partial T_2)^2 \end{bmatrix} \tag{21}$$

and the diagonal elements of $\bar{M}^{-1}$ are the lower bounds on the variances of the parameters C and $T_2$.

Next we generalize the above mentioned models of a PS experiment to a model of a PS experiment with multiple waiting times tw(i),i=1,...,nw and multiple echo times te(j),j=1,...,ne:

$$\underline{w}_{i,j} = g(tw(i),te(j);(\rho,T_1,T_2)^T) + \underline{v}_{i,j} \qquad i=1,...,nw; j=1,...,ne \tag{22}$$

$$\text{where: } g(tw(i),te(j);(\rho,T_1,T_2)^T) = \rho(1-\exp(-tw(i)/T_1))\exp(-te(j)/T_2) \tag{23}$$

This experiment enables a simultaneous determination of $\rho$, $T_1$ and $T_2$. The derivatives of g to the parameters $\rho$, $T_1$ and $T_2$ follow from eq. 23:

$$\partial g_{i,j}/\partial C = (1-\exp(-tw(i)/T_1))\exp(-te(j)/T_2) \tag{24}$$

$$\partial g_{i,j}/\partial T_1 = -(\rho/T_1^2).tw(i).\exp(-tw(i)/T_1)\exp(-te(j)/T_2) \tag{25}$$

$$\partial g_{i,j}/\partial T_2 = (\rho/T_2^2)(1-\exp(-tw(i)/T_1)).te(j).\exp(-te(j)/T_2) \tag{26}$$

where $g(tw(i),te(j))$ has been abbreviated to $g_{i,j}$. The information matrix becomes:

$$\tilde{M} = \sigma^2 \begin{bmatrix} \sum\limits_{i=1}^{nw}\sum\limits_{j=1}^{ne}(\partial g_{i,j}/\partial\rho)^2 & \sum\limits_{i=1}^{nw}\sum\limits_{j=1}^{ne}(\partial g_{i,j}/\partial\rho)(\partial g_{i,j}/\partial T_1) & \sum\limits_{i=1}^{nw}\sum\limits_{j=1}^{ne}(\partial g_{i,j}/\partial\rho)(\partial g_{i,j}/\partial T_2) \\ \sum\limits_{i=1}^{nw}\sum\limits_{j=1}^{ne}(\partial g_{i,j}/\partial\rho)(\partial g_{i,j}/\partial T_1) & \sum\limits_{i=1}^{nw}\sum\limits_{j=1}^{ne}(\partial g_{i,j}/\partial T_1)^2 & \sum\limits_{i=1}^{nw}\sum\limits_{j=1}^{ne}(\partial g_{i,j}/\partial T_1)(\partial g_{i,j}/\partial T_2) \\ \sum\limits_{i=1}^{nw}\sum\limits_{j=1}^{ne}(\partial g_{i,j}/\partial\rho)(\partial g_{i,j}/\partial T_2) & \sum\limits_{i=1}^{nw}\sum\limits_{j=1}^{ne}(\partial g_{i,j}/\partial T_1)(\partial g_{i,j}/\partial T_2) & \sum\limits_{i=1}^{nw}\sum\limits_{j=1}^{ne}(\partial g_{i,j}/\partial T_2)^2 \end{bmatrix} \tag{27}$$

The diagonal elements of $\tilde{M}^{-1}$ are the minimum variance bounds on the parameters $\rho$, $T_1$, and $T_2$. As stated before, the method employed for the calculation of the MVB is equally valid for other types of NMR experiments.

## PRECISION OF $\rho$, $T_1$ AND $T_2$ AS A FUNCTION OF SEQUENCE TYPE AND SEQUENCE TIMINGS

Once the MVB on the precision has been adopted as a criterion for achievable precision, it is a straightforward task to explore the efficacy of various experimental set-ups in realizing certain parameter estimation objectives. Sequence type and timings which yield a specified precision in $\rho$, $T_1$ and $T_2$ or which provide optimum precision in a specified measurement time can now in principle be determined. Not surprisingly the general lay-out of such a study is largely similar to the lay-out of such studies in conventional NMR relaxation measurements (see e.g. Weiss et al.,1980). Minor adaptations are only necessary to accommodate for data acquisition by spin echoes and the stringent time constraints characteristic of clinical NMR.

In designing a practical experiment many choices have to be made, such as the total measurement time, sequence type and sequence timings, number of echoes, echo times and the range of $T_1$ and $T_2$ values for which optimum precision is desired. This large number of degrees of freedom makes it virtually impossible to study the effect of experiment design in complete generality. We therefore restrict our attention to the type of experiments commonly utilized in quantitative NMR imaging. In order to allow a comparison of experiments in terms of precision in the parameters achieved per unit time, a fixed measurement time is assumed for the collection of the source images. Further the noise in the source images is assumed to be independent of the type of experiment and all comparisons are made for equal signal to noise ratios, only corrected for the number of times that an experiment can be repeated in the allotted amount of time. The different experimental set-ups are evaluated for the clinically relevant ranges of $T_1$ and $T_2$ ($T_1$: 200-1800ms, $T_2$: 50-150ms).

### Precision of the parameter $T_1$, estimated from PSSE, IRSE or MS experiments

The parameter $T_1$ can be calculated from various sets of NMR experiments, e.g. a partial saturation spin echo (PSSE) experiment, an inversion recovery spin echo (IRSE) experiment or a mixed sequence (MS). For these experiments the minimum variance bound on the precision of $T_1$ can be calculated as explained for the PS sequence in a previous section (eq. 15).

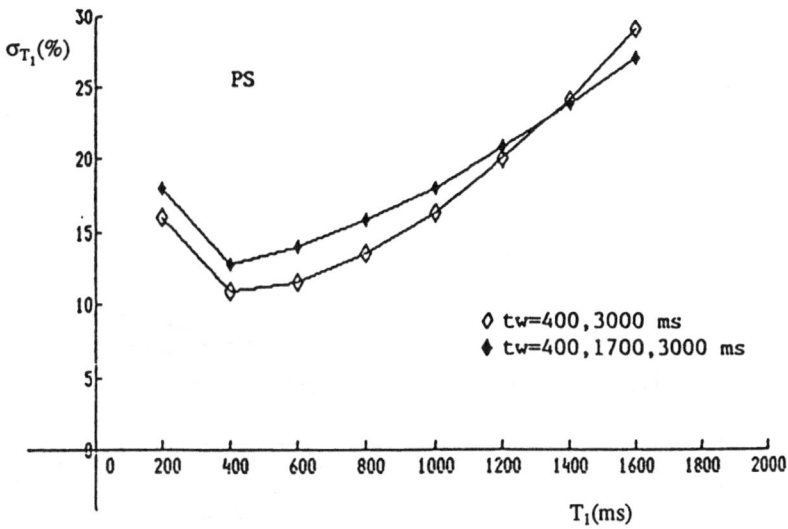

Figure 1: The Cramer-Rao lower bound on the relative precision of $T_1$ as a function of $T_1$ for PSSE experiments with different sets of waiting times.

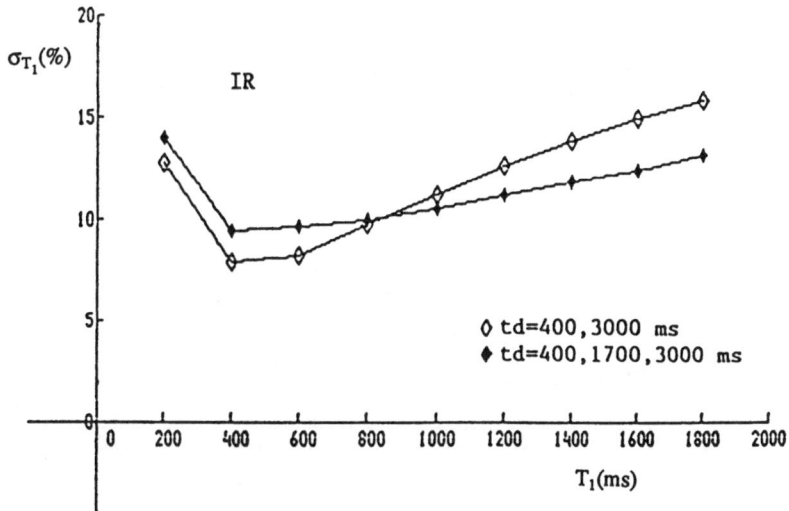

Figure 2: The Cramer-Rao lower bound on the relative precision of $T_1$ as a function of $T_1$ for IRSE experiments with different sets of delay times. The waiting time is: tw=3000ms.

In case of the PSSE experiment the waiting time tw is the independent variable. We choose the longest waiting time to be a few times the largest relevant $T_1$ value, i.e. when relaxation is nearly complete and the signal to noise ratio is nearly maximal. This remark is also valid with regard to the choice of the waiting times in the IRSE and MS experiments. As illustrated by figure 1 the shortest waiting time of the PSSE experiment determines the $T_1$ value, for which the standard deviation is minimal. Figure 1 further shows that choosing three waiting times instead of two gives only a slight broadening of the range of $T_1$ values for which the experiment is optimal. Improvement of the precision by choosing more waiting times is offset by the fact that the number of times

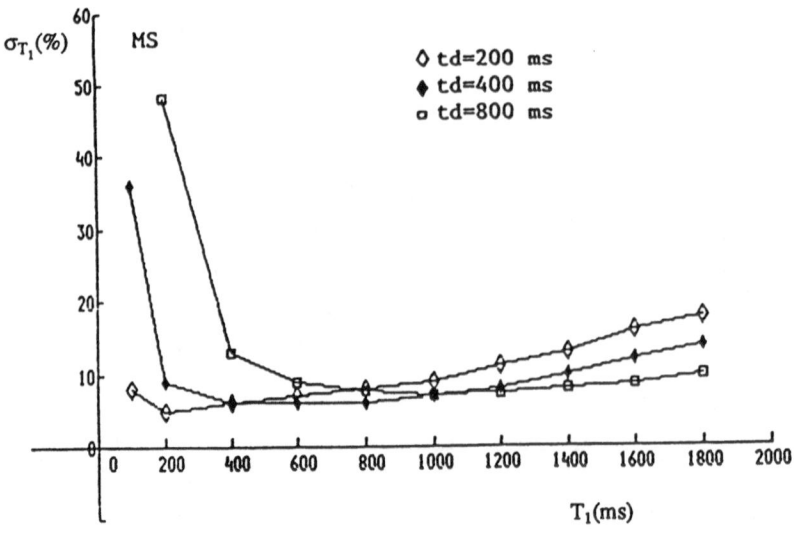

Figure 3: The Cramer-Rao lower bound on the relative precision of $T_1$ as a function of $T_1$ for MS experiments with different delay times. The waiting times are: tw1=1000ms and tw2=3000ms.

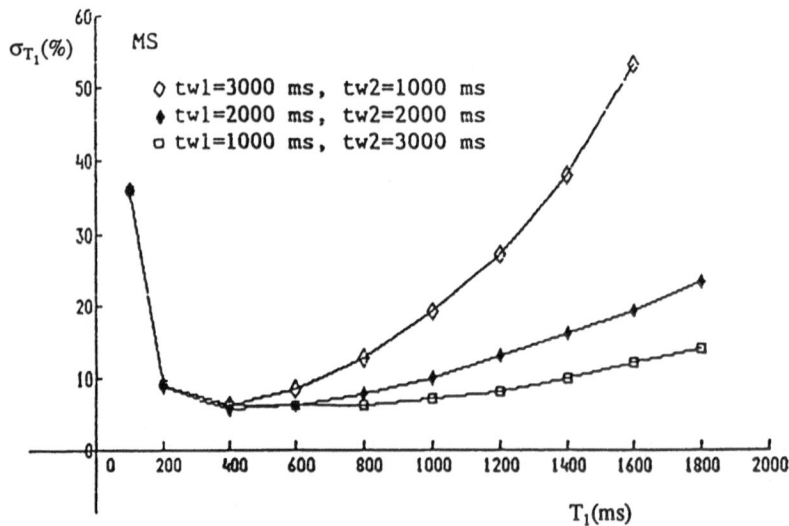

Figure 4: The Cramer-Rao lower bound on the relative precision of $T_1$ as a function of $T_1$ for MS experiments with different sets of waiting times. The delay time is: td=400ms.

that a set of experiments can be repeated in the allotted amount of measurement time is reduced.

In case of the IRSE experiment two parameters, the delay time td and the waiting time tw, can be varied (see table 1). Figure 2 illustrates the effect of varying the delay times. The experiments are optimal for a range of $T_1$ values around 400ms, which is the value of the shortest delay time. Choosing three delay times instead of two produces a broadening of the range of $T_1$ values for which the experiment is optimal.

490

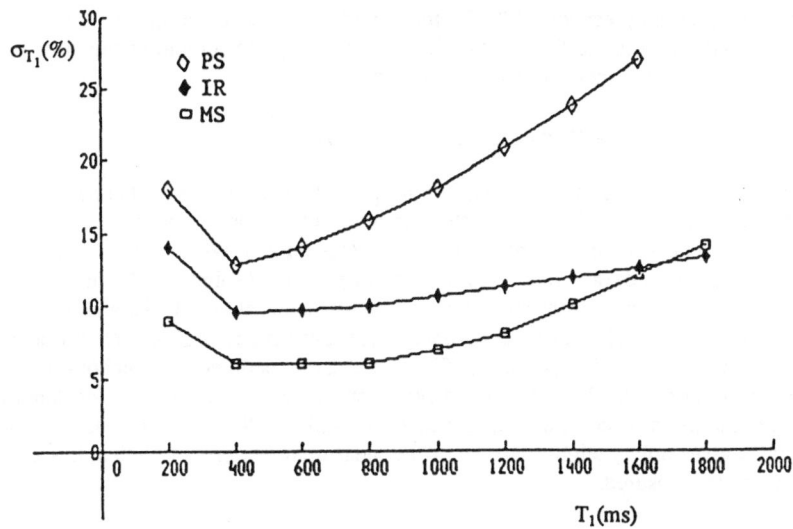

Figure 5: The Cramer-Rao lower bound on the relative precision of $T_1$ as a function of $T_1$ for a PSSE, an IRSE and a MS experiment.
(◊)PSSE/tw=400,1700,3000ms,
(♦)IRSE/td=400,1700,3000ms/tw=3000ms
(◻)MS/td=400ms,tw1=1000ms,tw2=3000ms

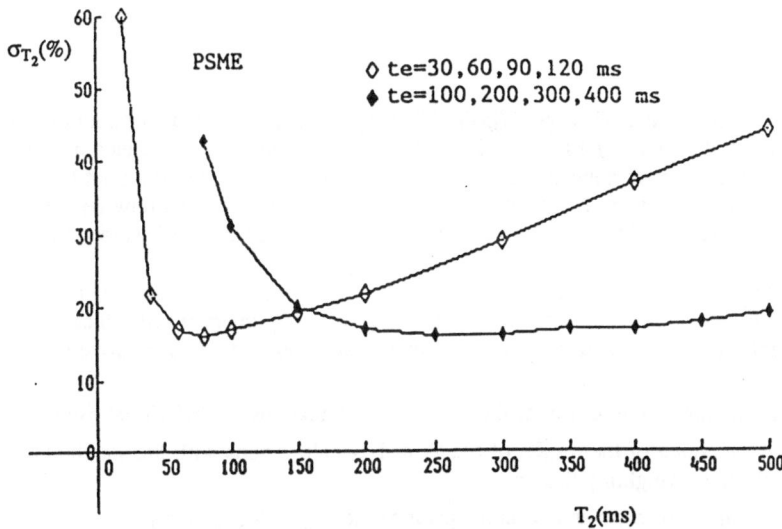

Figure 6: The Cramer-Rao lower bound on the relative precision of $T_2$ as a function of $T_2$ for two PSME experiments with different echo times. The waiting time is: tw=3000ms.

In case of the MS experiment there are three parameters which can be varied independently. These parameters are the delay time td in the IR-part of the sequence and the waiting times tw1 and tw2 (see table 1). Figure 3 illustrates the effect of the delay time td. The range of $T_1$ values with minimal standard deviation shifts to larger $T_1$ values as the delay times increase. For the range of relevant $T_1$ values between 200 and 1800ms td=400ms appears a reasonable choice. The precision of $T_1$ for several ratios of tw1 and tw2 is depicted in figure 4, which illustrates that the ratio tw2/tw1 equal to 3 is about optimal.

491

In figure 5 we plot the precision of $T_1$ for the experiments discussed above. The figure illustrates that, in comparison with the PSSE and IRSE, the MS experiment allows the most precise estimation of the parameter $T_1$ per unit experiment time.

## Precision of the parameter $T_2$, estimated from a PSME experiment

The parameter $T_2$ can be calculated from a multiple echo sequence. For this purpose the PS experiment is most efficient. We have calculated the minimum variance bound of $T_2$ for this experiment with one particular waiting time and four echoes (see eq 21). We restrict ourselves to equidistant echoes, because these are commonly used in practice. In figure 6 the precision of the estimated parameter $T_2$ achieved from an experiment with echoes at 30, 60, 90 and 120ms is compared to the precision achieved from an experiment with four echoes at 100, 200, 300 and 400ms. For the range of clinically relevant $T_2$ values (50-150ms) the experiment with echoes at 30, 60, 90 and 120ms is the better choice. To improve the precision for longer $T_2$ values (body fluids) one could extend the number of echoes, e.g. eight echoes at 30,60,...,240ms. The extension of the number of echoes gives only a slight increase of the measurement time. In clinical practice usually up to four echoes are measured.

## PRECISION IN $\rho$, $T_1$ AND $T_2$ AS A FUNCTION OF DATA ANALYSIS METHOD

In clinical practice $\rho$, $T_1$ and $T_2$ images are usually obtained from a set of partial saturation, saturation recovery or inversion recovery experiments with multiple echoes and multiple repetition times. For a partial saturation experiment with multiple echoes te(j),j=1,...,ne and multiple waiting times tw(i)=trep(i)–te(ne),i=1,...,nw, for instance , the relation between the source images is expressed by:

$$S(i,j)=\rho(1-ew(i))e(j) \tag{28}$$

with ew(i)=exp(–tw(i)/$T_1$) and e(j)=exp(–te(j)/$T_2$). This type of experiment, a slight modification is required for saturation recovery and inversion recovery experiments, thus yields a ne x nw matrix of images in which the rows contain the $T_2$ information and the columns bring out the $T_1$ dependence of the signal amplitudes. $T_1$, $T_2$ and their estimated uncertainties can now be calculated for each column and each row in the datamatrix by applying a two parameter least-squares fit.

In practice, $T_1$ and $T_2$ are usually calculated from the row and the column with the highest signal to noise ratio. Obviously this procedure does not produce optimum results since only part of the available information is utulized. Several methods can be envisaged to improve upon this situation:

I.    Simple averaging of the results of the $T_1$ and $T_2$ calculations for individual rows and columns

II.   Weighted averaging of the results of the $T_1$ and $T_2$ calculations with the standard errors of the individual fits as weighting factors

III.  Simple averaging of rows and columns prior to the regression analysis

IV.   Weighted averaging of rows and columns prior to the regression analysis

V.    A simultaneous three-parameter fit to the ne x nw observed signal values for each pixel

For a given experimental set-up the improvement in the precision of the $T_1$ and $T_2$ calculations resulting from methods I through V can be evaluated quantitatively (Bakker and De Graaf,1987) and compared with the reference method discussed above. Figure 7 shows the results for the $T_1$ calculation from a partial saturation experiment with ne=4 and nw=5. Weighted averaging of source images prior to regression analysis (method IV), weighted averaging of intermediate results (method II) and a simultaneous three-parameter fit (method V) provide optimum precision for the calculation of $T_1$ and $T_2$ in all cases. Under the assumption of normally distributed noise N(0,$\sigma$) it can be shown that the least squares estimators of methods II, IV and V are maximum likelihood

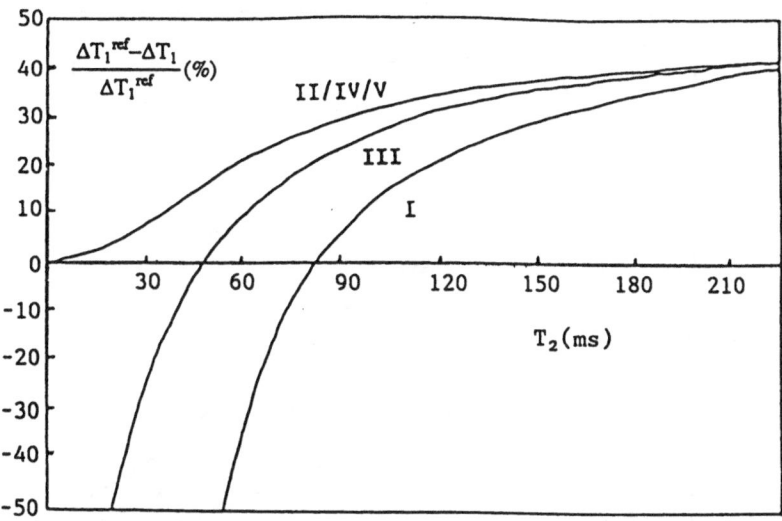

Figure 7: Improvement of the precision of the $T_1$ calculation as a function of $T_2$ for the data reduction methods I-V for a PS experiment with 5 waiting times and 4 echoes.

estimators, which achieve the minimum variance bound (see eq. 27). The differences in performance of the methods is most conspicious for short $T_2$ and long $T_1$ values. Although mathematically equivalent to methods II and V, method IV is the method of choice for computational efficiency and robustness. Since averaging is performed prior to data reduction, low signal levels at long echo times or short repetition times do not corrupt the precision of the results in this method. A distinct advantage of the three parameter fit is the calculation of $\rho$ on equal footing with $T_1$ and $T_2$.

ISO-PRECISION DISPLAY OF PARAMETER IMAGES

In clinical NMR, attention is usually focused on the soft tissues (intermediate $T_1$ and $T_2$ values). In consequence, the set-up of quantitative studies is generally chosen such as to provide greatest precision for this intermediate range of values to the detriment of longer and shorter $T_1$ and $T_2$ values (fluid collections, fatty tissues). This practice is exemplified by figure 8 showing the estimated precision $p_{T_1} = 1/\Delta T_1$ of $T_1$ calculated from a double spin-echo experiment with echo times te(1)=30 and te(2)=90ms and waiting times tw(1)=500 and tw(2)=2000ms (the so-called minimal dataset). As expected, greatest precision is achieved in the soft tissue range with deteriorating results towards longer and shorter values.

The question now arises how to take full advantage of the type of information supplied by figure 8 in displaying parameter images. Obviously this information is completely ignored when $T_1$ or $T_2$ images are displayed linearly. A better approach would therefore be to define a gray scale $g=g(\Theta)$ in which the density of the gray levels is proportional to the precision of the displayed parameter values:

$$dg(\Theta)/d\Theta = p(\Theta) \tag{29}$$

The appropriate gray scale transformation is readily found by numerical integration of eq. 29. Figure 9 shows the result $g(T_1)$ for the minimal dataset defined above, assuming $T_1$ equal $10 \cdot T_2$. This transformation indeed stretches the gray scale for the relatively precise intermediate $T_1$ values while

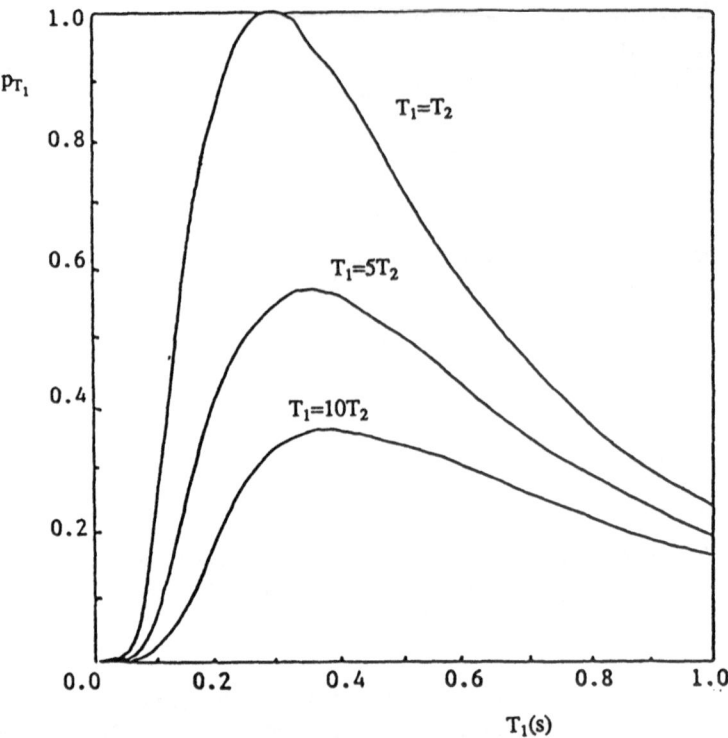

Figure 8: Normalized precision of $T_1$, calculated from the minimal dataset, as a function of $T_1$ for various $T_1/T_2$ ratios.

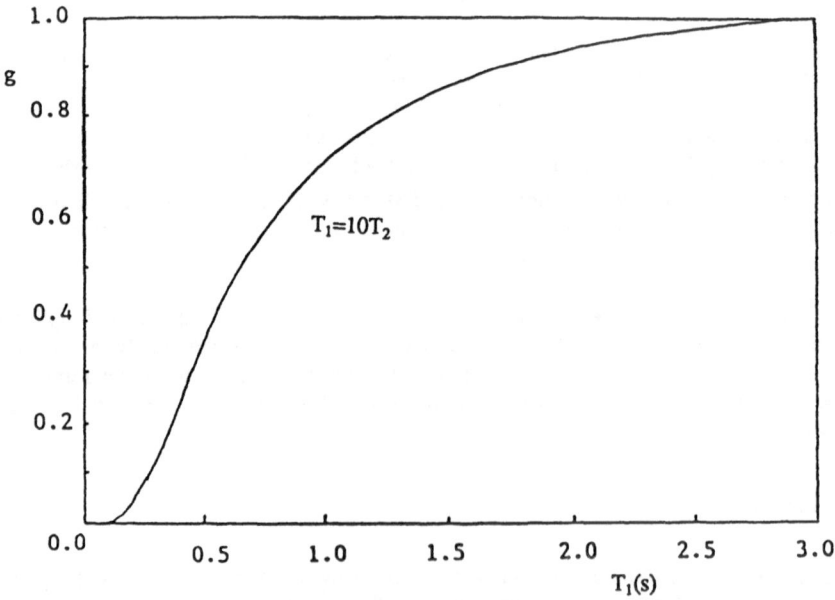

Figure 9: Gray scale in arbitrary units for iso-precision display of $T_1$ images obtained from the minimal dataset (assuming $T_1=10.T_2$).

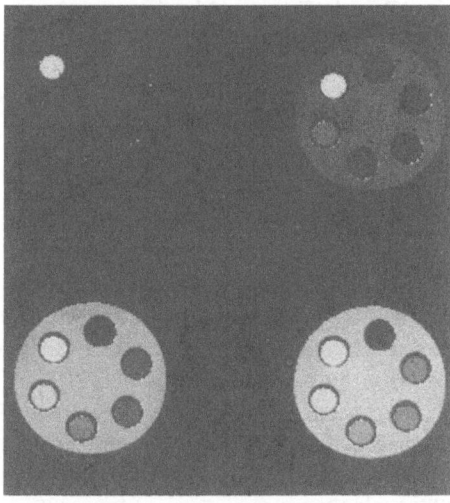

Figure 10: Windowed linear (upper left 0-100, upper right 0-50, bottom left 0-20) and iso-precision display of a $T_2$ image of a phantom containing tubes with $Mn^{2+}$ doped aqueous solutions with $T_2$ values ranging from 100 to 400ms and a tube of pure water.

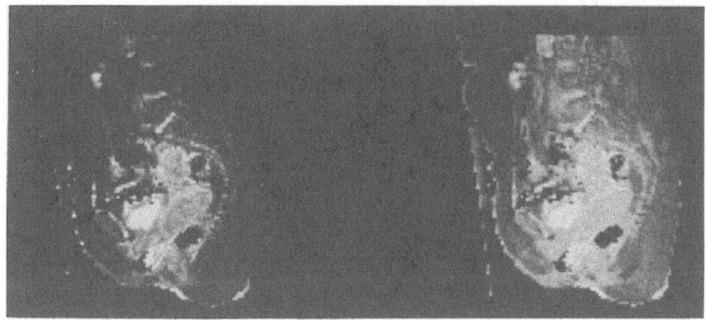

Figure 11: Linear and iso-precision display of a $T_1$ image of a sagittal slice of a patient with a carcinoma of the cervix uteri.

compressing it for longer and shorter $T_1$'s.

Figure 10 shows the linear and iso-precision display of a $T_2$ image of a phantom containing 4 tubes with $Mn^{2+}$ doped aqueous solutions with $T_2$ values ranging from 100 to 400ms, a tube with pure water and an empty tube. As shown by the figure upper left the range of $T_2$ values is too large to allow differentation of low $T_2$ values from the background and from each other when displayed linearly. Interactive window and level control (upper right and bottom left) improve upon this situation, but introduce a subjective element. Iso-precision display (bottom right) allows visualization of any significant differences of $T_2$ within an object in a single image. Figure 11 shows the linear and iso precision display of a $T_1$ image of a sagittal slice of a patient with a carcinoma of the cervix uteri as an example from clinical practice.

From figure 8 it is clear that the proposed gray scale transformation merely takes into account precision in an approximate way. Due to the $T_2$ dependence of the $T_1$ analysis and the $T_1$

dependence of the $T_2$ analysis, $\Delta T_1$ and $\Delta T_2$ can not be determined uniquely unless an additional assumption about the $T_1/T_2$ ratio is provided.

Currently it is being investigated how the iso-precision representation of parameter images advocated here should be weighed against other display strategies.

REFERENCES

Bakker, C.J.G. and De Graaf, C.N. (1987). Precision in calculated $\rho$, $T_1$ and $T_2$ images as a function of data analysis method, Magn. Res. Imaging, 5, in press.

Bos, A. van den (1982). Parameter Estimation, in: Handbook of Measurement Science, P.H. Sydenham (ed.), John Wiley & Sons Ltd., London, 331-377.

Lee, J.N. and Riederer, S.J. (1986). A modified saturation recovery approximation for multiple spin-echo sequences, Magn. Res. Med., 3, 132-134.

Lende, O. R. van der (1985). Enkele numerieke en statistische aspecten van de bepaling van de longitudinale relaxatietijd $T_1$ uit IR metingen, Internal Report Technical University Delft, Delft

Weiss, G.H., Gupta, R.K., Ferretti, J.A. and Becker, E.D. (1980). The Choice of Optimal Parameters for Measurement of Spin-Lattice Relaxation Times. I. Mathematical Formulation, Journ. Magn. Res., 37, 369-379.

# Applications 2: Nuclear Medicine, SPECT, PET

# THE REALITY AND MEANING OF PHYSIOLOGICAL FACTORS

Martin Šámal, Helena Sůrová, Miroslav Kárný, Eva Maříková,
Petr Pěnička, and Zdeněk Dienstbier

Charles University
and the Czechoslovak Academy of Sciences
Prague, Czechoslovakia

## INTRODUCTION

The term "physiological factor" was introduced by Bazin et al. (1979) for a time-activity curve detected above the separate compartment of a radio-pharmaceutical in the body. Considering formally the elementary time-activity curves recorded in dynamic radionuclide study as vectors then the physiological factors can be regarded as a non-orthogonal base of the corresponding vector space. Under certain restrictive conditions this base can be found by the methods of factor analysis.

An alternative idea of physiological factor representing the image of the separate compartment was introduced by our group in 1985 to overcome some drawbacks of the former conception (Šámal et al., 1986 a; 1987). Although formally equivalent (the physiological factors are considered to form a non-orthogonal base in vector space of vectors-images) the latter idea offers several advantages in practice: the classic procedures of factor analysis can be applied more conveniently, the limiting conditions formulated more strictly and the interpretation of results carried out more clearly.

The aim of our contribution is to analyse the concepts of physiological factors from two points of view: (1) what features in fact are represented by factors, and (2) what precision can be expected in their estimation. The relevance of these criteria was emphasized by Goris (1982) who stated that: "It is preferable to think of functional or parametric images as particular forms of image processing that share one common characteristic: the procedure involves feature enhancement or information extraction of the original dynamic data and of necessity leads to concomitant information loss. Generally, the success of the operation depends on the value of the extracted features and the precision by which it can be computed." The following problems will be discussed in order to evaluate the reality and meaning of physiological factors: an underlying model, data preparation, the extraction and rotation of factors and their interpretation.

## BASIC MODEL

A basic model of factor analysis, its relation to dynamic radionuclide studies and possible interpretations are discussed in this section.

## Factor Analysis

Factor analysis is based on an assumption that the variables measured on a set of objects are the external manifestation of latent variables called factors. Formally, each variable can be expressed as a linear combination of factors

$$Z = G F + \overline{E} \tag{1}$$

where Z is the data matrix (m,n) containing measurements of m variables on n objects, G is the matrix (m,k) of coefficients relating m variables to k factors (k is less than m), and F is the matrix (k,n) of factors. The entries of an error matrix $\overline{E}$ express both the noise and the modelling errors. By factor analysis the number of factors affecting the real data can be estimated, the relationship between latent factors and measured variables specified and the values of factors on each object computed (Harman, 1960; Überla, 1971).

## Factor Analysis of Dynamic Radionuclide Study

The dynamic radionuclide study can be regarded as the (m,n) data matrix Y containing m images having n pixels each. The entries of Y are formed by count rates detected in time-interval i (i = 1, ..., m) and picture element (pixel) j (j = 1, ..., n). The formal equivalence of rows and columns in data matrix Y allows for choice either the time-activity curves or the images to be measured as variables. In the former case the objects are represented by individual time intervals (images) while in the latter the objects correspond to the individual pixels. Both of these ways are seemingly equal and lead to equivalent factors in an errorless case. Nevertheless, in practice the problems to be solved during factor analysis and the factors extracted by respective methods differ from each other.

In a compact way the data matrix can be expressed as a linear combination

$$Y = C V + \overline{E} \tag{2}$$

where C is the matrix (m,k) containing concentrations of a radionuclide in time interval i per unit volume of the compartment s (s = 1, ..., k), and V is the matrix (k,n) containing information about the volume of the compartment s under the area of pixel j. The equations (1) and (2) are formally equal so that the model of factor analysis can be used to analyse the dynamic study without further transformation.

Due to the product form of the model the factors are considered to be homogeneous. It means that the spatial structures corresponding to factors (regardless of their form of images or time-activity curves) express the same temporal variation of count rate at all their points. The postulated homogeneity of compartments is the only and reasonable price paid for the simplicity of the model after which the analysis can be executed without some stronger preliminary assumptions usually inaccessible in practice. The interpretation of (2) given above fits better for non-equilibrium studies in which the radionuclide concentration is the time-dependent variable. However, considering entries of C as formal coefficients reflecting the volume changes of compartments, the model (2) can be accepted also for equilibrium studies. As it was shown by Pavel and Briandet (1983), even in the pixels on the periphery of cardiac ventricles the time-activity curves do not follow an "all or nothing" response but reveal a similarity to the global ventricular curve.

In real conditions the decomposition (1) of the data matrix Z cannot be performed completely. The differences between the measured data and those reconstructed with the help of matrices G and F are contained in an (m,n) residual matrix E. In contrast to analysis of principal components, in factor analysis each residual is presumed to be composed of two distinct parts: the true measurement error and the specificity of each variable which cannot be explained by factors. In factor analysis of single dynamic study the specificity of variables is considered to be zero. By other words, it is presumed that the substantial portion of variance of each variable is shared by factors and the residuals are both randomly distributed and not correlated mutually nor with the factors. From this point of view the factor analysis of single dynamic study can be regarded as a special case of factor analysis which is very close to the analysis of principal components.

## Descriptive Applications of Factor Analysis

The factor analysis has been often performed on a series of dynamic studies in order to extract time-activity curves reflecting more general features corresponding to physiologically normal function and to the different degrees of pathological conditions (Schmidlin, 1979; Oppenheim and Appledorn, 1979; Houston et al., 1979). In principle, the physiological factors cannot be found by this approach mainly for two reasons: (1) it does not take into account the specific factors (i.e. the factors specific for respective individual studies), and (2) it does not transform primary factors to the position suitable for interpretation. However, the method offers good results useful for the purposes of data reduction, formal description and classification of time-activity curves.

## DATA PREPARATION

In principle, no special preparation of dynamic study data is necessary for factor analysis. This is due mainly to the fact that all the variables (regardless of their form of the images or time-activity curves) are measured in the same units of count rate per pixel and time interval. Therefore the direct decomposition of data matrix can be performed to find both its basic structure and primary factors (Horst, 1965; Jöreskog et al., 1976). However, in practice the data are transformed either by centering and/or by normalization of variables in order to facilitate the execution of some steps during analysis.

## Standardization of Variables

The most frequent procedure used for preliminary transformation of data in factor analysis is their standardization

$$z(i,j) = [y(i,j) - \overline{y}(i)]/s(i) \tag{3}$$

where $\overline{y}(i)$ is the arithmetic mean of variables $y(i,.)$ and $s(i)$ is the corresponding standard deviation. Mean values of standardized variables are equal to zero and their standard deviations are equal to unity. If the factor analysis is performed on the correlation matrix containing the correlations between the variables (as it is carried out by us) the standardization (3) is made automatically. The procedure gives greater weights to variables with lower variance. However, the results of factor analysis have been shown to be invariant to this transformation (Jöreskog, 1963; Blahuš, 1985).

An addition of a constant to all the values of one variable or the multiplication of its values by a constant does not change the standardization and therefore does not alter the results of factor analysis. Considering the variables as the images, the spatially homogeneous background count rate does not modify the results of analysis regardless of its temporal variance. However, when the spatially heterogeneous but temporally constant background

501

is simulated by tissue crosstalk (as it is usual in equilibrium studies) only its minimum level can be considered as the additive constant while the greater values of background enter the factor analysis.

## Benzécri's Normalization

The character of scintigraphic data (their non-negativity and discreteness) makes them suitable especially for the normalization given by Benzécri (1969). This procedure suppresses the differences between the variables and objects. It converts count rates $y(i,j)$ into the fractions $y(i,j)/S$ where S is the sum of all the elements in data matrix. These fractions can be treated formally as the probabilities. Using this transformation, Benzécri modified the factor analysis to so-called analysis of correspondences which was formerly used for the evaluation of both static and dynamic radionuclide studies (DiPaola et al., 1975; Schmidlin and Rösel, 1975; Schmidlin, 1979; Houston, 1986). The procedure is convenient for descriptive purposes. It is suitable also for the data reduction and noise filtration while the possibility of objective interpretation of extracted factors can hardly be expected.

## Normalization of Curves

The procedures of factor analysis based on the concept of variables and factors as time-activity curves use their normalization either to the unit sum of their elements (Barber, 1980; DiPaola et al., 1982; Houston, 1986) or to the unit length of the vector formed by their elements (Nijran and Barber, 1985). The former procedure is further completed by an additional subtraction of the mean normalized curve in order to reduce the dimensions of the examined vector space by one and to allow the function of the so-called apex-seeking algorithm. In fact this step corresponds to the centering of rows in the data matrix with previously normalized columns.

The normalization of curves to the unit sum of their elements is not influenced by the multiplication of curves by a constant. All the other changes in the original data including an addition of a constant either to rows or columns enter into the factor analysis. The procedure may sometimes give too much weight to the curves containing no significant information. Occasionally, improper curves must be removed before the analysis (Cavailloles et al., 1984).

## Preliminary Reduction of Data and Noise Rejection

In dependence on the nature of factors the analysis of matrices $Z Z'$ or $Z' Z$ is to be performed (in this paragraph, Z is considered to be a general normalized data matrix). Both of the matrices given above have the same positive eigenvalues. Consequently, in an errorless case, they contain an equivalent information about the data structure. However, the matrices differ from each other with respect to noise-rejection properties, the matrix $Z' Z$ of the order n making the results more sensitive to errors. Moreover, this matrix is too large to be suitable for direct decomposition. The problem is solved by an artificial reduction of data (Bazin et al., 1979): the pixels are grouped into rectangles of different size (but, obviously, of the same size in one study) which are then regarded as the elementary areas. The advantages of this solution are considerable shortcut of computational demands and increased robustness of the procedure. However, the new vectors of curves are found in arbitrary positions given by clustering of pixels. Although the factors forming the base of corresponding vector space can be considered to be the same regardless of clustering, their estimation in practice will differ in different vector spaces. On the other hand, our approach leads naturally to analysis of the (m,m) matrix $Z Z'$ which is more robust with respect to errors, easier for computation and independent of subjective clustering.

# FACTOR EXTRACTION

The common procedure used for extraction of factors is the method of principal components. In this section, its theoretical background is given and the problems of number of factors to be extracted and that of the factor enhancement are discussed.

## Basic Structure of Matrix

The solution of equation (1) can be performed using the concept of basic structure or singular analysis of a matrix (Eckart and Young, 1936; Johnson, 1963; Jöreskog at al., 1976). A brief review will help us to understand better the solved problems. Let H be (m,n) matrix with m less than n and with the rank r (naturally less than or equal to m). Such a matrix can be explicitly expressed as

$$H = K D M' \tag{4}$$

where K and M are (m,r) and (n,r) matrices respectively, satisfying relations

$$K'K = I, \quad M'M = I$$

where I is the identity matrix of the order r. The matrix D is the (r,r) diagonal matrix. Its diagonal elements d(s,s) are called the singular values of matrix H. It can be shown that both of the products H H' and H'H have r identical positive eigenvalues

$$d(1,1)^2, d(2,2)^2, \ldots, d(r,r)^2$$

with corresponding eigenvectors represented by columns of matrices K and M respectively. From the point of view of factor analysis the most important consequence of the relation (4) is that the new matrices $\bar{H}$, $\bar{H}\bar{H}'$ and $\bar{H}'\bar{H}$ with the rank k less than r can be computed using only the first k columns of matrices K and M and the first k rows and columns of D

$$\bar{H} = \bar{K}\bar{D}\bar{M}' , \quad \bar{H}\bar{H}' = \bar{K}\bar{D}^2\bar{K}', \quad \bar{H}'\bar{H} = \bar{M}\bar{D}^2\bar{M}' \tag{5}$$

each representing the best approximation in the sense of the least squares of the original matrices H, H H' and H'H respectively. Another important consequence related to our discussion is that the matrix $\bar{M}$ can be found using the matrices $\bar{K}$, $\bar{D}$ and H

$$\bar{M} = H'\bar{K}\bar{D}^{-1} \tag{6}$$

which makes analysis of matrix H'H of the order n unnecessary.

## Principal Components

Analysis of principal components is the most widely accepted method for the extraction of primary factors. In our procedure, the orthogonal principal components of the correlation matrix

$$R = Z Z'/(n-1) \tag{7}$$

are determined to fulfill the relation

$$\bar{R} = U U' \tag{8}$$

where $\bar{R}$ is the best least square k-rank approximation of R and U is the (m,k) matrix of coefficients of the first' k significant principal components. Each element u(i,s) of this matrix is determined to be

$$u(i,s) = a(i,s) \, [b(s)]^{1/2}, \quad i = 1, \ldots, m, \quad s = 1, \ldots, k \qquad (9)$$

where a(i,s) is i-th element of s-th normalized eigenvector and b(s) is s-th eigenvalue of the matrix R. The principal components themselves are computed using the matrix U and data Z

$$W = (U'U)^{-1} U'Z \qquad (10)$$

where W is the matrix (k,n) of principal components. The final result of transformation (10) is that the information content of the original study is compressed into a few principal components (Fig. 1). The other components containing predominantly the noise are neglected.

There are several ways of selecting the number of factors to be extracted from the dynamic study. Providing the number of compartments is known in advance and verified to be really reflected in data it can be substituted for the number of factors. Sometimes it is useful to extract one additional factor if some pathology is expected. Another way is to select a minimum threshold of relative variance which must be exceeded by extracted factors. This limit should not be less than the relative variance of one original image (e.g. if 20 images are processed the threshold should be at least 1/20 or 5% of total variance). This condition prevents the extraction of factors weighting less than one original image. However, the limit should not be evaluated in principal components but after their orthogonal transformation to varimax factors (Überla, 1971).

Factor Enhancement

Sometimes the threshold for factor extraction is too high to be overcome by factors corresponding to relatively small structures or those with relatively short transit time. Providing such factors should be extracted for diagnostic reasons the input data must be reduced in order to suppress unimportant but strong factors and to intensify those relatively weak but interesting. This procedure (in spatial domain called "masking") has been successfully used to extract the factors corresponding to the intrahepatic bile ducts and portal blood flow in dynamic cholescintigraphy (Herry et al., 1982; Sámal et al., 1986 b) and to increase the resolution in the detection of the regional wall motion abnormalities in gated equilibrium ventriculography (Pavel et al., 1984; 1986). While the routines for factor extraction and rotation are fixed by choosing a respective method, the selection of input data is fully in hands of operator. From this point of view the principle of factor enhancement should be respected in practice as the results of factor analysis naturally reflect the input data.

FACTOR ROTATION

The ultimate goal of factor analysis of dynamic radionuclide studies is the interpretation of factors as real physiological objects. Principal components represent the primary factors which fulfill some useful formal requirements but which usually are not suitable for physiological interpretation. Therefore a new position of coordinate axes must be found in which the factors can be interpreted. Up to now, three different methods have been developed in factor analysis of dynamic studies to satisfy the optimal position of factors in vector space of the original variables.

504

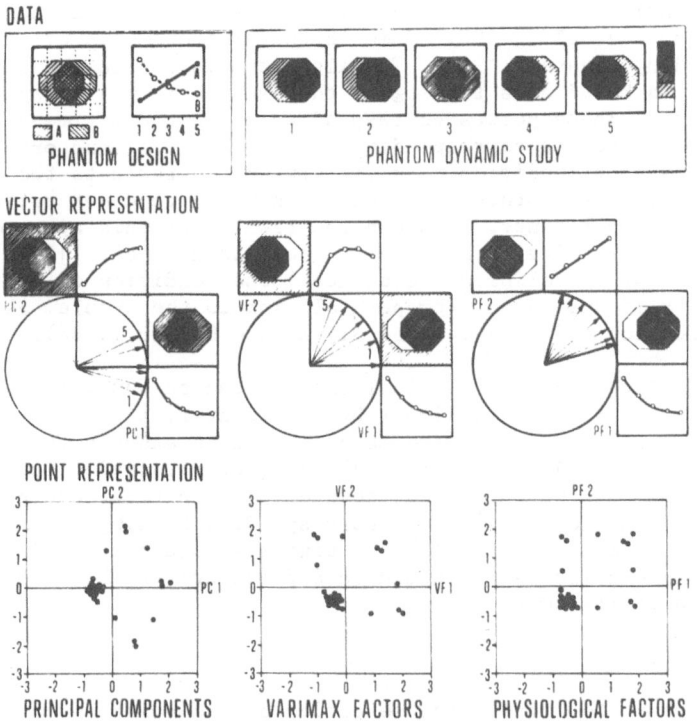

Fig. 1. Phantom dynamic study No. 1. The phantom consists of two partially
overlapping octagonal structures A and B in the 5 x 5 image matrix.
The correlation of factors, i.e. that of the images of separate
structures A and B is r(A,B)=0.529. The time-activity curves simulated in A and B are given in the standardized scale (with zero mean
and unit standard deviation), as well as the approximate sketches
of five images forming the phantom study. Three different factor solutions are demonstrated in both their vector and point representations. The vector representation demonstrates five vectors (normalized to the same unit length) representing five original images
projected into a plane of two factors. The cosine of the angle between any two of the vectors is equal to the correlation coefficient
of the corresponding images. Factors are represented also in the
form of images. Factor dynamics is reflected by standardized time-
-activity curve attached to every image. The point representation
demonstrates the standardized pixel values of factors. For the sake
of simplicity the coordinate axes of physiological factors are
presented as to be orthogonal although the factors in fact are in
a non-orthogonal position already. In the orthogonal configuration
the layout of points specified as the simple structure (represented
by the balanced background values in factors) can be recognized more
clearly. The abbreviations PC, VF and PF are used for principal
components, varimax factors and physiological factors respectively.

## Apex-Seeking Procedure

The first method of finding the physiological factors (time-activity curves) was described by Bazin et al. (1979). An algorithm more efficient in practice was suggested by Barber (1980). This algorithm has been further developed by Bazin and DiPaola (1982) and its final form was described in detail by DiPaola et al. (1982). Some further improvements of the method were suggested by Houston (1986). The algorithm is called the apex-seeking procedure. It is based on a finding of the extreme points in space of principal components. These points correspond to the extreme time-activity curves in the study. The points corresponding to physiological factors are then extrapolated using a condition of positivity which reflects the nature of measured variables  and states that only non-negative count rates are acceptable in single compartments. Although the results of this approach are rather good from the qualitative point of view (see Bazin et al. (1984) and Cavailloles (1984) for clinical references) the condition of positivity does not by itself guarantee a proper solution to the problem as it was shown recently by Houston (1984; 1986) and Nijran and Barber (1986).

Theoretically, the physiological factors can be found in the vector space of time-activity curves simply by the identification of factors with the extreme vectors of curves. The method based on exactly the same principle has been described by J. Imbrie (see Jöreskog et al. (1976) for references). Three conditions must be satisfied, however, to use this concept in practice: (1) elementary time-activity curves corresponding to single compartments must exist in the data matrix, (2) the pixels should not be clustered, and (3) the signal-to-noise ratio should be sufficiently high at least in the extreme time-activity curves.

## Intersection Method

In an attempt to improve the selection of the position of physiological factors the further limitations on factors have been introduced by Barber and Nijran (1982) and Nijran and Barber (1985; 1986). Their solution is based on a hypothesis about the expected shape of the factor (time-activity curve) to be extracted. The curve is expressed analytically and an appropriate vector space is formed by many theoretical curves. These curves are generated by changing the parameters of the function in some reasonable limits. Then the least square estimate of physiological factor forming an intersection between the theoretical and real study space is found. The method is dependent on a preliminary knowledge of the suitable mathematical description of examined physiological function and at present it makes possible to extract just a single factor. On the other hand, it is the only method able to extract the factor if it is overlapped totally by other dynamic structures in the image matrix.

## Rotation to Simple Structure

Considering variables and factors as the images, the true position of factors can be found using the strengthened condition of positivity. This condition admits only the homogeneous background values in factor images (Figs 1-3). It has been shown already that an additive constant does not contribute to correlations between images and thus it does not enter the factor analysis. In each factor image the homogeneous background (i.e. the area not covered by factor structure) thus can be expected. The corresponding configuration of background points reflecting the equalized minimum values in factors was called the simple structure in the point representation of factors (Šámal et al., 1987). This configuration of scintigraphic data can be regarded as their characteristic which can be used for the location of physiological factors thus resembling the similar notion of classic factor analysis (Thurstone, 1947).

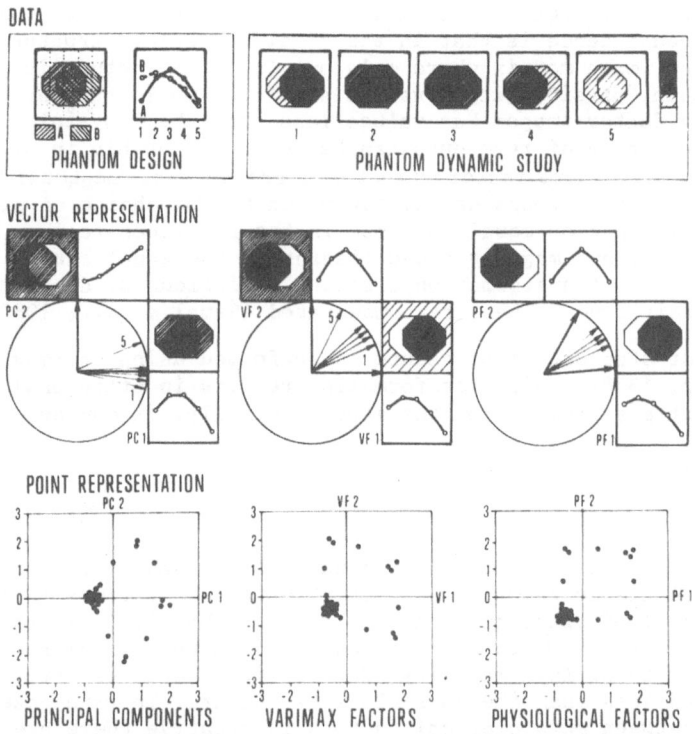

Fig. 2. Phantom dynamic study No. 2. The structures A and B are the same as
in Fig. 1 while the simulated time-activity curves are different.
The different dynamics is reflected by the different position of
vectors representing the original images. By other words, the examined configuration of vectors is given by the dynamics of factors. It
is in contrast to the methods using the clustering of pixels preliminary to the factor analysis because after the clustering, the position of vectors to be examined is arbitrary. The simple structure of
physiological factors is achieved by the suitable correction of varimax factors. This correction consists in equalizing of the minimum
values found in the varimax factors with the values found in pixels
localized outside the dynamic factor structures. In this phantom,
the count rate in the structure B falls down to zero in the last
image of the study. Therefore, this image is directly proportional to
the physiological factor corresponding to the image of structure A.

In practice, the homogeneity condition can be introduced in two steps:
(1) the pixels belonging only to the background in factor images (i.e.
those not belonging to the dynamic factor structures) must be found, and
(2) the values in background pixels must be equalized. The first step is
equivalent to finding of the images the correlation of which is less then
that of the true factors. Such images may fulfill the condition of positivity
but generically do not fulfill the condition of background homogeneity. In
these images, due to the lower correlation, the pixel values found in the
originally overlapped structures are smaller while those in the areas where
only one factor structure was originally present are greater than true factor
values. The consequence is that in the specific factor structure (i.e. in
the area of an image matrix where only one factor structure is projected)
the higher than "physiological" values are found while the same area in the
complementary factor images has values less than the "physiological" ones.
Providing the region of reference can be selected roughly in original images
indicating an area where factor structures are absent, the total area of background in each factor image can be estimated by the choice of pixels which
values are less than or equal to those in the reference region. Then the
transformation of an image is found leading to the equalization of background
values. During the transformation also the deviations of dynamic factor structures from their true values are compensated (Šámal et al., 1986 a; 1987).

The first step of the procedure is performed using varimax transformation (Kaiser, 1958). This transformation results in orthogonal factors similar to the extreme images from the study. Formally, it can be expressed by

$$Q = U \, T1 \tag{11}$$

$$P = T1' \, W \tag{12}$$

where U and W are the matrices from equations (8) and (10), Q is the matrix
(m,k) of coefficients relating m variables to k varimax factors and P is
the matrix (k,n) of orthogonal varimax factors. Matrix T1 is the orthogonal
transformation matrix which is designed to maximize the variance within the
columns of matrix Q. In a majority of real situations the varimax factors
are correlated less than the physiological factors. In rare cases where
correlation between physiological factors is negative there are several
possibilities for suitable modification of the varimax solution. One of these
methods is demonstrated in Fig. 4 and 5.

The final transformation to simple structure and physiological factors
can be expressed as

$$F = T2 \, P \tag{13}$$

$$G = Q \, T2^{-1} \tag{14}$$

where F is the matrix (k,n) of physiological factors (images) and G is the
matrix (m,k) of physiological factor coefficients. The regular (k,k) matrix
T2 is the transformation matrix designed to minimize k expressions

$$[t(s,.) \, P(s) - fBG(s)] \, [t(s,.) \, P(s) - fBG(s)]' = min. \tag{15}$$

where $s = 1, \ldots, k$, $t(s,.)$ is the s-th row of the matrix T2 and $P(s)$ is
the submatrix $(k,n(s))$ of P from (12) containing $n(s)$ (less than n) columns
of P. These columns are selected by evaluating the pixel values of the s-th
varimax factor. Only the pixels with values $p(s,j)$ less than or equal to
the 95th percentile of values found in the reference background area in
the respective factor image are taken into account and considered to form
the factor background. The $fBG(s)$ is the vector $(1,n(s))$ with constant
elements corresponding to the constant background level of respective s-th

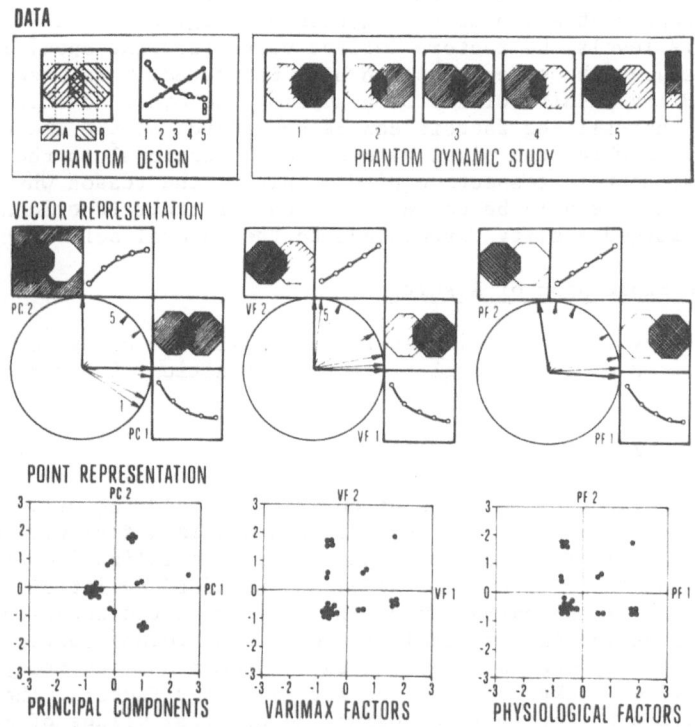

Fig. 3. Phantom dynamic study No. 3. The structures A and B and their time-
-activity curves are the same as in Fig. 1 while their superposition
is considerably smaller corresponding to the lower correlation
between factors in this phantom. The correlation coefficient r(A,B)=
=-0.114 reflects nearly orthogonal position of physiological factors,
however, the angle of corresponding vectors is greater than 90 degrees. Consequently, the vectors of the orthogonal varimax factors
lie inside the angle contained by the vectors of physiological factors and the usual transformation to the simple structure cannot be
performed directly. The varimax factors with zero correlation are
correlated more positively in this phantom than the physiological
factors having negative correlation. It results in the contamination
of varimax factors by the dynamic structures of other factors and in
the occurrence of minimum values in pixels outside the area of unification of the varimax factor structures.

factor. This factor-specific constant can also be found during the minimization of (15) which is performed using the methods described by Bierman
(1977) and Kárný (1982).


INTERPRETATION OF FACTORS

The concept of physiological factor can hardly be expressed strictly
in physical or mathematical terms. The factors on all the levels of their
extraction represent a linear combination of original variables. However,
on respective levels the factors reflect very different specific features.
In our procedure, these features can be interpreted. This makes useful even
the intermediary results of factor analysis. The other advantage of our
approach is that all the factors can be considered as the images of different
compartments in which the pixel values are proportional to the local volume
of the compartment in respective pixel. This is the reason why reading of
the factor images should be easier than that of other functional images
because the imaged quality corresponds to the natural scintigraphic measure.

## Quantitative Expression of Results

Considering factors as images the original data of dynamic study can
be reconstructed on every level of factor extraction. The reconstructed data
$\overline{Z}$ then are

$$\overline{Z} = U\,W, \quad \overline{Z} = Q\,P\,, \quad \overline{Z} = G\,F \tag{16}$$

using the complementary matrices of coefficients and factors. Both factors
and reconstructed data are expressed in standardized form with zero mean and
unit standard deviation. The straightforward denormalization of factors is
not possible as their true mean values and standard deviations are unknown.
However, an useful approximation can be made using the equation (3). The
data Y corresponding to the single factor can be reconstructed under the
condition that only one factor is actually present in the study substituting
the minimum (i.e. background) values for all other factors. Then the single
factor study can be denormalized using the original values of means and
standard deviations. Even the background data can be reconstructed substituting the minimum values for all the factors. The mean background value
$\overline{x}BG(i)$ in i-th image is then

$$\overline{x}BG(i) = s(i) \sum_{s=1}^{k} g(i,s)\, fBG\,(s) + \overline{y}(i) \tag{17}$$

where $i = 1, \ldots, m$, E is used for the sum over the factors from $s = 1$ to $k$,
$\overline{y}(i)$ and $s(i)$ is the mean and standard deviation of the image $i$, $g(i,s)$
is the i-th coefficient of factor $s$ and $fBG(s)$ is the minimum value of
factor $s$. The mean time-activity curve of the factor $s$ after the background subtraction is

$$\overline{x}(i,s) = -s(i)\, g(i,s)\, fBG(s) \tag{18}$$

where $\overline{x}(i,s)$ represents i-th mean value of the factor $s$. Finally, the
factor images or even the complete factor study can be reconstructed without
the background using

$$x(i,j,s) = s(i)\, g(i,s)\, [f(s,j) - fBG(s)] \tag{19}$$

where $x(i,j,s)$ is the reconstructed value of factor $s$ in j-th pixel of
i-th image and $f(s,j)$ is the standardized value of the factor $s$ in pixel
$j$. However, due to the homogeneity of factors, the factor images

510

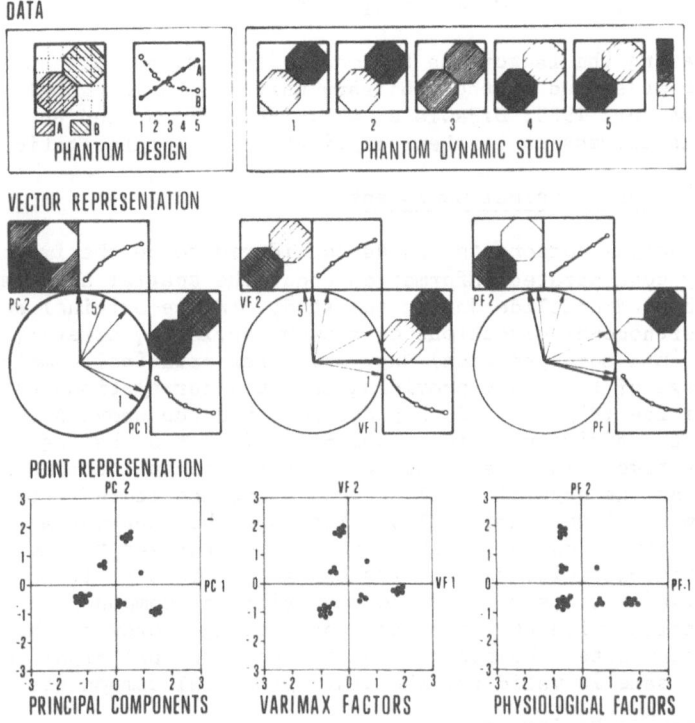

Fig. 4. Phantom dynamic study No. 4. The structure A and B and their time-
-activity curves are the same as in Fig. 1 while their superposition
is zero in this phantom and the correlation coefficient is r(A,B)=
=-0.423. The contamination of varimax factors by complementary structures is evident. In order to achieve the intermediary factors suitable for the finding of simple structure (i.e. those correlating mutually less than the physiological factors) the virtual dynamic study
is considered consisting of the same structures as the real one but
having the positive correlations between all its images. This study
is generated only in the vector space of principal components by
the proportional narrowing of the vectorial bundle of the original
images as it will be demonstrated in Fig. 5. The varimax factors of
the virtual study then correspond to the sought intermediary factors of the real study. They are suitable for the detection of minimum values in the area of unification of dynamic factor structures
and for the final transformation to the simple structure.

reconstructed by this way differ from each other by the multiplication constant only. The total sum of background data and respective factor studies is then equal to the study reconstructed directly as

$$x(i,j) = s(i) \; \overline{z}(i,j) + \overline{y}(i) \tag{20}$$

where $x(i,j)$ is the value reconstructed in pixel $j$ of the $i$-th image. The mean curves given by (18) can be further processed using procedures computing the descriptive curve parameters, deconvolution, etc. (Gremillet et al., 1986; Villanueva-Meyer et al., 1986).

Considering the factors as time-activity curves the results of factor analysis are presented in the arbitrary units emphasizing only their dynamic character (Barber, 1980; DiPaola et al., 1982; Nijran and Barber, 1986). However, this expression further complicates the interpretation of factors.

## Interpretation of Principal Components

The principal components can be considered to be the images containing an extremely concentrated information about the spatial and temporal distribution of the radionuclide during the study. In the original data they represent the orthogonal directions of maximum variance, however, they can be interpreted in a more practical way. The first principal component is simply the mean image of the study providing that the correlations between images are all positive (Fig. 6). If they are not then the above statement is valid for the first positive principal component (i.e. that having all its coefficients positive). In this sense, the first principal component may be interpreted as the physiological structure because it reflects the total distribution space of the radionuclide. Its image has the maximum correlations with all the study images and its pixel values reflect the mean values of elementary time-activity curves. Its own mean time-activity curve reflects the mean curve of the study. The second principal component can be interpreted by analogy with the first one considering, however, the residual study remaining after the subtraction of the first principal component. Obviously, the same is valid for the other principal components.

## Interpretation of Varimax Factors

Varimax factors represent the orthogonal images which are in close proximity to extreme images of the original study. Provided the correlations between the original images are all positive then the varimax factors enhance the areas specific for the extreme images and reduce those which are common to a greater number of images. If there are also negative correlations between the images in the study the varimax factors should be transformed to be correlated less than the physiological factors, however, their orthogonality is then lost. The correlations between the varimax factors and original images are either very high or very low in different time intervals.

The structures imaged on the varimax factors are as different as possible with regard to respective data in both space and time domain. In contrast to the feature imaged by principal components which can be called the "communality" of the pixel dynamics, the feature imaged by varimax factors can be called the "specificity" or "singularity" of it. While the former term reflects the measure of belonging of the pixel dynamics to the common dynamics characteristic for the study the latter terms reflect the measure of belonging of each pixel to the extreme different dynamics found in the study.

It should be emphasized that the use of both the principal components and varimax factors is not limited to dynamic radionuclide studies. They can be applied with benefit as the general image processing methods in conditions

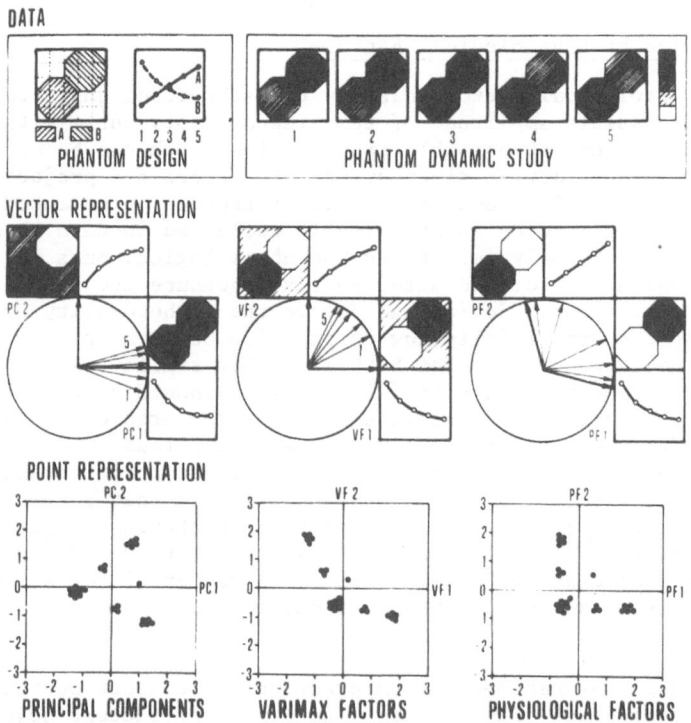

Fig. 5. Phantom dynamic study No. 5. This phantom corresponds to the virtual
dynamic study consisting of the same physiological factors as the
phantom study examined in Fig. 4. The only difference observed between the images of real and virtual studies is the enhanced contrast
in the images of virtual study between the area of unification of
dynamic factor structures and the remaining background area. The
principal components of both studies are the same and the varimax
factors fulfill the criteria for the transformation to the simple
structure. The physiological factors are presented in relation to
the images of the original phantom study from Fig. 4. If the correlation between the extreme images of the study approaches the value
of -1 (i.e. if one image becomes the photographic negative of the
other one) the first principal component still represents the direction of maximum variance in geometric representation of the original
data, however, its physical interpretation is different. The angle
between the vectors of extreme images approaches 180 degrees and the
vectors themselves are very close to the positive and negative orientation of the first principal component. Then the second one or even
further principal component having all its coefficients positive
must be selected to represent a physically acceptable mean image of
the study.

when several features are mixed gradually in original images as it is usual in dynamic computer tomography, nuclear magnetic resonance imaging, digital subtraction radiography and positron emission tomography. In every of these methods the evaluation of communalities and singularities may be helpful both for the image analysis and image processing (e.g. for contrast enhancement, reconstruction of images reflecting the respective relaxation times, etc.).

## Interpretation of Physiological Factors

The physiological factors display the structures characterized by the maximum possible amplitude of the time-activity curve with the uniform phase shift and longest possible transit time which can be derived from the given data considering given number of factors and projected on a homogeneous background. Provided the number of factors is selected properly and the physiological structures are clearly reflected in data then the imaged compartments are closely related to the physiological ones (Fig. 7). In fact, the physiological factors computed by our procedure are the varimax factors after the correction of deviations due to the orthogonality or, more generally, due to the artificially low correlation between the varimax factors. Therefore the interpretation of both is rather similar. Nevertheless, for physiological factors, the term "singularity" should be substituted by the term "proportionality", as the values within the area of background and active factor structures reach their true proportions. The resulting images conforming to a condition of simple structure are positive and correlated. The resulting correlation of factors is less than that between the extreme images from the original study because the structures of different factors contaminating the extreme images are absent. The term "proportional images" has been used already by Barber (1980) in a rather different sense for the images with the pixel values proportional to the local weight of factor curves.

There are many reasons why in practice the factors deviate from images of true physiological compartments. The number of factors selected improperly and low signal-to-noise ratio in the original images belong to the most important and most frequent ones. The compartment to be displayed as factor and the dynamics of this compartment must affect input data significantly. Therefore a concept of factor enhancement should be kept in mind using the method. Another class of deviations arises from the presence in original images of areas having a higher constant count rate during the study (and, consequently, the zero amplitude of time-activity curve). These areas are taken as being composed of the dynamic factors regardless of the fact that their origin may be also different. Having the extreme positive values in all the original images they contaminate proportionally all the extracted factors and deviate their time-activity curves. In the non-equilibrium studies this way of treatment is quite acceptable while in the equilibrium ones (where the true compartments with zero amplitude of time-activity curve may exist) it can make some troubles. On the other hand, this drawback is probably responsible for the better "sensitivity" of factor over the phase analysis in detecting the kinetic abnormalities of cardiac walls (Fig. 8). The analysis of noise in the area of zero amplitude (i.e. the distribution of actual random values among the factors) contributes also to the phenomenon described above. The effect of zero amplitude of time-activity curves can hardly be corrected formally as we are not able to separate in advance the pixels in which the analysis should be done from those in which it should not. After all, the differentiation of pixel dynamics is the merit of the method.

Another problem in the interpretation of physiological factors is represented by the local motion artifacts which, of course, contaminate the factors according to their extent and contribution to local amplitudes. In non-equilibrium studies they indicate usually the motion of a patient and can

514

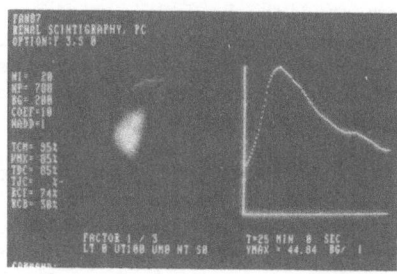 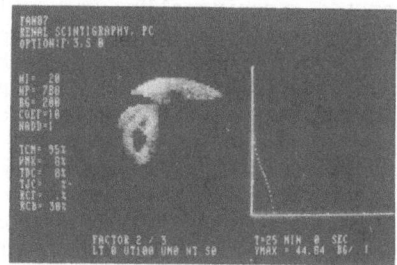

a                                b

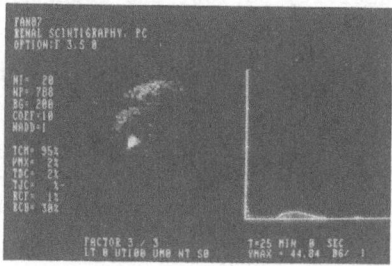

c

Fig. 6. Principal components extracted from the dynamic renal study (99mTc-
-EDTA) in a patient with normal function of the left kidney.
The first principal component (a) covers 85% of total variance of
20 original images selected from the study.

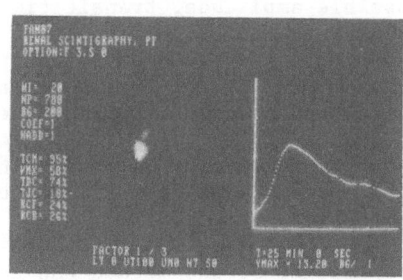 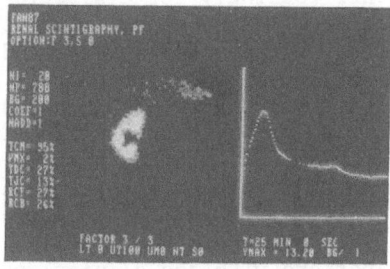

a                                b

c

Fig. 7. Physiological factors resulting from transformation of principal
components presented in Fig. 6 by means of the varimax procedure and
rotation to simple structure.

be interpreted unequivocally. In equilibrium studies, however, they can complicate the interpretation of factors considerably, reflecting the translational motion of the heart during the contraction and the bellows-like contraction of the right ventricle. The problem is not that of the factor analysis itself and, at least in some cases, can be corrected in principle.

Considering the factors as time-activity curves their interpretation is more difficult with the exception of the method of Nijran and Barber (1986) in which the character of the extracted factor is given in advance. The difficulty of interpretation in other methods is given predominantly by the method of data normalization, arbitrary clustering of pixels and arbitrary termination of apex-seeking procedure. Under the optimal conditions, i.e. if the physiological factors can be identified with the clusters of real extreme elementary time-activity curves, the meaning of factors converges with that of factors considered to be images.

Finally, it should be mentioned that the time scale in dynamic study can be substituted by energy spectrum and a data matrix containing the images recorded in different energy windows can be processed by factor analysis. This way is useful both for the analysis of multiple isotope studies (Soussaline et al., 1975; DiPaola et al., 1975) and the routine quality control of scintigraphic cameras (DiPaola et al., 1985).


CONCLUSIONS

The physiological factors, regardless of their character of images or curves, can be extracted from the dynamic study provided their existence is reflected significantly in the input data for factor analysis. In general, for the reasons stated above, we consider the concept of factors as images to be more suitable for computation and interpretation of factors. Regardless of their biological identity, the physiological factors reflect the structures characterized by terms of maximum possible amplitude, transit time and uniform phase shift of corresponding time-activity curves, which can be extracted under the given conditions from respective dynamic data, and projected into a matrix with the homogeneous background. The correspondence between the physiological factors derived from the dynamic study and their real biological counterparts can be achieved in practice by the convenient data acquisition and preparation and by the proper use of the method. The communality and singularity as the qualities imaged by principal components and varimax factors can be used also in other imaging modalities.

In a clinical routine, the operator dependence of the method can be minimized substantially by a standardization (both organ- and study-specific) of procedures in order to avoid misinterpretation of factors. In general, the method can be used either routinely for evaluation of factors themselves or as a preliminary processing of data before the further analysis of factor curves (dynamic renal studies, first-pass cardiac studies, etc.) or it can be used in selected cases only as a final procedure e.g. after the equivocal results of phase analysis have been found. The procedure described above for factor analysis of dynamic studies has been verified in both of these ways and was found to be useful. However, its further improvement can still be made e.g. by avoiding the necessity to select the reference background area and its substitution by the area with the minimum pixel values in the first principal component, etc. This one and other modifications are currently being tested but do not interfere with the clinical evaluation of the method as they do not modify the character of extracted factors.

The factor analysis of dynamic radionuclide studies provided it is designed and used properly provides information on both the dynamics and volumes of physiological compartments minimizing the influence of their projection overlap. From this point of view, the method can be regarded as a procedure of image processing which represents a useful tool of information extraction, in fact forming the interstage between the functional imaging and tomography.

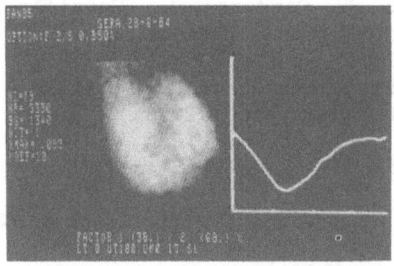
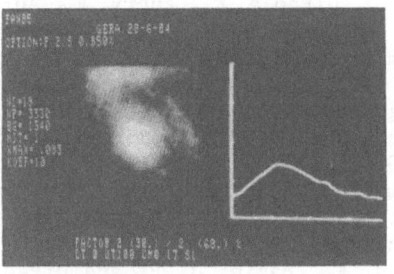

a                                                      b

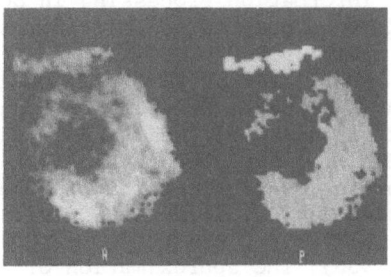

c

Fig. 8. The result of analysis of gated equilibrium ventriculography (99mTc-
-RBC) in a child suffered from the massive tricuspid regurgitation.
The physiological factors (a, b) presented with their time-activity
curves demonstrate the maximum amplitude in the area of atrioventri-
cular superposition. In all the original images this area is characterized by a high constant count rate as it corresponds to the projection of rather great volume of blood pulsating between the right
atrium and ventricle in the direction perpendicular to the image
plane. Consequently, both the amplitude (A) and phase (P) images demonstrated in (c) indicate the zero amplitude describing exactly
the time-activity changes in data. Considering this fact, the result
of factor analysis can be regarded as the artificial one. However,
from both the physiological and diagnostic points of view this
result is useful because it reflects exactly the underlying conditions. On the other hand, the image of the left ventricular residual
volume which is the "true compartment" with constant count rate is
also decomposed into two parts. While the part in the factor image
with ventricular dynamics is hidden, that one in the second factor
image with the atrial dynamics simulates the contrapulsating structure in the area of left ventricle.

517

# REFERENCES

Barber, D. C. (1980). The use of principal components in the quantitative analysis of gamma camera dynamic studies, Phys. Med. Biol.,25, 283-292.

Barber, D. C. and Nijran, K. S. (1982). Factor analysis of dynamic radionuclide studies, in: Nuclear Medicine and Biology, C. Raynaud, ed., Pergamon Press, Paris, 31-34.

Bazin, J. P., DiPaola, R., Gibaud, B., Rougier, P. and Tubiana, M. (1979). Factor analysis of dynamic scintigraphic data as a modelling method. An application to the detection of metastases, in: Information Processing in Medical Imaging, R. DiPaola and E. Kahn, eds., INSERM 88, Paris, 345-366.

Bazin, J. P. and DiPaola, R. (1982). Advances in factor analysis applications in dynamic function studies, in: Nuclear Medicine and Biology, C. Raynaud, ed., Pergamon Press, Paris, 35-38.

Bazin, J. P., DiPaola, R., Aubry, F., Aurengo, A., Capderou, A., Cavailloles, F., Cinotti, L., Herry, J. Y. and Lumbroso, J. (1984). Factor analysis of dynamic structures, Informatek Users Group Newsletter, 1, 3-15.

Benzécri, J. P. (1969). Statistical analysis as a tool to make patterns emerge from data, in: Methodologies of Pattern Recognition, S. Watanabe, ed., Academic Press, New York, 35-74.

Bierman, G. J. (1977). Factorization Methods for Discrete Sequential Estimation, Academic Press, New York.

Blahuš, P. (1985). Factor Analysis and its Generalization (in Czech), SNTL, Prague.

Cavailloles, F., Bazin, J. P. and DiPaola, R. (1984). Factor analysis in gated cardiac studies, J. Nucl. Med., 25, 1067-1079.

DiPaola, R., Penel, C., Bazin, J. P. and Berche, C. (1975). Factor analysis and scintigraphy, in: Information Processing in Scintigraphy, C. Raynaud and A. Todd-Pokropek, eds., Proceedings of the IVth International Conference, Orsay, 91-123.

DiPaola, R., Bazin, J. P., Aubry, F., Aurengo, A., Cavailloles, F., Herry, J. Y. and Kahn, E. (1982). Handling of dynamic sequences in nuclear medicine, IEEE Trans. Nucl. Sci., NS-29, 1310-1321.

DiPaola, R., Boudet, F., Bazin, J. P., Aubert, B. and Ricard, M. (1985). Factor analysis in routine quality control of gamma camera energy correction, Poster Presentation, European Nuclear Medicine Congress, London.

Eckart, C. and Young, G. (1936). The approximation of one matrix by another of lower rank, Psychometrika, 1, 211-218.

Goris, M. L. (1982). Functional or parametric images, J. Nucl. Med., 23, 360-362.

Gremillet, E., Herrmann, T., Essabah, H., Rusch, P., Champailler, A. and Healy, J. C. (1986). New non-invasive method for assessment of 99mTc-RBC cerebral transit: a quantitative use of factorial analysis, Nuklearmedizin, Suppl. 22, 21-22.

Harman, H. H. (1960). Modern Factor Analysis, University of Chicago Press, Chicago.

Herry, J. Y., Bazin, J. P., Bourguet. P., DiPaola, M. and DiPaola, R. (1982). Factor analysis of dynamic structures. Application to kinetics of hepatobiliary traces, in: Nuclear Medicine and Biology, C. Raynaud, ed., Pergamon Press, Paris, 2240-2243.

Horst, P. (1965). Factor Analysis of Data Matrices, Holt, Rinehart and Winston, New York.

Houston, A. S. (1984). The effect of apex-finding errors on factor images obtained from factor analysis and oblique transformation, Phys. Med. Biol., 29, 1109-1116.

Houston, A. S. (1986). The use of set theory and cluster analysis to investigate the constraint problem in factor analysis in dynamic structures, in: Information Processing in Medical Imaging, S. L. Bacharach, ed., Martinus Nijhoff Publishers, Dordrecht, 177-192.

518

Houston, A. S., MacLeod, M. A. and Sampson, F. D. (1979). Principal component analysis as an aid to classification of renal dynamic studies, Eur. J. Nucl. Med., 4, 295-299.

Johnson, R. M. (1963). On a theorem stated by Eckart and Young, Psychometrika, 28, 259-263.

Jöreskog, K. G. (1963). Statistical Estimation in Factor Analysis, Almquist and Wiksell, Uppsala.

Jöreskog, K. G., Klovan, J. E. and Reyment, R. A. (1976). Geological Factor Analysis, Elsevier Scientific Publishing Company, Amsterdam.

Kaiser, H. F. (1958). The varimax criterion for analytic rotation in factor analysis, Psychometrika, 23, 187-200.

Kárný, M. (1982). Recursive parameter estimation of regression model when the interval of possible values is given, Kybernetika (Prague), 18, 37-49.

Nijran, K. S. and Barber, D. C. (1985). Towards automatic analysis of dynamic radionuclide studies using principal component factor analysis, Phys. Med. Biol., 30, 1315-1325.

Nijran, K. S. and Barber, D. C. (1986). Factor analysis of dynamic function studies using a priori physiological information, Phys. Med. Biol., 31, 1107-1117.

Oppenheim, B. E. and Appledorn, C. R. (1979). Functional renal imaging using factor analysis, in: Information Processing in Medical Imaging, R. DiPaola and E. Kahn, eds., INSERM 88, Paris, 321-334.

Pavel, D. G. and Briandet, P. A. (1983). Quo vadis phase analysis, Clin. Nucl. Med., 8, 564-575.

Pavel, D. G., Briandet, P. A., Fang, R. B., Zolnierczyk, K. and Sychra, J. (1984). The normal heart: patterns for various functional images obtained from radionuclide gated equilibrium studies, in: Informatioín Processing in Medical Imaging, F. Deconinck, ed., Martinus Nijhoff Publishers, Boston, 250-265.

Pavel, D. G., Sychra, J., Olea, E., Kahn, C., Virupannavar, S., Zolnierczyk, K. and Shanes, J. (1986). Factor analysis: its place in the evaluation of ventricular regional wall motion abnormalities, in: Information Processing in Medical Imaging, S. L. Bacharach, ed., Martinus Nijhoff Publishers, Dordrecht, 193-206.

Šámal, M., Sůrová, H., Maříková, E., Kárný, M. and Dienstbier, Z. (1986 a). Improved precision, quantitative expression and enhancement of physiological factors in factor analysis of dynamic studies, Nuklearmedizin, Suppl. 22, 649-650.

Šámal, M., Sůrová, H., Kárný, M., Maříková, E., Michalová, K. and Dienstbier, Z. (1986 b). Enhancement of physiological factors in factor analysis of dynamic studies, Eur. J. Nucl. Med., 12, 280-283.

Šámal, M., Kárný, M., Sůrová, H., Maříková, E., and Dienstbier, Z. (1987). Rotation to simple structure in factor analysis of dynamic radionuclide studies, Phys. Med. Biol., 32, 371-382.

Schmidlin, P. (1979). Quantitative evaluation and imaging of functions using pattern recognition methods, Phys. Med. Biol., 24, 385-395.

Schmidlin, P. and Rösel, F. (1975). Application of factor analysis for scintigraphic picture processing, in: Information Processing in Scintigraphy, C. Raynaud and A. Todd-Pokropek, eds., Proceedings of the IVth International Conference, Orsay, 80-90.

Soussaline, F., Todd-Pokropek, A. E., DiPaola, R. and Bazin, J. P. (1975). Techniques for combining isotopic images obtained at different energies, in: Information Processing in Scintigraphy, C. Raynaud and A. Todd-Pokropek, eds., Proceedings of the IVth International Conference, Orsay, 17-42.

Thurstone, L. L. (1947). Multiple Factor Analysis, University of Chicago Press, Chicago.

Überla, K. (1971). Faktorenanalyse (in German), Springer Verlag, Berlin.

Villanueva-Meyer, J., Philippe, L., Cordero, S., Marcus, C. S. and Mana, I. (1986). Use of factor analysis in the evaluation of left to right cardiac shunts. J. Nucl. Med., 27, 1442-1448.

# THE IMPORTANCE OF CONSTRAINTS IN FACTOR ANALYSIS OF DYNAMIC STUDIES

K S Nijran[+] and D C Barber[++]

[+]Department of Nuclear Medicine,
 Charing Cross Hospital, London, U.K.

[++]Department of Medical Physics,
 Royal Hallamshire Hospital, Sheffield, U.K.

## INTRODUCTION

A dynamic radionuclide study provides a description of the way the administrated tracer behaves in the several separate structures in the body. The usual aim of dynamic study analysis is to attempt to isolate the information from one or more important structures from the rest of the study. Because of the way the images of structures overlap it is rarely possible to derive the variation of tracer concentration within a single structure directly from the dynamic study. The common approach to this problem is to define a region (a region-of-interest (ROI)) around the structure of interest and compute the curve representing the variation of activity within that region and then attempt to estimate and remove from this curve the contribution from the surrounding and overlapping structures (background structures). An estimate of this component of activity is usually obtained from a second ROI over a region in the study indicative of the background activity in the region of the structure of interest.

The problems associated with the above approach are well known. The need to carefully select appropraite ROI's, the use of a background correction which is not strictly valid, and furthermore the method is subject to operator influence on the result, are some of the major drawbacks to this method. In order to provide some measure of consistency, analysis is commonly restricted to a few or even a single person ensuring that if the results are in error at least they are systematically in error. Use of an automatic method of region selection, if possible, may remove operator variability but may not reduce error.

This paper will show how some of these problems may be solved using principal components factor analysis.The description of dynamic radionuclide data in terms of physiological factors and corresponding factor images is a powerful one. The use of principal components factor analysis to extract these factors from a dynamic study involves obtaining the principal components and then exploring the space (the study space S) defined by these components for the physiological factors. These factors can only be found by the application to this space of constraints provided by other knowledge. Several methods have been proposed. Each elemental activity time curve (a dixel) in the study plots as a point in the study space. The earliest approach (FADS- factor analysis of dynamic structures) involved identifying the physiological factors with extrema in the distribution of dixels in study space. In addition positivity constraints could also be applied to the physiological factors and the corresponding factor images (Barber, 1980; Bazin et al., 1982). Although fairly successful FADS often fails to produce pure uncontaminated physiological factors. Houston (1986) has considered some of the properties of these methods and suggested some techniques to generate better factors.

An alternative approach is to explore study space using mathematical models of the physiological factors being sought. Nijran and Barber (1984) showed that by finding the intersection of the study space and a space (the theory space T) derived from a general model of one of the factors it was possible to extract this specific physiological factor from the study. This intersection method (IM) did not directly generate a factor image but Nijran and Barber (1986) later showed that it could be combined with FADS to produce an improved full factorisation of a dynamic study.

All the above methods have applied constraints in the temporal domain. Much less attention has been given to constraints in the spatial domain. This paper will show how spatial constraints can also be used to extract physiological factors from a dynamic study.

## METHOD

In order to make sense of a dynamic study and extract useful information from it, it is often necessary to make some important assumptions about the nature of the objects being imaged, although these assumptions have generally been implicit rather than explicit. The most important idea is that the study can be partitioned into discrete compartments. In compartmental analysis a compartment is usually taken to be the mathematical abstraction of a (possibly transient) storage unit and a similar idea shall be adopted here. However in compartment analysis the contents of a compartment may not be open to inspection whereas in many dynamic studies this is not the case. A further restriction therefore on the definition of a compartment is that it is homogeneous. By this is meant that the behaviour of tracer with time in any small volume within the compartment is the same at all points in the compartment. In practice real structures may be combination of several interconnecting compartments (the kidney is an example) yet it may be convenient to treat such a structure as a single entity. In this paper there will be a clear distinction between a compartment and a structure. In theory it may not be possible to exactly divide structure into a small number of discrete compartments. However in practice the fact that data is noisy will often ensure that only a limited number of discrete compartments within a structure can be clearly identified. A compartment is essentially defined by the concept of homogeneity whereas a structure is often a more informal concept. In some sense the whole of the body is a single structure. In practice it often makes sense to divide the body into several discrete and interconnecting structures.

Associated with each compartment is a curve representing the variation of tracer concentration with time in that compartment. This curve will be called the factor curve (or physiological factor) for that compartment. Recognising the discrete nature of dynamic radionuclide data both in space and time the curve associated with the ith compartment in a study will be represented in vector notation as $f_i$ (in the following mathematical description vectors are represented by bold characters). The variation of tracer concentration within a structure will then be represented by a linear sum of the curves associated with the compartments contained within the structure

$$g = \Sigma a_i.f_i \tag{1}$$

Although the weights $a_i$ will depend on the relative sizes of the compartments within the structure they will also depend on the measurment configuration. Whereas the shape of each $f_i$ (but not necessarily the amplitude) will be the same no matter from what direction the structure is viewed or what conditions of attenuation and scatter prevail, the shape of $g$ will depend on these factors. Given the above comments it is clear that direct extraction of $g$ from a structure by conventional methods such as ROI analysis is essentially an imprecise activity.

Each pixel within the study defines an elemental ROI. The variation of activity within a pixel represents an elemental tracer concentration curve called a dixel. In each dixel contains a contribution from several compartments and may be written as a linear summation of the curves associated with, say M such compartments e.g.

$$d_j = \Sigma \; a_{ij}.f_i \tag{2}$$

For the ith compartment the values $a_{ij}$ form an image which will be called the factor image. If there are J pixels in each image of the study and N images in the study then the matrix D whose N rows are the images in the study is called the data matrix. It is related to the factor images and the factor curves by the relationship

$$D = F.A \tag{3}$$

F is the (N x M) matrix of factor curves and A the (M x J) matrix of factor images.

Equation 2 assumes that the study only contains M factors. In fact D will contain noise which means that this equation cannot be exactly satisfied. Rewriting this equation as

$$D_M = F.A \tag{4}$$

recognises that the data matrix reconstructed from the factors only has a rank of M rather than N.

The important analytical problem here is generally the extraction of one or more of the factor curves. Note that there is generally no direct solution to the above equation for F since neither F and A are known. Most solutions to the extraction of F rely on the use of one or more constraints discussed above.

A symmetric matrix C, the covariance matrix, may be derived from the data matrix D by multiplying this matrix with its transpose.

$$C = D.D^t \tag{5}$$

This matrix may be diagonalised by its eigenvectors

$$U^t.C.U = R \tag{6}$$

and its has been shown elsewhere that these eigenvectors form the set of orthogonal vectors which can most efficiently reconstruct the columns of D (i.e. the dixels of the study). Each dixel may be represented as a linear sum of the columns of U

$$d_j = \Sigma^N \; c_{ij}.u_i \tag{7}$$

where $u_i$ is the ith column of U, the principal components of this study and the $c_{ij}$ are the coefficients which reconstruct the jth dixel. The principal

$$\mathbf{d}_j = \Sigma^M c_{ij}.\mathbf{u}_i \tag{8}$$

is (averaged over all the dixels) the best estimate of $\mathbf{d}_j$ obtained from a reconstruction using $M$ orthogonal vectors. It is easily shown that

$$E(c_{ij}^2) = R_i \tag{9}$$

where $R_i$ is the ith diagonal element of the matrix $\mathbf{R}$. Given this result it is easy to see that the full matrix form of equation 7 can be written as

$$\mathbf{D} = \mathbf{U}.\mathbf{R}^{\frac{1}{2}}.\mathbf{V}^t \tag{10}$$

where the matrix of coefficient vectors has been written as $\mathbf{R}^{\frac{1}{2}}.\mathbf{V}^t$ i.e. the rows of the matrix $\mathbf{V}^t$ have been normalised such that their norm is unity. Taking the transpose of the above equation

$$\mathbf{D} = \mathbf{V}.\mathbf{R}^{\frac{1}{2}}.\mathbf{U}^t \tag{11}$$

and premultiplying equation 11 by equation 10 gives

$$\mathbf{D}^t.\mathbf{D} = \mathbf{V}.\mathbf{R}^{\frac{1}{2}}.\mathbf{U}^t.\mathbf{U}.\mathbf{R}^{\frac{1}{2}}.\mathbf{V}^t \tag{12}$$

which reduces to

$$\mathbf{B} = \mathbf{D}^t.\mathbf{D} = \mathbf{V}.\mathbf{R}.\mathbf{V}^t \tag{13}$$

and hence to

$$\mathbf{V}^t.\mathbf{B}.\mathbf{V} = \mathbf{R} \tag{14}$$

$\mathbf{B}$ is the column covariance matrix of the data matrix and $\mathbf{V}$ the matrix of its eigenvectors. Note that, provided $J > N$ there are only $N$ of these eigenvectors because of the rank of $\mathbf{B}$ will only be $N$. Diagonalisation of both $\mathbf{B}$ and $\mathbf{C}$ produce the same matrix of eigenvalues.

Equation 10 represents the singular value decomposition (SVD) of the data matrix $\mathbf{D}$.

If the data matrix has a rank $M$ which is smaller than $N$ because the data is constructed from only $M$ factors (equation 2) then only the first $M$ diagonal elements of $\mathbf{R}$ will be non zero and $\mathbf{U}$ and $\mathbf{V}$ will each have only $M$ columns. Because of noise in practice it is unlikely that any diagonal elements of $\mathbf{R}$ will be truly zero, but many will be small and in some cases it may be possible to determine $M$ by inspection of these values.

The first $M$ columns of $\mathbf{U}$ define the study space $S$ of Nijran and Barber and all the dixels and the factor curves lie in this space. As reviewed above most attempts to find the factor curves have concentrated on a constrained search of $S$ space. Equation 3 suggests that an alternative possibility is to identify the factor images and then use them to derive the factor curves. Apex seeking algorithms, including positivity constraints, should work in this space and provide results similar to the use of the same algorithm in $S$ space.

A compartment, as part of a structure, is usually limited in spatial extent. The factor image of this compartment will therefore also be limited in extent. This simple fact may be used as a powerful constraint for locating factor images of such a compartment. This factor image can be expanded in terms of the columns of $\mathbf{V}$.

$$\mathbf{f} = \Sigma^M b_i.\mathbf{v}_i \tag{15}$$

In order to determine $\mathbf{f}$ it is necessary to determine the $b_i$. But many of the elements of $\mathbf{f}$ are zero and therefore, provided more than M elements meet this condition there are more than enough equations in the equation set represented by equation 15 to solve for the $b_i$.

Let $\mathbf{f_z}$ be the vector of zero elements (positionally) selected from $\mathbf{v_i}$. If $\mathbf{0}$ is the null vector then

$$\mathbf{f_z} = \mathbf{0} = \Sigma \ b_i.\mathbf{v_{zi}} \tag{16}$$

the trivial solution $b_i = 0$ is avoided by fixing $b_1 = 1.0$. Then

$$\mathbf{v_{z1}} = - \ \Sigma^M \ b_i.\mathbf{v_{zi}} \tag{17}$$

where the summation is from i=2,M. In matrix notation this becomes

$$\mathbf{v_{z1}} = - \ \mathbf{V_{z-1}}.\mathbf{b_i} \tag{18}$$

where $\mathbf{V_{z-1}}$ is $\mathbf{V_z}$ with the first column removed, and $\mathbf{b}$ is the vector of the $b_i$ from i=2,M. This equation is solved by premultiplying by the transpose of $\mathbf{V_{z-1}}$.

$$\mathbf{V^t_{z-1}}.\mathbf{v_{z1}} = - \ \mathbf{V^t_{z-1}}.\mathbf{V_{z-1}}.\mathbf{b} \tag{19}$$

$$= \mathbf{Z}.\mathbf{b}$$

and then inverting Z and premultiplying by its inverse

$$\mathbf{Z^{-1}}.\mathbf{V^t_{z-1}}.\mathbf{v_{z1}} = -\mathbf{b} \tag{20}$$

The zero elements are selected by an ROI. From the above derivation it can be seen that provided the number of elements in $\mathbf{f_z}$ is greater than M the solution should be independent of the detailed selection of the zero elements. While the presence of noise will strictly invalidate this result it can be expected that the extraction of the factor image should not be unduly sensitive to the way the zeros ROI is drawn.

One component which cannot be treated in this way is the background component. In order to extract factor image for the background component it may be necessary to model this factor image. Nijran and Barber (1984) described an analogous approach in S space for extracting a factor curve, the intersection method. In the present example an appropriate model for the background might be a polynomial function

$$g(x,y) = p_0 + p_1 x + p_2 y + \dots \tag{21}$$

Higher order square and cubic terms may be added as required. In Barber and Nijran (1981) a non-linear model was used so an iterative solution had to be used to match the model to S space. However equation 21 is linear in the coefficients $p_i$ and so a direct matrix solution is possible. In matrix notation 21 may be written as

$$\mathbf{g} = \mathbf{X}.\mathbf{p} \tag{22}$$

where the matrix $\mathbf{X}$ is of the form

$$\begin{bmatrix} 1 & x_1 & y_1 & \dots \\ 1 & x_2 & y_2 & \dots \\ & & & \\ 1 & x_j & y_j & \dots \end{bmatrix}$$

Then

$$\mathbf{X.p} = \mathbf{V.b} \qquad (23)$$

Although the columns of $\mathbf{X}$ are not orthogonal they are independent and define a theory space as defined by Nijran and Barber. Following their paper equation 23 may be solved for $\mathbf{p}$ and $\mathbf{b}$ by rewriting this equation as

$$
\begin{bmatrix} v_{11} \\ v_{21} \\ \\ \\ \\ v_{J1} \end{bmatrix}
=
\begin{matrix} = \\ = \\ \\ \\ \\ = \end{matrix}
-
\begin{bmatrix} v_{12} & v_{13} & \dots & v_{1M} & -1 & -x_1 & -y_1 & \dots \\ v_{22} & v_{23} & \dots & v_{2M} & -1 & -x_2 & -y_2 & \dots \\ \\ \\ v_{J2} & v_{J3} & \dots & v_{JM} & -1 & -x_J & -y_J & \dots \end{bmatrix}
\begin{bmatrix} b_1 \\ b_2 \\ \\ b_M \\ p_1 \end{bmatrix}
$$

which is of the form

$$\mathbf{t} = \mathbf{K.s} \qquad (24)$$

This may be solved for the elements of $\mathbf{s}$ in a manner similar to equation 18. The first $M-1$ elements of $\mathbf{s}$ are the coefficients $\mathbf{b}$ for $i=2,M$ ($b = 1.0$) and the remaining elements are the coefficients $p_i$ of the polynomial expansion. The factor image is reconstructed from the product.

$$\mathbf{f} = \mathbf{V.b}$$

Because in both the zero fitting and the model fitting example one coefficient had to be selected arbitrarily the scale of the reconstructed factor images is also arbitrary.

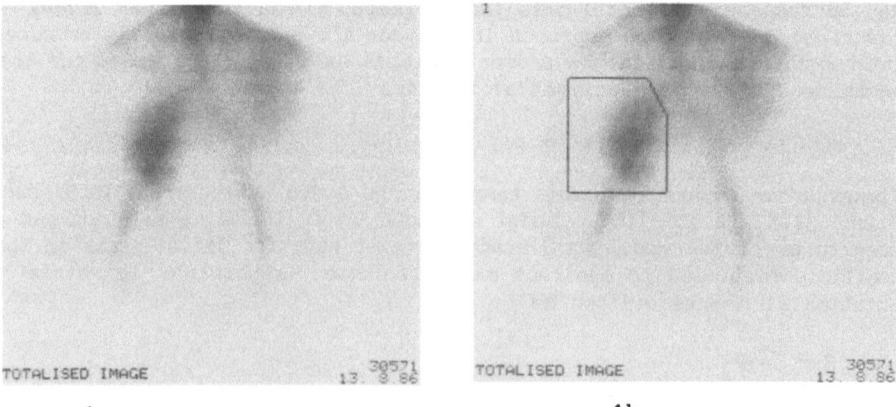

1a            1b

Figure 1a Totalised image for the first 30 seconds of a renal transplant study.

Figure 1b A region defining the dixels used for constructing study space.

## RESULTS

Figure 1a shows a totalised image for the first 30 seconds of a renal transplant study, representing the total of 20 frames, each of 1.5 seconds duration. It is assumed that three factors are to be extracted from this study, a kidney factor, an arterial factor and a background factor. Figure 1b shows the same image with a region defining the dixels selected for construction of the study space in this example. Figure 2a shows the zero elements for the kidney factor image and Figure 2b the factor image itself. Figure 3a shows the zero elements for the arterial factor image and figure 3b the factor image for this compartment. Finally figure 4 shows the background factor extracted using a model given by equation 21 in which the first three terms are retained. The normalised factor images are used to solve equation 3 for the factor curves and the normalised factor curves are fitted to the study curve to compute the correct scaling factors. Figure 5 shows the final factor curves.

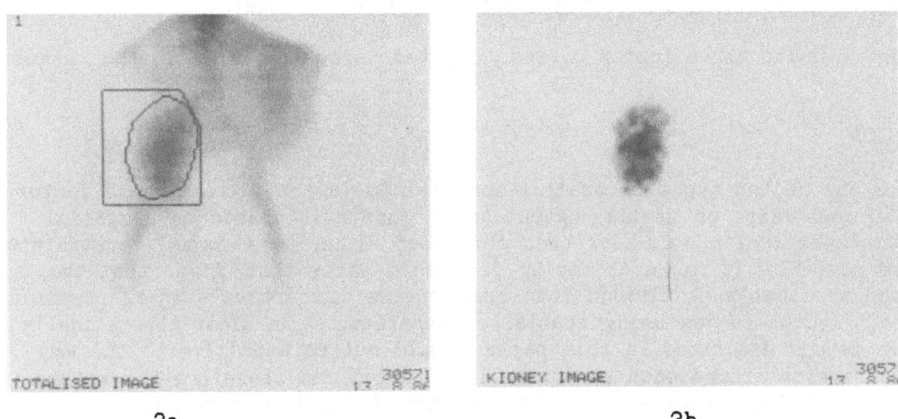

2a                    2b

Figure 2a The zero elements selected for the kidney factor image.

Figure 2b The kidney factor image computed.

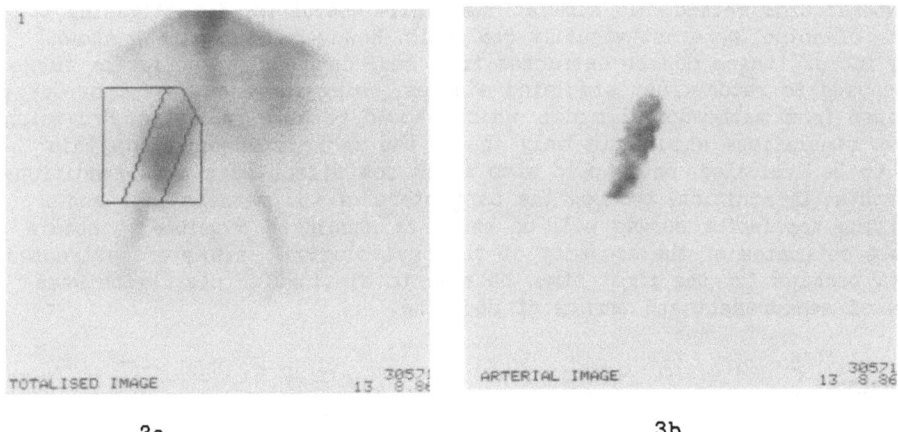

3a                    3b

Figure 3a The zero elements selected for the arterial factor image.

Figure 3b The arterial factor image computed.

527

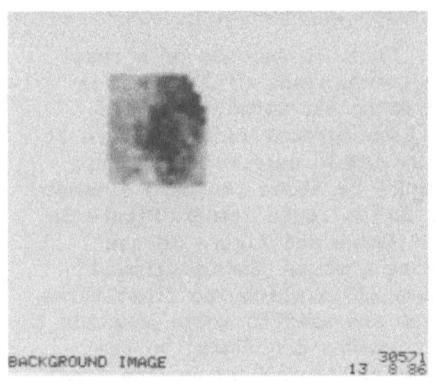 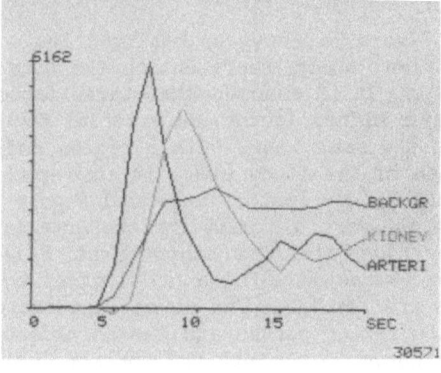

| 4 | 5 |

Figure 4 The background image extracted using a model.

Figure 5 The three factor curves computed using the three factor images.

## DISCUSSION

The use of two types of spatial constraints in the extraction of factor curves, a constraint on spatial extent and a constraint based on a spatial domain mathematical model, have been described. Other less formal constraints are also possible. It is worth noting from this paper that, given that the study can reasonably be divided into homogeneous compartments it is possible to extract factor curves using spatial constraints. It is clear theoretically that the method described in this paper should not be sensitive to the way the zeros region around each structure is selected and therefore the method should be much less dependent on the operator. The method automatically removes cross-correlation between compartments. Further work is envisaged in which the possibility of using jointly temporal and spatial constraints is considered. Inevitably with any new technique the question of validation arises. Pure clinical validation is not appropriate since there is rarely any independent validation of the hypothesis that the physiological parameter being estimated is indeed a good indicator of clinical prognosis. Nijran (1984) used simulated dynamic study data to investigate the performance of the intersection method. His simulations, while useful for investigating the effects of noise, were not visually realistic. However, as has been shown above, factor images can be extracted from real data and these factor images may be used to reconstruct simulated studies, using for example factor curves generated from mathematical model, which should be more realistic. Provision of such simulations should not only enable the methods described in this paper to be evaluated, but should also allow comparison with more traditional approaches. In addition, because the parameters of the mathematical model generating the factor curves will be known it should be possible to obtain reliable estimates of the accuracy of the physiological parameters extracted, and so, perhaps for the first time, be able to distinguish clearly between errors of measurement and errors of medicine.

## REFERENCES

Barber,D.C. (1980).The use of principal components in a quantitative analysis of gamma camera dynamic studies, Phys. Med. Biol. 25, 283-292.
Barber,D.C. and Nijran,K.S. (1981). Factor analysis of dynamic radionuclide studies, in: Information Processing in Medical Imaging, M.Goris (ed.), Univ. Stanford, Stanford, 13-28.

Bazin,J.P. and Di Paola,R. (1982). Advances in factor analysis application in dynamic function studies, in: Proc. 3rd World Congr. of Nuclear Medicine and Biology, C.Raynauld (ed.), Pergamon, Paris, Vol 1, 35-38.

Houston,A.S. (1986). The use of set theory and cluster analysis to investigate the constraint problem in factor analysis in dynamic structures (FADS), in: Information Processing in Medical Imaging, S.Bacharach (ed.), Martinus Nijhoff, 177-192.

Nijran,K.S. (1984). Analysis of dynamic radionuclide studies using principal components factor analaysis, Ph.D. thesis, University of Sheffield, Sheffield.

Nijran,K.S. and Barber,D.C. (1984). Analysis of dynamic radionuclide studies using factor analysis- a new approach, in: Information processing in medical imaging, F.Deconinck (ed.), Martinus Nijhoff, 30-45.

Nijran,K.S. and Barber,D.C. (1986). Factor analysis of dynamic function studies using a priori physiological information, Phys. Med. Biol. 31, 1107-1117

# INTELLIGENT TRIGGERING OF MULTIGATED STUDIES

Valentin Fidler, Milan Prepadnik, Peter Rakovec, Jurij Fettich, Sergej Hojker, Ciril Grošelj and Miran Porenta

University Clinic of Nuclear Medicine
Ljubljana, Yugoslavia

## ABSTRACT

The object of the work is the development of universal triggering method for multi-gated studies, so that several different representative cycles can be acquired simultaneously. The commonly used method takes the physiological signal (e.g.ECG, respiratory movement, EMG, etc), it electronically detects the most significant structure (R-wave, inspirium peak, etc) and triggers the computer acquisition of scintigraphic data. Using existing commercial systems, differentiation among different events is based on their time duration and it is impossible to resolve timely similar cycles.

In our laboratory, the computer controlled triggering was developed. By means of an additional microprocessor the physiological signal is structure analysed and the trigger code for a chosen shape is sent to scintigraphic acquisition system. For ECG recognition in equilibrium gated radionuclide ventriculography a two-parametric (interval derivative and area) image was created from short record and the limit area for each differentiable ECG structure was selected and used in real time scintigraphic data triggering.

Currently, the intelligent gated list-mode acquisition is used for separate reconstruction of representative heart cycles of regular sinus beats, ventricular and/or supraventricular extrasystoles and postextrasystolic beats.

## INTRODUCTION

Multi-gated studies, specially radionuclide ventriculography, are among the most frequent nuclear medicine procedures. Clinically, the differentiation between normal and pathological heart cycles is very important in estimating the global and regional functional indexes and the contraction-conduction wave patterns for each kind of cycle. Accordingly, the nuclear stetoscope with the capability of real time categorizing the heart pump function, would be an improvement in continuous patient monitoring.

The conventional method (Adam et al., 1979; Bitter et al.,1979) of the gating technique divides the physiological cycle into time segments,each presented by an image. The gate signal comes to acquisition system from a physiological signal recorder at the beginning of each functional cycle (electrical end diastole, inspirium, etc).The criterion for cycle selection is average cycle interval +- tolerance measured before the acquisition starts and taken as a constant during the acquisition. The problem with this method is rejection of large number of cycles in patients with arrhythmias. An improvement of this technique was made by Ioannou et al.(1981), who introduced the changing of average cycle interval by taking the average of the last four normal cycle intervals. He also decreased the rejection of cycles by combining the ejection part of the too short current cycle with the filling part of the previously accepted cycle. The method is preferred to others because of short acquisition time and small computer storing memory. For patients with arrhythmias the gated list-mode acquisition (Kalff et al.,1982) was developed, which stores the spatial coordinates for each detected gamma ray along with the time and gate marks on big mass storage media. From these data and the histogram of gate-to-gate intervals the representative cycle is reconstructed for each chosen part of histogram. The latest improvement of this method is an integration of a semi-automated ECG analysis system with the list-mode acquisition system (Houle et al.,1987) and reconstruction of representative cycle is based on gate-to-gate interval and beat classification code. The disadvantage of this method is a very long acquisition time (20-30 minutes) and large mass storage capacity (more than 30 Mbytes).

In our work we have tried to find solutions to intelligent triggering for existing acquisition systems with different software limitations and we are proposing a model of a universal acquisition system.

METHODS

Ideal acquisition system

Ideally, the acquisition system should work as shown schematically in fig.1a. Every physiological cycle should be recognized and categorized in the appropriate representative sequence of images in real time acquisition. None of the heart cycles would be lost. For such acquisition technique the study time would be short and the physiological conditions equal for all kind of representative cycles. The computer hardware configuration would be the following (fig.1b). Spatial x and y data go directly (DMA) into the temporary buffer and after completing a cycle it is added according to the cycle duration into the appropriate buffer, what is determined and coded by microprocessor analyser of physiological signal.

Two-parametrical shape analyser

Microprocessor physiological analyser should be able to do the following functions in real time monitoring: analog to digital conversion, pattern recognition and sending the coded information to scintigraphic acquisition system. The method of physiological shape differentiation should be fast enough. We have tried several standard methods of pattern recognition as: cross correlation, difference and gradient methods (Abboud and Sadeh, 1984; Akker et al.,1982; Wartak et al.,1970).None of them was fast enough to differentiate the QRS shapes in real time successfully.

(a)

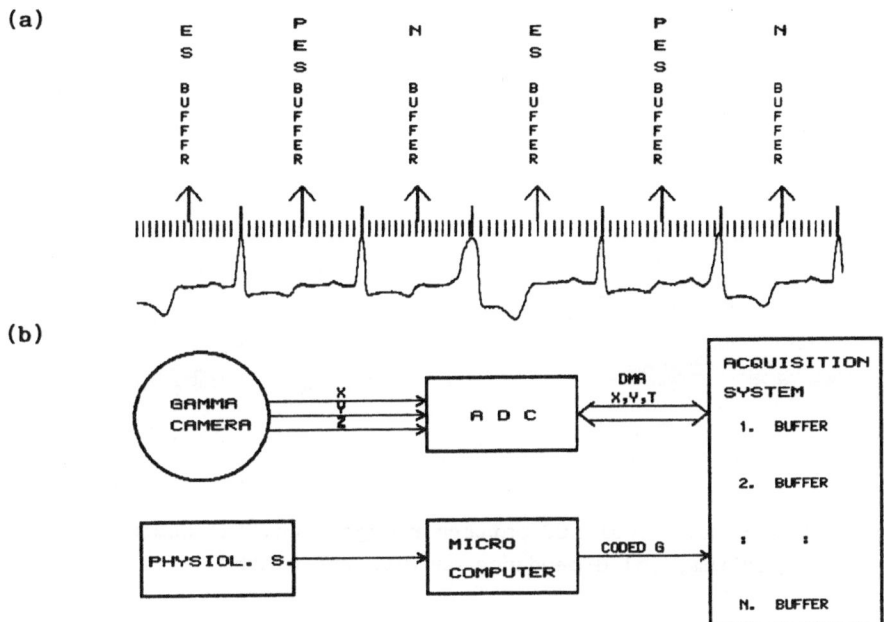

(b)

Fig.1. Schema of the ideal multi-gated acquisition system.(a) Beat-to-
beat categorizing the  scintigraphic data;(b) hardware configuration.


The method we have introduced in ECG recognition is based on two-parametric information of ECG shape. We have found that the most  significant
shape parameters are the interval  area between ECG and its baseline and
the interval arc, approximated by the sum of successive derivatives (fig.
2a).  The interval width N is responsible for a positioning of ECG structures in two-parametric space. Small N (N < 5) makes large differences
between normal and pathological structures in arc's direction and vice
versa, large N (N > 4) makes large differences in area's direction (fig.
2b). For an easier R-wave maximum detection the small N (N=2 or 3) is
preferred.

At the beginning of the study the "learning" ECG record has to be analysed and from two-parametrical diagram the limit range for interval area
and arc has to be chosen manually (fig.3a). The  chosen regions should
not overlap. When real time monitoring is applied, the interval area and
arc are computed for every ECG sample and compared to the predefined

(2a)

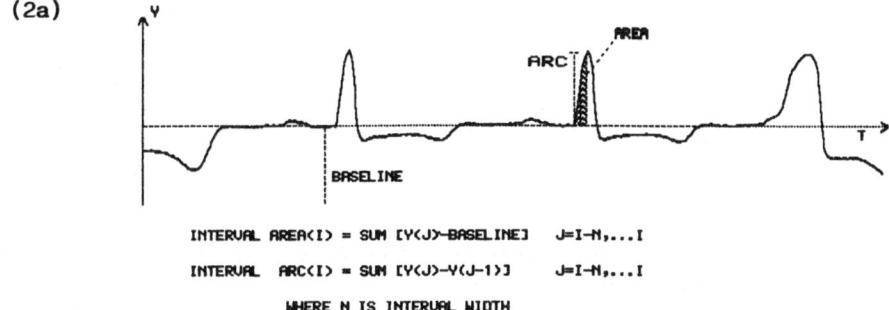

2b

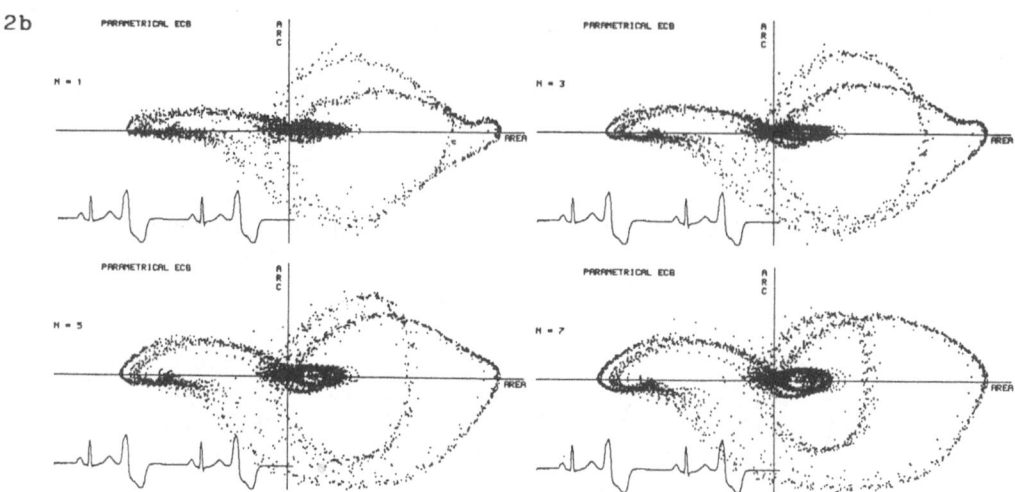

Fig. 2. Two-parametrical ECG pattern recognition. (a) Computation
algorithm; (b) dependance on interval width.

(a)

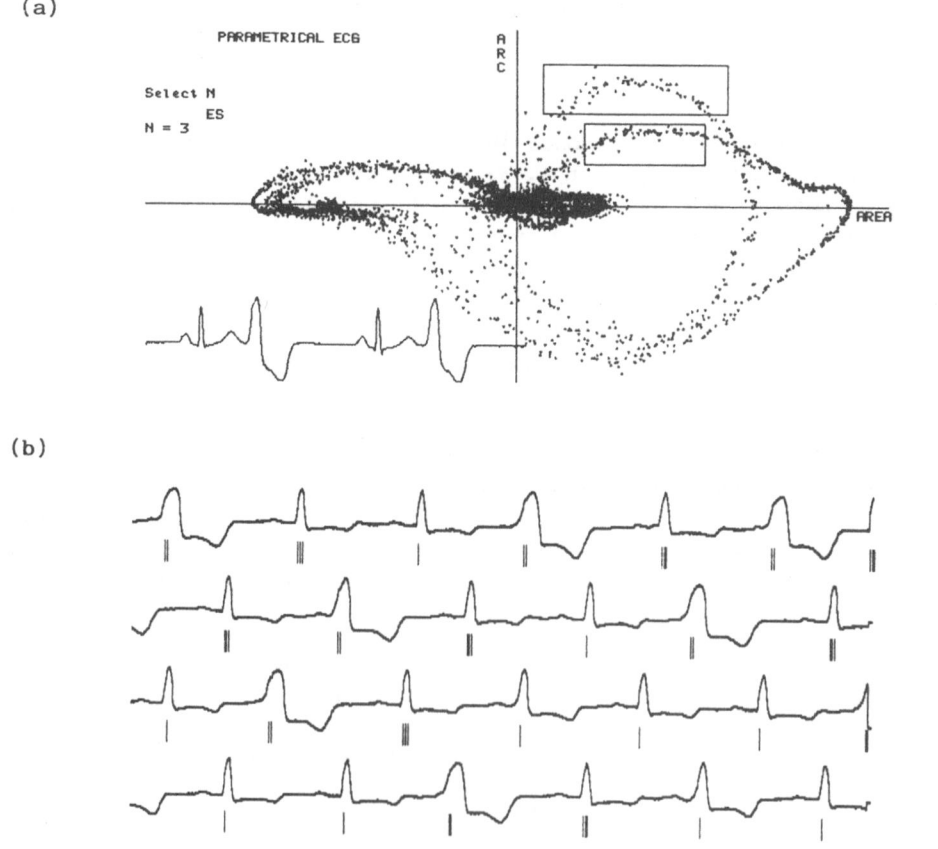

(b)

Fig. 3. Selection of two-parametric limit range (a) and an example of
trigger pulse sequence (b).

values of the chosen QRS shapes. The appropriate code is formed and sent to the scintigraphic acquisition system. An example of ECG monitoring and QRS coding is shown in fig. 3b. The method of two-parametric pattern recognition can also be applied to other physiological signals.

## Classification of acquisition system for multi-gated studies

Gated histogram mode acquisition is mostly applied for regular and uniform ECG signal. Principally, there are two kinds of such acquisition softwares. We called them "past" and "future" systems.

The "past" system (Ioannou et al., 1981) acquires scintigraphic data in the temporary buffer from latest R-wave to the currently detected R-wave. If R-to-R interval is within tolerance, then the sequence of images from temporary buffer is added to the representative cycle in the accumulating buffer. The "future" systems start acquiring the scintigraphic data at currently detected R-wave on condition that the time interval in the last cycle was within tolerance.

For ECG forms as shown in fig. 4 we are unable to acquire the scintigraphic data properly. The upper Ecg has unacceptable R-to-R average cycle time for gated histogram mode. For such ECG type with a large difference in the R-to-R interval between normal and extrasystole cycles we can acquire data in gated list mode. The lower one has an acceptable average R-to-R interval, but normal and extrasystole cycles are mixed in one representative cycle. Because of both R-to-R intervals overlapping we cannot use gated list mode.

## RESULTS

### Solutions to intelligent triggering of existing acquisition systems

For "past" gated histogram acquisition mode systems the intelligent triggering can be applied consecutively (fig. 5). First the normal cycles are acquired, then extrasystole and at last postextrasystole cycles. Microprocessor ECG analyser sends only two trigger signals, at the beggining and end of the proper cycle. Before the acquisition starts, the system is "adapted" to the proper average R-to-R interval. This is determined by the ECG microprocessor analyser and the regular train of trigger code is sent to the acquisition system.

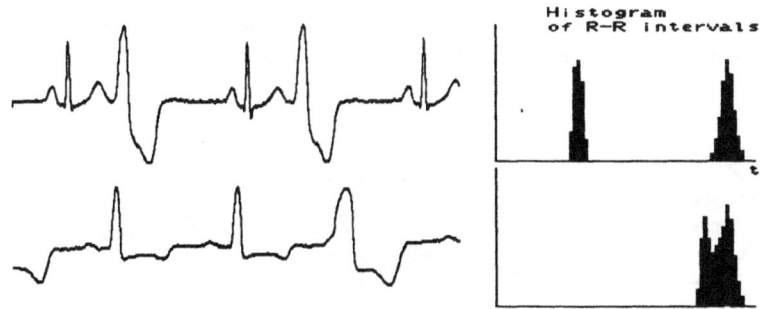

Fig. 4. ECG patterns with well separated (upper) and overlapping (lower) R-to-R cycle times for normal and extrasystole heart beats.

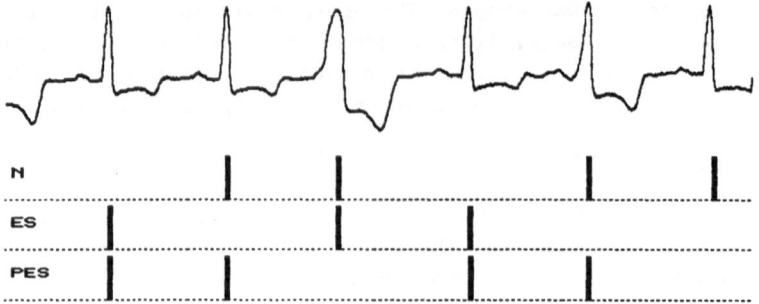

Fig. 5. Consecutive acquisition in "past" gated histogram systems.

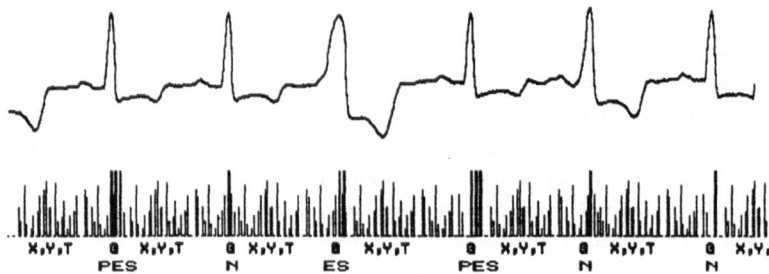

Fig. 6. Intelligent gated list-mode acquisition in systems with no "gate-to-gate" time limit.

In "future" gated histogram mode systems one can solve the triggering problem only by using a modified gated list mode acquisition. If the system has no gate-to-gate limitation, the following trigger code, as shown in fig.6, can be applied to mark different cycles.

Most of the systems, also GAMMA 11, have a gate-to-gate interval limitation. The solution to intelligent scintigraphic data acquisition is coding the "z" impulse (fig. 7a). After each extrasystole R-wave the "z" impulse is electronically disconnected for a short time (2 mseconds) and after postextrasystole R-wave for double period (fig. 7b). From recorded gate and "z" marked list mode scintigraphic data all types of representative cycles can be reconstructed. It takes approximately 2 to 3 hours of processing time for 20 million data in high computer language.

(7a)

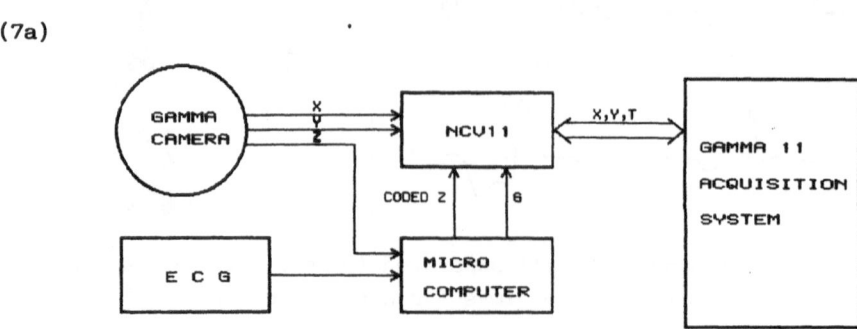

(7b)

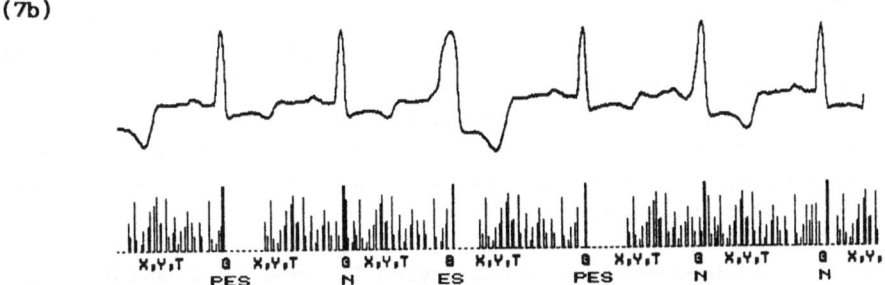

X,Y,T    G   X,Y,T    G   X,Y,T    G   X,Y,T    G   X,Y,T    G   X,Y,T    G   X,Y,
PES        N        ES        PES        N        N

Fig. 7. Intelligent gated list-mode acquisition in systems with "gate-
to-gate" time limitation. (a) Hardware modification; (b) software modification of system.

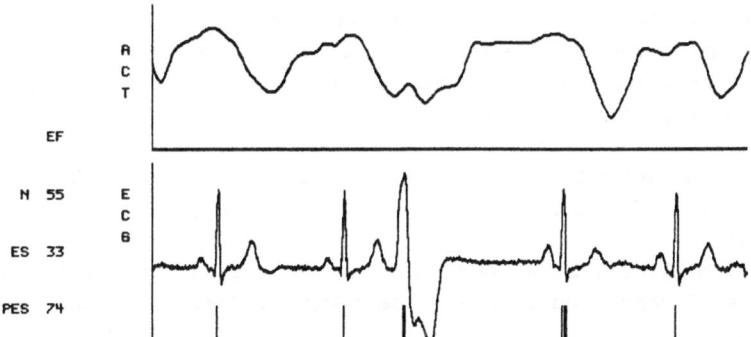

Fig. 8. Real time categorizing of ejection fraction with nuclear stetoscope.

Elegantly, the ECG pattern recognition and cycle categorizing has been
applied to nuclear stetoscope where real time classifying of ejection
fraction becomes possible (fig.8).

With the described hardware and software modifications for the last
type of systems we successfully tested the system on several patients
with contraction-conduction abnormalities.

DISCUSSION AND CONCLUSIONS

The developed intelligent gated list-mode acquisition and proposed
solutions to other systems make possible the acquisition in patients who
have any kind of arrhythmia. The average cycle time is not sufficient for
the selection of the physiologically different cycles. Additionally, characteristic shape criteria for physiological signal are introduced in
creating the trigger code for categorizing the scintigraphic data. This
new feature in multi-gated acquisition is gained by parallel real time
processing of physiological signal by use of an additional microprocessor
Unfortunately, the proposed modifications of commercial systems are cumbersome because of time acquisition and processing inefficiency and large
storage needs. An ideal intelligent system is proposed with short acquisition time, several accumulating buffers and no reconstruction needed.

# REFERENCES

Adam, W. E., Tarkowska, A., Bitter, F. et al. (1979). Equilibrium (gated) radionuclide ventriculography, Cardiovasc. Radiol. 2, 161–173.

Bitter, F., Adam, W. E., Geffers, H. et al. (1979). Synchronized steady state heart investigations, in : Ultrasound, Dose Planning and Nuclear Medicine, 3, J. Garsou, W. Gordenne, and G. Merchie (eds.), Presses Univ., Liège, 9.1–9.5.

Ioannou, B., Kearns, D. S., LaRosa, J., Applegate, R. (1981). Cardiac Module II. A microprocessor-based device for on-line determination of cardiac ejection fraction, Picker J. Nucl. Instr., 2, 1, 6–13.

Kalff, V., Pitt, B., Rabinovitch, M. and Thrall, J. (1982). The use of list-mode radionuclide ventriculography, Software (MDS), 10 (2), 1982, 6–11.

Houle, S., Yip, T-C-K., Friedman, F., Berland, G., Herscovici, Liu, P. (1987). An integrated ECG analysis and list mode processing system for gated blood pool studies, J. Nucl. Med., 28 (4), 618.

Abboud, S. and Sadeh, D. (1984). The use of cross-correlation function for the alignment of ECG waveforms and rejection of extrasystoles, Comput. Biomed. Res. 17, 258–266.

Van Den Akker, T. J., Ros, H. H., Koeleman, A. S. and Dekker, C. (1982). An on-line method for reliable detection of waveforms and subsequent estimation of events in physiological signals, Comp. Biomed. Res. 15, 405–417.

Wartak, J., Milliken, J. A. and Karchmar, J. (1970). Computer Program for Pattern Recognition of Electrocardiogram, Comput. Biomed. Res. 4, 344–374.

# MULTI-PARAMETRIC CLASSIFICATION IMAGES

## OF CARDIAC LV RWMA IN NUCLEAR MEDICINE

JJ Sychra(*), DG Pavel(*), and  E Olea(**)

(*)  University of Illinois, Chicago, U.S.A.
(**) University of Chile, Santiago, Chile

## INTRODUCTION

It is often difficult to extract information of interest from multiple radiological images as they may contain an overwhelming amount of information ( and noise ) that is only remotely or not at all related to the diagnostic information we are seeking.  This problem led to the development of parametric images, representing 2-D spatial distributions of a single physical ( or statistical ) variable describing certain features of physiological functions ( hence "functional images" ). However, the current parametric images do not suggest directly how the input image data should be interpreted diagnostically. The processes and algorithms generating the current parametric images do not use information that is available outside the input image data of the studied single case ( for example, diagnostically labeled image data of previous patients and the frequency of their occurrence in the patient population ) and other diagnostically important information  ( results of diagnostic tests, age, sex, medical history, ... ).

In order to overcome this shortcoming we have developed two new types of parametric  images : regression and discriminant classification images. The new images directly suggest a diagnosis of the regional wall motion abnormalities (RWMA) when presented with normal or RWMA data, and are void of the information not relevant to the intended diagnostic effort. The computer "learns" the patterns characteristic for diagnostic classes of interest from already diagnosed  images, and then expresses in the classification images of a new patient the presence of these patterns. While the actual development has been tuned to the image data generated by radionuclide equilibrium gated cardiac studies and to the problem of the diagnosis of the LV RWMA, the concept is a general one and can be readily applied to a variety of other imaging problems in radiology.

## MATERIALS AND METHODS

### Image Data Base

The used data base contains image data from 16 normals and 51 patients with various degrees and localization of left ventricular (LV) RWMA, 67 cases in total. The normal cases were determined by clinical examination, ultrasound echo evaluation and by phase (Pavel et al., 1984, 1983) and factor analysis (Cavailloles et al., 1985, Pavel et al., 1984, 1986, Harman, 1977). The RWMA cases were confirmed in addition by biplane contrast angiography. Every case was acquired on the SOPHA Simis-4 computer as a time sequence of 64 images representing an average heart cycle, each image 32x32 pixel large. The input image data were preprocessed before the feature extraction took place : the input image sequences were corrected for the data loss (Bitter et al., 1979, Byrom et al., 1981), zoomed by bi-linear interpolation with the zoom factor of 2 and subsequently the number of images was reduced to 16 by summing images of subsequent image quartets in the time domain. In the next step the region of interest (ROI) of the LV at the end of diastole was established as well as a sample of the background domain (Byrom et al., 1981). The image data were then transferred on the VAX computer for the final analysis.

Using the combination of diagnostic procedures mentioned above, the second and the third author of this article classified LV pixels into one of the following 8 classes : (1) **normal #1** ( pixels from normal cases ), (2) **normal #2** ( normal pixels from RWMA cases ), (3) **mildly hypokinetic**, (4) **hypokinetic**, (5) **hypo-akinetic**, (6) **akinetic**, (7) **akinetic-dyskinetic** and (8) **dyskinetic**. Questionable pixels - mostly at the base of the LV ROI - were not used in the training set. The resulting "ideal" classification images of the data base contain approximately ten thousand labeled pixels.

### Feature Space

To "teach" the computer by the LV pixels already classified by a physician into RWMA classes, each LV pixel was described to the computer by its feature vector $\mathbf{f} = [ f_1, f_2, \ldots, f_n ]$, composed by features $f_i$. The derived features can be separated into the following categories :

**Relative location of pixels.** As LVs differ by location, size, shape and overall orientation from case to case, the column-row pixel coordinates are practically useless as features to the classification process. To compare the pixels' feature values and to take into consideration the **relative** locations of pixels in the LV as well, we have developed a simple "LV-ROI-invariant" coordinate system. Its origin is located at the center of gravity of the LV ROI and its coordinate axes are parallel to the eigenvectors of the covariance matrix of the original column-row coordinates of the LV pixels. The metric of the new coordinate system is then given by the normalization by the square roots of the eigenvalues, i.e. the covariance matrix of the new coordinates of the LV pixels is the identity matrix. The pool of the used coordinate features also include polar coordinates of the LV pixels in the new coordinate system.

**Normalized time activities.** The time activities ( count rates ) depend on the size of the LV, on the concentration of the radioactive material in the blood and on the background level. We have used the following types of time activity (TA) normalization :

(1)    normalization by the local TA span ( $c' = (c-c_{min})/(c_{max}-c_{min})$ , where $c_{min}$ and $c_{max}$ are the pixel's extreme activities, and $c$, $c'$ are the pixel's TA before and after the normalization, respectively ),

(2)    normalization by the mean LV TA span ( $c' = (c-c_{min})/(C_{max}-C_{min})$, where $C_{min}$ and $C_{max}$ are pixels' extreme activities averaged over the whole LV ), and

(3)    normalization by the span of "95%-tile" of TA extremes over the

whole LV ( $c' = (c-c_{min})/(D_{max}-D_{min})$, where $D_{min}$ and $D_{max}$ are 5%-tile and 95%-tile of the LV pixels' minima and maxima, respectively, i.e. just 5% of all TA minima in a given LV are smaller than $D_{min}$, and just 5% of all TA maxima of the LV pixels are greater than $D_{max}$ ).

**Quartiles, moments and extremes of the pixel's TA curve.** Let us normalize the pixels's TA so that its new minimum is 0 and its maximum 1. The quartiles are then the relative times, normalized by the length of the RR interval and measured from the time of the maximal TA, when the normalized TAC reaches its .75, .50 and .25 heights, respectively. In addition, the normalized TAC levels at relative times .25, .50 and .75. have been also used as pixel features. The TAC moment features are the values of the central moments of the inverted pixel's TAC. The TAC extremes features are the times when the pixel's TAC and its time derivatives reach their extreme values.

**TA span features.** These features are measures of the amplitude ( or minimum ) of the pixel's TA, related to the variability of the activity over the whole LV. They include

(i)     the pixel's TA amplitude normalized by the mean LV TA span, i.e. the used feature value is $(c_{max}-c_{min})/(C_{max}-C_{min})$;

(ii)    the pixel's TA amplitude normalized by "95%-tile" of the TA span over the whole LV, i.e. the used feature value is $(c_{max}-c_{min})/(D_{max}-D_{min})$;

(iii)   the pixel's minimal TA level normalized by the mean LV TA span, i.e. the used feature value is $(c_{min}-C_{min})/(C_{max}-C_{min})$;

(iv)    the pixel's minimal TA level normalized by the "95%-tile" of TA, i.e. the used feature value is $(c_{min}-D_{min})/(D_{max}-D_{min})$;

(v)     the regional and differential regional ejection fractions, and

(vi)    the TAC amplitude normalized by the LV-mean ejection fraction.

**Fourier features.** The computed Fourier features of the TAC consist of the first three phases and normalized amplitudes of the Fourier expansion of the pixel TAC. The second and the third amplitude are normalized by the first one, which is then normalized by its LV-mean. For the continuity reasons we are also using sines and cosines of the phase angles. The phase angle features are measured relative to the vector-mean phase angles over the whole LV, i.e. the mean value of sines of the pixel phases over the whole LV becomes zero and the mean value of cosines is equal to one ( we will add mode-referenced phase measures at a later data )

**Global features.** The global features are constant for all pixels of the same LV. Those derived from the image data express global measures of the LV TA, for example, ratios of different measures of the TA scatter, such as LV-mean TA span $C_{max}-C_{min}$, standard deviation over LV of the pixel TA span and percentiles of the pixel distributions of TA spans ($D_{max}-D_{min}$). The rest of the global features originates outside the input image data : age, sex and heart rate.

It must be stressed that **the features listed above do not depend on the amount of blood inside the LV, the concentration of the radioactive material in the blood or on the background level** ( the only exception are the ejection fraction related features, which depend on the accuracy of our estimates of the background radiation level ).

## Regression Analysis

As the RWMAs can be ordered according to their severity, one can assign to every applicable pixel k an integer regression value $c_k$, the degree of the RWMA. We have used the regression scale from 1 ( pixels from normal cases ) to 8 ( dyskinetic pixels ) - see the class list above. Using the training set's pixel feature vectors $\mathbf{x}_k$ and the corresponding RWMA classifications $c_k$, where $k = 1,2,...,m$ and m is the size of the training set, the regression analysis (Seber, 1977, Draper and Smith, 1966) is then used to derive the "RWMA function" $f(\mathbf{x})$. This analytical function f of the pixel feature vector $\mathbf{x}$ approximates the associations $\{\mathbf{x}_k;c_k\}$ of the pixel feature vectors $\mathbf{x}_k$ with the corresponding RWMA classes $c_k$, i.e., the function $f(\mathbf{x})$ approximates the diagnostician's classification optimaly under the conditions imposed by the type of the used regression analysis. The type of the sought-after function $f(\mathbf{x})$ is chosen beforehand. Once the function $f(\mathbf{x})$ is known, regression images of new, undiagnosed LVs can be generated, with pixel intensities corresponding to the estimated local degree of the RWMA.

The presented regression images are based on the results of the linear regression analysis with the least squares condition on a selected feature subset, i.e. we have searched for the function

$$f(\mathbf{x}) = \mathbf{a}\mathbf{x} + b, \tag{1}$$

with constants $\mathbf{a} = [a_1,a_2,...,a_n]$ and b minimizing the mean regression error $\epsilon$ :

$$\epsilon^2 = (1/n) \sum_{k=1}^{k=n} w_k [ f(\mathbf{x}_k)-c_k ]^2 , \tag{2}$$

where n is the number of the selected features and $w_k$ are regression weights. We have also investigated the minimizing of the mean absolute error $\epsilon'$ :

$$\epsilon' = (1/n) \sum_{k=1}^{k=n} w_k | f(\mathbf{x}_k)-c_k | , \tag{3}$$

but did not find a significant improvement in the corresponding regression images, especially after images of the both type were submitted to a noise suppressing filter. While the process of minimizing $\epsilon'$ usually took approximatelly twenty times longer than the minimization of $\epsilon$, the value of $\epsilon'$ decreased only about 1% from that obtained by the minimization of $\epsilon$.

As it is usual in the regression analysis, one has to compromise between the "best feature subset" and the "best regression equation". For practical reasons we have limited the number of features used to generate regression images to the "best" 16 features. Because of the computational time constraints, the used 16-feature subset had to be selected in a sub-optimal manner : the exhausting evaluation of all 16-feature subsets from the available pool of 136 features would require an evaluation of $2.6 \times 10^{20}$ of feature subsets. To do that, even a supercomputer spending only one second on each evaluation would require more than $8 \times 10^{12}$ years. The term "best" is then subjective as there is no unique statistical method for the corresponding feature selection. Consequently, the selection of the method is a question of personal judgment. In our case we have restricted the available feature pool by selecting the best 32 features for the 8 classes by Wilks' $\lambda$ and Rao's $\mathbf{V}$ tests (Montgomery and Peck, 1982, Finn, 1974). Starting with the best 12 features - in the Wilks and Rao sense - we

## TABLE 1. The "best" 16 regression features, excluding age, sex and heart rate

| Feature | Wilks' $\lambda$ | Rao's V |
|---|---|---|
| global "95%-tile" TA span normalized by the mean pixel's TA span ( $(D_{max}-D_{min})/(C_{max}-C_{min})$ ) | .597 | 6480 |
| cosine of pixel's 1st phase angle | .414 | 11088 |
| sine of pixel's 1st phase angle | .332 | 14350 |
| global "95%-tile" TA span normalized by the LV-mean standard deviation of pixels' TA | .292 | 16028 |
| modified longitudinal pixel's coordinate | .264 | 17597 |
| normalized pixel's minimum of TA | .242 | 18796 |
| pixel's 14-th TA normalized by the global "95%-tile" TA span | .230 | 19553 |
| pixel's 1st Fourier amplitude | .208 | 20829 |
| pixel's 1st Fourier amplitude / ejection fraction | .190 | 22533 |
| pixel's 14-th TA normalized by LV-mean TA amplitude | .182 | 23219 |
| pixel's 1st TA normalized by pixel's TA amplitude | .176 | 23830 |
| pixel's 7-th TA normalized by LV-mean TA amplitude | .171 | 24268 |
| pixel's 4-th TA normalized by LV-mean TA amplitude | .168 | 24489 |
| pixel's 4-th TA normalized by pixel's TA amplitude | .163 | 25104 |
| pixel's 3rd Fourier amplitude | .161 | 25354 |
| pixel's 4-th TA normalized by the global "95%-tile" TA span | .158 | 25525 |

have searched by the stepwise regression for additional 4 features. In the next steps we have repeatedly eliminated features by a backward search, and then searched again by the stepwise regression for the needed features to complete the 16-feature set. This process was stopped after the mean error $\epsilon$ could not be decreased more than 0.1% by an additional eliminate/add cycle. The selected feature subsets were also tested and favored by the Mallows' $C_p$ statistics (Seber, 1977).

As we have mentioned above, our pool of available features contains the global features age, sex and heart rate. When a training set represents well the applicable patient population, the inclusion of these features is justified and desirable. One can even go further and stress the importance of certain groups of patients ( for example certain age categories ) by assigning greater values to their weights $w_k$. However, the sets of normals and patients used to build our present training set are relatively small. Consequently, the training set may be a biased representation of the diagnosis seeking population ( the age and sex distributions and our insistence on using only catheterized patients are the most probable sources of a bias ). While the used training set is acceptable for an illustration of the method, it may need a further enlargement before it can be used **routinely** for clinical diagnosis. For this reason, and also to illustrate the additional classification improvement by inclusion of the global features, we have developed two main types of regression images. The first category is generated from features derived from input image data only; the second category includes age, sex and heart rate. In both cases the error $\epsilon$ was minimized with unit weights $w_k$. The selected features are listed in order of selection by Wilks' $\lambda$ in the Tables 1 and 2 together with their cumulative Wilks' $\lambda$ and Rao's V.

## Discriminant analysis

When the regression analysis is applied to the classification of the individual LV pixels, we are taking advantage of the fact that the RWMAs can be ordered according their severity. However, in a general diagnostic

TABLE 2. The "best" regression features

| Feature | Wilks' $\lambda$ | Rao's $\mathbf{V}$ |
|---|---|---|
| age | .585 | 6806 |
| global "95%-tile" TA span normalized by the mean pixel's TA span ( $(D_{max}-D_{min})/(C_{max}-C_{min})$ ) | .363 | 15669 |
| cosine of pixel's 1st phase angle | .253 | 20324 |
| sine of pixel's 1st phase angle | .203 | 23742 |
| sex | .165 | 27480 |
| modified longitudinal pixel's coordinate | .149 | 28923 |
| pixel's 1st TA normalized by pixel's TA amplitude | .142 | 29799 |
| pixel's 7-th TA normalized by LV-mean TA amplitude | .136 | 30566 |
| longitudinal pixel's coordinate | .132 | 31184 |
| normalized pixel's minimum of TA | .126 | 31901 |
| pixel's 9-th TA normalized by the global "95%-tile" TA span | .122 | 32479 |
| heart rate | .117 | 33045 |
| pixel's 7-th TA normalized by the global "95%-tile" TA span | .115 | 33423 |
| pixel's 3rd Fourier amplitude | .113 | 33624 |
| 1st phase angle minus the time of TA minimum | .112 | 33789 |
| time of the 1st 25% TA quartile | .110 | 34233 |

case such an ordering is not possible, and a more general classification approach must be taken. As an alternative to the regression analysis, we have investigated an application of the Fisher's discriminant analysis (Hand, 1981) to the classification of LV RWMA.

During the first step, the "best" 25 features in the Wilks and Rao sense were selected ( they include almost all features selected for the regression analysis ). In the next step seven linear Fisher's discriminant functions, corresponding to the eight RWMA classes, were defined. As a result, the 25-D classification problem has been reduced to a 7-D problem, with the resulting 7-D space of discriminant functions providing optimal separation of the classes in the sense of the Fisher criterion ( maximizing the ratio of distances of the sample means and the standard deviation within the samples ). The generation of the discriminant functions and the observation of the resulting data suggest approximately normal distribution of the class samples in the discriminant function space. In the next step unit priors were used to derive the corresponding normal classifier in the space of the discriminant functions. Besides the indication of the discriminant power of individual input features, the discriminant analysis resulted in the following four types of the pixel descriptors :

*(i)*     discriminant functions,

*(ii)*    the probability with which a pixel belongs in RWMA classes,

*(iii)*   the $\chi^2$ measure of the departure from a class sample centroid, and

*(iv)*    the identification of the class into which the pixel is classified.

### Generation of classification images

The used training set consists of approximately 10000 pixels. The classification images were derived for two "optimal" feature subsets, one without the global features age, sex and heart rate, and one including the three global features.

**Regression images.**     The regression transforms were derived for the "best" 16-features, selected in the manner described above. The regression values were computed for all LV pixels and piece-wise linearly mapped on the pseudocolor scale. The regression images can be presented in two different modes : the "continuous scale" regression images, obtained by the just described process and shown in Fig.1, and the discrete scale "class" regression images. The "class" images are obtained from the former ones by rounding the regression values to the nearest class identifying value.

**Discriminant images.** The corresponding classification rules for eight classes of pixels were derived using the "best" 25 features in Wilks $\lambda$ sense. While the method permits to generate a variety of discriminant analysis images, only the predicted class membership images were generated for this manuscript, as they are easy to compare with the regression images and the "ideal" classification images drawn by the physician.

The noise in the resulting images was suppressed by a conditional 3x3 median filter : a pixel value was replaced by the median when the pixel value differed from the median more than a given threshold difference.

## RESULTS AND DISCUSSION

To illustrate how the proposed methods handle new, "unknown" cases, we have selected an object set of six typical cases and removed them from the above training set. The corresponding regression coefficients **a** and b of (1) and classification rules were then found, and the matching regression and discriminant images were computed.

First, we have found in preliminary analyses that - measured by the time activity behavior, by the regression values and by the clustering of the first four discriminant function values - the hypokinetic pixels are much closer to the "normal" pixels from abnormal cases than to the pixels from normal cases. Therefore, we have divided the pixels classified by the human experts as normal into the corresponding classes : **normal** 1 ( from normal cases, represented by the 2nd darkest grey ) and **normal** 2 ( from abnormal cases, represented by the 3rd darkest grey ). The classification images further add a weight to this observation ( see Fig. 1, rows 3 to 5 ) : most of the pixels of the normal cases were classified by the computer into the **normal** 1 class, and practically all "normal" pixels of the abnormal cases into the **normal** 2 class. We have also observed that adding the age, sex and heart rate information improved the classification of pixels from normal and slightly abnormal cases, which may be in a part influenced by the age distribution in our data base.

As the diagnostician's confidence in his own pixel classification varies with the degree of mutual agreement among information provided by phase and factor analyses, echocardiography and biplane contrast angiography, we have decided to declare computer classifications into a RWMA class next to the "ideal" one as correct. The quality of the obtained classification results can be evaluated at two different levels : the LV and the pixel RWMA diagnosis, respectively. The rating at the LV level may be desirable, but is very subjective and not quite compatible with the method used to generate the classification images : the regression and discriminant analyses were used to classify individual pixels, not the whole LVs. Nevertheless, the classification images generated on the full training set were found in good agreement with the diagnosis previously arrived at by physicians. When the location of abnormality, its extent and its maximum degree were evaluated, the correlation was found to be very good in 67% of the cases, and in 29% of the cases the regression images were judged acceptable. The remaining 4% were debatable, but even in these cases none was falsely positive or falsely negative.

## TABLE 3. Mean regression errors of the training set

( the mean absolute error $\epsilon'$ is based on the least
square error $\epsilon$; the mean actual pixel error $\epsilon''$
is $\epsilon'$ after conditional median filtering )

| Feature sets | $\epsilon$ | $\epsilon'$ | $\epsilon''$ |
|---|---|---|---|
| 16-features without age,sex and heart rate | 1.20 | .96 | .75 |
| 16-feature including age,sex and heart rate | 1.13 | .88 | .70 |

Pixel classification errors provide more objective evaluation of the obtained results. The regression analysis errors $\epsilon$ and $\epsilon'$ are listed in the Table 3, which also shows that the mean absolute error of the regression image pixel values decreases about 20% due to the filtering by the conditional median filter. In the case of normal pixels the errors $\epsilon$, e' and $\epsilon''$ are approximately 25% lower, and in the akinetic/dyskinetic pixels 64% higher, than the averages given in Table 3. The classification accuracy of the discriminant analysis classifier on the training set is presented in the form of confusion matrices in Tables 4 and 5, respectively. As the severe misclassifications rarely occur in large clusters, they are usually suppressed on the image level by the conditional median filter ( most of the time the misclassifications seem to be caused by either noise or erroneous delineation of the LV border ).

As we have mentioned above, to illustrate the diagnostic quality of the regression images of "new", "unknown" cases, the typical cases were removed from the training set, and then their regression images were derived ( Fig. 1.). The first two columns represent two normal cases, and the remaining four columns are images of the LVs of four patients with various degrees of RWMA. The continuous grey scale wedge on the left side is applicable to the 1st to 4th image row, respectively, while the discrete scale wedge on the right side is used for the rest of the picture ( its darkest grey segment is applicable only to the lowest image row where it represents unclassified portions of left ventricular images ). The top image row contains the distribution of the best TA feature, the normalized 6th input intensity. The second row contains a powerful linear combination of 25 input features, the 1st Fisher discriminant function. The next four rows contain regression ( rows # 3 and 4 ) and discriminant ( rows # 5 and 6 ) images, not including ( rows # 3 and 5 ) and including ( rows # 4 and 6 ) age, sex and heart rate information. The "ideal" classification images drawn by physicians on the basis of all available information ( before the first regression results were known ) are displayed in the bottom row. The regression and classification errors of this set of six cases are roughly 4 to 7% higher than when they are included in the training set.

## TABLE 4. Training set classification based on 25 features
( sex, age and heart rate not used )

| actual group | predicted by computer (% of classified pixels) | | | | | | | |
|---|---|---|---|---|---|---|---|---|
| | norm_1 | norm_2 | m_hypo | hypok | h_akin | akinet | a_dysk | dyskin |
| normal 1 | 89 | 6 | 1 | 2 | 0 | 2 | 0 | 0 |
| normal 2 | 15 | 31 | 25 | 21 | 4 | 3 | 1 | 0 |
| mild hypokin. | 10 | 18 | 44 | 17 | 5 | 4 | 1 | 1 |
| hypokinetic | 7 | 8 | 13 | 42 | 13 | 13 | 3 | 1 |
| hypo-akinetic | 1 | 8 | 6 | 19 | 41 | 17 | 6 | 2 |
| akinetic | 3 | 1 | 6 | 11 | 18 | 48 | 10 | 3 |
| aki-dyskinet. | 0 | 0 | 0 | 4 | 9 | 13 | 62 | 13 |
| dyskinetic | 0 | 0 | 0 | 3 | 4 | 20 | 14 | 59 |

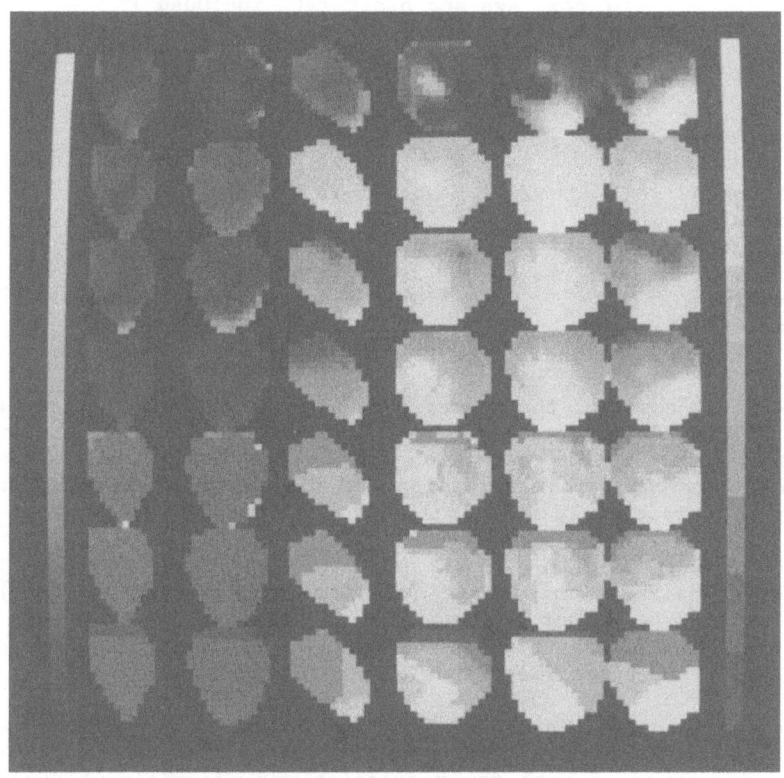

**FIG. 1.** Classification images of the left ventricle

**Columns 1 and 2** : two normal cases;
**columns 3 to 6** : four RWMA cases.
**Row 1** :    normalized 6th input activity, selected by the
             Wilks' $\lambda$ and Rao's **V** tests test as the most
             powerful single TA feature ( the color scale range
             of values is <0; 0.6>;
**row 2** :    the first discriminant function, including age,
             sex and heart rate information;
**row 3** :    continuous regression measure of RWMA based on 16
             features, not including age, sex and heart rate (
             blue corresponds to the normal regional wall
             motion, white to the highly dyskinetic one );
**row 4** :    same as row 3, but age, sex and heart rate
             features were included in the regression analysis;
**row 5** :    classification images based on the discriminant
             analysis ( 25 features ), not using age, sex and
             rate information;
**row 6** :    as in row 5, but the feature pool contained age,
             sex and heart rate features;
**row 7** :    the "ideal" classification drawn by physicians,
             based on all available information.

**The continuous grey scale** is used in rows 1 to 4.
**The discrete grey scale** used in rows 5 to 7, from bottom up
: not classified, normal 1, normal 2, slightly hypokinetic,
hypokinetic, hypo-akinetic, akinetic, aki-dyskinetic, and
dyskinetic ( white ).

TABLE 5. **TABLE 5. Training set classification based on 25 features ( sex, age and heart rate included )**

| actual group | predicted by computer (% of classified pixels) | | | | | | | |
|---|---|---|---|---|---|---|---|---|
| | norm_1 | norm_2 | m_hypo | hypok | h_akin | akinet | a_dysk | dyskin |
| normal 1 | 94 | 5 | 0 | 0 | 1 | 0 | 0 | 0 |
| normal 2 | 12 | 34 | 24 | 23 | 3 | 3 | 0 | 0 |
| mild hypokin. | 4 | 24 | 46 | 17 | 5 | 3 | 1 | 1 |
| hypokinetic | 1 | 11 | 15 | 47 | 8 | 14 | 2 | 2 |
| hypo-akinetic | 0 | 8 | 5 | 13 | 50 | 16 | 6 | 2 |
| akinetic | 1 | 2 | 5 | 18 | 10 | 50 | 11 | 3 |
| aki-dyskinet. | 0 | 0 | 0 | 4 | 7 | 17 | 59 | 13 |
| dyskinetic | 0 | 0 | 1 | 2 | 4 | 19 | 10 | 64 |

The **first case** and the **second case** are normal cases and are as such recognized by the classification images. While there is a suggestion of slight hypokinesia in the regression images not using the age, sex and heart rate information, the regression and discriminant images using this information are practically identical with the "ideal" images drawn by the physician.

The classification images of the **third case** demonstrate a remarkable ability to detect and localize the small akinetic domain at the apex. The probable overestimation of the area of mild hypokinesia is acceptable as it satisfies the criterion postulated above.

The **fourth case** is a challenging one - even to a physician - as one may guess from the complexity of the corresponding "ideal" image. The only significant departure of both the regression and discriminant images from the "ideal" image is the shift of the most severe RWMA toward the septum. This shift is also demonstrated in the images of the 1st and the 2nd row.

In the **fifth case**, the classification images are in a good agreement with the physician. However, the regression images not using age, sex and heart rate information overestimate the degree of the RWMA from the LV center toward 3 to 4 o'clock. The regression images also overestimate the RWMA in the apex domain, while discriminant images have a tendency to underestimate the RWMA in the vicinity of the septum. Nevertheless, these slight departures from the ideal image satisfy the acceptance criteria formulated above.

The **last case** is an example of an overall good agreement between the regression images and the human expert's classification. However, the regression images may be pushing the transition hypokinetic region too close to the base of the LV in the segment at 1 to 2 o'clock, especially when age, sex and heart rate information is included.

The strength of the developed classification images is in their ability to extract from a large image data base multiparametric information, to use supplementary information provided by other means and to "learn" from image data already classified by a consensus of human experts, who based their decisions on information from several diagnostic procedures. Consequently, the regression and discriminant images tend to offer a robust and objective diagnosis of RWMA. However, the process of building a good training set is usually time consuming. To further improve the obtained classification results - we expect to at least halve the present regression errors and misclassification by the discriminant analysis - we are at present developing new features, enlarging our image data base and making it more representative of the patient population diagnosed in our department.

# REFERENCES

Bitter, F., Adam, W. E., and Geffers, H., 1979, Synchronized steady state heart investigations, in: "Proceeding symposium on fundamentals in technical progress : ultrasound, dose planning and nuclear medicine", J. Garsou, W. Gordenne, G. Merchie, eds., Presses Universitaires de Liege, Lieage.

Byrom, E., Pavel, D., Swiryn, D., and Meyer-Pavel, C., 1981, Phase images of gated cardiac studies: a standard evaluation procedure, in: "Functional Mapping of Organ Systems and Other Computer Topics", Society of Nuclear Medicine, New York.

Cavailloles, F., Bazin, J. P., and DiPaola R., 1985, Factor analysis in gated cardiac studies, J. Nucl. Med. 25:1067.

Draper, N., and Smith, H., 1966, "Applied regression analysis", John Wiley & Sons, New York.

Finn, J. D., 1974, "A general model for multivariate analysis", Holt, Rinehart and Winston, New York.

Hand, D. J., 1981, "Discrimination and classification", John Wiley & Sons, New York.

Harman, H. H., 1977, "Modern factor analysis", The University of Chicago Press, Chicago.

Montgomery, D.C., and Peck, E.A., 1982, "Introduction to linear regression analysis", John Wiley & Sons, New York.

Pavel, D. G., Briandet, P. A., Fang, R. B., Zolnierczyk, K., and Sychra, J., 1984, The normal heart : patterns for various functional images obtained from radionuclide gated equilibrium studies, in: "Information Processing in Medical Imaging", F. Deconinck, ed., Martinus Nijhoff, Brussels.

Pavel, D. G., Sychra, J., Olea, E., Kahn, C., Virupannavar, S., Zolnierczyk, K., and Shanes J., 1986, Factor analysis : its place in the evaluation of ventricular regional wall motion abnormalities, in: "Information Processing in Medical Imaging", Bacharach, ed., Martinus Nijhoff, Boston.

Pavel, D. G., Byrom, E., Lam, W., Meyer-Pavel, C., Swirin, S., and Pietras R., 1983, Detection and quantification of regional wall motion abnormalities using phase analysis of equilibrium gated cardiac studies, Clin. Nucl. Med. 8:315.

Seber, G. A. F., 1977, "Linear regression analysis", John Wiley & Sons, New York.

TWO DIMENSIONAL MAPPING OF THREE DIMENSIONAL SPECT DATA:  A PRELIMINARY

STEP TO THE QUANTITATION OF THALLIUM MYOCARDIAL PERFUSION SINGLE PHOTON

EMISSION TOMOGRAPHY

Michael L. Goris

Division of Nuclear Medicine
Stanford University School of Medicine
Stanford, CA  94305-5105

ABSTRACT

A method is presented by which tomographic myocardial perfusion data
are prepared for quantitative analysis.  The method is characterized by an
interrogation of the original data which results in a size and shape normalization.  The method is analogous to the circumferential profile methods
used in planar scintigraphy, but requires a polar to cartesian transformation from three to two dimensions.  As was the case in the planar situation,
centering and reorientation are explicit.  The degree of data reduction is
evaluated by reconstructing "idealized" three-dimensional data from the
two-dimensional sampling vectors.

The method differs from previously described approaches, by the absence
in the resulting vector of a coordinate reflecting cartesian coordinate in
the original data (slice number).

INTRODUCTION

Planar Thallium Myocardial scintigraphy has been quantified by radial
sampling, starting from the center of the cavity, towards the periphery
(Vogel et al., 1979; Burrow et al., 1979; Mead et al., 1978).  The effect
of this approach has been a reduction of a two-dimensional image, to a one-
dimensional vector, which is not affected by size and shape of the ventricle, but only by the angular orientation (Goris et al., 1981).  This (size
and shape) normalized vector allows the intercomparison of images from different patients, and a quantitative analysis based on the definition of
"normal" count distribution vectors (Goris et al., 1985; Garcia et al.,
1981).

In this paper we present an analogous approach for three-dimensional
data sets, obtained by single photon emission tomography.  Our approach,
which produces a two-dimensional sampling vector is again characterized by
a size and shape normalization, which reduces topographical information to
angular locations, and differs from previously described methods, in which
the radial distance in the polar vector represents a slice number (Mullani
et al., 1986; Caldwell et al., 1984; Garcia et al., 1985).

Tomographic data are acquired in 32 (over 180 degrees) or 64 (over 360 degrees) 64x64 digitized projection images. Tomographic reconstruction is performed by filtered back projection, and results in the production of a 64 cubed digitized reconstruction volume.

Preprocessing includes interactive recentering of the data around the center of the left ventricular cavity. Zooming the centered image by a factor of 2 is optional, if the myocardium appears too small (e.g. when large field of view cameras are used). The zooming of the three-dimensional image is purely a display function, in contradistinction to zooming during acquisition, where the limiting factor is the necessity to have the object (the patient's thorax) recorded in toto in all projection images.

The next step is a thresholding step, in which a single threshold value is subtracted from all pixels in the reconstructed image. This value is interactively selected by the operator, but based on the maximal count rate within the myocardial structure, and in our cases was selected as 33% of the maximum pixel value in the myocardium.

Finally, the data are reoriented, again interactively and under visual control as follows: The operator is presented with the central transverse slice (X,Y,32), central sagittal slice (32,Y,Z) and central coronal slice (X,32,Z), each shown in one screen quadrant. Additionally, three of the remaining four sixteenths of the screen are occupied with an image representing the reprojection of the data on the (XY), (XZ) and (YZ) surface of the cube representing the reconstruction volume. The reprojection consists of a summation of all pixel values along x to produce the reprojection image (YZ), along y to produce the reprojection image (XZ) and along z for (XY).

The rotations which are implicitly performed in a fixed sequence, are, until the last moment simply address correspondence searches. The rotation in one plane would be performed as follows:

A 64x64 vector CART contains the index indicating the corresponding address in a 32x256 vector POL, following a polar transform:

The word in location $n=(y-1)*64+x$ in CART contains a value $m=(I-1)*32+R$, where $I=ARCTAN[(y-31.5)/(x-31.5)]$, expressed in units of 360 degrees/256 and $R=SQRT[(x-31.5)**2+(y-31.5)**2]$. Similarly the word in location $m=(I-1)*32+R$ in POL contains the index $n-(Y-1)*64+x$, where $y=R*sin(I*360/256)+31.5$ and $x=cos(I*360/256)+31.5$.

If $(x,y)'$ are the coordinates of a point in a frame rotated by an angle $I*360/256$ degrees, then the data corresponding to this location in the original frame $(x,y)$ are defined as follows: $(x,y)'$ defines the location $n'$ in CART, where one finds the index $m'$ in POL. In location $m=m'+32*I$ in POL, one finds $n=(y-1)*64+x$ where the data for pixel $(x,y)'$ are to be found. This follows from the fact that cartesian rotations are polar translations (Goris et al., 1981).

Oblique slices are defined as orthogonal slices in a volume which would have resulted from the rotation A,B,C around 31.5,31.5,31.5. As was the case for planar rotation, the operation consists of address equivalence searches, from destination to origin. The address defined by coordinates x",y",z" in the original reconstruction cube of the value belonging in coordinate x,y,z of the reoriented cube is found by three ordered planar rotations. The first rotation A, around the axis 32,32,z yields x',y',z and is a rotation in the zth transverse section (XY). A second rotation B

around the axis 32,Y,32 yields x'',y',z' and is a rotation in the newly
defined y'th frontal plane (X',Z). A third rotation C around x,32,32 yields
x'',y'',z'' and is a rotation in the newly defined x''th sagittal plane
(Y',Z').

The angles A,B, and C are individually and incrementally modified
using the keyboard. At each incrementation the orthogonal slices (X,Y,32),
(X,32,Z) and (32,Y,Z) in the virtually, but not actually, rotated volume
are shown. Images in the right lower quadrant illustrate the individual
rotations along the three axes.

When the operator validates a particular set of angles, the whole
volume is rotated. The goal of the rotation (and preliminary centering) is
to have the ventricular long axis along the (32,32,z) axis of the reoriented
image volume.

The final interaction is the search for the center of the three-dimensional radial sampling and the limits of the sampling volume. Quadrants 1
and 2 display central long axis slices in the (X,32,Z) and (32,Y,Z) planes.
In overlay 3 lines indicate the zero angle Phi parallel to the long axis
(to correspond to the apex) and the Phi angles +/- 135 degrees. Under visual
control the operator moves this overlay until the 0 angle radius intersects
the apex, and one of the 270 degree radii becomes tangent to the edge of
the myocardial wall at the valve plane, while the other does not intersect
the myocardial wall. The motion of the Y-shaped overlay is controlled in
three planes (X,Y) along y and z seen in quadrant 1 and x and z seen in
quadrant 2. At validation, the origin of the three radii becomes the center
of the recentered reconstruction volume and is not necessarily the center
of the left ventricular cavity.

The limits illustrated by the two Y-shaped overlays are those of a
partial sphere centered around (31.5,31.5,31.5), which defines the sampling
volume Phi, Theta, Rho with Rho going from 0 to 31 (in units of voxels),
Theta going from 0 to 255 in units of 360/256 degrees, and Phi from 0 to 31
in units of 180/48 degrees.

Sampling is performed along the surface of the circular cone defined
by an origin at (31.5,31.5,31.5) and the solid angle Phi for the 32 values
of Phi. The surface is sampled along a radial value Rho from 0 to 31 for
the angle Theta from 0 to 255. To compensate for the undersampling (when
Rho reaches the value 31) (Goris et al., 1981) sampling is, however, performed along three lines defined in the volume by Phi-1, Phi, and Phi+1.
The resulting sampling values are the maximum value (count rate density)
along the radius (MAX(Phi,Theta), and the integrated value (sum of all count
rate densities) TOT(Phi,Theta).

The resulting values are placed in two 64x64 arrays, one for MAX and
one for TOT, which are originally initialized (all values are zero). The
sampling values MAX(Phi,Theta) are placed in location (x,y) of the corresponding array, where x is defined as Phi*cos(Theta)+31.5 and y=Phi*sin-
(Theta)+31.5. Since the mapping is many to one (32x256 into 64x64), the
stored value is the larger of the value in place and the newly defined value.

Sampling results therefore in the generation of two 64x64 images,
obtained by a polar to cartesian transformation. In this cartesian representation the distance from the center represents the value of the angle
Phi or longitude, and the angle represents the value of Theta or latitude
(Bull's-eye representations). The two Bull's-eye images are further normalized to 256 for MAX and (256*6) for TOT.

To display the data reduction inherent in this approach, idealized

volume data are reconstructed as follows:  The density values
MAX(Phi,Theta) are placed in a 64x64x64 image volume in the pixels defined
by (Phi,Theta,R1) to (Phi,Theta,R2), where R1=16 and R2=16+TOT(Phi,Theta)/
MAX(Phi,Theta).  The count rate density in this idealized image represents
therefore the maximum sampling value at each angle, while the wall
thickness (R2-R1) is defined by the relation between total counts and
maximum counts.

To test to what extent the method is indeed insensitive to the effect
of the target's size, we processed 11 randomly selected cases, but before
and following tri-dimensional zooming.  The resulting Bull's-eye vectors
are compared either to an "average" Bull's-eye vector, or a comparison is
made between the vector obtained from the stress image and the one obtained
from the redistribution image.  In both cases the comparison yields a
single positive value, which is the integrated negative difference.

The value should be nearly identical regardless of the zooming, but
is to some degree influenced by the reproducibility of centering, and discretisation "errors" due to data reduction in a discrete space.

All processing is performed on a Motorola 68010 based microprocessor,
with a 256 kilobyte programming memory, and a 1 megabyte image memory.


RESULTS AND DISCUSSION

In this paper the analysis of reconstructed tomographic data, rather
than the reconstruction itself, is described.  One assumes only that the
reconstructed data have maintained spatial coherence, i.e. that slices are
one pixel wide, and in their natural order, while the reconstructed volume
is mapped in a 64x64x64 cube.

Since all images are sampled into a 32x256 vector, in which the coordinates correspond to angular location, and in which the radial coordinate
Rho does not appear, there is an implicit size and shape normalization:
The reduction of all topographical information to angular coordinates nor-
malizes the shape, the elimination of the Rho coordinate eliminates the
effect of size (Goris et al., 1981).

It is worth noting that the origin of the polar coordinate system is
defined as a location on the long axis of the ventricle, further defined by
a fixed angle between two vectors tangent to the base of the myocardium, an
approach which appeared to us to be more easily consistent than an unaided
definition of the center of the cavity.

To make the vectors comparable within a patient study, or between
patient studies, one nevertheless needs a normalization of the origin of
Phi and Theta.  In our case this is achieved by the reorientation on the
basis of three angles (A,B, and C), in contradistinction to reorientations
by two rotations, which makes further definition of the origin of Theta
necessary (Mullani et al., 1986).

The undersampling inherent for small values of Phi in the polar to
cartesian transformation which creates the Bull's-eye image, is compensated
by the oversampling along Theta, in the circular cone surface, when Phi is
small.

The choice of MAX and TOT as sampling values is somewhat arbitrary,
but in line with published quantitation methods, where in general the maximum value along a radius is the only value sampled (Vogel et al., 1979;
Burrow et al., 1979; Mead et al., 1978;  Garcia et al., 1981; Calwell et

al., 1984; Garcia et al., 1985). Some have restricted the sampling to the line integral (Mullani et al., 1986), which seems to have a better rationale, assuming that one tries to identify global perfusion for each sampling angle. For planar data the analysis has also been based on sampling for the maximum value, the line integral, and the average value, from which one can derive the wall thickness (Goris et al., 1981; Goris et al., 1985). But in planar data the analysis is complicated by the concatination of volume and concentration effects (Goris, 1979). Theoretically the count rate densities in tomographic data represent concentrations only, and wall thickness can independently be determined.

In this approach we choose to derive the wall thickness from the (arbitrary) ratio of TOT/MAX, but we keep MAX and TOT for further quantitative analysis.

Thresholding remains critical. We assume in the case of tomography that a single threshold is rational, since one intends to interrogate the data about the presence or absence of a sufficient tracer concentration in the target organ. A variable threshold, by which one attempts to accommodate the effect of volumes superimposed on the target (Goris et al., 1976) is not critical. The criteria for this threshold remains, however, to be determined by experience.

In contradistinction to the published Bull's-eye methods (Mullani et al., 1986; Caldwell et al., 1984; Garcia et al., 1985), in which the distance from the origin corresponds to a slice number, in our method the sampling is wholly angular. The distinction is necessary, since one would, in the former method, need an additional normalization for the number of slices and the slice thickness. This could be done by compression (Caldwell et al., 1984; Garcia et al., 1985) but assumes that the original number of slices between upper upper and lower limits is an integral multiple of the number of compressed slices, or requires a method of interpolation.

Additionally, when parallel slices are used for the analysis of SPECT or PET data, the problems of slices tangential to the myocardial wall, and, wholly or partially cutting through them must be accommodated. This problem is only partially overcome by the addition of slices parallel to the long axis, for the analysis of the apex (Garcia et al., 1985), an approach which requires a separate determination of the region "assigned" to the apex, and which, in the presented form, arbitrarily assigns a sampling direction to the apex.

The comparison between the results in the case of zoomed versus unzoomed images was performed by linear regression. For the absolute comparison, that is with an "average" Bull's-eye vector, the regression yielded:

$$Y = 0.9659 \ X - 162$$

where Y is the integrated difference for unzoomed data, and X for zoomed data. The average value of Y was 4071, and of X 4383. The standard error of the estimate was 884, and the F-ratio 945. In a paired difference analysis the average difference was -311 +/- 269.

This compares well with the relative comparison (stress versus redistribution) where size does not play a role, but reproducibility of centering and discretisation do. In this case the regression yielded:

$$Y = 0.866 \ X + 57$$

with an average value for Y of 1322 and for X of 1459. The standard error of the estimate was 305 and the F-ratio 96. The average paired difference was found to be -137 +/- 98.


CONCLUSION

The reduction of tomographic data to a set of sampling vectors, represents a first step for quantitative analysis. There are three fundamental aspects to this reduction: First, to allow inter-patient comparison, the analysis has to include size and shape normalization, and a reorientation normalization. Our results indicate that the size normalization works, since the variation between results due to different sizes of the image do not seem to significantly add to the variation caused by lack of centering reproducibility.

Second, one needs to evaluate the degree of data or information loss resulting from the reduction. This is done by recreating idealized images, and judging whether they are a fair representation of the original data. Finally, even though thresholding in tomographic data is a simpler problem than in planar imaging, a standardized approach will have to be determined.

But, once the sampling vectors are defined, tomographic myocardial perfusion studies can be analyzed in manners analogous to the methods used in planar scintigraphy (Goris et al., 1985; Garcia et al., 1981). The two dimensions in the sampling vector do however maintain proximity relations which existed in the three dimensions.

REFERENCES

Vogel, R.A., Kirch, D.L., Lefree, M.T., Rainwater, P.O., Jensen, G.P., and Steele, R.P. (1979). Thallium-201 myocardial perfusion techniques, Am J Cardiol, 43 , 787-793.

Burrow, R.D., Pond, M., Schafer, A.W., and Becker, L. (1979). "Circumferential profiles": A new method for computer analysis of Thallium-201 myocardial perfusion images, J Nucl Med, 20, 771-777.

Mead, R.C., Bamrah, V.S., Horgan, J.D., Ruetz, P.P., Kronenwetter, C., and Yeh, E-L. (1978). Quantitative methods in the evaluation of Thallium-201 myocardial perfusion images, J Nucl Med, 19, 1175-1178.

Goris, M.L., Sue, J., and Johnson, M.A. (1981). A principled approach to the "circumferential" method for Thallium myocardial perfusion scintigraphy quantitation, in: "Functional Mapping of Organ Systems and Other Computer Topics," P.D. Esser, ed., Society of Nuclear Medicine.

Goris, M.L., Gordon, E., and Kim, O. (1985). A stochastic interpretation of thallium myocardial perfusion scintigraphy, Invest Radiol, 20, 253-259.

Garcia, E., Maddahi, J., Berman, D., and Waxman, A. (1981). Space/Time quantitation of Thallium-201 myocardial scintigraphy, J Nucl Med, 22, 309-317.

Mullani, N.A., Ranganath, M.V., Adler, S., Goldstein, R.A., Volkow, N., and Gould, K.L. (1986). 3-D surface mapping of functional PET images for the heart and the brain, J Nucl Med, 27, 918 (abstract).

Caldwell, J.H., Williams, D.L., Harp, G.D., Stratton, J.R., and Ritchie J.L. (1984). Quantification of size of relative myocardial perfusion defect by single-photon emission computed tomography, Circulation, 70, 1048-1056.

Garcia, E.V., Van Train, K., Maddahi, J., Prigent, F., Friedman, J., Areeda, J., Waxman, A., and Berman, D.S. (1985). Quantification of rotational Thallium-201 myocardial tomography, J Nucl Med, 26, 17-26.

Goris, M.L. (1979). Non-target activities: Can we correct for them? J Nucl Med, 20, 1312-1314
(Teaching editorial).
Goris, M.L., Daspit, S.G., McLaughlin, P., and Kriss, J.P. (1976).
Interpolative background subtraction, J Nucl Med, 17, 744-747.

# SIMULTANEOUS EMISSION AND TRANSMISSION TOMOGRAPHY

D.L. Bailey and B.F. Hutton

Department of Nuclear Medicine
Royal Prince Alfred Hospital
Sydney. Australia

## INTRODUCTION

Single Photon Emission Computed Tomography (SPECT) has the capability of providing quantitative information about in-vivo radionuclide activity distribution using a rotating gamma camera, which is now available to most nuclear medicine departments. This quantitative potential has been limited largely because of the inability to accurately correct for the effects of photon attenuation. Researchers are becoming increasingly aware that knowledge of attenuation coefficients is necessary to implement accurate attenuation correction, particularly in the thorax. However, this normally necessitates an extra study. This paper proposes a method which overcomes this limitation by measuring the attenuation of the body with a transmission scan concurrent with the measurement of radiopharmaceutical distribution. The accuracy of the method when applied to iterative post-reconstruction attenuation correction is examined.

Essentially two problems are considered. Firstly, there is the simultaneous acquisition and subsequent separation of attenuation and emission data, and secondly, the methodology in which these data are used for reconstructing quantitatively accurate emission scans. As the emphasis is on accurate attenuation correction, the problem of scatter correction in the emission photopeak is not addressed in this paper.

## SCATTER SUBTRACTION IN SIMULTANEOUSLY RECORDED TRANSMISSION AND EMISSION DATA

### Transmission Scanning

The use of transmission scanning to delineate anatomy has been in use in nuclear medicine for over 20 years (Kuhl et al, 1966; Anger et al, 1968; Sorenson et al, 1969). More recently, the incorporation of transmission computed tomography (TCT) data into attenuation correction protocols has been proposed. Webb et al (1983) suggest that transmission scanning would overcome the attenuation correction problem in principle, but consider the increase in scanning time unacceptable. Moore (1982), using X-ray TCT, and Malko et al (1986), using an external flood source and a

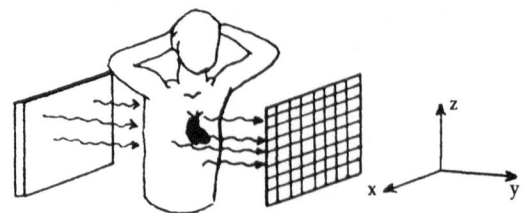

Figure 1. Geometry of transmission scanning

gamma camera, have both described attenuation correction using transmission data. The geometry of the transmission source and detector is shown in figure 1. This co-ordinate system will be used throughout the paper to describe both emission and transmission imaging.

Both methods still suffer from the need for separate studies of emission and transmission and the associated problems, such as increased scanning time and difficulty in patient re-alignment.

To use a transmission scan for correction, the acquired planar transmission data are converted to attenuation data which are then suitable for backprojection. The conversion is done by solving for the attenuation coefficient ($\mu$) in the equation

$$N_t(x,z) = N_o \exp\left(- \sum_{i=1}^{d} \mu_i(x,z)\Delta y\right) \tag{1}$$

giving

$$\sum_{i=1}^{d} \mu_i(x,z) = \frac{\ln(N_o/N_t(x,z))}{\Delta y} \tag{2}$$

where $N_t$ is the transmitted count rate, $N_o$ is the unattenuated count rate from the source, and d is the distance from the source to the detector. The constant $\Delta y$ is equivalent to the size of a pixel, and the attenuation of photons in air is assumed to be negligible.

After this conversion, convolution backprojection is performed in the usual manner. The resultant tomographic slices contain the attenuation coefficients per pixel.

To overcome the difficulties expressed by the above authors, the method proposed is that the transmission scan be acquired at the same time as the emission tomogram. This does introduce other problems, however, which will be discussed in the following sections.

Simultaneous Acquisition of Transmission and Emission Data

The concurrent imaging of transmission and emission data requires that the two sets of data can be separated by some means. It would be difficult to separate the data if photons of the same energy were used for both studies. Separation can be accomplished by the use of a transmission source of different photon energy to the emission source, to permit discrimination by pulse height analysis. Another consideration is that the transmission imaging procedure should not interfere with the emission data, so it is desirable to use a transmission source of lower photon energy than the emission source. The lower energy transmission window will however contain scatter from the upper energy emission radionuclide in this situation which will require correction.

AIR                                    SCATTER

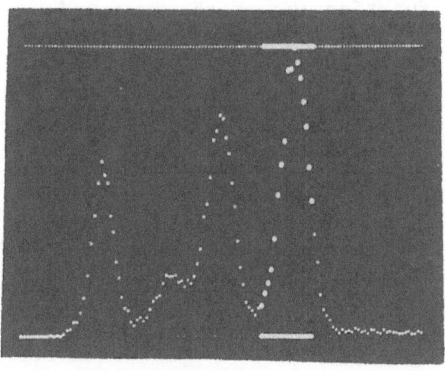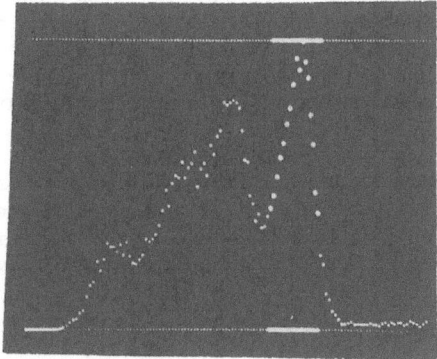

Figure 2.  Energy Spectra for Gd-153 and Tc-99m. The
upper peak is the 140keV Tc-99m peak, and lower two
peaks are from Gd-153 (the lowest is an Eu-153 X-ray).


We have concentrated on Tc-99m as the emission source and so a transmission source of < 140 keV is required. The transmission source used at
present is Gd-153($t_{\frac{1}{2}}$=242d, $E_\gamma$=98 and 103 keV).  The long half-life gives
an effective source life of approximately 1 year, and the 100keV photons
give adequate photopeak separation for NaI(Tl) spectroscopy. The source is
readily available and is inexpensive. Figure 2 shows the combined Gd/Tc
energy spectrum recorded on a gamma camera in both air and in 10 cm of
scattering media (water).

The Gd-153 is used as a flood source which is attached to the rotating
gammma camera by means of a metal frame, so that the source is always on
the opposite side of the subject to the detector. The flood source is not
collimated as this gives attenuation coefficients more appropriate for the
broad-beam imaging case.

Having selected Tc-99m and Gd-153 as the radionuclides for emission
and transmission respectively, a dual radionuclide tomographic study (of
64 angles, over 360°, and typically for 20 secs/angle) is acquired with
photopeak windows of 140keV±10% and 100keV±10%.  This results in two sets
of images, one for each photopeak.


Dosimetry

Any significant increase in radiation dose to the patient must always
be weighed against the potential value of the test.  In the case of this
technique, the greatest proportion of the dose comes from the internal
radionuclide, which the patient would receive for a routine scan.

The radiation exposure from the Gd-153 source was measured with a
hand-held survey monitor at a distance of 1 metre from the source.  The
estimated dose for a 30 minute exposure (a study takes about 25 minutes
normally) was less than 100 µGy for a source activity at its maximum of
1.5GBq (soon after production). This contribution is considered virtually
negligible compared with the radiopharmaceutical dose.


Image Separation

The gamma camera can be considered to be a spatially and temporally

invariant linear system for a point source located at a distance from the
detector (Beck et al, 1973). The transfer function (h) of the system does
depend however on the distance the point is from the detector, the surrounding (attenuating) media, the characteristics of the collimator selected,
the pulse height analyser (PHA) window selected, and the energy of the
photons being imaged. A general linear systems model of the process is
shown in figure 3.

This model is valid for both emission and transmission imaging with
the gamma camera, and for various photopeak windows with variation of h to
suit. As the system is spatially invariant the transfer function is independent of x and z and is therefore only a function of y, that is, the
distance from the detector.

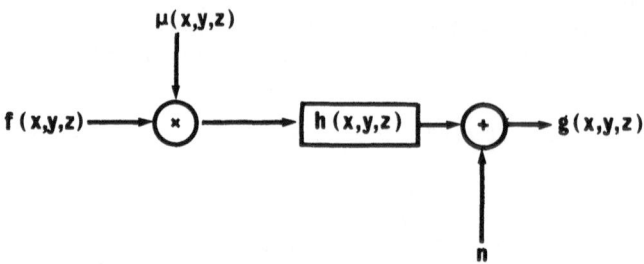

where f is the object distribution
       $\mu$ is the attenuation by the media
       h is the transfer function for the given conditions
       n is additive Poisson noise
       g is the image distribution
and + and x are additive and multiplicative procedures respectively.

Figure 3. General model for imaging system including attenuation

The terminology used in this paper will be that the subscript u
refers to the upper energy window, ul refers to the upper energy object as
seen in the lower energy window, and t refers to the transmission image.

The model of the simultaneous imaging method proposed is shown in
figure 4. The images recorded in a dual energy collection are $g_u$ and $g_o$.
The problem is one of removing the scatter image ($g_{ul}$), which is unknown,
from the lower window observed image ($g_o$) to leave an estimate of the
transmission image ($\hat{g}_t$).

Scatter Removal

As the scatter image ($g_{ul}$) is not known, some method of producing an
estimate of scatter is required. A scatter function (s) may be defined as
the function which, when convolved with the upper energy image, gives the
distribution of the upper energy radionuclide as seen in the lower energy
window ($g_{ul}$), i.e.,

$$g_{ul} = g_u * s \tag{3}$$

where * indicates two-dimensional convolution.

562

The scatter function can either be found by the deconvolution of $g_{ul}$ with $g_u$, or by empirical curve fitting. This is equivalent to the solution of deconvolving $h_{ul}$ by $h_u$:

$$S = \frac{G_{ul}}{G_u} = \frac{F_u \times H_{ul}}{F_u \times H_u} = \frac{H_{ul}}{H_u} \tag{4}$$

where upper case characters refer to the frequency space representation of the real space function.

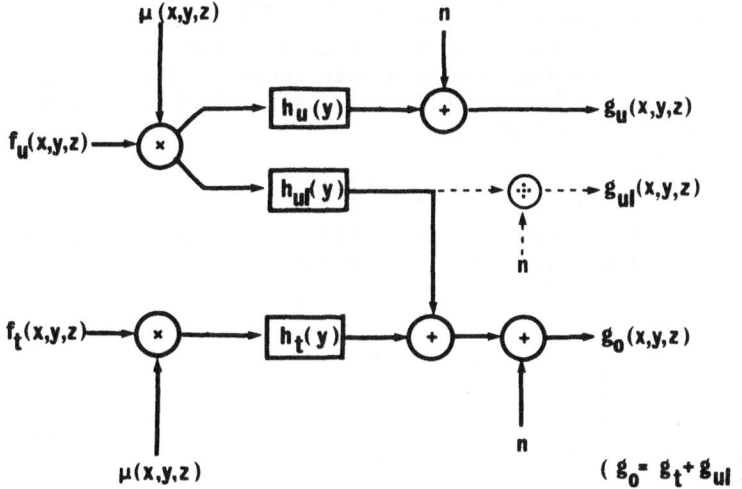

where $g_o$ refers to the observed lower energy window image

Figure 4. Linear systems description of simultaneous emission/transmission imaging

For a planar image, however, the scatter function is highly dependent on the depth of the source in the medium. To minimise this geometric mean (GM) images have been employed. The geometric mean of opposing views has previously been reported as being relatively insensitive to changes in depth for both resolution and sensitivity. (Tothill et al, 1971; Filipow et al, 1979; Larsson, 1980; Axelsson et al, 1984). Further investigation has shown that this depth independent quality is not only limited to photopeak counts, but applies over a good deal of the entire energy spectrum. (Hutton et al, 1987) In particular, the number of counts in a lower (scatter) window is relatively constant for changes in depth. This provides a means of estimating the number of scatter counts expected in the lower energy PHA window. Figure 5a shows three of the energy spectra

recorded for Tc-99m contained in a 150ml ellipsoid at various depths in a
water filled tank (dimensions 30x20x20cm). The decrease in photopeak
counts is clearly seen along with a corresponding increase in the relative
number of scatter counts. Figure 5b shows the mean GM energy spectrum for
the same data, that is, with complementary depths' geometric means calculated. The curve seen is the fit to the data points with the error bars
indicating ±1 standard deviation of the data. For 20% energy windows set
over the Tc-99m and Gd-153 photopeaks the ratio of counts in the lower
window ($C_{ul}$) to the counts in the upper window ($C_u$), termed the scatter
ratio (k), was found to be 0.58±0.012.

The use of GM images therefore allows the number of counts scattered
into the lower window (corresponding to the transmission photopeak) to be
estimated independent of the source depth. The ratio k will vary slightly
for different attenuators and radionuclide distributions, but a mean k is
applicable, in general, to a section of the body (eg. thorax, head, abdomen).

These properties of the geometric mean result in system transfer
functions ($h_u$, $h_{ul}$) which are independent of <u>depth</u> as well as being two-
dimensional spatially invariant. Therefore, as an approximation, a single
transfer function can be employed to predict the spatial distribution of
scatter (ie. $g_{ul}$) in two-dimensional planar images. The scatter function
has been found by empirically modelling it as a radially symmetric bi-
exponential function of the form,

$$s(r,\theta) = Ae^{-br} + e^{-cr} . \tag{5}$$

This was found to give a superior prediction of scatter over solutions
found by deconvolution methods as the deconvolution severely compromised

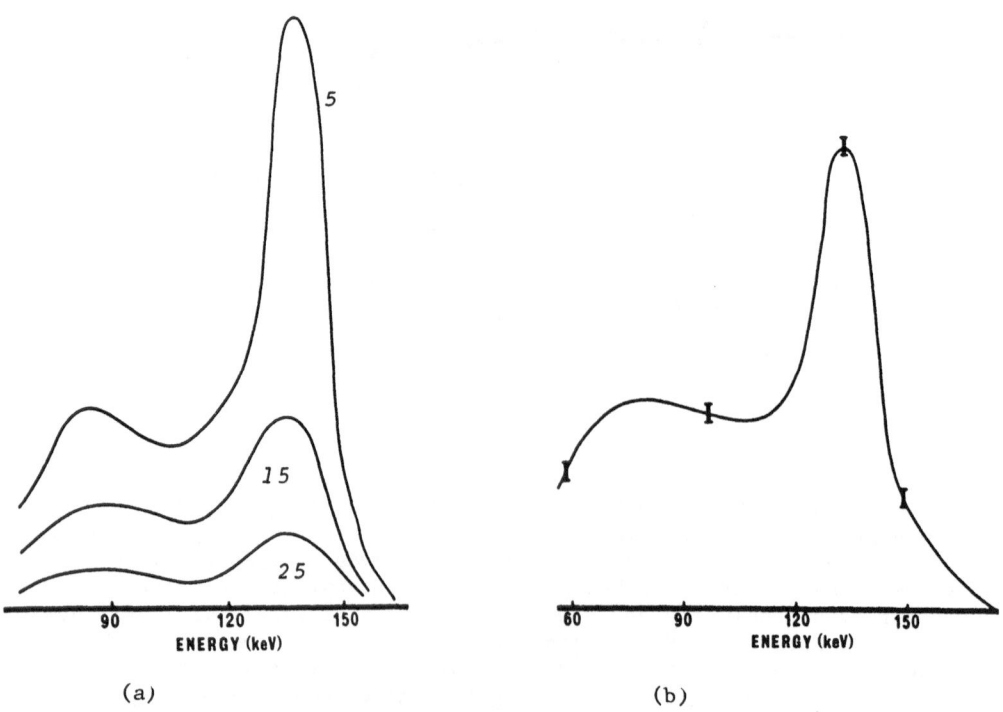

(a)                                             (b)

Figure 5. (a) Tc-99m energy spectra at the depths
              indicated (cm) in a water tank,
          (b) Mean geometric mean energy spectrum of
              the data

the sharp central peak in the solution (Jayasinghe, 1984). The scatter function is convolved with the photopeak GM images ($g_u$) to give the estimated scatter images ($\hat{g}_{ul}$). These images are then scaled (by k) and subtracted from the observed GM lower window images to leave the estimated transmission images, which, from equation (2) can be reconstructed as indicated earlier. An overview of the method is shown in figure 6.

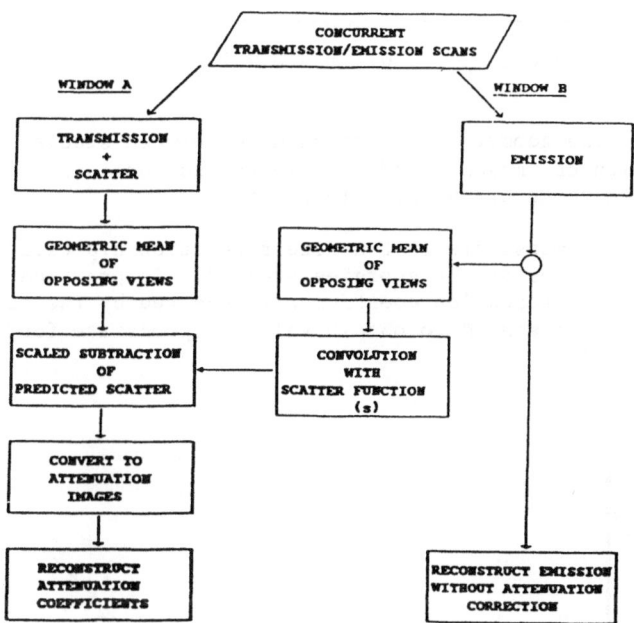

Figure 6. Method for obtaining emission and scatter
subtracted transmission studies

Attenuation at Different Photon Energies

The use of radionuclides with different photon energies raises questions about whether the attenuation coefficients measured by one radionuclide are applicable to another radionuclide with a different photon energy. As Gd-153 has a lower energy than Tc-99m, the coefficients measured by Gd-153 should be higher (ie. more severely attenuated) than for Tc-99m.

To examine this, an attenuation phantom consisting of a number of components of differing densities, and a human volunteer, were both studied by transmission tomography with Tc-99m and Gd-153 transmission sources.

Table 1.  Attenuation coefficients at different
photon energies

A.  Attenuation Phantom

| Component | $\mu_{Gd}$ (cm$^{-1}$) | $\mu_{Tc}$ (cm$^{-1}$) |
|---|---|---|
| Sawdust | .010 | .004 |
| Wood | .043 | .034 |
| Paper Book | .075 | .068 |
| Water | .110 | .093 |
| Perspex | .129 | .120 |

B.  Human Thorax

| Component | $\mu_{Gd}$ (cm$^{-1}$) | $\mu_{Tc}$ (cm$^{-1}$) |
|---|---|---|
| Lung | .039 | .030 |
| Heart | .135 | .122 |
| Chest Wall | .138 | .128 |
| Spine (Bone) | .146 | .140 |
| Aorta | .145 | .129 |

$$\mu_{Tc} = 0.97\mu_{Gd} - 0.007; \quad r = 0.997$$

In each case, the geometry was not changed between studies, allowing direct comparison of images in transverse reconstructions.  The results from table 1 are shown graphically in figure 7.

The results demonstrate that a linear relationship exists between the attenuation of photons at the energies studied.  In practical terms, this suggests that the attenuation coefficients measured by the gadolinium source can easily be scaled to obtain values appropriate for technetium.

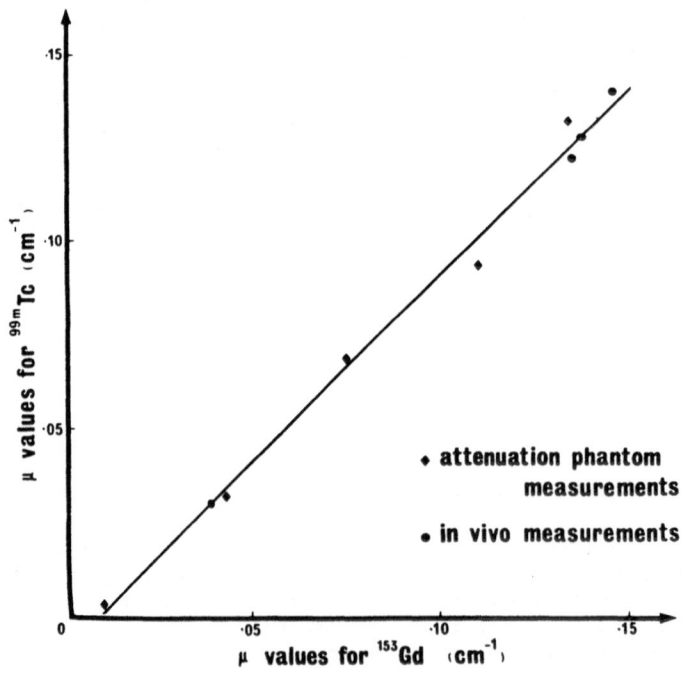

Figure 7. Attenuation coefficients at different energies

The accuracy of the reconstructed attenuation coefficients derived from scatter subtracted transmission imaging will depend on the relative countrates recorded for transmission and emission (which may vary from subject to subject, or over time as the flood source decays), the ability of a single scatter function to predict scatter, and the amount of noise introduced into the reconstruction by the subtraction process. These factors will ultimately determine the extent to which the data can provide accurate reconstructions of radioactivity distribution.

All nuclear medicine images are subject to statistical variations giving rise to uncertainties in measured values. This is amplified in the reconstruction of tomographic sections as the convolution performed before backprojection enhances higher spatial frequency components in the image, one of which is noise. The processing of attenuation data acquired from the simultaneous emission/transmission technique increases the noise in the reconstructions due to the subtraction of estimated scatter.

The scatter subtracted transmission image is given by

$$\hat{g}_t = g_o - \hat{g}_{ul} \tag{6}$$

The image $\hat{g}_{ul}$ is essentially noiseless and so the absolute value of the standard deviation of the final image $g_t$ is the same as for $g_o$, resulting in a poorer signal to noise ratio. The standard deviation of the reconstructed attenuation image has previously been shown to be (Rutherford et al, 1975),

$$\sigma(\mu) = \frac{\sigma(C_t)}{C_t} \times \frac{1}{a\sqrt{12}\sqrt{M}} \tag{7}$$

where $C_t$ = transmitted counts, a = sampling interval(cm), and M = number of projections. For the situation of scatter subtracted transmission the standard deviation in this equation will be replaced by the standard deviation of the image $g_o$ (of count $C_o$),
i.e.,

$$\sigma(\mu) = \frac{\sigma(C_o)}{C_t} \times \frac{1}{a\sqrt{12}\sqrt{M}} \tag{8}$$

To investigate the effects of scatter, a subject had separate transmission and emission scans recorded, so that a true scatter scan ($g_{ul}$) could be acquired as well as the usual emission scan. This true scatter scan was scaled to different count levels, the noise was adjusted appropriately, and then added to the transmission image to simulate different amounts of administered radioactivity. The change in the noise level in the reconstructed images with increasing scatter counts is shown in figure 8. The images shown are from a perfusion lung study (Tc-99m/MAA). The ratio $C_e$:$C_t$ refers to the upper energy window (emission) countrate relative to the transmission countrate for a geometric mean anterior/posterior image, measured over the organ of interest. The $C_e$:$C_t$ ratio of 4.4 is equivalent to twice the routine dose administered in this department.

The average reconstructed u values and their standard deviations for specific areas in the reconstruction are shown in table 2.

The results show that the ability to reconstruct accurate attenuation coefficients is maintained over a range of relative scatter countrates, which for this example is up to twice that expected from a routine study. This is similar to the case where the transmission source has decayed over one half-life and a normal routine dose of radioactivity is used. This then provides the basis for attenuation correction using measured attenuation data.

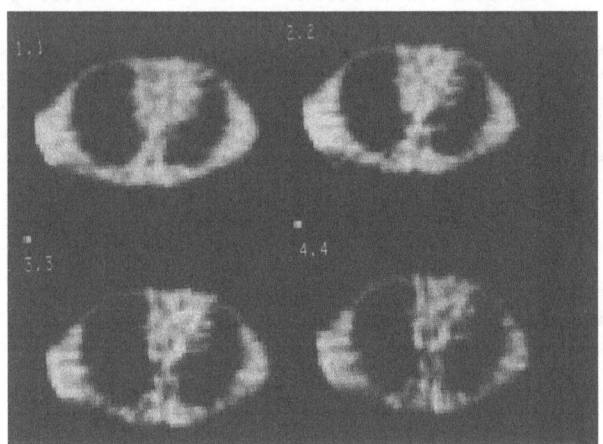

Figure 8.   Attenuation sections from a perfusion lung study for different amounts of scatter. The numbers correspond to the $C_e$:$C_t$ ratio described in the text.

Table 2. Attenuation coefficients reconstructed from scatter subtracted transmission tomography

| Ratio $C_e$:$C_t$ | Attenuation Coefficients (cm$^{-1}$) | | |
|---|---|---|---|
| | Lung $\mu$ (SD) | Heart $\mu$ (SD) | Spine $\mu$ (SD) |
| 0* | .041 (.021) | .134 (.021) | .149 (.021) |
| 1.1 | .042 (.028) | .131 (.039) | .140 (.040) |
| 2.2 | .043 (.028) | .140 (.052) | .134 (.037) |
| 3.3 | .041 (.031) | .137 (.053) | .150 (.049) |
| 4.4 | .037 (.035) | .135 (.068) | .130 (.072) |

* A $C_e$:$C_t$ ratio of zero indicates a transmission study without any emission scatter present.

## IMPLEMENTATION OF SCATTER SUBTRACTED TRANSMISSION DATA IN ITERATIVE ATTENUATION CORRECTION

### Outline of the Problem

Photons emitted from an internally distributed radionuclide undergo attenuation by the surrounding tissues. The reconstructed countrate detected from the point $(x,y)$ in figure 9 is given by,

$$N'_e(x,y) = N_e(x,y) \left[ \frac{1}{M} \sum_{i=1}^{M} \exp(-\mu l(x,y,\theta_i)) \right] \qquad (9)$$

where $N'$ is the attenuated countrate, $N$ is the true (unattenuated) count rate, the subscript $e$ refers to the emission case, $\mu l$ is the sum of attenuation coefficients from the point $(x,y)$ to the detector for the angle $\theta_i$, and $M$ is the number of acquired projection angles.

An approximate post-processing correction can be performed by calculating the inverse of the term enclosed in brackets in (9). In most cases, the $\mu$ values are not known, and the assumption of a constant mean $\mu$ value for all tissues is made. The accuracy of this correction, especially for studies in the chest where there is a large variation in $\mu$ values, is greatly improved if the actual $\mu$ values are used.

In our department, the approach has been to use actual $\mu$ values rather than assume a constant $\mu$ for use in correction. To implement this in a _practical_ protocol has necessitated the development of dual measurement of transmission and emission data.

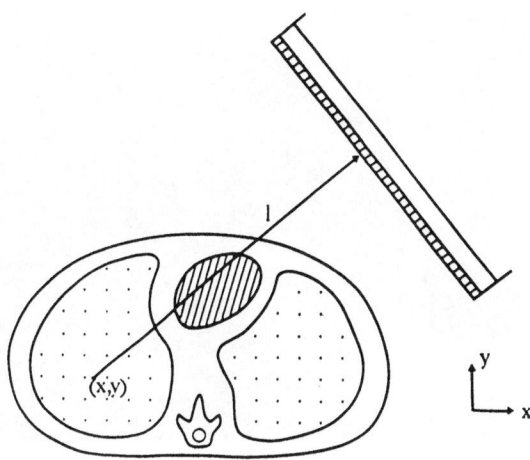

Figure 9. Attenuation of emitted photons

First Order Attenuation Correction Using Measured
Attenuation Coefficients

In order to implement attenuation correction using a post reconstruction method, a first order correction based on that originally suggested by Chang (1978) has been employed. This consists of calculating, at each point, a mean attenuation correction factor,

$$C(x,y) = \left[ \frac{1}{M} \sum_{i=1}^{M} \exp{-\left( \sum_{r=1}^{l(x,y,\theta_i)} \mu(x+r\cos\theta_i, y+r\sin\theta_i)\Delta r \right)} \right]^{-1} \quad (10)$$

where C is the correction factor to be applied at the point (x,y), M is the number of projection angles used to calculate the attenuation term, l is the distance to the detector, and the $\mu$ values are summed for each interval $\Delta r$ over the total length $l(x,y,\theta_i)$.

The reconstructed emission scan is simply multiplied by the resultant attenuation correction map. An example is shown in figure 10. The figure shows the reconstruction, the map of attenuation correction factors (from equation 10), and the error in the correction factors compared with the correction map obtained from a transmission study which was acquired prior to the administration of the radiopharmaceutical.

The correction factor map produced is inherently smooth because of the averaging which occurs in calculating the raysum for each point over 360°. In our implementation, the number of projection angles M is 60.

The accuracy of first order correction was studied by reconstructing emission tomograms of known amounts of radioactivity. A thorax phantom consisting of flasks containing either water or sawdust with Tc-99m added, and immersed in a water tank, was examined. The amount of activity in the flasks varied in the range 35.5 - 83.5 MBq (N=4). A dual emission/transmission study was acquired and processed in the usual manner. The final

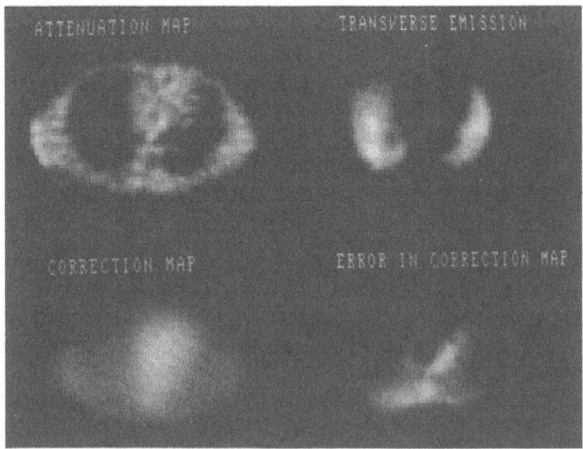

Figure 10.  Example of First Order Correction

Table 3. First-order correction of flasks containing
         radioactivity

| Flask Contents | Calibrated Activity (MBq) | Measured Activity (MBq) | % error |
|---|---|---|---|
| Sawdust | 77.9 | 76.5 | -1.8 |
| Sawdust | 83.5 | 80.3 | -3.8 |
| Water | 52.5 | 52.8 | +1.0 |
| Water | 35.5 | 36.0 | +1.4 |

activity was calculated from the equation,

$$A = \frac{1}{E} \times \frac{\sum_{i=1}^{N} C_e(x,y,z_i)}{\text{Frame time} \times M} \tag{11}$$

where A=total activity, E=system efficiency (Cts/sec/MBq), $C_e$ is the sum
of counts for slice i in a region of interest for each flask, and M is
the number of acquired projections. The emission data was corrected for
decay and reconstructed with a ramp filter. No scatter correction of the
emission data was performed. The results are given below.

For comparison, a first-order Chang correction using a constant $\mu$
value (appropriate for the thorax) gave an overestimate of activity of
around 15%. This is mostly due to the overestimation of the correction
factors in the lungs. However, a recent report has pointed out that the
inconsistency in the acquired projection data in the thorax will lead to
an overestimate in the backprojection procedure as well (Manglos, 1987).
This error is not accounted for in any first order correction method.

These results were found for a simple geometric arrangement which
contained only two materials, and hence two attenuation coefficients, and
are probably better than would be expected in a clinical study. The
difficulty with assessing the technique in patient studies is to know
accurately the amount of radioactivity in an organ. To this end we have
combined the use of patient studies and computer simulations to reconstruct
and compare accurately known amounts of activity by this procedure.

Iterative Attenuation Correction Using Measured Attenuation Coefficients

A significant improvement in the correction procedure can be achieved
by extending the technique to include a single iteration such as described
by Walters et al (1981) and Moore et al (1982). This consists of estimating
projection data by forward projecting the 1st order corrected emission
data using the map of attenuation coefficients, derived from transmission
tomography, to account for attenuation on each angular profile. Errors
$E(x,z,\theta_i)$ for each projected angle are calculated as the difference between
estimated ($P_e$) and true (recorded) profile data (P), i.e.,

$$E(x,z,\theta_i) = P(x,z,\theta_i) - P_e(x,z,\theta_i) \tag{12}$$

These error profiles are reconstructed using filtered back projection
to form an error map which is subsequently first order attenuation corrected and then used to modify the uncorrected estimate.  The basis for this
approach is that differences between estimated and true profiles must be
due to the inaccuracy in the first order attenuation correction method.
This method has previously been shown by Moore (1982) to give accurate
quantitative reconstructions of the emission radioactivity. The entire
procedure is shown below.

In order to assess the quantitative accuracy of iterative attenuation
correction using simultaneously recorded emission/transmission data the
following method was used.  Separate transmission and dual energy emission
data were recorded for patient studies (i.e., photopeak and true scatter).
Both lung perfusion and red blood cell (RBC) studies were acquired for the
thorax.  Different proportions of emission scatter were added to the
transmission data to simulate various emission/transmission count ratios

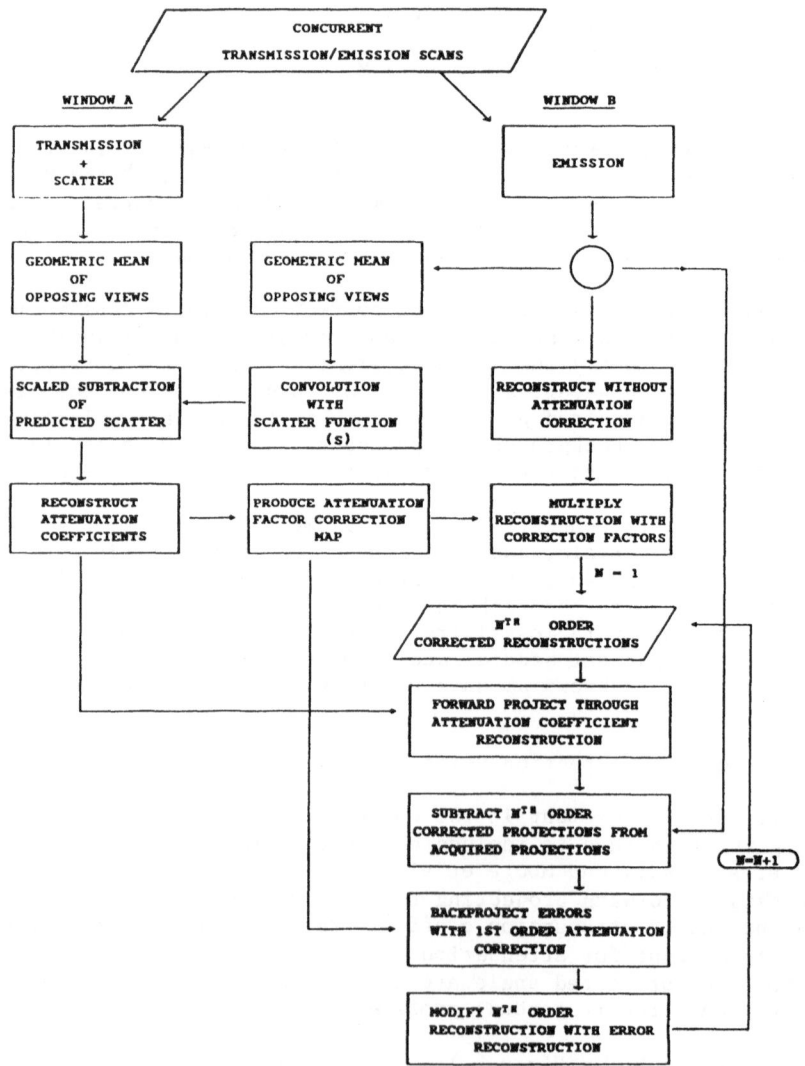

Figure 11. Procedure for using scatter subtracted
transmission data in iterative correction

(i.e., simulating simultaneous emission/transmission acquisitions under different conditions). Scatter subtraction was performed and the resulting transmission scans used to derive attenuation correction factor maps. Results could be compared directly with a best estimate using scatter-free transmission data or a worst estimate assuming elliptical body outline and constant u. In order to assess quantitatively the error in applying these maps using 1st and 2nd order correction, the patient data were used as the basis of a computer generated activity distribution with realistic simulation of counts in heart, lung and background. These data were forward projected through the "true" attenuation coefficient map to provide profiles at each angle which were subsequently reconstructed without attenuation correction. The resultant tomograms were attenuation corrected and compared to the "known" activity distribution for estimation of correction accuracy. This approach permits assessment of quantitative errors in attenuation correction independent of other factors (scatter within the photopeak or resolution variation with depth). Figure 12 shows the starting "known" activity section, and the uncorrected, 1st, and 2nd order corrected reconstructions for a RBC heart study (the $C_e:C_t$ ratio is 7.2).

Table 4 shows the quantitative results from this approach. The ratio $C_e:C_t$ is the same as was used in assessing the accuracy in reconstructed $\mu$ values. Ratios typical of clinical studies using a 1.5GBq transmission source are 2.2 for lung perfusion and 7.2 for RBC studies. The % error is then calculated from the first or second order correction as the difference between the known original counts and the reconstructed counts for the organ of interest. A negative value indicates undercorrection in the reconstructed image, and a positive value indicates overcorrection.

The reason for the inability of the technique to accurately correct for attenuation as scatter increases is because the profiles formed after the 1st order correction are projected through an attenuation map which contains errors due to under and over subtraction of scatter in the planar transmission images. This would be improved by improving the prediction of scatter by the use of a spatially variant scatter function. However,

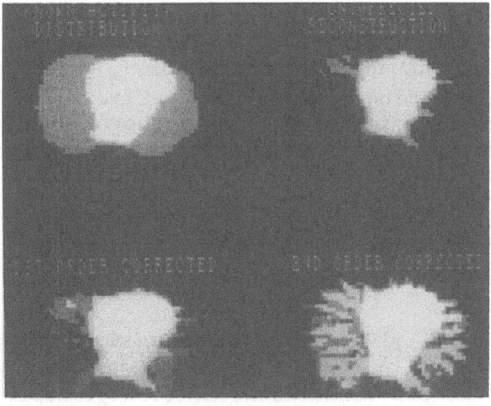

Figure 12. Example of simulated activity distribution, uncorrected, 1st, and 2nd order corrected reconstructions

Table 4.  Accuracy of 1st and 2nd Order corrections of
         known count distributions for different
         amounts of scatter

| Ratio $C_e{:}C_t$ | Lung (%) | | Ratio $C_e{:}C_t$ | Heart (%) | |
|---|---|---|---|---|---|
| | 1st Order | 2nd Order | | 1st Order | 2nd Order |
| 0 | −5.4 | −0.9 | 0 | +8.3 | +1.1 |
| 1.1 | −5.1 | −0.6 | 3.6 | +5.8 | −1.7 |
| 2.2 | −3.8 | +0.6 | 7.2 | +8.0 | +1.4 |
| 3.3 | −1.1 | +3.2 | 10.7 | +8.6 | +3.6 |
| 4.4 | +0.3 | +4.4 | 14.2 | +10.2 | +5.5 |

the method still corrects well under very high scatter conditions. In
practice, a damping factor is applied to the error estimate (Moore, 1982),
but noise amplification in the 2nd order correction still occurs. This is
being examined further.

The overestimate of counts in areas of low attenuation as reported by
Manglos will be compensated for in the 2nd order correction, as the overestimate in the backprojection will appear as an error in the forward
projected profiles. In our studies, we have found that the extra counts
seen in low attenuation areas are misplaced counts shifted from areas of
greater attenuation. Therefore, the errors profiles formed will take this
mispositioning due to backprojection into account.

The determination of individual attenuation coefficients for correction may not be considered necessary in the head or the abdomen, but the
method described still offers anatomical reference images which are helpful in qualitative viewing, and accurate body contours within which to
apply a correction based on a mean constant $\mu$ value. In the head, however,
we have noted that while a mean $\mu$ value is applicable for a particular
slice, the value increases towards the top of the cranium, probably reflecting a higher calvarial to cerebral mass ratio with increasing skull
thickness (Bailey, 1986).

Conclusions

The technique described presents a practical approach to accurate
quantitative SPECT.  The simultaneous acquisition method eliminates the
problems of re-positioning and data translation, which arise when using an
X-ray TCT device to determine attenuation coefficients. This method seems
particularly appropriate for studies of the thorax, and the future introduction of Tc-99m myocardial perfusion agents will have direct applications
for the technique.

REFERENCES

Anger, H.O. and McRae, J. (1968). Transmission Scintiphotography, J.Nucl.
    Med. 9, 267–269.
Axelsson, B., Msaki, P. and Israelsson, A. (1984). Subtraction of Compton
    scattered photons in SPECT, J.Nucl.Med. 25, 490–494.
Bailey, D.L. (1986). Towards Quantitation in SPECT: A Dual Radionuclide
    Approach. M.App.Sc. thesis, NSWIT, Sydney.

Beck, R.N., Zimmer, L.T., Charleston, D.B. et al (1973). Advances in Fundamental Aspects of Imaging Systems & Techniques, in Medical Radionuclide Scintigraphy Vol I, pp 3-45, IAEA, Vienna.

Chang, L.T. (1978). A Method for Attenuation Correction in Radionuclide Computed Tomography, IEEE Trans.Nucl.Sci. NS-25, 638-643.

Filipow, L.J., Macey. D.J. and Munro, T.R. (1979). Measurement of the Depth of a Point Source of a Radioisotope from Gamma Ray Spectra, Phys.Med.Biol. 24, 341-352.

Hutton, B.F., Jayasinghe, M.A.C., Bailey, D.L. et al (1987). Artefact Reduction in Dual Radionuclide Subtraction Studies, Phys. Med. Biol. 32, 477-493.

Jayasinghe, M.A.C. (1984). Possibe improvements for the subtraction imaging technique in radio-imunodetection of cancer (RID), M.Sc. thesis, UNSW, Sydney.

Kuhl, D.E., Hale, J. and Eaton, W.L. (1966). Transmission Scanning: A Useful Adjunct to Conventional Emission Scanning for Accurately Keying Isotope Deposition to Radiographic Anatomy, Radiology 87, 278-284.

Larsson, S.A. (1980). Gamma Camera Emission Tomography, ACTA Radiologica Supplementum 363, pp24-30, Stockholm.

Malko, J.A., Van Heertum, R.L., Gullberg, G.T. et al (1986). SPECT Liver Imaging Using an Iterative Attenuation Correction Algorithm and an External Flood Source, J.Nucl.Med. 27, 701-705.

Manglos, S.H., Jaszczak, R.J., Floyd, C.E. et al (1987). Non-Isotropic Attenuation in SPECT: Phantom Tests of Quantitative Effects and Compensation Techniques, J.Nucl.Med. (in press).

Moore, S.C. (1982). Attenuation Compensation, in Computed Emission Tomography, Ell P.J. and Holman B.L.(Eds.), pp 339-360, Oxford University Press.

Moore, S.C., Brunelle, J.A. and Kirsch, C-M. (1982). Quantitative Multi-Detector Emission Computerized Tomography Using Iterative Attenuation Compensation, J.Nucl.Med. 23, 706-714.

Rutherford, R.A., Pullen, B.R., Goddard, J. et al (1975). Quantitative Information from the EMI scanner, in Information Processing in Scintigraphy, pp 353-376, Todd-Pokropek A. and Raynaud C.(Eds.), Orsay.

Sorenson, J.A., Briggs, R.C. and Cameron, J.R. (1969). $^{99m}$Tc Point Source for Transmission Scanning, J.Nucl.Med. 10, 252-253.

Tothill, P. and Galt, J.M. (1971). Quantitative Profile Scanning for the Measurement of Organ Radioactivity, Phys.Med.Biol.16, 625-634.

Walters, T.E., Simon, W., Chesler, D.A. et al (1981). Attenuation Correction in gamma emission tomography, J.Comput.Assist.Tomogr.5, 89-94.

Webb, S., Flower, M.A., Ott, R.J. et al (1983). A comparison of attenuation correction methods for quantitative single photon emission computed tomography, Phys.Med.Biol. 28, 1045-1056.

QUANTITATION WITH THE HIDAC POSITRON CAMERA

D.Townsend[1], R.Clack[2], M.Defrise[3], H-J.Tochon-Danguy[1],
P.Frey[1], S.Kuijk[3], and F.Deconinck[3]

[1] Division of Nuclear Medicine, Geneva University
   Hospital, Geneva, Switzerland
[2] Department of Mathematics, Dalhousie University
   Halifax, Nova Scotia, Canada
[3] Division of Nuclear Medicine, VUB, Brussels
   Belgium

INTRODUCTION

    An important goal of positron emission tomography (PET) is
the measurement of regional tissue concentrations of
positron-emitting radionuclides.  Such measurements are obtained
from local count densities in PET images which have been
corrected for background due to random coincidences and
scattered photons.  Photons which scatter and are undetected
give rise to attenuation effects and hence an underestimation of
the regional tissue concentration at depth. Conversely,
uncorrected image background from scatter and randoms results in
an overestimation of the concentration.  The relationship
between the true tissue concentration and the PET measurement
depends upon the extent to which background and attenuation
effects can be corrected.  Inaccuracies in the count density
estimate will influence the precision of the parameters (e.g.
rate constants) obtained by subsequent physiological modelling.

    In conventional, crystal-based, ring cameras, attenuation
and randoms are corrected by measuring their effect on the data:
an out-of-time randoms map is subtracted from the sorted
coincidence data (sinogram) to correct for random coincidences,
and the necessary coefficients to correct for attenuation are
obtained from a transmission scan.  The distribution of scatter,
however, cannot in general be measured and consequently a number
of scatter compensation procedures have been proposed (Bergstrom
et al., 1983;  Endo et al, 1984). These procedures are based on
the deconvolution from the measured projection data of the
scatter distribution for a line spread function. In practice,
ring cameras are designed to minimise the fraction of scattered
photons in the image by a careful choice of ring diameter,
inter-crystal septa and shielding, and by applying a lower
energy threshold. A commercial PET camera consists of multiple
rings (typically up to 8) of BGO crystals, the ring diameter
being in the range 75 to 100 cm. For the ECAT camera, each ring

comprises 512 crystals 5.6 mm wide by 12.9 mm high and 30 mm deep, yielding a spatial resolution of 5 to 6 mm and a direct plane sensitivity of 6,000 cps/μCi/ml for the standard 20 cm diameter phantom. At a singles rate of 1.5 MHz, the true coincidence rate is 44 kHz with 3% randoms (5 nsec time resolution) and 3.8% dead time. The lower limit of the energy window is set around 300 keV.

PET imaging with the High Density Avalanche Chamber (HIDAC) positron camera presents a rather different situation. The HIDAC camera consists of dual area detectors, 30 cm x 30 cm in size, rotated around the patient to acquire a complete data set for three-dimensional reconstruction of the positron distribution. The camera performance is characterised by a reconstructed spatial resolution of 3 mm full-width at half-maximum (FWHM) in all three directions, a coincidence resolving time of 40 nsecs and a volume sensitivity of about 15,000 cps/μCi/ml for a standard 20 cm diameter phantom, 18.5 cm in length. Due to the nature of the photon conversion process (Jeavons et al., 1983), no explicit energy measurement is possible. Therefore, as a consequence of these operating characteristics, both transmission and emission imaging with the HIDAC camera may involve significant amounts of scatter and randoms, and low overall image statistics. Different approachs to those used in conventional PET cameras are required to correct the HIDAC camera data properly for scatter and randoms.

Compared with the two-dimensional slice reconstruction, a different approach is also required to the three-dimensional reconstruction problem as a consequence of the unavailability of the projection data (the sinograms). The number of line integrals potentially sampled by area detectors such as the HIDAC may exceed $2^{33}$, and hence it is impractical to store the data in such a form, given that the number of coincidences acquired in a typical study may be $2^{21}$ or less. Instead, the data must be stored in list mode and the first step in the reconstruction procedure is back-projection into the image volume. Thus, as the data are never explicitly available in the form of projections, techniques which operate directly on the projections, either for reconstruction or scatter correction, cannot be applied to the HIDAC camera.

This paper examines some of the problems associated with obtaining quantitative images from the HIDAC camera. The effect of scatter is investigated both by computer simulation and with images from a prototype HIDAC camera. To correct for attenuation, a scaling procedure is presented that provides an approximate solution and is particularly robust in the presence of high levels of background. The prospects for full image quantitation with the HIDAC camera will be summarised.

HIDAC IMAGE QUANTITATION: THEORETICAL CONSIDERATIONS

PET is used to provide *in vivo* measurements of blood flow, blood volume, oxygen metabolism, glucose consumption, and a number of other physiological parameters, particularly for the brain and the heart. In order to make these measurements, the PET images, from which the necessary count densities are extracted, must be properly corrected for attenuation effects and free of distortions due to the background effects outlined above. In this section, potential sources of quantitation error are considered in detail with particular reference to the HIDAC camera.

## Random Coincidences

Random coincidences arise as a consequence of accepting two uncorrelated photons as a coincident pair. The line joining the two photons intersects the imaging volume along a random channel. The rate of such random coincidences (R) may be estimated from the well-known equation:

$$R = S_1 S_2 (2\tau) \tag{1}$$

for $\tau \ll 1/S_1$ and $1/S_2$, where $S_1$ and $S_2$ are the singles rates on the two detectors and $2\tau$ is the coincidence resolving time. It is important to minimise the randoms rate by keeping the resolving time as short as possible. Typically, for the HIDAC camera with 450 µCi of activity in a 20 cm diameter cylinder (18.5 cm long), the singles rates are 90 kHz for a coincidence rate of 1.1 kHz and a randoms rate of 29%.

Two standard methods are available with commercial cameras to correct the projection data for random coincidences. One approach is to estimate the randoms rate from eqn.1, and then to subtract the corresponding level uniformly from the projection data. A second approach is to actually measure a random coincidence map by introducing a delay into the coincidence signal from one detector. The delay is sufficient to ensure that no true coincident events can occur within the time window. The randoms map may require smoothing before being subtracted from the projection data to reduce statistical fluctuations in the measurements.

Similar approaches may be used with the HIDAC camera data by applying the correction to the back-projection rather than the projections, since the latter are unavailable. It is worth noting that the correction applied to each voxel will be small even though the total randoms rate may be as high as 30% or 40%. For the remainder of this study, it will be assumed that the data have been corrected for random coincidences.

## Scattered Coincidences

In a typical brain imaging study, as little as 20% of the emitted photon flux emerges from the head unscattered. When one or both of a pair of annihilation photons scatter and are detected by the camera, the line joining the two points of detection does not pass through the original annihilation point. A positron event is therefore removed from one coincidence channel (attenuation) and incorrectly assigned to a different channel (scatter background). Attenuation depends only on the energy of the photons and on the distribution of the attenuating medium, whereas scatter depends also on the radioactive source distribution and on the detection process. A significant scatter background leads to reduced image contrast and overestimation of local tissue concentrations.

Since scattered photons lose energy in the scattering process, they can, in principle, be identified in the detector. However, crystal-based cameras have energy resolutions of typically 25% to 30% at 511 keV and are operated with a lower energy threshold of 300 keV to 350 keV. The scatter fraction is minimised by the large detector separation, the small septa opening and additional lead shielding. Scatter fractions for the standard 20 cm diameter phantom are about 15%, some two-thirds of which comes from scatter within the plane.

Intrinsically, the effects of attenuation and scatter are compensatory: scatter replaces some of the photons lost through attenuation. In general, the distributions and rates of the two effects differ since, for example, the scatter fraction depends on the detection process (the energy resolution of the detector), whereas the attenuation effect does not. Thus, an attempt to correct for attenuation without prior scatter compensation will usually result in over-correction. This over-compensation can be somewhat artificially reduced by using values for the linear attenuation coefficient ($\mu$) which are less than the true value, a procedure sometimes employed to correct for attenuation in single photon tomography (SPECT). Clearly, a more satisfactory approach is to first correct the projection data for scatter and then use the true value of $\mu$ in the attenuation correction.

A number of scatter compensation procedures have been proposed which attempt to remove the scatter component from the measured projection data before reconstruction. The techniques are based on estimating the scatter in the projection by a convolution of the measured data with a filter function. The filter function is obtained either from measurements of the line spread function in various scatter situations (King et al., 1981; Bergstrom et al., 1983), or from a Monte Carlo scatter model (Endo et al., 1984). It is found that the projection of a line spread function in a scatter medium has tails which may be satisfactorily modelled by a simple exponential. The appropriate filter is thus obtained from a two-parameter fit to the scatter tails. One problem with these methods is that they do not correct fully for the non-stationarity of the scatter component. However, any approach which takes non-stationarity fully into account will require point source measurements for all voxels within the field of view, and such an approach is not, in general, practicable. Significant reduction in the scatter background has nevertheless been achieved by the methods mentioned above, resulting in improved image contrast and reduced quantitation error.

The HIDAC detectors are shielded to some extent from radiation originating outside the field of view, but as with any area detector, they are open to scattered radiation within their angular acceptance. As mentioned above, the effect of this scatter on the reconstructed image will depend upon the scatter medium, source distribution, and the response of the detectors to lower energy photons. This response has been measured (Jeavons et al., 1983), and shows the expected decreasing efficiency with decreasing photon energy as fewer of the photoelectrons escape from the lead into the holes of the converter. However, since the image reconstruction is performed directly on the list mode data and the projection data (sinograms) are never explicitly available, the techniques used to correct scatter in ring systems cannot easily be applied to the HIDAC camera data. The behaviour of the scatter background has been investigated for the HIDAC camera both experimentally and by computer simulation, and some of the results will be presented in the next section.

## Attenuation Correction

Three different procedures are used to correct for photon attenuation in conventional PET cameras:

(a) A correction based on a transmission scan to provide the line integrals of the attenuation coefficients that are required to correct the projection data. This is the standard procedure when a high statistics transmission scan is available.

(b) A calculated correction based on an operator-positioned body outline, or edge-detection algorithm, and a mean value for $\mu$. The body dimensions could also be obtained from the patient's MRI or CT image, if available.

(c) A hybrid approach combining the above two methods; the transmission data are used to provide the body contour, while the actual projection correction factors are obtained using a constant attenuation coefficient.

In all cases the correction factors are used to weight the projection data before filtering and back-projection, thereby compensating for photon attenuation. The above methods are, however, either difficult or impossible to apply to the HIDAC camera data. This is because:

(1) The number of projection channels for the HIDAC camera is very large and the acquisition of sufficient statistics in a transmission scan to provide reliable estimates of the correction factors would be impossible. The use of erroneous correction factors may result in serious artifacts in the image.

(2) The determination of the patient outline is crucial in order to estimate the correct attenuation weights. However, such an outline is difficult to obtain either from the PET data or from an independent measurement such as the use of small point sources or the CT or MRI scan.

(3) In a conventional camera, the high-statistics transmission scan can be reconstructed, as for CT, to provide an image of the attenuation coefficients at 511 keV; the image can be used to provide a reliable body contour. For the HIDAC camera, the extremely small number of counts acquired for each projection would exclude such a reconstruction procedure.

For these reasons, a post-reconstruction scaling method has been developed and tested. The method corrects for the average attenuation effect at each point in the reconstructed image. It is assumed that the reconstruction from uncorrected projection data does not contain serious artifacts, an assumption that is reasonably well satisfied, especially for sources near the centre of the attenuating medium. Thus,

$$f_r(\underline{x}) \approx \alpha(\underline{x}).f(\underline{x}) \qquad (2)$$

where $f_r$ and $f$ are the uncorrected and corrected

reconstruction, respectively. The weighting factors $\alpha(\underline{x})$ represent the average attenuation at a point $\underline{x} = (x,y,z)$, defined by:

$$\alpha(\underline{x}) = \iint_\Omega \exp\{-\int\mu(\underline{x}+\lambda\underline{n})\,d\lambda\}\,d\omega \;/\; \iint_\Omega d\omega \qquad (3)$$

where the solid angle $\Omega$ includes all possible projection

directions $\underline{n}$, and $d\omega = \cos\phi\,d\phi\,d\theta$ is an element of solid angle. The inner integral represents the integration of $\mu$ along one of the directions within $\Omega$ through the point $\underline{x}$. The overall weighting factor $\alpha(\underline{x})$ is then the sum of line weights for all lines through $\underline{x}$ and within $\Omega$.

The advantage of the approach represented by eqn.2 is that, as a result of the angular averaging in eqn.3, the $\alpha(\underline{x})$ are less affected by low statistics than the individual exponential attenuation factors; the disadvantage is that the relationship (eqn.2) is an approximation. The validity of this approximation will be examined later.

In practice, the $\alpha(\underline{x})$ are obtained by a method similar to that used for the exponential channel correction factors in the usual measured PET attenuation correction. Two additional scans are necessary: a blank transmission scan without the patient in position, and a normal transmission scan with the patient positioned exactly as for the emission scan. The data from each scan are back-projected to form a blank scan back-projection $b_0(\underline{x})$ and a patient transmission scan back-projection $b_t(\underline{x})$; $\alpha(\underline{x})$ can be shown to be the point-wise ratio:

$$\alpha(\underline{x}) = b_t(\underline{x}) \;/\; b_0(\underline{x}) \qquad (4)$$

However, in practice, after correction for randoms, $b_0(\underline{x})$ will include scatter from the detectors, and $b_t(\underline{x})$ will include scatter from both the detectors and the patient. The effect of scatter in the transmission scan will be more serious than for an emission scan because the number of true coincidence lines back-projected in a given channel will be small, and may even be comparable with the number of scattered photon lines. Thus, the scaling factors given by eqn.4 will be incorrect unless the scatter background is first subtracted. Unfortunately, neither the level nor the structure of this background is known *a priori*.

Transmission studies with an area detector can be performed by mounting positron-emitting flood sources on one or both detectors, so as to make maximum use of their large angular acceptance. The sources rotate around with the detectors, and data are acquired in exactly the same way as for an emission scan. However, in order to estimate the *level* of scatter as required by the algorithm, the transmission scans are performed with a small lead cylinder (diameter around 7 cm) in the field of view. In the absence of scatter, the average voxel contents in a region-of-interest in the centre of this cylinder should be essentially zero due to the high attenuation. Hence the average voxel contents actually found can be used as a measure of the contribution due to scatter; this average value is then subtracted from all voxels in the back-projection. Clearly, the procedure contains two major assumptions:

- that the scatter background in the transmission scan is approximately uniform and only the level needs to be determined.
- that the scaling factors obtained from transmission scans including the lead cylinder are the same as those that would be obtained from scatter-free scans without the cylinder, i.e. the presence of the cylinder does not seriously distort the scans.

Experimental evidence in support of the validity of these two assumptions will be presented in the next section.


RESULTS

The influence of scatter and attenuation in HIDAC camera images has been investigated both by Monte Carlo simulation and by actual measurements made with a prototype camera. Except for very simple phantoms such as a line source, the background due to scatter cannot be measured, and a good Monte Carlo model is required to study the effects. Such a model has been developed for the HIDAC camera (Defrise et al., 1985). For the purposes of this investigation, the prototype HIDAC camera used for the measurements (Townsend et al., 1987a) has been simulated. It consists of dual detectors, 30 cm x 30 cm in size, rotating around the patient in 20 angular positions. The separation of the detectors is 54 cm. Positron range and photon acolinearity are not simulated; the intrinsic detector resolution is 1 mm. An important parameter for the realistic simulation of scatter is the energy response of the detectors. This has been simulated by introducing an energy-dependent detection efficiency $\varepsilon(E)$ given by:

$$\varepsilon(E) \ = \ 0.17 - 0.49 \ e^{-.0074E} \tag{5}$$

where the incident photon energy E is expressed in keV. This empirical function is based on the form of the measured energy response curve (Jeavons et al., 1983). A lower energy cut-off is applied at 200 keV.

Simulations and measurements have been made for two

phantoms:

- a line source, 5 cm long and 0.5 mm internal diameter.
For the measurement, the source is a steel needle (to eliminate
effects due to positron range) containing $^{68}$Ga. It is
positioned along the axis of rotation of the camera.
- a short cylinder, 20 cm in diameter and 2 cm long
containing three cylindrical cold regions, 5 cm, 3 cm and 1 cm
in diameter. The cylinder is positioned centrally with its axis
coincident to the axis of the camera. For the measurement, the
cylinder is filled with a solution of 500 μCi of $^{68}$Ga.

The attenuating medium is a 20 cm diameter, water-filled
cylinder, 20 cm in length, positioned so as to effectively
extend the active cylinder 10 cm in each direction. For the
study of the attenuation correction, measurements have also been
made with a short uniform cylinder with the same dimensions as
the cold-spot cylinder. The transmission scans were made by
fixing uniform flood sources containing 100 μCi of $^{68}$Ge to the
front face of each HIDAC detector.

For the line source, 400,000 coincidences were simulated in
air and in the scatter medium. In the latter case, 167,000
events were scattered. Profiles through the reconstructed line
source with and without scatter are essentially
indistiguishable. The FWHM is 3 mm, in agreement with the
measurement of the same source published previously (Townsend et
al., 1987b). There is little difference between the profiles
even at the level of the full-width at tenth maximum (FWTM).

A simulation including the effect of attenuation was
performed in order to generate, for the cold-spot cylinder, a
data set with one million positron coincidences; 388,000 of the
events were detected to be scattered. A reconstructed
transverse section through the phantom is shown in fig.1a with a
voxel size of 3.5 mm. Attenuation has been corrected using
method (b) above, with the weights calculated from the known
size and position of the attenuating cylinder and assuming the
true value at 511 keV of the linear attenuation coefficient
(0.097 cm$^{-1}$). The reconstructed distribution of scattered
events is shown in fig.1b, normalised to the contents of the
maximum voxel. The reconstruction of the same phantom imaged in
the HIDAC camera is shown in fig.1c, with the attenuation
corrected by method (b). The background within a
region-of-interest (ROI) inside the 5 cm cold spot is 12% for
the simulation and 15% for the measured data.

The behaviour of the calculated attenuation correction
(method (b) above) is demonstrated for the cold spot cylinder
phantom in fig.2. Firstly, for comparison, fig.2a shows a
transverse section through the reconstruction of a cylinder for
which the simulation did not include attenuation. The effect of
including attenuation in the simulation is shown in fig.2b, and
the result of correcting for this attenuation using method (b)
is shown in fig.2c. The same procedure was used to attenuation
correct the measurements in fig.1c. Since this correction
procedure depends on a knowledge of the shape and position of
the attenuating medium, fig.2d shows the consequence of making a
2 cm error in the position of the centre of the cylinder.

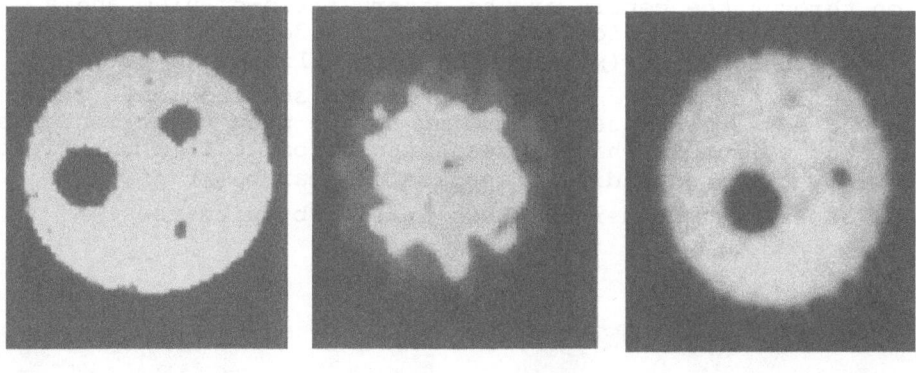

(a) Simulation    (b) Scattered events    (c) Measurement

Fig. 1. A 20cm diameter cylindrical cold-spot phantom

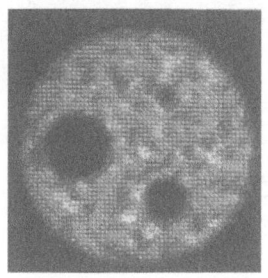
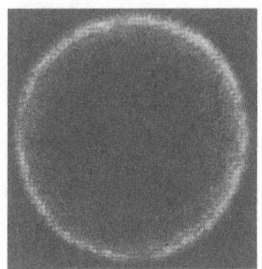

(a) Without attenuation    (b) With attenuation

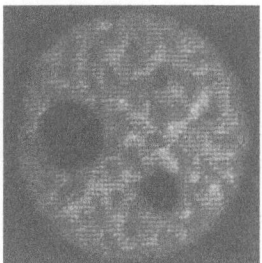
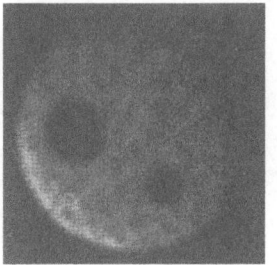

(c) Attenuation corrected    (d) Cylinder mispositioned

Fig. 2. Simulation of a 20cm diameter cold spot phantom

The results of the alternative correction procedure based
on a transmission scan is shown in fig.3 for the measurement of
a uniform cylinder of activity. In each case, both a transverse
section through the centre of the camera field-of-view and a
profile across the section are shown. Fig.3a shows the blank
scan back-projection $b_0(\underline{x})$ with the lead cylinder in place,
before (left) and after (right) background subtraction. The
background level is chosen according to the mean voxel contents
in the lead cylinder, which appears at bottom left in the field
of view. The corresponding transmission scan $b_t(\underline{x})$ of the
uniform activity cylinder is shown in fig.3b, with the

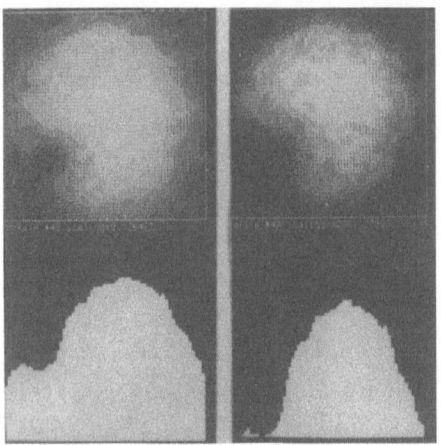
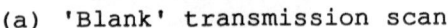
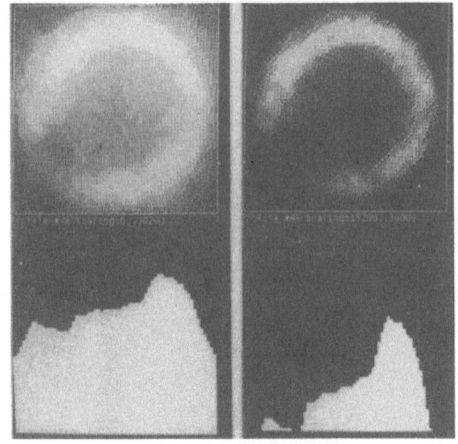

(a) 'Blank' transmission scan     (b) Object transmission scan

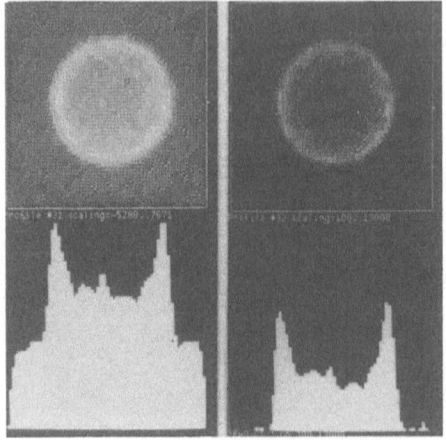
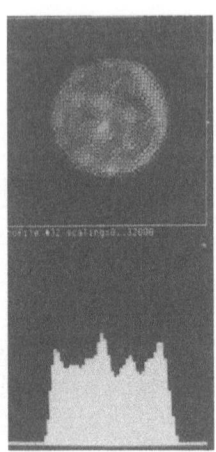

(c) Uncorrected emission scan     (d) Corrected emission scan

Fig. 3. Post-reconstruction scaling to correct for attenuation

background level determined as for fig.3a. The emission scan, uncorrected for attenuation, is shown in fig.3c; the background is estimated from a ROI outside the cylinder and subtracted from all voxels in the image (fig.3c, right). After rescaling with the factors obtained from the two transmission scans according to eqns.2 and 4, a section through the uniform cylinder is shown in fig.3d.


DISCUSSION

It is seen from measurements with a line source that scattered photons contribute a low-frequency, low-level background to the image. The FWHM and FWTM of the line source profile are unaffected by the presence of the surrounding scatter medium. The apparent increase in the FWTM reported in Townsend et al. (1987b) was found to be due to the positron range effect which has been suppressed in this study by the use of a steel rather than glass needle. This result differs from the effect found in ring systems where scatter tends to increase the FWTM by the introduction of significant tails into the line spread function. The difference may be due to the distribution of the scatter for area detectors into three dimensions which tends to average out potential structure. In ring systems, most of the scattered events in a transverse section come from scatter within the plane. The uniform nature of the scatter background in the HIDAC images is confirmed for the cold spot phantom in fig.1. The measurement (fig.1c) agrees reasonably well with the simulation (fig.1a); the slight increase in the measured scatter level is most likely due to positron penetration of the cold spot, an effect which was not included in the simulation. The conclusion from this study, therefore, is that, to a reasonable degree of approximation, the scatter background is uniform even for a structured source distribution.

In a given imaging situation, the background level due to the scattered photons has to be measured. Although, a more satisfactory approach to that of simple thresholding would be to adopt a deconvolution technique such as the one suggested by Bergstrom et al. (1983), which would correct automatically for any level of scatter, the fact that this and other such procedures operate on the projection data excludes them from use with the HIDAC camera. In a HIDAC emission image, one way to estimate the level of scatter is to use a post-reconstruction region of interest technique outside the known source volume. The average number of counts in the background provides an estimate of the level of scatter. However, this procedure assumes that the reconstruction of data which includes scatter does not result in serious artifacts.

Attenuation correction is an important procedure even without the requirement of accurate image quantitation. Correction factors at the centre of a 20 cm diameter cylinder increase the voxel contents by as much as a factor of eight, and thus even qualitative image interpretation is unreliable on uncorrected images. Calculated attenuation correction factors (method (b)) are usually adequate for the head, provided an outline of the skull (or scalp) is obtained from the emission or transmission image. However, a measured attenuation correction from a transmission scan (method (a)) is essential when imaging the heart or the liver. As expected, method (b) works well in situations of constant, or near constant, $\mu$ with an accurately-known object contour, as shown in fig.2. However, when the object contour is incorrectly positioned, serious distortions in the reconstructed activity distribution can arise (fig.2d).

The procedure described above and illustrated in fig.3 corrects well for attenuation, provided that the scatter background is fairly uniform and the transmission scan with the object in place is not seriously distorted by the presence of the lead cylinder to define the zero level. However, since the scaling factors are determined from the ratio of two scans both of which include the lead cylinder, the effect of the latter should be correctly taken into account. The scaling factors within the field of interest of the emission scan should, therefore, be unaffected by the presence of the lead. Thus, the method should be effective, providing the high $\mu$ cylinder is not placed too close to the emission source. For a uniform cylinder, the results are comparable to those obtained with the attenuation correction method (b), without requiring the knowledge of position and outline of the attenuating medium. Work is continuing to evaluate the validity of the new method in clinical imaging situations such as $^{68}$Ga-colloid studies of the liver.

CONCLUSION

This paper has presented a preliminary study of the scatter background in HIDAC camera images using both simulated and measured phantom data. A post-reconstruction scaling method has been suggested to correct for attenuation using a low statistics transmission scan rather than a calculated attenuation correction. The method is based on the assumptions that the scatter background is rather uniform and that its level can be determined experimentally by introducing an area of high attenuation into the transmission scan. The method has been shown to work well for a uniform cylinder of activity.

Nevertheless, for a number of reasons the method cannot be expected to provide true image quantitation. Firstly, the lead cylinder may interfere slightly with the scaling factors for the emission image, and in any case post-reconstruction scaling is only an approximation to exact procedures using exponential back-projection weights (methods (a) or (b)). Secondly, a proper scatter correction should ideally be applied *before* reconstruction, rather than the simple thresholding used here which, to be effective, must ensure complete background removal. Finally, a reconstruction that does not correct for the effect of attenuation does not necessarily yield an artifact-free attenuated version of the true image from which the true image can be recovered by simple scaling. Therefore, given the current performance characteristics of these area detectors, it is difficult to see how more accurate procedures can be implemented in order to yield improved quantitative accuracy.

While work is continuing to assess the limits of

quantitation to be expected from this type of camera in clinical studies, it may be that a major application field for such a high resolution PET camera will be animal imaging. Among other advantages, these studies would avoid the problems of scatter and attenuation which dominate the human clinical applications, and thus true image quantitation would be a realistic possibility.


## ACKNOWLEDGEMENTS

This work is supported by the Fonds National suisse under grant number 3.853-0.85. M.D. and S.K. are respectively Research Associate and Research Assistent of the Belgium National Foundation for Scientific Research. R.C. wishes to thank Professor A.C.Thompson of Dalhousie University Mathematics Department for his encouragement and support of this work. We are grateful to Mr Antoine Geissbühler who programmed the attenuation correction and provided the display routines. Dr. Gerry Bennett of the Medical Department, Brookhaven Laboratory, USA provided the flood sources for the transmission studies.


## REFERENCES

Bergstrom, M., Eriksson, L., Bohm, C., Blomqvist, G., and Litton, J. (1983). Correction for scattered radiation in a ring detector positron camera by integral transformation of the projections, J. Nucl. Med., 7,42-50.

Defrise, M., Deconinck, F., Kuijk, S. (1986) Methodology for predicting the performances of different PET camera designs, in: Information Processing in Medical Imaging, S.L. Bacharach (ed.), Martinus Nijhoff, Dordrecht, 455-474.

Endo, M., and Iinuma T.A. (1984). Software correction of scatter coincidence in positron CT, Eur. J. Nucl. Med., 9,391-396.

Jeavons, A.P., Hood, K., Herlin, G., Parkman, C., Townsend, D.W., Magnanini, R., Frey, P.E., Donath, A., (1983). The high-density avalanche chamber for positron emission tomography, IEEE Trans. Nucl. Sci., NS-30(1),640-645.

King, P.H., Hubner, K., Gibbs, W., Holloway, E., (1981). Noise identification and removal in positron imaging systems, IEEE Trans. Nucl. Sci., NS-28(1),148-151.

Townsend, D.W., Clack, R., Magnanini, R., Frey, P.E., Donath, A., Schorr, B., Jeavons, A.P., Herlin, G., and Froidevaux, A., (1983). Image reconstruction for a rotating positron tomograph, IEEE Trans. Nucl. Sci., NS-30(1),594-600.

Townsend, D.W., Frey, P.E., Jeavons, A.P., Reich, G., Tochon-Danguy, H-J., Donath, A., Christin, A., Schaller, G., (1987a). The HIDAC positron camera, To appear in J. Nucl. Med.

Townsend, D.W., Frey, P.E., Reich, G., Christin, A., Tochon-Danguy, H-J., Schaller, G., Donath, A., Jeavons, A, (1987b). The quantitative imaging potential of the HIDAC positron camera, in: Mathematics and Computer Science in Medical Imaging, M.A.Viergever and A.E.Todd-Pokropek (eds.), Springer, Berlin.

# REGION OF INTEREST DETERMINATION FOR QUANTITATIVE EVALUATION OF

# MYOCARDIAL ISCHEMIA FROM PET IMAGES

R. Wanda Rowe, Michael E. Merhige, Bernard Bendriem,
and K. Lance Gould

Positron Diagnostic and Research Center
University of Texas Health Science Center at Houston
6431 Fannin St., Houston, TX 77030, USA.

## INTRODUCTION

Positron Emission Tomography (PET) of the heart permits non-invasive identification of myocardial ischemia and infarction through metabolic and perfusion imaging. Ischemic tissue is characterized by reduced perfusion and appears as a defect when 13-N ammonia is used as the imaging agent because this tracer is taken up in the myocardium in proportion to blood flow (Schelbert et al., 1981). Within the ischemic zone, viable tissue can be differentiated from non-viable or infarcted tissue by the presence of persistent metabolic activity which can be imaged with 18-F deoxyglucose (18-FDG) (Schwaiger et al., 1985). Of particular clinical importance is the non-invasive measurement of the fraction of the total left ventricular (LV) volume which is infarcted or ischemic. We have developed two approaches to accurately recover the fraction of LV myocardium involved in the ischemic process directly from PET images of myocardial perfusion, metabolism, and the LV bloodpool.

Because of partial volume, scatter and positron range effects, accurate measurement of the myocardial volume from PET images is difficult by conventional region of interest (ROI) generation techniques such as hand-drawing, simple thresholding (Tauxe et al., 1982), histogram analysis (Chow and Kaneko, 1972), filtering (Raff, Stroud, and Hendee, 1986) or gradient searching (Trivedi, Herman and Udupa, 1986). Our approaches to ROI generation attempt to compensate for partial volume effects through accurate edge detection and are designed to lead to reproducible, automated outlines of myocardial tissue in the LV. The first, we have named the adjacent edge rollback (AER) technique, while the second is based on adaptive thresholding. Although these methods are presented in the context of cardiac imaging with PET, the principles involved can be applied to other imaging modalities such as SPECT where structures being imaged are smaller than two or three resolution distances.

## THE ADJACENT EDGE ROLLBACK TECHNIQUE

Myocardial ischemia occurs when coronary blood flow is unable to meet metabolic demands. Under these circumstances, superimposition of flow and metabolic scans of the heart permits identification of ischemic, yet viable portions of the LV. The volume of normally perfused LV can be recognized by

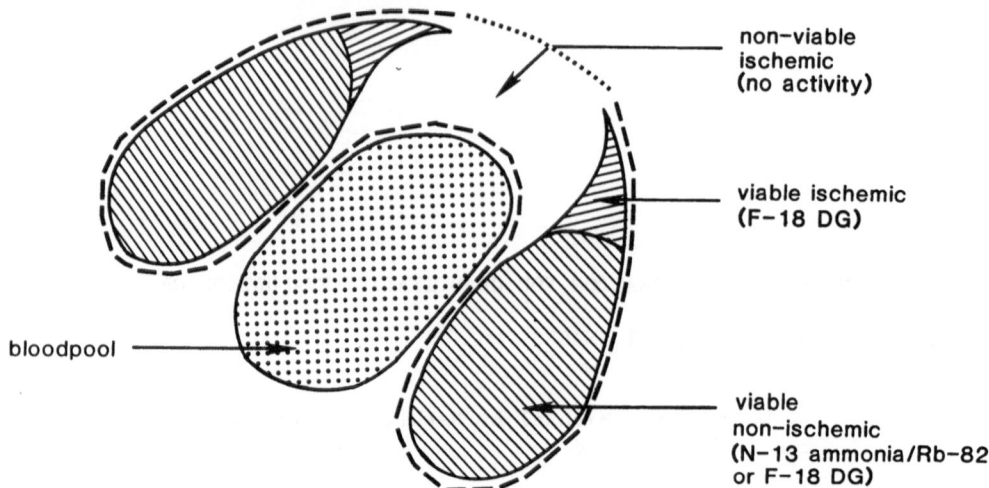

non-viable
ischemic
(no activity)

viable ischemic
(F-18 DG)

bloodpool

viable
non-ischemic
(N-13 ammonia/Rb-82
or F-18 DG)

Fig. 1.  Diagram of region of interest generation by Adjacent Edge
Rollback technique.  PET images of LV myocardial flow, metabolism and bloodpool are thresholded at AER separation intensity and formed into composite image.  ROI boundary bisects
resulting gap between bloodpool and LV wall and maintains a
constant distance from edge of myocardium.  Boundary of
infarcted area is completed by criteria of symmetry and
distance from bloodpool.

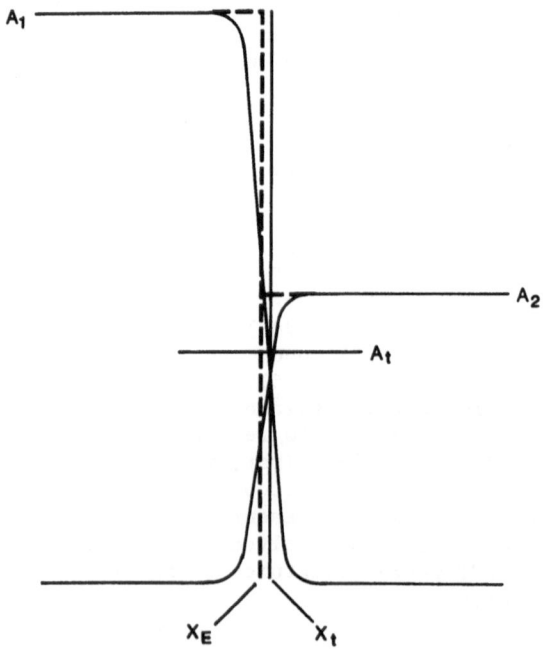

Fig. 2.  Diagram of Adjacent Edge
Rollback technique.  Bisection of
gap between adjacent distributions
separated by thresholding yields
small error in edge location.

avid uptake of 13-N ammonia. In contrast, in ischemic tissue, uptake of these tracers is reduced but 18-FDG will accumulate if the tissue is still viable. Infarcted tissue is not imaged since it has both severely reduced blood supply and has no metabolic activity. Thus the myocardial edge in infarcted regions is not defined. However, the endocardial edge of the LV is the junction of the bloodpool and the myocardial tissue. The bloodpool can be imaged with 15-0 labeled carbon monoxide (CO-15), which labels red blood cells. Thus the boundary between bloodpool and myocardial flow or metabolic distributions can be used to give further edge information which permits identification of the endocardial LV boundary (fig. 1). The AER technique utilizes properties of adjacent edges and their spread functions to identify the true LV boundaries from combined bloodpool, flow and metabolic images.

## Theory

Consider two adjacent uniform distributions whose edges are blurred due to the resolution of the imaging system. Fig. 2 shows the superimposed spread functions resulting from step edges of height $A_1$ and $A_2$ respectively, imaged with a Gaussian impulse response function typical of a positron camera with circular detectors. The true edge location is marked by the dashed line in fig. 2. Thresholding of the two edge images to retain only pixels with values above some intensity such as $A_t$ causes a gap to appear between the two superimposed distributions (hence the term adjacent edge rollback). A pixel which is at the center of this gap lies close to the true edge point as indicated by the solid vertical line. By choosing $A_t$ to just cause separation of the two distributions, the error in location of the edge is minimized. The precise threshold level above which a gap will appear in the image is dependent on the ratio of the intensities on either side of the edge, as shown in Fig. 3(a). The error in edge location resulting from this optimal thresholding is demonstrated in Fig. 3(b) for an imaging system with a Gaussian point spread function with a full width at half maximum (FWHM) of 15mm. As the difference in intensity between the distributions increases, the threshold which just produces separation decreases from 50% of the higher intensity. For intensity ratios between 1 and 3, the separation threshold can be approximated by a linear function of the logarithm of the intensity ratio. The edge location error increases linearly with the logarithm of the intensity ratio and depends on the shape and width of the edge blurring function of the imaging system. In PET, the width of the edge spread is determined by the resolution of the detectors, the reconstruction filter, positron range, and the amount of scattered radiation. For typical PET systems imaging adjacent LV bloodpool and myocardium, the optimum threshold is between 45% and 50% yielding an error in edge placement of less than 1mm. This degree of error in edge detection is of no practical consequence in clinical cardiac PET imaging.

## Implementation

In order to validate the ability of the AER method to produce an endocardial edge directly from PET images of the myocardium and LV blood-pool, 4 dogs were imaged with 13-N ammonia and CO-15. Peak activity in the myocardium and bloodpool was measured in mid-ventricular slices and the ratio of these values was computed. Each image was then thresholded at the corresponding separation threshold level shown in Fig. 3(a) as predicted by the mathematical simulation described above. Simultaneous display of bloodpool and flow distributions was achieved by compressing the intensities in each thresholded image to one half of the dynamic range of the display system. Where more than one distribution was represented in a pixel, the maximum of the competing values was selected for display. In each of the resulting composite images the endocardial edge was clearly seen as a single pixel wide black band with neither CO-15 nor 13-N activity. In these studies the ratio of the peak image value in the CO-15 bloodpool to the peak value

ADJACENT EDGE SEPARATION THRESHOLD
as function of intensity ratio

RELATIVE EDGE LOCATION ERROR
as function of intensity ratio

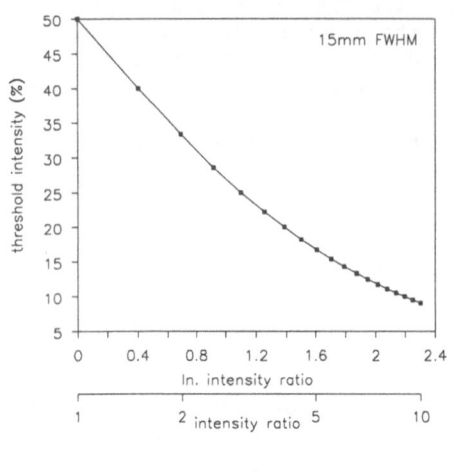

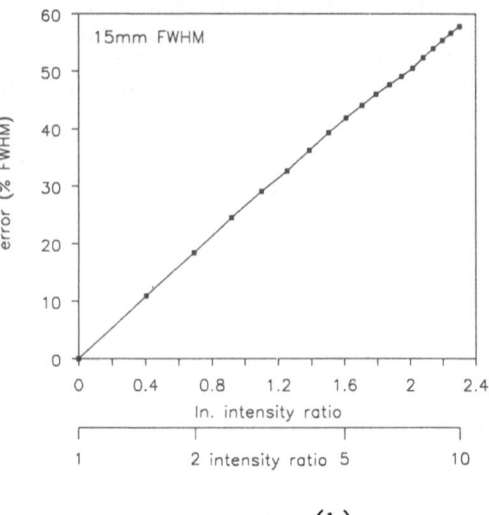

(a)

(b)

Fig. 3. (a) Threshold level (expressed as percentage of the higher intensity) above which separation of adjacent distributions occurs, plotted as a function of the ratio of intensities of the two distributions.
(b) Error in location of the edge between adjacent distributions (expressed as fraction of the FWHM of the imaging system) plotted as a function of the ratio of intensities of the two distributions.

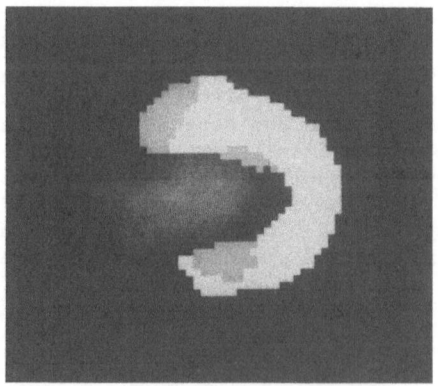

Fig. 4. Composite PET image of left ventricular bloodflow, metabolism, and bloodpool in a dog heart after AER thresholding.

in the myocardium in the flow image was found to range from 1.01 to 1.21, the mean value of $1.09 \pm 0.08$ corresponding to an optimal threshold of 48%.

The myocardial metabolic distribution of activity can similarly be thresholded and displayed in a composite image with the perfusion distribution and bloodpool image by compressing each distribution into one third of the available dynamic range. Fig. 4 shows an example of such a composite image. Bloodpool was displayed with the lower third of the color or grey levels, metabolism in the middle third, and flow in the highest third of the display scale.

In order to validate the ability of the AER method to measure the proportion of ischemic LV, coronary artery occlusions were surgically produced in dogs who were subsequently given CO-15 to label the bloodpool and 13-N ammonia to produce perfusion images of the myocardium. The images obtained during coronary occlusion were then thresholded using the AER method. Regions of interest defining the myocardium as shown in fig. 1 were then drawn by hand on the composite images using the following criteria. The endocardial boundary was drawn to bisect the gap between the bloodpool and myocardial flow distribution. The distance of the bisector from the myocardial distribution also defined the distance of the LV image boundary from the epicardial and bloodpool edges. For epicardial infarcted zones the edges must be generated by extrapolation from neighboring portions of the boundary using symmetry and distance from the bloodpool as guidelines. After drawing the myocardial boundaries, total LV volume was computed as the sum of all pixels within the drawn boundaries in all slices. The non-ischemic volume within the same boundaries was measured by summation of the number of remaining pixels in the flow distribution after thresholding. Thus the ischemic volume is the difference between the total LV and non-ischemic volumes and can be expressed as a percentage of the total LV volume. The percent LV ischemic volume by PET was compared with that obtained by in-vitro measurement of myocardial perfusion with 15 micron radio-labeled microspheres (Heymann et al., 1977). Ischemia was defined as the cumulative LV mass with absolute coronary perfusion less than 0.6 ml/min/g. The fraction of the LV involved in the ischemic process was determined by dividing this ischemic mass by the total mass of the LV. In 5 dogs in which both PET imaging of bloodpool and perfusion as well as micro-sphere analysis was performed during coronary occlusion, the correlation between the fractional ischemic volume measured by using AER generated ROIs no change microspheres was 0.93.

An automated implementation of the AER technique is under development. While the threshold computation and combined image formation can be easily performed automatically, tracing of the myocardial ROI without operator intervention requires the development of decision rules which determine which parts of the boundary follow the bloodpool and which parts follow the myocardial distributions.


ADAPTIVE THRESHOLDING

The width of the LV wall in both humans and dogs is smaller than the resolution of the current generation of PET cameras. Consequently, so-called partial volume effects pertain (Hoffman, Huang and Phelps, 1979), causing loss of peak activity and blurring of edges. Thus the dimensions of structures obtained from conventionally thresholded images may be signifi-cantly in error. We propose an adaptive thresholding technique which yields more accurate object dimensions by compensating for partial volume effects.

Theory

The response of an imaging system to an object distribution is given by the convolution of the system's impulse response function with the object distribution function (Lamberts, Higgins and Wolfe, 1958). Fig. 5 illus-trates in one dimension the response to a rectangular function (e.g. a cut through the LV wall) of decreasing width which results from a system

with a Gaussian point spread function (PSF). In case (a), the object width
is greater than twice the full width at half maximum (FWHM) of the PSF and
there are no partial volume effects; the peak measured intensity is the same
as the object intensity and the boundary of the imaged distribution crosses
the object distribution at the half peak intensity points. Thus for large
objects (such as the LV bloodpool), a 50% threshold will yield the true
object dimension. Case (b) pertains when the object width is between 1 and
2 FWHM. The peak intensity is now less than the object intensity and a
threshold at 50% of the measured maximum intensity will slightly overestimate the object width. Note that the true width will be given by a
threshold above 50% of the measured peak value and at 50% of the true object
intensity. For objects less than 1 FWHM, (case (c)), intensity recovery is
even less and the over-estimate of the object width resulting from a 50%

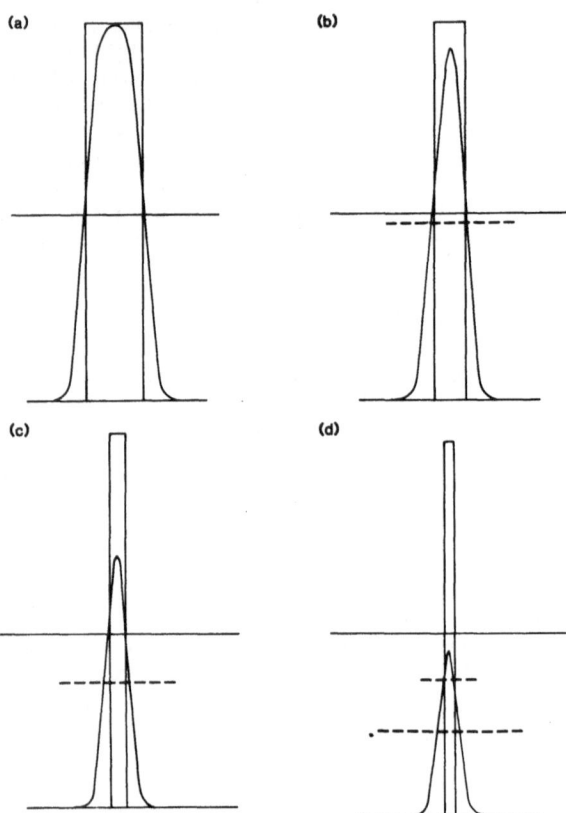

Fig. 5. Partial volume effects and thresholding illustrated for 1-D rectangular distributions of decreasing widths.
(a) Width > 2 FWHM; full recovery, 50%
threshold gives true width. (b) Width
1 to 2 FWHM; partial recovery, 50%
threshold over-estimates width, threshold giving true width > 50%. (c) Width
< 1 FWHM; significant loss of re-
covery, 50% threshold significantly
over-estimates width, threshold giving
true width > 50%. (d) Width << 1 FWHM;
recovery < 50%, 50% threshold significantly overestimates width, threshold
giving true width is close to 100%.

threshold is much greater. Eventually, as the object dimension becomes still smaller (case (d)), less than 50% of the true intensity is recovered, the width yielded by a 50% threshold can be several times the true width. The threshold giving the true width approaches 100% as the object becomes smaller.

If the imaged object is small with respect to the resolution of the imaging system in more than one dimension, then the loss of recovery and blurring are compounded. Fig. 6(a) plots the width measured from a 50% thresholded image as a function of the true dimension for a two-dimensional Gaussian spread function. Note that the width of the object must be more than 2.5 times the FWHM in order for a 50% threshold to yield the correct size. An object one FWHM in width has its size over-estimated by one half in a 50% thresholded image, while objects smaller than half the FWHM result in an error of 300% or more. Fig. 6(b) shows the threshold which must be applied in order to recover the correct width of the object distribution in the 2-D model. For an object one FWHM in size a 75% threshold is required, while objects smaller than half the FWHM require a threshold of 90% or more.

These observations suggest an adaptive thresholding scheme which can compensate for the partial volume effects which occur in a given imaging system. First, the object distribution must be simulated in various sizes and convolved with the system spread function to give an estimate of the imaged distribution. Ideally this should be done in three dimensions, but for many applications good accuracy can be achieved with a two-dimensional simulation. A 50% threshold is then applied to the simulated image and the dimensions of interest in the thresholded images, together with the threshold which will give the true dimensions, are stored as a function of the simulated object size. These parameters form a look-up table by which PET images can be correctly analyzed. For each dimension measured from a 50% thresholded image, the true dimension and the corresponding new threshold is extracted from the look-up table and applied to the original images. The dimension in the newly thresholded image will then be quite close to the true dimension.

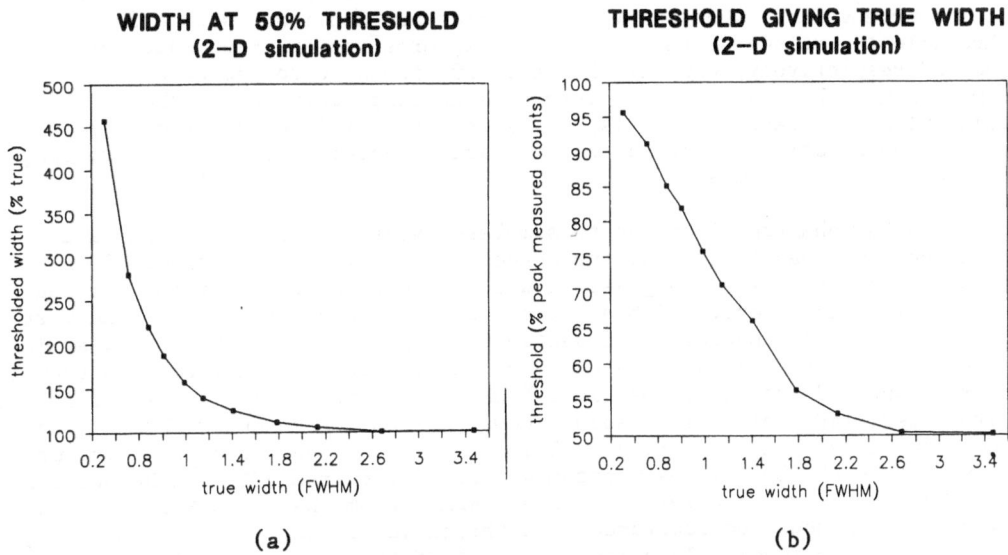

Fig. 6. (a) Width yielded by 50% threshold for 2-D distribution as function of true width. Imaged width can be several times true width.
(b) Threshold giving correct width as function of object size.

Table 1.  Volume recovery in sphere phantom by thresholding

| TRUE SIZE | | THRESHOLDED MEASUREMENTS | | |
| | | 50% threshold | Resolution dependent threshold | |
| Volume (cc) | Diameter (cm) | Volume recovery (pixels/cc) | Threshold (%) | Volume recovery (pixels/cc) |
| --- | --- | --- | --- | --- |
| 20.2 | 3.4 | 12.5 | 51.5 | 12.1 |
| 11.3 | 2.8 | 12.9 | 53.0 | 12.4 |
| 5.4 | 2.2 | 15.6 | 58.0 | 12.2 |

Implementation and results

The ability to recover accurate object dimensions using the thresholding concepts presented above was tested on PET scans of phantoms.  Three hollow spheres of diameters 2.3, 1.9, and 1.5 times the camera system FWHM, respectively were filled with the same concentration of 18-F and imaged inside a water-filled 20cm diameter cylindrical tank until 30 million counts had been acquired.  A threshold at 50% of the maximum imaged value in each sphere was applied and the total number of pixels for each sphere in all slices in the thresholded images was computed.  New thresholds obtained from the graph in Fig. 6(b) were then applied and the number of pixels in each sphere was again computed.  Table 1. illustrates the improvement in volume recovery, as measured by the ratio of the number of pixels in each sphere to its true volume, when optimal thresholds are applied.  With a 50% threshold the volume of the two smaller spheres was over-estimated by 7.5% and 30% respectively, causing the ratio of pixels/cc to increase with diminishing sphere diameter.  After thresholding according to the 2-D simulation, the ratio of pixels/cc was essentially independent of object size, demonstrating correction of the partial volume effect and permitting recovery of true volumes.

Another phantom, intended to simulate myocardial flow or metabolic distributions, was imaged and subjected to adaptive thresholding.  This phantom consisted of a wineglass in which a 50cc laboratory flask was suspended, leaving a cavity with a horseshoe shaped cross-section in the vertical direction and annular cross-sections along horizontal cuts, similar in shape and size to the LV.  The width of the chamber varied from less than 1 FWHM on one side to approximately 2 FWHM on the other.  The flask was filled with water, 149cc of an 18-F solution was placed in the outer chamber, and the phantom was imaged until 40 million counts had been acquired.  The mean width of the chamber of the phantom was estimated from 50% thresholded images to be 8 pixels or 1.3 times the system FWHM.  From the 1-D simulation, the average width would be recovered by a threshold of 56%.  After eliminating all pixels with image values less than 56% of the peak 'midwall' value, a total of 1733 pixels remained giving a pixel to true volume ratio of 11.6 pixels/cc.  This figure is slightly lower than the value obtained with the spheres.  This can be explained by the considerable loss of activity from the thinnest regions of the phantom which caused even the highest activity in those regions to fall below the applied threshold. Thus these regions disappeared from the image after thresholding. Such drop-out of very small structures can be prevented by computing the optimum threshold on the basis of an accurate 2-D model of the shape of each of the sections of the phantom which were imaged. Alternatively, the thresholds from the 1D model could be applied to perpendicular cut-lines through the simulated myocardial wall. Two and three dimensional simulations are also being performed to more accurately generate the optimal thresholds for objects with complex shapes such as the heart.

We have begun to develop an automated thresholding algorithm which involves the following steps. First a 50% threshold is applied to each slice and the the centroid of the resulting distribution is computed. Then the boundary pixels are identified and the width of the imaged distribution is computed along radial lines emananting from the centroid at 1 degree intervals. Revised widths along these radial lines are obtained using the thresholds predicted by the simulation in order to compensate for partial volume blurring. This new threshold is assigned to every pixel within the 50% thresholded image along the radial line. Pixel threshold values lying between the radial lines are computed by interpolation between neighboring values. Thus a complete pixel threshold map can be generated. The peak measured value along each of the radial lines is also computed and the threshold level stored in each pixel as a fraction of the peak value. The thresholding is finally performed on a pixel by pixel basis such that only pixels whose value is greater than the value stored in the threshold map are retained.

Discussion

The adaptive thresholding algorithm described above will work well for circular or annular shaped distributions, but for non-circularly symmetric objects, the radial lines originating from the centroid are not perpendicular to the object boundaries. Provided the same radial lines are used to measure the widths in the object simulation, then the technique should also work for any arbitrary object distribution. An alternative approach for the myocardium would be to compute the perpendiculars to the midwall at narrowly spaced intervals.

CONCLUSIONS

Two methods have been presented for quantitating the fractional volume of ischemic tissue in the myocardium in the presence of coronary insufficiency, directly from PET images. By modeling the effects of the resolution of the imaging system, true volume recovery is possible even in the presence of partial volume effects. The principles established apply also to other imaging techniques such as single photon emission tomography where partial volume effects occur. Similarly, the results of the adaptive thresholding experiments can be applied to improve the threshold optimization in the AER technique by further compensating for partial volume errors. We are pursuing a synthesis of the two techniques.

While the primary goal of this work was generation of accurate myocardial boundaries, an important end point is minimization of operator intervention and, ultimately, complete automation. The adaptive thresholding concept lends itself readily to automation, at least for objects with simple shapes. Automatic tracing of regions on composite images created by the AER method is more difficult and may require the application of artificial intelligence techniques.

Further validation and calibration of both the AER and the adaptive thresholding techniques using phantoms of known volume as well as in-vivo studies in dog hearts are under way. We anticipate that these techniques will be applied in routine diagnostic PET imaging procedures to non-invasively measure the ischemic zone at risk in the human heart.

REFERENCES

Chow, C.K. and Kaneko, T. (1972). Automatic Boundary Detection of the Left Ventricle from Cineangiograms, Comput. Biomed. Res., 5, 388-410.

Heymann, M.A., Payne, B.D., Hoffman, J.I.E., and Rudolph, A.M. (1977). Blood Flow Measurements With Radionuclide-labeled Particles, Progress in Cardiovascular Diseases, XX(1), 55-79.

Hoffman, E.J., Huang, S-C, and Phelps, M.E. (1979). Quantitation in Positron Emission Computed Tomography: 1. Effect of Object Size, J. Comput. Assist. Tomogr., 3(3), 299-308.

Lamberts, R.L., Higgins, G.C. and Wolfe, R.N. (1958). Measurement and Analysis of the Distribution of Energy in Optical Images, J. Opt. Soc. America, 48(7), 487-490.

Schelbert, H.R., Phelps, M.E., Huang S-C, MacDonald, N.S., Hansen, H., Selin, C., and Kuhl, D.E. (1981). N-13 Ammonia as an Indicator of Myocardial Blood Flow, 63(6), 1259-1272.

Schwaiger, M., Schelbert, H.R., Ellison D., Hansen, H., Yeatman, L., Vinten-Johansen, J., Selin, C., Barrio, J., and Phelps, M.E. (1985). Sustained Regional Abnormalities in Cardiac Metabolism after Transient Ischemia in the Chronic Dog Model, J.A.C.C., 6(2), 336-47.

Raff, U., Stroud, D.N., and Hendee, W.R. (1986). Improvement of Lesion Detection in Scintigraphic Images by SVD Techniques for Resolution Recovery, IEEE Trans. Medical Imaging, MI-5(1), 35-44.

Tauxe, W.N., Soussaline, F., Todd-Pokropek, A., Cao, A., Collard, P., Richard, S., Raynaud, C. and Itti, R. (1982). Determination of Organ Volume by Single-Photon Emission Tomography, J. Nucl. Med., 23(11), 984-987.

Trivedi, S.S., Herman, G.T., and Udupa, J.K. (1986). Segmentation Into Three Classes Using Gradients, IEEE Trans. Medical Imaging, MI-5(2), 116-119.

# IMAGE ANALYSIS OF PET DATA WITH THE AID OF CT AND MR IMAGES

Chin-Tu Chen[$+], Charles A. Pelizzari*, George T.Y. Chen*, Malcolm D. Cooper[$+] and David N. Levin[+]

[$]PET Center, The Franklin McLean Memorial Research Institute and
[+]Department of Radiology; *Michael Reese/University of Chicago Center for Radiation Therapy. The University of Chicago, Chicago, IL., U.S.A.

## ABSTRACT

A new technique that takes into account variations in subject position, orientation, pixel size and slice thickness has been developed for the registration of brain images from different modalities. This method uses surface-fitting algorithms which minimize the mismatch between models of the external surface as constructed from each scan. An advantage relative to techniques that have been previously reported is the absence of the requirement for identification of either internal or external landmarks. Models of the external surface of the head are derived from transmission scans in positron emission tomography (PET) and from images obtained by using X-ray computed tomography (CT) and magnetic resonance (MR). The surface models are constructed from multiple external contours determined on various transverse slices. The fitting procedure yields a set of transformation parameters that represent the translation, rotation and linear scaling factors between two sets of images. Results from preliminary studies indicate that registration accuracy of 2-3 mm can be achieved between PET and CT or MR images.

## INTRODUCTION

Quantitative analysis of brain images obtained in positron emission tomography (PET) requires delineation of multiple regions-of-interest (ROIs) on each transverse slice in order to extract functional information associated with particular brain structures. Techniques for the definition of ROIs must be objective, accurate and reproducible. Therefore, it is desirable to employ morphological images such as those from a standard atlas, or those produced in X-ray computed tomography (CT) and magnetic resonance (MR), to aid in defining ROIs based on individual structural information. This approach requires precise image correlation in three dimensions.

A number of methods have been developed to improve the accuracy with which such correlations may be made. One well-established technique involves the use of a stereotactic frame fixed to the patient so that a three-dimensional reference coordinate system can be established to map structures from a standard atlas of normal brain anatomy onto the PET images (Fox et al., 1985). Another method, which incorporates patient-specific rather than standardized anatomic information, involves warping of CT images to maximize the correlation between a number of point pairs tentatively identified as representing the same anatomical loctions in CT and PET images (Maguire et al., 1985). Stereotactic frames that are visible both in PET and in CT and/or MR have been developed to derive the coordinate transformation between a PET scan and a CT or MR scan (Oliver et al., 1987). Once the transformation is known, anatomical structure outlines, ROIs and the image data themselves may be mapped from one scan onto another. Similar techniques using externally applied fiducial markers visible in PET and in CT or MR have also been reported (Martin et al., 1987).

We have developed a method (Pelizzari and Chen, 1987; Pelizzari et al., 1987) based on computer matching of surfaces as identified in multiple imaging scans which allows registration of any number of scans from single or multiple modalities. This technique has several important practical advantages: (1) No stereotactic frame or external fiducial markers are required. This simplifies image acquisition considerably, and more importantly, allows retrospective correlation using data acquired in routine clinical practice. (2) Patient-specific anatomy rather than standardized normal anatomy is used. This is of particular importance in studies involving patients with anatomic abnormalities, e.g. for planning and evaluation of cancer radiation therapy or of neurosurgical or radiosurgical procedures. (3) No identification of internal anatomical landmarks is required. The need for an expert observer to make such identification is thus eliminated. (4) The surfaces used are characterized by many hundreds of points; thus uncertainties in the location of individual points are of minimal importance.

Using the coordinate transformation between scans derived by the surface-matching algorithm, information from one scan may be integrated with that from the another in several ways: (1) Volumes-of-interest (VOIs) defined by outlining on multiple slices of one scan may be transformed and sliced along the planes of the second scan, yielding contours which can be overlaid on the second scan. For example, a tumor region well visualized in an MR image may be mapped onto a CT image for radiotherapy planning; a three-dimensional anatomical structure from CT or MR images may be sectioned along the planes of a PET scan. These images may then be displayed side by side, allowing anatomical ROIs to be defined on CT or MR images and simultaneously shown in PET images. Regional functional information from the PET images may then be extracted using the ROIs defined in CT or MR images. (2) Resliced images as described above may be merged, for example, by adding a translucent pseudocolored PET image to a greyscale CT or MR image so anatomy and functional activity may be seen simultaneously. (3) Views orthogonal or oblique to the original scans may be produced; for example, the distribution of PET functional activity on a sagittal or coronal CT section can be determined and displayed simutaneously.

METHOD

The steps required to register two scans are described briefly as follows. The example given here is for the correlation of a PET scan and a CT or MRI scan. When more than two scans are to be correlated, they are processed in pairs (for example, both CT and MR scans can be correlated with a PET scan respectively, and possibly also with each other). The surface to be matched is nearly always the external head surface; but any other surfaces, in principle, can be used also. This surface is identified on both scans by outlining the external contours on all available slices. For PET, images from transmission scan, normally acquired for the purpose of attenuation correction, are used to define the external surface. This operation is performed using an automatic edge finding algorithm based on threshold following. In the case of PET transmission images, it is useful to first perform an edge enhancement, using for example a Sobel operator, since the edges tend to be rather soft and noisy. Figure 1 demonstrates an example of the resulting external contours from this edge finding operation. A pair of three- dimensional models of the surface can then be generated from multiple contours determined on the serial slices of both scans, respectively and independently.

The essence of the remaining steps is to find the geometric transformation which brings these models most nearly into congruence. A useful analogy to this procedure is the fitting of a rigid, form-fitting hat onto a head (this hat-head concept is used throughout the following discussions). The "head" model is derived from the scan covering the larger volume of the patient; this is nearly always CT or MR rather than PET. This "head" model is represented as a stack of disks, each with cross-section determined by one of the contours from the serial images, and with thickness and vertical position appropriate to the known slice thickness and scanner longitudinal coordinate. In the case of CT, correction for gantry tilt is also made if appropriate. The "hat" is represented as a list of three-dimensional points, which need not define complete closed contours. Figure 2 illustrates a "head" from MR (wire loops) and a "hat" from PET (isolated points).

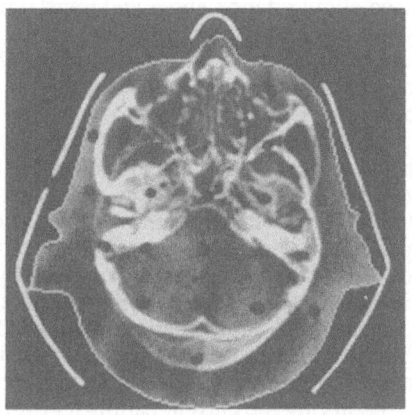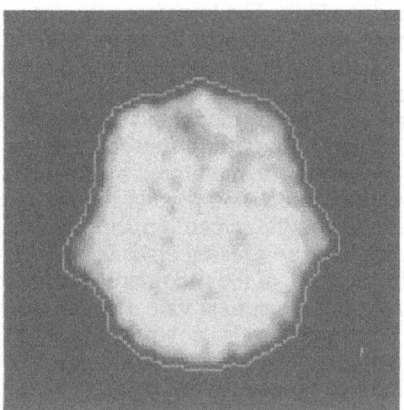

Fig. 1. External contours outlined by automatic edge finding; left: PET, right: CT.

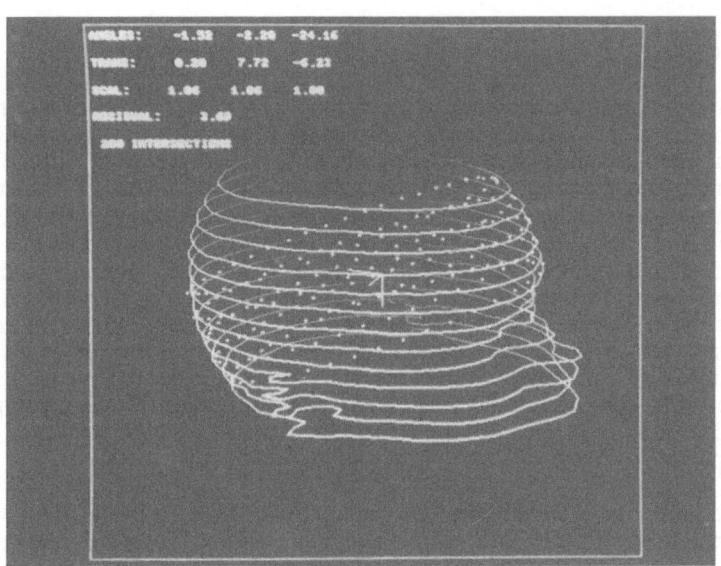

Fig. 2. Surface-fitting of two models: a "head" from MR (wire loops)
and a "hat" from PET (isolated points).

To determine the transformation which brings the "hat" most closely into congruence with the "head", both models are first scaled by their respective pixel sizes, then translated so their centroids lie at the origin of the resulting "world" coordinate system. A standard algorithm (Press et al., 1986) for minimization of a nonlinear function of several variables is then used to find the coordinate transformation which minimizes the average distance between "hat" points and "head" surface. The transformation parameters used allow rotation about and translation in three orthogonal directions. In addition to rigid-body rotation and translation, linear scaling factors are also included to account for minor uncertainties in pixel size, possible suboptimal choice of a threshold level for defining external contours, and possible distortions in MR images. For typical cases, a "head" model has about 1500 total points on 12-15 parallel contours and a "hat" 200-300 points. This fitting step requires several minutes of CPU time on a VAX-11/750. The fitting process may be monitored by displaying the "head" and "hat" at each iteration of the minimization procedure. As shown in Figure 2, current values of the transformation parameters are also illustrated on the screen (upper left corner). In addition, the current mean misfit value defined as the average squared distance between "hat" points and "head" surface is displayed to indicate the progress of the fitting process. The procedure may be interrupted at any point by an operator to alter the current values of the transformation parameters and the fitting is then resumed. The operator also controls which of the nine transformation parameters are allowed to vary at any stage of the process. A skilled operator can speed the process by judicious choice of initial parameter estimates and by recognizing situations where the minimization algorithm may not be searching the parameter space most efficiently, modifying the current parameter estimates and "steering" the fitting process in the right direction.

Transformation parameters derived from this surface-fitting process can be used to reslice CT or MR image data set in order to produce anatomical templates for PET emission scans. These anatomical templates can be displayed simultaneously with functional PET images to facilitate the appreciation of changes or abnormalities. In addition, regional quantitative information can be extracted from functional PET images using ROIs delineated on these anatomical templates.

VALIDATION

We have evaluated the accuracy of the method for PET/CT correlation using scans of an anthropomorphic phantom (Alderson "Rando" head). The phantom is of molded plastic in the shape of a human head and is sectioned into 25 mm slices. A matrix of 5 mm diameter holes on a 30 x 30 mm grid extends through the phantom normal to the slices. PET scans were made with the University of Chicago PETT-VI scanner using normal procedures, with a $^{68}$Ga transmission scan taken first, followed by an emission scan. Polyethylene tubes of 0.5 mm wall thickness containing a dilute solution of $^{68}$Ga doped EDTA were placed into eight of the holes within the phantom. The tubes were of three different lengths, and all had one end aligned with the superior end of the holes. With this arrangement the tubes appear as a matrix of bright spots in the emission scan, which ideally should register with the images of the holes in CT. CT scans were made with a Siemens Somatom DR3 scanner, without the radioactive linesources in place. Pixel sizes were 2.5 mm for PET, 1.15 mm for CT. The CT slice spacing used was 4 mm, PET slice spacing 14 mm. Two CT scans were made, with gantry angles of 0 and -14 degrees respectively.

As outlined in the METHOD section above, the "head" for surface fitting was derived from external surface contours in the CT scans. The "hat" was defined by sampling the external contours of the PET transmission scans with a suitable number of selected points (experience has shown that 200-300 "hat" points can produce good results). The fitting procedure was allowed to run without guidance from an operator, and arrived at a final mean misfit value of 3.3 mm$^2$ per "hat" point. This has proven typical for PET/CT and PET/MR fits with pixel sizes of 2.5 mm for PET and about 1 mm for CT or MR.

Using the transformtion parameters thus determined, oblique sections through the volume of CT data along the planes of the PET slices were produced. This is accomplished simply by transforming the coordinates of the corners of each slice expressed in the PET coordinate system into the CT coordinate system (this is exactly the same transformation applied to the "hat" points by the fitting procedure) and sampling along the plane so defined. The CT slices thus produced are nominally aligned along the same planes, and have the same pixel size as the PET images. They may therefore be directly overlaid with the PET slices; and the bright images of the line sources in PET should appear superimposed on the dark images of the empty holes in CT.

Figure 3 shows an overlay of the emission PET and interpolated CT images for a typical slice of the phantom scan. In this example, the upper left quadrant is the emission PET image, the upper right the interpolated CT image, and the lower left a colorwash in which the PET intensity at each pixel controls the hue as in an ordinary pseudocolor encoding, while the CT intensity at the same pixel controls the color intensity. By this means light and dark areas in the CT remain visible, with color varying to indicate local PET intensity. The color pallette is shown in the lower right quadrant of this Figure. The hot spots in PET register with the dark hole images in CT with an accuracy of 2-3 mm (recall the hole diameter is 5 mm). However, the effect of the colorwash, which is a powerful tool for use in interpreting the correlated images, cannot be fully demonstrated by this monochrome rendition. As a further check on the registration, we have generated sagittal PET slices and corresponding oblique CT sections. A sample section across the center of the PET scan is shown in Figure 4. The registration of the bright lines in PET with the dark holes in CT is fairly good, indicating the rotational part of the derived coordinate transformation is satisfactory. Only the results for the CT scan with zero gantry angle are shown here; those for the tilted gantry scan show a similar level of registration accuracy.

EXAMPLES

Figures 5 and 6 show results from the image correlation study of a patient with left frontal aspergilloma. The upper halves in these two Figures illustrate results from the PET/MR correlation, while the lower halves represent the PET/CT correlation. PET images shown here represent regional cerebral glucose metabolic rate derived from [18]FDG scans. A large area of lesion and edema appears white in the MR image, and the PET image demonstrates a marked lack of metabolic activity in the left frontal region (Fiqure 5). This abnormality is less apparant in the corresponding CT image. Fiqure 6 illustrates correlated images of a lower slice in which some features such as cerebellum lobes can be used for evaluation of the accuracy of the registration. Both Figures 5 and 6 reveal that excellent image correlation has been achieved in the present case. The "head" and "hat" configuration near the end of the fitting process for the case of PET/ MR correlation is shown in Figure 1. The residual misfit per "hat" point in this example is 3.4 $mm^2$ which is similar to the value obtained in the phantom study discussed earlier.

One application of the PET/CT or PET/MR correlation is to employ the structural information provided by morphological images (from CT or MR) to aid in data analysis of functional images (from PET). For example, one can delineate ROIs on the resliced CT or MR images and overlay these outlines onto the PET images for extracting quantitative functional information. To demonstrate this application, an anatomy expert was asked to outline multiple ROIs on the PET images and the corresponding resliced CT and MR images. The task was performed by working on one type of images at a time without referring to any other types of images; therefore, inferences from different sets of images are much reduced. Figure 7 illustrates two sample ROIs that were drawn on the same slices as shown in Figures 5 and 6. The left column shows the boundaries, as seen by the expert in individual images, of the abnormality. It is obvious that the MR image gives a clear indication of the extent of the abnormality (the largest area outlined by the brightest boundary). However, the expert decided to choose a much smaller frontal area in the PET image for its drastically reduced metabolic activity (the smallest area outlined by the darkest boundary). The abnormal structure is less apparent in the CT image, and the area judged by the expert as abnormal is shown to be of intermediate size. The average regional glucose metabolic rate (in mg/100g/min) within each of these three boundaries is: PET = 4.56; CT = 4.84; MR = 6.46. The higher value from MR indicates that some regions may be morphologically abnormal but fuctionally still relatively active. The right column in Figure 7 is the case of right cerebellum. Both areas outlined by the boundaries based on the CT (line of intermediate brightness) and MR (brightest line) images are somewhat larger than that based on the PET image (darkest line). The average metabolic rate within each of these ROIs is: PET = 7.2; CT = 6.05; MR = 5.97. It can be noted that the value from PET is about 20% higher than those from CT and MR, probably because the latter two have slighter larger areas that include some regions

605

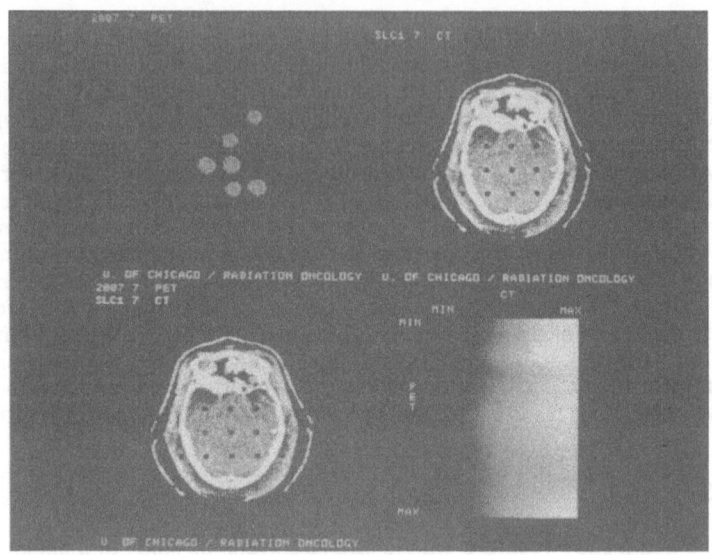

Fig. 3.  PET/CT correlation of an Alderson "Rando" head phantom

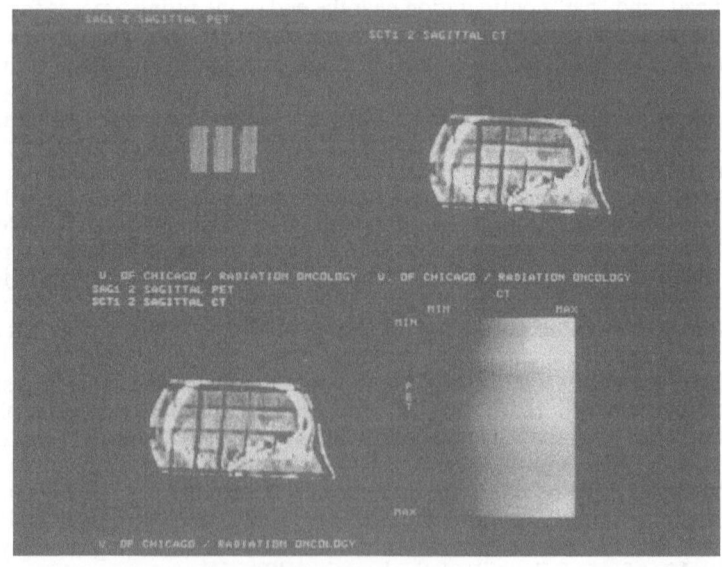

Fig. 4.  Sagittal sections of the correlated PET and CT scans from the phantom study.

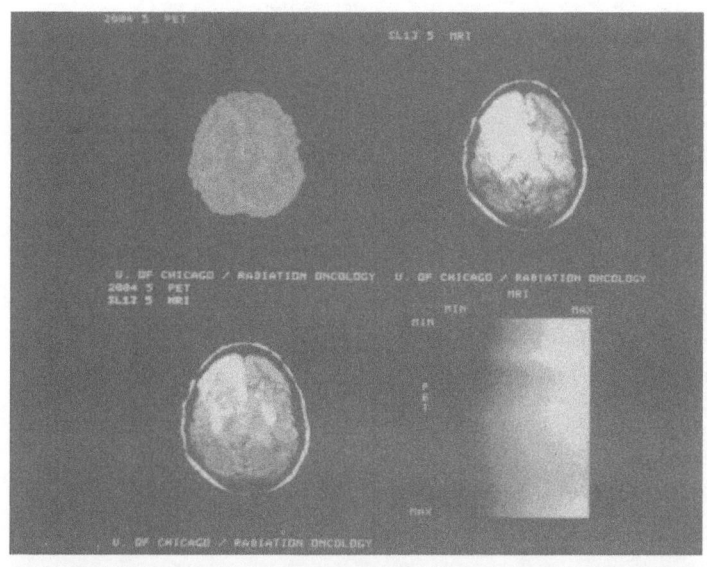

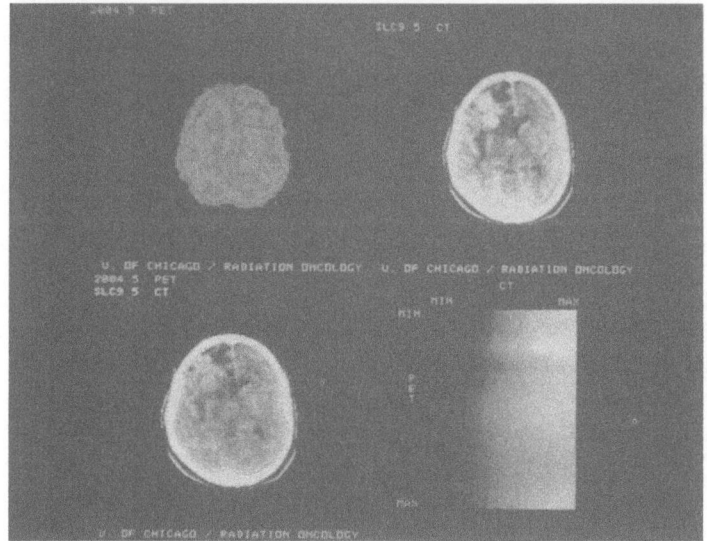

Fig. 5.  Correlated images; upper: PET/MR, lower: PET/CT.

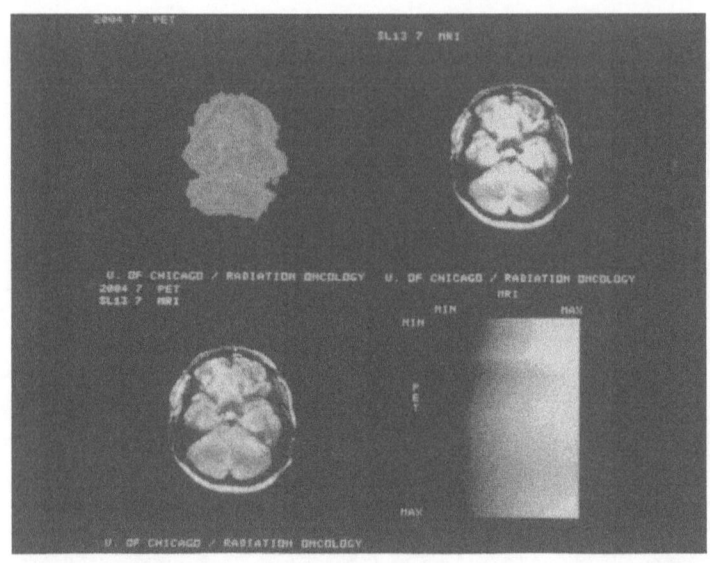

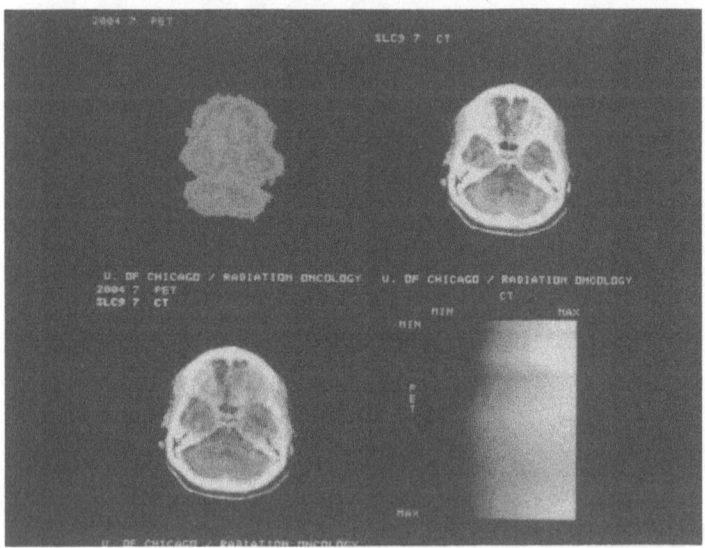

Fig. 6. Correlated images; upper: PET/MR, lower: PET/CT.

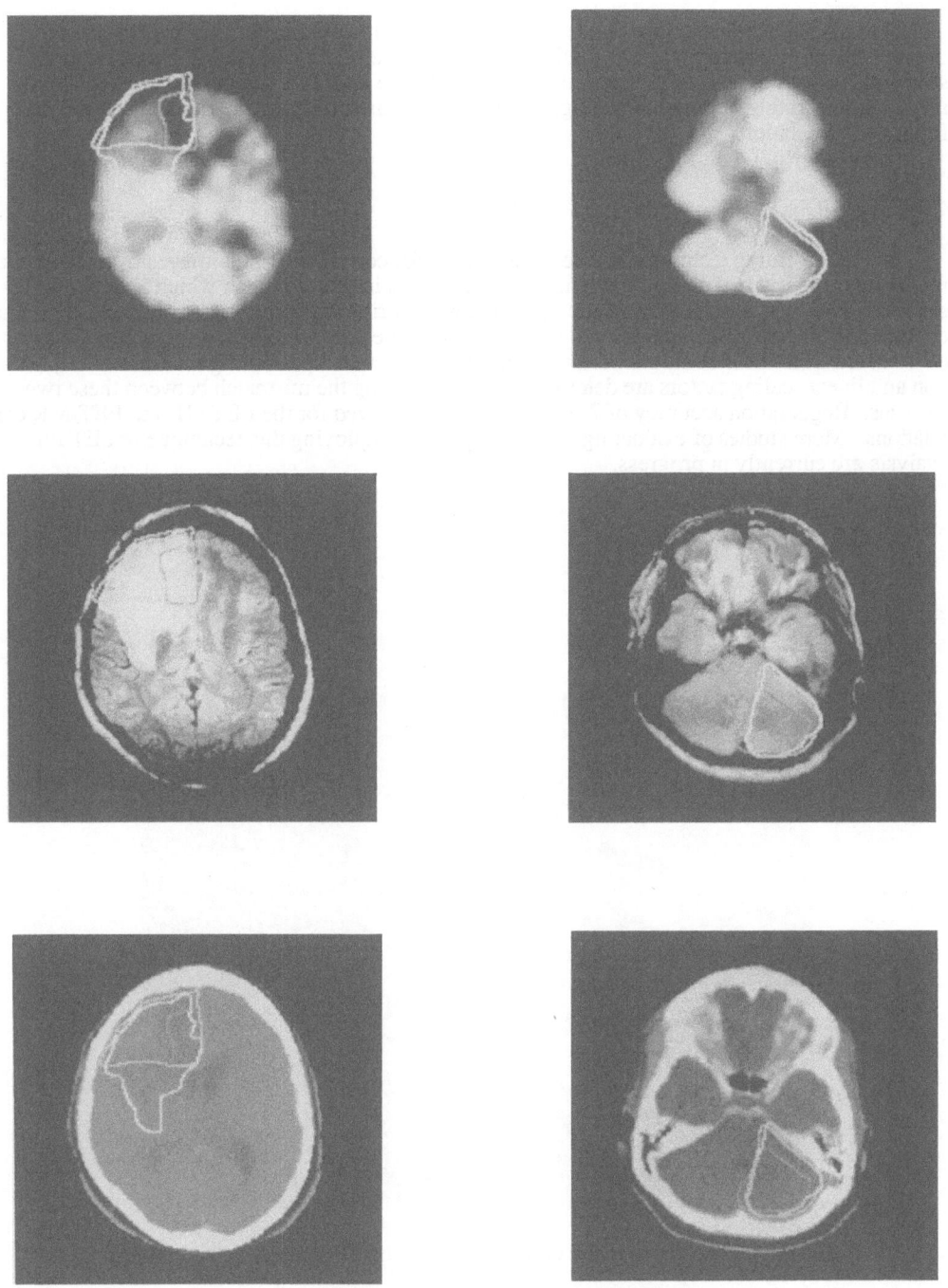

Fig. 7. Correlated images with delineated ROIs.

exhibiting apparent low metabolic activity. Notice also that the ROIs delineated in the CT and MR images and the metabolic rates associated with these two regions are nearly identical, indicating relatively accurate image registration. More comparison studies are currently in progress to assess the full impact of this approach.

As indicated earlier, image data sets can be resliced in any orientation for examination. Figure 8 shows an example of a sagittal section across the midline of the PET scan. It can be seen that the boundaries of the ventricular space in the PET and CT images are in good agreement, demonstrating once again the high accuracy that this surface-fitting method can provide for image correlation.

CONCLUSION

A surface-fitting technique has been developed for correlating brain images from different modalities. No internal or external landmark is required in this approach which also allows retrospective correlations. An automatic edge finding algorithm is employed to outline the external contours on all available slices in both scans that are to be correlated. Two surface models are constructed from these contours. Transformation parameters representing the translation, rotation and linear scaling factors are determined by minimizing the mismatch between these two surfaces. Registration accuracy of 2-3 mm has been achieved for the PET/CT and PET/MR correlations. More studies of evaluating the full impact of employing this technique in PET image analysis are currently in progress.

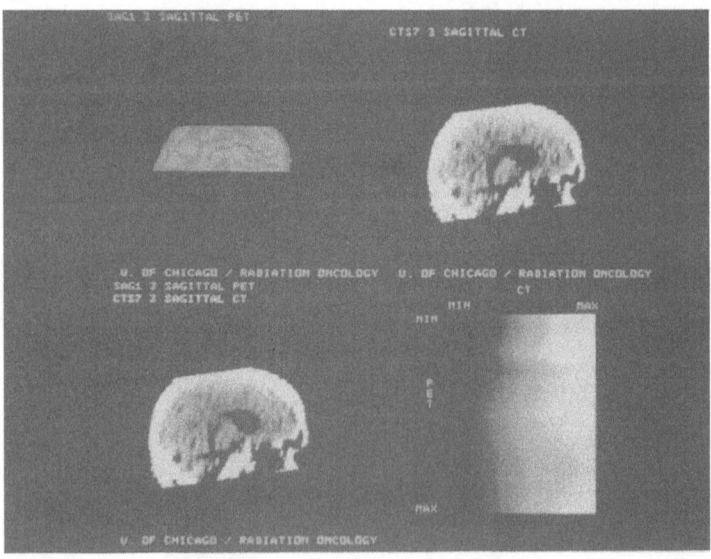

Fig. 8. Sagittal sections of the correlated PET and CT scans of a human brain.

## ACKNOWLEDGEMENTS

We wish to thank N. Yasillo and M. Dowd for performing the phantom experiments, M. Diamond for identification of the ROIs and D. Cop for secretarial assistance.

## REFERENCES

Fox, P.T., Perlmutter, J.S. and Raichle, M.E. (1985). A stereotactic method of anatomical localization for positron emission tomography, J. Comput. Assist. Tomogr., 9, 141-153.

Maguire, G.Q., Noz,M.E., Lee, E.M. and Schimpf, J.H. (1986). Corrleation methods for tomographic images using two and three dimensional techniques, in: Information Processing in Medical Imaging (Proceedings of the Ninth IPMI Conference), S.L. Bacharach, ed., Martinus Nijhoff, Dordrecht. pp. 266-279

Martin, W.R.W., Grochowski, E., Palmer, M., and Pate, B.D. (1987). Correlation of structural and functional images in the same patient, J. Nucl. Med., 28:634.

Oliver, A., Peters, T.M., Clark, J.A., Marchand, E., Mawko, G., Bertrand, G., Vanier, M., Ethier, R., Tyler, J. and deLotbiniere, A. (1987) Intergration de l'angiographie numerique, de la resonance magutique, de la tomodensitometrie et de la tomographie par emission de positrons en stereotaxie, Rev. E.E.G. Neurophysiol. Clin., 17, 25-43.

Pelizzari, C.A. and Chen, G.T.Y. (1987). Registration of multiple diagnostic imaging scans using surface fitting. Proceedings of the 9th ICCR, (in press).

Pelizzari, C.A., Chen, G.T.Y. Halpern, H., Chen, C.T. and Cooper, M.D. (1987). Three dimensional correlation of PET, CT and MRI images. J. Nucl. Med., 28, 682.

Press, W.H., Flannery, B.P., Teukolsky, S.A. and Vetterling, W.T. (1986). Numerical Recipes: The Art of Scientific Computing. Cambridge University, Cambridge.

# Participants

B.P. Alblas
Institute for Perception TNO
Kampweg 5
3769 DE Soesterberg
THE NETHERLANDS
+31-3463-1444

C.R. Appledorn
Division of Nuclear Medicine
Indiana University School of Medicine
926, West Michigan Street
Indianapolis IN 46223
USA
+1-317-274-1802

J.D. Austin
University of North Carolina
Department of Computer Science
Sitterson Hall 083A
Chapel Hill NC 27514
USA
+1-919-962-1747
jda@unc.cs.edu

S.L. Bacharach
NIH
Building 10, Rm 1C401
Bethesda MD 20592
USA
+1-301-496-5675

E. Backer
Delft University of Technology
Dpt. of Electrical Engineering
Mekelweg 4
Delft
THE NETHERLANDS
+31-15-786176

D.L. Bailey
Royal Prince Alfred Hospital
Department of Nuclear Medicine
Camperdown N.S.W. 2050
AUSTRALIA
+61-2-5166171

D.C. Barber
University of Sheffield
Dept of Medical Physics
Royal Hallamshire Hospital
Sheffield S10  JF
UNITED KINGDOM
+44-742-304717

H.H. Barrett
University of Arizona
Optical Sciences Center
Tucson AZ 85721
USA
+1-602-621-4425

J. Behets
Elscint Benelux Operations
Excelsiorlaan 35 (B.2)
B-1930 Zaventem
BELGIUM
+32-2-7209246

V. Bencivelli
Clinical Physiology Institute
Via Savi 8
I.56100 Pisa
ITALY
+39-50-47231
lfchp1@icnucevm

U. Bittner
Siemens AG, Medical Division
Department RDEK 21
Henkestr. 127
D-8520 Erlangen
WEST GERMANY
+49-9131-846283

Y. Bizais
Projet DIMI, HGRL
CHR Nantes, BP1005
44035 Nantes CEDEX 01
FRANCE
+33-40-483685

I. Bloch
Ecole des Mines de Paris
Centre de Morphologie Mathématique
35 rue St.Honoré
77305 Fontainebleau
FRANCE
+33-164-224821

J.A.K. Blokland
Akademisch Ziekenhuis Leiden
Div. of Nuclear Medicine
Bldg. 1, C4 - Q
Rijnsburgerweg 10
2333 AA Leiden
THE NETHERLANDS
+31-71-263485
blokland@hlerul54.bitnet

F.L. Bookstein
University of Michigan
300 North Ingalls Building
Ann Arbor MI 48109
USA
+1-313-764-2443
fredl.bookstein@um.cc.unich.edu

W.R. Breckon
Dept. of Computing and Math. Sciences
Oxford Polytechnic
Oxford OX3 OBP
UNITED KINGDOM
+44-865-819677
wrbreckon@uk.ac.oxpoly.a

A.B. Brill
Brookhaven National Lab
Medical Dept.
Upton NY 11973
USA
+1-516-282-3240

C.T. Chen
FMI, Box 433
5841 South Maryland Ave.
The University of Chicago
Chicago IL 60637
USA
+1-312-702-6269

J. van Cleynenbreugel
K.U.Leuven E.S.A.T.
De Croylaan 52B
B-3030 Heverlee
BELGIUM
+32-16-286211 ext 2250

A. Colchester
Guys Hospital
Dept. Neurology
London Bridge
London SEI 9 RT
UNITED KINGDOM
+44-1-407-7600 ext 2228

Dechamps
Agfa Gevaert
Septestraat 27
B2510 Mortsel
BELGIUM
+32-3-4443837

F. Deconinck
AZ-VUB
Laarbeeklaan 101
1090 Brussels
BELGIUM
+32-2-4784890 ext 4404
frank@primis.vub.uucp

M. Defrise
Akademisch Ziekenhuis
Dienst Radioisotopen
Laarbeeklaan 101
1090 Brussels
BELGIUM
+32-2-4784890 ext 4404

Degueldre
Universite de Liege
Centre de Recherches du Cyclotron
Batiment B-30 Sart-Tilman
B-4000 Liege 1
BELGIUM
+32-41-562986

J.S. Duncan
Yale University
Dept. of Diagnostic Radiology
Yale University
333 Cedar Street (BML 327)
New Haven CT 06510
USA
+1-203-785-6322

A.A. van Est
Philips Medical Systems Division
Postbus 10000
56 DA  Best
THE NETHERLANDS
+31-40-762858

V. Fidler
University Clinic for Nuclear Medicine
Univerzitetna Klinika za nukl.med.
Zaloska C.7
61000 Ljubljana
YUGOSLAVIA
+38-61-316855

J.M. Fitzpatrick
Vanderbilt University
Box 80 Station B
Vanderbilt Yniversity
Nashville TN 37235
USA
+1-615-322-2365

J.S. Fleming
Dept. of Nuclear Medicine
Southampton General Hospital
Southampton SO9 4XY
UNITED KINGDOM
+44-703-777222 ext 4248

J. Gauch
University of North Carolina
Route 5, Box 325 B
Chapel Hill NC 27514
USA
+1-919-942-1033

A. Geissbühler
Hopital Cantonal Universitaire
Division de médecine nucleaire
1200 Geneva
SWITZERLAND
+41-22-226553

P. Gerlot
Ecole Nat. Sup. de Mecanique
L.A.N., ENSM, 1 Rue de la Noc
44072 Nantes Cedex
FRANCE
+33-40-483607

M.L. Goris
Division Nuclear Medicine Rm CO22
Stanford University Medical Center
300 Pasteur Drive
Stanford CA 94305-5105
USA
+1-415-723-6881

C.N. de Graaf
Institute of Nuclear Medicine
Un Hospital Utrecht, room 73038
Catharijnesingel 101
3511 GV Utrecht
THE NETHERLANDS
+31-30-372846
mcvax!accumv!azung!kees

G.T. Gullberg
The University of Utah
Department of Radiology
AC-213 Medical Center
Salt Lake City UT 84132
USA
+1-801-581-8410

B.M. ter Haar Romeny
Univ. Hospital Utrecht
Dept. of Radiology
Catharijnesingel 101
3511 GV Utrecht
THE NETHERLANDS
+31-30-372164
gcnrome%hutruu0
(.bitnet@relay.cs.net)

H.J.A.M. Heijmans
C.W.I.
Kruislaan 413
1098 SJ Amsterdam
THE NETHERLANDS
+31-20-5924118

C. Herscovici
Elscint Haifa
Advanced Technology Center
Haifa 31004
ISRAEL
+972-4-540540

K.H. Höhne
Universtitäts-Krankenhaus Eppendorf
Institut für Mathematik und Daten-
    verarbeitung in der Medizin
Martinistrasse 52
2000 Hamburg 20
B.R.DEUTSCHLAND
+49-40-468-3698
f58uke@dhhdesy3.bitnet

A. Hoekstra
Institute of Nuclear Medicine
University Hospital Utrecht
Catharijnesingel 101
3511 GV Utrecht
THE NETHERLANDS
+31-30-372847
mcvax!accumv!azung!anne

A.S. Houston
Department of Nuclear Medicine
Royal Naval Hospital Haslar
Gosport, Hants PO12 ZAA
UNITED KINGDOM
+44-705-584255 ext 2416

J.C. van Houwelingen
Dept. of Medical Statistics,
University of Leiden
P.O.Box 9512,
2300 RA Leiden
THE NETHERLANDS
+31-71-277026

B.F. Hutton
Royal Prince Alfred Hospital
Department of Nuclear Medicine
Camperdown N.S.W. 2050
AUSTRALIA
+61-2-5166171

M.F. Insana
Univ. of Kansas Medical Center
Dept. of Diagnostic Radiology
39 th and Rainbow Blvd.
Kansas City KA 66103
USA
+1-903-588-6820

C. Jennison
School of Mathematical Sciences
University of Bath
Bath, BA2 7AY
UNITED KINGDOM
+44-225-826468

G. Jonkers
Koninklijke/Shell Laboratorium
Dept.AG/43
Badhuisweg 3
1031 CM Amsterdam
THE NETHERLANDS
+31-20-303509

M. Jubb
University of Bath
School of Mathematic Sciences
Claverton Down
Bath BA2 7AY
UNITED KINGDOM
+44-225-826826 ext 5991

M. Jungke
Deutsche Klinik f. Diagnostik
Aukammallee 33
D-6200 Wiesbaden
W.-GERMANY
+49-6121-577552

K. Knesaurek
KB "Dr.M.Stojanovic"
Vinogradska 29
41000 Zagreb
YUGOSLAVIA
+38-41-574666 ext 541

A. Koenderink - van Doorn
Dpt. of Medical Physics
University of Utrecht
Princetonplein 5
Utrecht
THE NETHERLANDS
+31-30-533985


S. Kuijk
VU Brussel
Dienst VUCY, VUB
Laarbeeklaan 103
1090 Brussel
BELGIUM
+32-2-4784890 ext 7117
mcvax!vub!sytse
sytse@vub.uucp


P. Levin
NRCN
P.O.Box 9001
Beer Sheva
84191 ISRAEL
+972-57-968219


L. Lifshitz
Biomedical Imaging Group
University of Mass, Medical School
Worcester MA
USA


J. Llacer
University of California
Lawrence Berkeley Laboratory
Building 29
Berkeley CA 94720
USA
+1-415-486-5898


V. Lokner
Klinika za Nuklear Medizin
    i Onkologija
Bolnica Dr.M.Stojanovic
Vinogradska 29
41000 Zagreb
YUGOSLAVIA
+38-41-574666 ext 541


I. Magnin
INSA bat. 502
20 Ave. A.Einstein
69621 Villeurbanne
FRANCE
+33-78-948112 ext 8607


G.Q. Maguire Jr.
Columbia University
Dept. of Computer Science
500 West. 120 Street
New York NY 10027- 7031
USA
+1-212-280-8106
maguire@cs.columbia.edu


J.T. Marcus
TNO Institute of Perception
Kampweg 5
Soesterberg
THE NETHERLANDS
+31-3463-1444


R. Mattheus
Radiology and Medical Imaging
AZ-VUB
Laarbeeklaan 101
B-1090 Brussel
BELGIUM
+32-2-4784890


M.A. Moerland
University Hospital Utrecht
Department of Radiotherapy
Catharijnesingel 101
3511 GV  Utrecht
THE NETHERLANDS
+31-30-372900


W. Müller-Schauenburg
Strahleninstitut
Röntgenweg 11
D-7400 Tübingen
W.GERMANY
+49-7071-296029


J. Newell
Dept. of Medical Physics
Queen Elisabeth Hospital
Edgbaston
Birmingham B15 2TH
UNITED KINGDOM
+44-21-4721311 ext 3141
newellja@uk.ac.bham


K.S. Nijran
Dept.Nuclear Medicine
Charing Cross Hospital
Fulham Palace Road
London W6
UNITED KINGDOM
+44-1-7482040 ext 2412


M.E. Noz
NEW YORK University
Dept. of Radiology
550 First Ave
New York NY 10016
USA
+1-212-340-6371
noz@nyu.arpa
cmcl2!nucmed1!noz


O Ying Lie
Institute of Nuclear Medicine
Un Hospital Utrecht, room 73038
Catharijnesingel 101
3511 GV  Utrecht
THE NETHERLANDS
+31-30-372846
mcvax!accumv!azung!ying


W.R. Oliver
University of North Carolina
Dept. of Pathology
North Carolina Memorial Hospital
Chapel Hill NC 27514
USA
+1-919-966-4131


D.A. Ortendahl
USF-RIL
400 Grandview Dr.
South San Francisco CA 94705
USA
+1-415-952-1372

D.L. Parker
Un of Utah, LDS Hospital
325 Eighth Avenue
Salt Lake City UT 84143
USA

J.H. Peters
Philips Medical Systems
P.O.Box 10000
5680 DA Best
THE NETHERLANDS
+1-40-762380

M.K. Pidcock
Dept. of Computing and Math. Sciences
Oxford Polytechnic
Oxford OX3 OBP
UNITED KINGDOM
+44-865-819668
mkpidcock@uk.ac.oxpoly.a

S.M. Pizer
University of North Carolina
Department of Computer Science
Sitterson Hall 083A
Chapel Hill NC 27514
USA
+1-919-962-1785
pizer@cs.unc.edu

R.A. Robb
Mayo Foundation/Clinic
200 First Street Southwest
Rochester MN 55905
USA
+1-507-284-4937

C.C. Robilotta
Instituto de Fisica
Universidade de Sao Paulo
Caixa Postal 20516
Sao Paulo - 01498 - SP
BRASIL
+55-11-815-5599 ext 217

J.B.T.M. Roerdink
Centrum v. Wiskunde en Informatica
Kruislaan 413
1098 SJ Amsterdam
THE NETHERLANDS
+31-20-5924120

S. Rosenberg
CHS Beauregard, Bourges
91, rue Louis Mallet
18000 Bourges
FRANCES
+33-48-211208 ext 434

R.W. Rowe
University of Texas Medical School
Positron Diagnostic and Research Center
6431 Fannin St.
Houston TX 77
USA
+1-713-792-5178

M. Samal
Institute of Biophysics
   and Nuclear Medicine
Faculty of Medicine
Charles University
Salmovska 3
120 00 Praha 2
Czechoslovakia
+42-2-201375

P.J.W. Sirba
Institute of Nuclear Medicine
Un Hospital Utrecht, room 73043
Catharijnesingel 101
3511 GV Utrecht
THE NETHERLANDS
+31-30-372844
mcvax!accumv!azung!paul

C. Solomon
Royal Marsden Hospital
Downs road
Sutton, Surrey, SM2 SPT
UNITED KINGDOM
+44-1-642-6011 ext 242

F. Soussaline
Ecole des Mines de Paris
Centre de Morphologie Mathématique
35 rue St.Honoré
77305 Fontainebleau
FRANCE
+33-164-224821

H. Surova
Institute of Biophysics
   and Nuclear Medicine
Faculty of Medicine
Charles University
Salmovska 3
12000 Praha 2
Czechoslovakia
+42-2-201375

J.J. Sychra
University of Illinois Hospital
1740 West Taylor
Suite 2500
Chicago IL 60612
USA
+1-312-996-3969

E. Tanaka
Nat. Institute of Radiological Sciences
9-1, Anagawa-4-chome
Chiba-shi 260
Japan
+81-472-51-2111

U. Tiede
Institut für Mathematik und Daten-
   verarbeitung in der Medizin
Martinistr. 52
D-2000 Hamburg 20
WEST GERMANY
+49-40-4683933

A. Todd-Pokropek
Dept. of Medical Physics
University College London
Gower St.
London WCIE 6BT
UNITED KINGDOM
 +44-1-387-9300 ext 5319
 rmap221@uk.ucl.euclid

A. Toet
Dpt. of Medical Physics
University of Utrecht
Princetonplein 5
Utrecht
THE NETHERLANDS
 +31-30-533985

P. Tofts
Institute of Neurology
Queen Square
London WC 1N 3BG
UNITED KINGDOM
 +44-1-837-3611

D. Townsend
Division of Nuclear Medicine
University Hospital of Geneva
24 ave Micheli-du-Crest
1211 Geneva 4
SWITZERLAND
 +41-22-226549

J. Vanregemorter
Vrije Universiteit Brussel
Akademisch Ziekenhuis
Laarbeeklaan 101
1090 Brussels
BELGIUM
 +32-2-4784890 ext 4404
 jo@vub.uucp

J.T.M. Verhoeven
St.Radboudziekenhuis
Biofysisch Lab.-O.H.K.
Postbus 9101
6500 HB  Nijmegen
THE NETHERLANDS
 +31-80-515170
 ohkhv@hnykun51

M.A. Viergever
Delft University of Technology,
Dpt. of Mathematics and Informatics
P.O.Box 356
2600 AJ  Delft
THE NETHERLANDS
 +31-15-784114
 mcvax!dutinfd!dutinfh!maxv

R.C. Warren
Dept. of Medical Physics
The Middlesex Hospital Medical School
Cleveland street
London W1P 6DB
UNITED KINGDOM
 +44-1-380-9306

S. Webb
Joint Section of Physics.
Institute of Cancer Research and
 Royal Marsden Hospital
Downs Rd
Sutton Surrey  SMZ 5PT
UNITED KINGDOM
 +44-1-642-6011 ext 343

J.C. Yanch
Institute of Cancer Research and
 Royal Marsden Hospital
Physics Department
Downs Road
Sutton Surrey SMZ 5PT
UNITED KINGDOM
 +44-1-642-6011 ext 413

B. Zeeberg
George Washington Un Medical Center
Walter G. Ross Hall
2300 Eye Street N.W.
Washington DC 20037
USA
 +1-202-676-3371

K.J. Zuiderveld
University Hospital Utrecht
Dept. of Radiology
Catharijnesingel 101
3511 GV Utrecht
THE NETHERLANDS
 +31-30-372164
 gafheet%hutruu0
 (.bitnet@relay.cs.net)

M. Zwaan
Centre for Mathematics and Computer
 Science
Kruislaan 413
1098 SJ  Amsterdam
THE NETHERLANDS
 +31-20-5924122

# Index

## U

## V

## W

## X